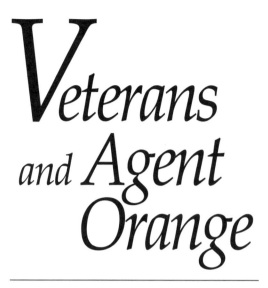

Veterans and Agent Orange

Update 2008

Committee to Review the Health Effects in
Vietnam Veterans of Exposure to Herbicides
(Seventh Biennial Update)

Board on Population Health and Public Health Practice

INSTITUTE OF MEDICINE
OF THE NATIONAL ACADEMIES

THE NATIONAL ACADEMIES PRESS
Washington, D.C.
www.nap.edu

THE NATIONAL ACADEMIES PRESS   500 Fifth Street, N.W.   Washington, DC 20001

NOTICE: The project that is the subject of this report was approved by the Governing Board of the National Research Council, whose members are drawn from the councils of the National Academy of Sciences, the National Academy of Engineering, and the Institute of Medicine. The members of the committee responsible for the report were chosen for their special competences and with regard for appropriate balance.

This study was supported by Contract No. V101 (93) P-2136, TO#15 between the National Academy of Sciences and US Department of Veterans Affairs. Any opinions, findings, conclusions, or recommendations expressed in this publication are those of the author(s) and do not necessarily reflect the view of the organizations or agencies that provided support for this project.

International Standard Book Number-13: 978-0-309-13884-0
International Standard Book Number-10: 0-309-13884-1

Additional copies of this report are available from the National Academies Press, 500 Fifth Street, N.W., Lockbox 285, Washington, DC 20055; (800) 624-6242 or (202) 334-3313 (in the Washington metropolitan area); Internet, http://www.nap.edu.

For more information about the Institute of Medicine, visit the IOM home page at: **www. iom.edu.**

Printed in the United States of America

The serpent has been a symbol of long life, healing, and knowledge among almost all cultures and religions since the beginning of recorded history. The serpent adopted as a logotype by the Institute of Medicine is a relief carving from ancient Greece, now held by the Staatliche Museen in Berlin.

Suggested citation: IOM (Institute of Medicine). 2009. *Veterans and Agent Orange: Update 2008*. Washington, DC: The National Academies Press.

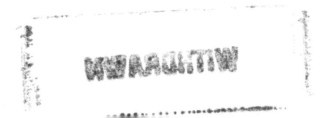

*"Knowing is not enough; we must apply.
Willing is not enough; we must do."*
—Goethe

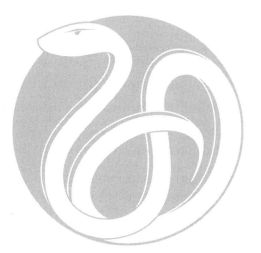

INSTITUTE OF MEDICINE
OF THE NATIONAL ACADEMIES

Advising the Nation. Improving Health.

THE NATIONAL ACADEMIES
Advisers to the Nation on Science, Engineering, and Medicine

The **National Academy of Sciences** is a private, nonprofit, self-perpetuating society of distinguished scholars engaged in scientific and engineering research, dedicated to the furtherance of science and technology and to their use for the general welfare. Upon the authority of the charter granted to it by the Congress in 1863, the Academy has a mandate that requires it to advise the federal government on scientific and technical matters. Dr. Ralph J. Cicerone is president of the National Academy of Sciences.

The **National Academy of Engineering** was established in 1964, under the charter of the National Academy of Sciences, as a parallel organization of outstanding engineers. It is autonomous in its administration and in the selection of its members, sharing with the National Academy of Sciences the responsibility for advising the federal government. The National Academy of Engineering also sponsors engineering programs aimed at meeting national needs, encourages education and research, and recognizes the superior achievements of engineers. Dr. Charles M. Vest is president of the National Academy of Engineering.

The **Institute of Medicine** was established in 1970 by the National Academy of Sciences to secure the services of eminent members of appropriate professions in the examination of policy matters pertaining to the health of the public. The Institute acts under the responsibility given to the National Academy of Sciences by its congressional charter to be an adviser to the federal government and, upon its own initiative, to identify issues of medical care, research, and education. Dr. Harvey V. Fineberg is president of the Institute of Medicine.

The **National Research Council** was organized by the National Academy of Sciences in 1916 to associate the broad community of science and technology with the Academy's purposes of furthering knowledge and advising the federal government. Functioning in accordance with general policies determined by the Academy, the Council has become the principal operating agency of both the National Academy of Sciences and the National Academy of Engineering in providing services to the government, the public, and the scientific and engineering communities. The Council is administered jointly by both Academies and the Institute of Medicine. Dr. Ralph J. Cicerone and Dr. Charles M. Vest are chair and vice chair, respectively, of the National Research Council.

www.national-academies.org

v

Reviewers

This report has been reviewed in draft form by individuals chosen for their diverse perspectives and technical expertise, in accordance with procedures approved by the National Research Council's Report Review Committee. The purpose of this independent review is to provide candid and critical comments that will assist the institution in making its published report as sound as possible and to ensure that the report meets institutional standards of objectivity, evidence, and responsiveness to the study charge. The review comments and draft manuscript remain confidential to protect the integrity of the deliberative process. We thank the following for their review of the report:

Rebecca Betensky, Department of Biostatistics, Harvard School of Public Health, Boston, Massachusetts

Linda Birnbaum, National Health and Environmental Effects Research Laboratory, US Environmental Protection Agency, Research Triangle Park, North Carolina

James Brophy, Royal Victoria Hospital, McGill University, Montreal, Quebec, Canada

Robert F. Herrick, Department of Environmental Health, Harvard School of Public Health, Boston, Massachusetts

Robert G. Holloway, Department of Neurology, University of Rochester Medical Center, Rochester, New York

Elaine S. Jaffe, Center for Cancer Research, National Cancer Institute, Bethesda, Maryland

Bernard M. Ravina, Department of Neurology, University of Rochester Medical Center, Rochester, New York

David A. Savitz, Disease Prevention and Public Health Institute, Mount Sinai School of Medicine, New York, New York

Robert D. Sparks, California Medical Association Foundation, El Dorado Hills, California

Jack Thompson, Northwest Center for Public Health Practice, Seattle, Washington

Hugh H. Tilson, Public Health Leadership Program, University of North Carolina, Chapel Hill, North Carolina

Bailus Walker, Jr., Department of Community Medicine, Howard University, Washington, DC

Mary K. Walker, College of Pharmacy, University of New Mexico, Albuquerque, New Mexico

Mary H. Ward, Division of Cancer Epidemiology and Genetics, National Cancer Institute, Rockville, Maryland

Although the reviewers listed above have provided many constructive comments and suggestions, they were not asked to endorse the conclusions or recommendations, nor did they see the final draft of the report before its release. The review of this report was overseen by **Kristine M. Gebbie**, School of Nursing, Hunter College, City University of New York, New York. Appointed by the National Research Council, she was responsible for making certain that an independent examination of this report was carried out in accordance with institutional procedures and that all review comments were carefully considered. Responsibility for the final content of this report rests with the authoring committee and the institution.

Preface

In 1991, Congress passed Public Law (PL) 102-4, the Agent Orange Act of 1991, to address the uncertainty about the long-term health effects on Vietnam veterans who during their service in Vietnam were exposed to herbicides—mixtures of 2,4-dichlorophenoxyacetic acid (2,4-D), 2,4,5-trichlorophenoxyacetic acid (2,4,5-T), and its contaminant 2,3,7,8-tetrachlorodibenzo-p-dioxin (TCDD), picloram, and cacodylic acid. That legislation directed the Secretary of Veterans Affairs to ask the National Academy of Sciences (NAS) to perform a comprehensive evaluation of scientific and medical information regarding the health effects of exposure to Agent Orange, other herbicides used in Vietnam, and the various chemical components of those herbicides, including TCDD. The resulting committee report, *Veterans and Agent Orange: Health Effects of Herbicides Used in Vietnam* (*VAO*), was published by the Institute of Medicine (IOM) in 1994. That report evaluated and integrated the scientific evidence regarding statistical associations between health outcomes and exposure to the herbicides and TCDD on the basis of published material that had accumulated by 1994.

As required by Public Law 102-4, the Secretary also asked that NAS conduct updates at least every 2 years for 10 years from the date of the first report to review newly available literature and draw conclusions from the overall evidence. The first of the updates, *Veterans and Agent Orange: Update 1996* (*Update 1996*), was published in March 1996. It was followed by *Veterans and Agent Orange: Update 1998* (*Update 1998*) in 1999, *Veterans and Agent Orange: Update 2000* (*Update 2000*) in 2001, *Veterans and Agent Orange: Update 2002* (*Update 2002*) in 2003, and *Veterans and Agent Orange: Update 2004* (*Update 2004*) in 2005.

PL 107-103, the Veterans Education and Benefits Expansion Act of 2001, extended the period for biennial updates to 2014. The first update after the new legislation was *Veterans and Agent Orange: Update 2006* (*Update 2006*), published in 2007. The present report is the second of this second 10-year period of evaluation.

The present update focuses on the scientific studies published since the release of *Update 2006*. To accomplish the review, IOM established a committee of 14 members representing a wide array of expertise to evaluate the newest scientific evidence and to consider it in light of the studies reviewed in *VAO, Update 1996, Update 1998, Update 2000, Update 2002, Update 2004*, and *Update 2006*. A link to the experience and expertise of previous committees was provided by recruiting six members from the committee responsible for *Update 2006*, two of whom had also served on the committees responsible for *Update 2004* and *Update 2006*. All committee members were selected because they are experts in their fields, have no conflicts of interest with regard to the matter under study, and have taken no public positions concerning the potential health effects of herbicides in Vietnam veterans or related aspects of herbicide or TCDD exposure. Biographic sketches of committee members and staff appear in Appendix C.

In this second decade of evaluation, the committee sought the most accurate information and advice from the widest possible array of knowledgeable sources for consideration. To be consistent with NAS procedures, the committee met in a series of closed sessions in which members could freely examine, characterize, and weigh the strengths and limitations of the evidence. The committee also convened three open meetings in March, June, and December 2008 to provide an opportunity for veterans and veterans service organizations, researchers, policy-makers, and other interested parties to present their concerns, review their research, and exchange information directly with committee members. The oral presentations and written statements submitted to the committee are listed in Appendix A. The committee thanks the persons who provided valuable insights into the health problems experienced by Vietnam veterans.

The committee is grateful to Mary Paxton, who skillfully served as study director for this project. The committee also acknowledges the excellent work of IOM staff members Jennifer Cohen, Tia Carter, David Butler, and Rose Marie Martinez. Thanks are also extended to Christie Bell, who handled the finances for the project; Norman Grossblatt, who provided editorial skills; and William McLeod, who conducted database searches.

The committee benefited from the assistance of several scientists and researchers who generously lent their time and expertise to give committee members insight into particular issues, provide copies of newly released research, or answer queries about their work. Steven Hawthorne, an environmental chemist at the University of North Dakota's Energy and Environmental Research Center, informed the committee about the ability of organic compounds to codistill during the production of potable water. Barbara Migeon, a professor at the Institute of Genetic Medicine at the Johns Hopkins University, and Michael Skinner, a professor at Washington State University, gave the committee an informative presentation on the nature of epigenetic mechanisms that may apply to dioxin. Vaughan Turekian, Chief International Officer of the American Association for the Advancement of Science and its representative to the US–Vietnam Dialogue Group on Agent Orange–Dioxin, discussed efforts toward cleanup and the possibility of conducting epidemiologic studies on the Vietnamese population cooperatively with the Vietnamese. Samuel Cohen, of the University of Nebraska Medical Center, was helpful in answering questions about the toxicity of organic arsenic. Christopher Reid, of the Charles Drew University of Medicine and Science, discussed Parkinson disease and herbicides sprayed in Vietnam. Joel Michalek, now of the University of Texas Health Center at San Antonio, joined us to discuss his long experience with the Air Force Health Study. And Douglas Wallace, a professor at the University of California, Irvine, described mitochrondial disruptions that might contribute to adverse health effects associated with Agent Orange.

Richard Fenske, PhD, MPH, *Chair*
Committee to Review the Health Effects
in Vietnam Veterans of Exposure to
Herbicides (Seventh Biennial Update)

Contents

ABBREVIATIONS AND ACRONYMS   xvii

SUMMARY   1
    Charge to the Committee, 2
    Committee's Approach to Its Charge, 3
    Evidence Reviewed by the Committee, 5
    The Committee's Conclusions, 6
    Committee Recommendations, 10

1   INTRODUCTION   13
    Charge to the Committee, 14
    Conclusions of Previous Veterans and Agent Orange Reports, 18
    Organization of This Report, 25
    References, 25

2   EVALUATING THE EVIDENCE   27
    Choice of Health Outcomes, 27
    Identification of Relevant Literature, 28
    Committee's Approach, 33
    Evaluation of the Evidence, 37
    References, 44

3   EXPOSURE TO THE HERBICIDES USED IN VIETNAM   46
    Military Use of Herbicides in Vietnam, 47
    TCDD in Herbicides Used in Vietnam, 49

Exposure of Vietnam Veterans, 51
Exposure of the Vietnamese Population, 55
New Models for Characterizing Herbicide Exposure, 56
Methodologic Issues in Exposure Assessment, 57
References, 61

4   INFORMATION RELATED TO BIOLOGIC PLAUSIBILITY   65
TCDD, 67
Phenoxy Herbicides: 2,4-D and 2,4,5-T, 81
Cacodylic Acid, 84
Picloram, 89
References, 92

5   EPIDEMIOLOGIC STUDIES—NEW CITATIONS AND
BACKGROUND ON REPEATEDLY STUDIED POPULATIONS   104
New Citations, 105
Relevant Populations: New Reports with Multiple Health Outcomes
     or with Results on Previously Studied Groups, 115
Vietnam-Veteran Studies, 115
Occupational Studies, 137
Environmental Studies, 158
References, 167

6   CANCER   202
Organization of Cancer Groupings, 204
Biologic Plausibility, 205
Oral, Nasal, and Pharyngeal Cancer, 209
Cancers of the Digestive Organs, 218
     Esophageal Cancer, 219
     Stomach Cancer, 223
     Colorectal Cancer, 233
     Hepatobiliary Cancers, 245
     Pancreatic Cancer, 252
Laryngeal Cancer, 259
Lung Cancer, 264
Bone and Joint Cancer, 275
Soft-Tissue Sarcomas, 279
Skin Cancer—Melanoma, 289
Skin Cancer—Basal-cell Cancer and Squamous-cell Cancer
     (Nonmelanoma Skin Cancers), 297
Breast Cancer, 301
Cancers of the Female Reproductive System, 311
Prostate Cancer, 317

Testicular Cancer, 328
Bladder Cancer, 332
Renal Cancer, 339
Brain Cancer, 345
Endocrine Cancers, 354
Lymphohematopoietic Cancers (Lymphomas and Leukemias), 358
    Hodgkin's Disease, 360
    Non-Hodgkin's Lymphoma, 368
    Multiple Myeloma, 385
    AL Amyloidosis, 392
    Leukemia, 394
        Chronic Lymphocytic Leukemia and Hairy Cell Leukemia, 406
Summary, 412
References, 414

7   REPRODUCTIVE EFFECTS AND IMPACTS ON FUTURE GENERATIONS   435
Biologic Plausibility of Reproductive Effects, 436
Endometriosis, 438
Fertility, 444
Spontaneous Abortion, 460
Stillbirth, Neonatal Death, and Infant Death, 465
Birth Weight and Preterm Delivery, 467
Birth Defects, 469
Childhood Cancer, 480
Effects Occurring Later in Offspring's Life or in Later Generations, 489
Summary, 494
References, 495

8   NEUROLOGIC DISORDERS   510
Neurobehavioral (Cognitive or Neuropsychiatric) Disorders, 512
Neurodegenerative Diseases, 515
    Parkinson's Disease and Parkinsonism, 515
    Amyotrophic Lateral Sclerosis, 527
Peripheral Neuropathy, 530
Summary, 536
References, 538

9   OTHER HEALTH EFFECTS   546
Chloracne, 547
Porphyria Cutanea Tarda, 549
Respiratory Disorders, 552
Immune-System Disorders, 566

Immune Suppression, 567
Allergy, 567
Autoimmune Disease, 568
Type 2 Diabetes, 571
Lipid and Lipoprotein Disorders, 587
Gastrointestinal and Digestive Disease, Including Liver Toxicity, 593
Peptic-Ulcer Disease, 593
Liver Disease, 594
Circulatory Disorders, 597
Hypertension, 620
Circulatory Diseases, 623
Synthesis, 627
Hypertension, 627
Ischemic Heart Disease, 628
Other Circulatory Disease, 631
Thyroid Homeostasis, 631
Summary, 636
References, 638

10 CONCLUSIONS AND RECOMMENDATIONS   **651**
Synopsis of Committee Conclusions, 651
Committee Recommendations, 655
References, 661

APPENDIXES

A Agendas of Public Meetings Held by the Committee to Review
    the Health Effects in Vietnam Veterans of Exposure to Herbicides
    (Seventh Biennial Update)   663
B Clarification of Cancer Groupings Used in Reporting Results,
    with Correspondence to NIOSH Cause-of-Death Codes and
    ICD Codes for Cancers   666
C Committee to Review the Health Effects in Vietnam Veterans of
    Exposure to Herbicides (Seventh Biennial Update) and Staff
    Biographies   676

Abbreviations and Acronyms

2,4-D	2,4-dichlorophenoxyacetic acid
2,4-DB	2-(2,4-diichlorophenoxy) butyric acid
2,4,5-T	2,4,5-trichlorophenoxyacetic acid
2,4,5-TCP	2,4,5-trichlorophenol
2,4,5-TP	2-(2,4,5-trichlorophenoxy) propionic acid or Silvex
ACC	Army Chemical Corps
ACS	American Cancer Society
AD	Alzheimer's disease
ADME	absorption, distribution, metabolism, and excretion
AFHS	Air Force Health Study
AH	aryl hydrocarbon
AHR	AH receptor
AHRE	AHR-responsive element of the canonical DNA recognition motif of the AHR/ARNT complex, also referred to as the dioxin-responsive element (DRE) or the xenobiotic-responsive element (XRE)
AHS	Agricultural Health Study
AHH	aryl hydrocarbon hydroxylase
AHRE	AHR-responsive element, which is the recognition motif of the AHR/ARNT complex (also called DRE or XRE)
AL	acute leukemia
AL amyloidosis	amyloid light chain form of amyloidosis in which the amyloid in deposits in various organs and tissues consists of antibody light chains

ALL	acute lymphocytic leukemia
ALS	amyotrophic lateral sclerosis (or Lou Gehrig's disease)
AOR	VA's Agent Orange Registry
ARNT	aryl hydrocarbon nuclear translocator
B[a]P	benzo[a]pyrene
bHLH	basic-helix-loop-helix
BIRLS	VA's Beneficiary Identification Record Locator Subsystem
BMI	body mass index
CALUX	assay for determination of dioxin-like activity in tissue samples
CAS No.	CAS Number is generated by the Chemical Abstracts Service and serves as unique identifier for every chemical
CDC	Centers for Disease Control and Prevention
CDD	chlorinated dibenzo-*p*-dioxin (usually preceded by indication of number of chlorine atoms substituted on chemical's rings)
CDF	chlorinated dibenzofuran (usually preceded by indication of number of chlorine atoms substituted on chemical's rings)
CI	confidence interval, as defined by lower (LCL) and upper confidence limits (UCL)
CLL	chronic lymphocytic leukemia (which is now regarded as being the same disease as small lymphocytic leukemia [SLL] and designated by some as CLL/SLL)
CNS	central nervous system
COIs	chemicals of interest to VAO series (i.e., TCDD, 2,4,5-T, 2,4-D, picloram, and cacodylic acid)
CVD	cardiovascular disease
CYP—	cytochrome P450 (individual type of these metabolizing enzymes are indicted by a number-letter-number suffix)
DEET	*N,N*-dietheyl-*m*-toluamide, insecticide
DEN	deep endometriotic nodule
dl	dioxin-like
DLC	dioxin-like compound (or chemical)
DMA	dimethyl arsenic acid
DMA^{III}	dimethyl arsenic acid of valency 3
DMA^{V}	dimethyl arsenic acid of valency 5; form of arsenic found in cacodylic acid
DOD	US Department of Defense
DRE	dioxin-responsive element, which is the recognition motif of the AHR/ARNT complex (also called AHRE or XRE)

ECG	electrocardiography
EE	ethynyl estradiol
EFMA	European Fertilizer Manufacturers Association
EPA	US Environmental Protection Agency
EU	European Union
fg	femtogram (10^{-15} gram)
FSH	follicle-stimulating hormone
GCT	germ-cell tumor
GD	gestation day
GERD	gastroesophageal reflux disease
GGT	γ-glutamyltransferase
GI	gastrointestinal
GIS	geographic information system
HbA1c	Hemoglobin A1c
HCL	hairy cell leukemia
HD	Hodgkin's disease (now referred to by some as Hodgkin's lymphoma)
HDL	high-density lipoprotein
HIV	human immunodeficiency virus
HLA	human leukocyte antigen
HOMA-IR	homeostasis-model assessment of insulin resistance
HpCDD	heptachlorodibenzo-*p*-dioxin, a dioxin congener with seven chlorines
HpCDF	heptachlorodibenzofuran, a furan congener with seven chlorines
HPV	human papilloma virus
HR	hazard ratio
hsp	heat shock protein
HxCDD	hexachlorodibenzo-*p*-dioxin, a dioxin congener with six chlorines
HxCDF	hexachlorodibenzofuran, a furan congener with six chlorines
IARC	International Agency for Research on Cancer
ICD-#	International Classification of Diseases, Revision # (# = version current for records being abstracted)
ICDO-II	International Classification of Diseases for Oncology, 2nd edition
IDL	intermediate-density lipoprotein
IH	industrial hygienist
IHD	ischemic heart disease

IgE	immunoglobulin E
IL-6	interleukin-6 (also called β2-interferon)
IRS	Internal Revenue Service
IU	international unit
IUGR	intrauterine growth retardation
JEM	job-exposure matrix
LCL	lower confidence limit
LD_{xx}	dose lethal to xx% of the animals exposed
LDL	low-density lipoprotein
LEL	lowest effect level
LH	luteinizing hormone
M	molar (concentration in a solution, molecules per volume)
MCPA	2-methyl-4-chlorophenoxyacetic acid
MCPP	2-(2-methyl-4-chlorophenoxy) propionic acid or Mecoprop
mg	milligram
MIP	macrophage-inflammatory protein
MMA	monomethyl arsonic acid
mmHG	millimeters mercury, for blood pressure measurements
MMP	matrix metalloproteinase
MOSC	Military Occupational Specialty Code
MPTP	1-methyl-4-phenyl-1,2,4,6-tetrahydropyridine
MTD	maximum tolerated dose
na	not applicable
NETRP	Neurotoxin Exposure Treatment Research Program
ng	nanogram (10^{-9} gram)
NHANES	National Health and Nutrition Examination Survey
NHL	non-Hodgkin's lymphoma
NIOSH	National Institute of Occupational Safety and Health
NK/T-cell	natural killer T-cell
NLS	nuclear-localization signal
NOEL	no-observed-effect level
NPC	nasopharyngeal carcinoma
nr	not reported
NRC	National Research Council
ns	not significant (usually refers to $p < 0.05$)
OCDD	octachlorodibenzo-*p*-dioxin (1,2,3,4,6,7,8,9-OCDT is the only dioxin congener with eight chlorines)

OCDF	octachlorodibenzofuran (1,2,3,4,6,7,8,9-OCDF is the only dioxin congener with eight chlorines)
OFFHS	Ontario Farm Family Health Study
OR	odds ratio
PAH	polycyclic aromatic hydrocarbons
PAS	Per-ARNT-Sim protein domain of amino-acid sequences related to sequences in ARNT and the *Drosophila melanogaster* genes *period* and *single minded*
PBPK model	physiologically-based pharmacokinetic model
PBDD	polybrominated dibenzo-*p*-dioxin
PBDF	polybrominated dibenzofuran
PCB	polychlorinated biphenyl
PCDD	polychlorinated dibenzo-*p*-dioxin
PCDD/F	dioxins and furans combined
PCDF	polychlorinated dibenzofuran
PCP	pentachlorophenol
PCT	porphyria cutanea tarda
PD	Parkinson's disease
PE	peritoneal endometriosis
PeCDF	pentachlorodibenzofuran, a furan congener with five chlorines
pg	picogram (10^{-12} gram)
picloram	4-amino-3,5,6-trichloropicolinic acid
PL	Public Law
PM	proportionate mortality
PMR	proportional mortality ratio
PND	postnatal day
PNS	peripheral nervous system
POP	persistent organic pollutant
ppb	parts per billion = ng/g
ppm	parts per million = mg/g
ppt	parts per trillion = pg/g
PSA	prostate-specific antigen
PtCDF	pentachlorodibenzofuran
PTD	preterm delivery, premature birth at less than 259 days (37 weeks gestation)
PTSD	post-traumatic stress disorder
RANTES	regulated on activation, normal T cell–expressed, and secreted
RDD	random-digit dialing

RH	Ranch Hand, member of Air Force unit primarily responsible for spraying herbicides in Vietnam
ROS	reactive oxygen species
RR	relative risk
SCE	sister chromatid exchange
SCL-90	Symptom Checklist-90-Revised
SEA	Southeast Asia
SEER	Surveillance, Epidemiology, and End Results
SES	socioeconomic status
SIR	Standardized Incidence Ratio
SLE	systemic lupus erythematosus
SLL	small lymphocytic lymphoma, which is now recognized as a different stage of CLL, rather than a separate disease
SMR	standardized mortality ratio
SPECT	single-photon emission computerized tomography
STS	soft-tissue sarcoma
SWHS	Seveso Women's Health Study
T3	triiodothyronine
T4	thyroxine
TCDD	2,3,7,8-tetrachlorodibenzo-*p*-dioxin
TCDF	tetrachlorodibenzofuran, a furan congener with four chlorines
TEF	toxicity equivalency factor, potency of a dioxin-like compound (DLC) relative to TCDD
TEQ	(total) toxicity equivalent quotient or cumulative toxic potency, sum of TEFs for a mixture of PCDDs, PCDFs, and PCBs
tetraCDD	tetrachlorodibenzo-*p*-dioxin, any of the dioxin congeners with four chlororines, including TCDD as defined above
TIPA	triisopropanolamine
TPA	12-*O*-tetradecanoylphorbol-13-acetate
TRH	thyrotropin-releasing hormone
TSH	thyroid-stimulating hormone
TWA	time-weighted average
UFW	United Farm Workers of America
VA	US Department of Veterans Affairs; previously, Veterans Administration
VEGF	vascular endothelial growth factor
VES	Vietnam Experience Study
VLDL	very-low-density lipoprotein

WBC   white blood cell
WHO   World Health Organization

XAP2   hepatitis B virus X-associated protein 2
XRE   xenobiotic-responsive element, which is the recognition motif
                 of the AHR/ARNT complex (also called DRE or AHRE)

Summary

From 1962 to 1971, the US military sprayed herbicides over Vietnam to strip the thick jungle canopy that could conceal opposition forces, to destroy crops that those forces might depend on, and to clear tall grasses and bushes from the perimeters of US base camps and outlying fire-support bases. Mixtures of 2,4-dichlorophenoxyacetic acid (2,4-D), 2,4,5-trichlorophenoxyacetic acid (2,4,5-T), picloram, and cacodylic acid made up the bulk of the herbicides sprayed. The herbicide mixtures used were named according to the colors of identification bands painted on the storage drums; the main chemical mixture sprayed was Agent Orange (a 50:50 mixture of 2,4-D and 2,4,5-T). At the time of the spraying, 2,3,7,8-tetrachlorodibenzo-p-dioxin (TCDD), the most toxic form of dioxin, was an unintended contaminant generated during the production of 2,4,5-T and so was present in Agent Orange and some other formulations sprayed in Vietnam; it is important to remember that Agent Orange is not synonymous with TCDD or dioxin.

In 1991, because of continuing uncertainty about long-term health effects of the sprayed herbicides in Vietnam veterans, Congress passed Public Law (PL) 102-4, the Agent Orange Act of 1991. That legislation directed the Secretary of Veterans Affairs to ask the National Academy of Sciences (NAS) to perform a comprehensive evaluation of scientific and medical information regarding the health effects of exposure to Agent Orange, other herbicides used in Vietnam, and the various components of those herbicides, including TCDD. The legislation also instructed the Secretary to ask NAS to conduct updates every 2 years for 10 years from the date of the first report to review newly available literature and draw conclusions from the overall evidence.

In response to the first request, the Institute of Medicine (IOM) convened

1

a committee, whose conclusions IOM published in 1994 in *Veterans and Agent Orange: Health Effects of Herbicides Used in Vietnam (VAO)*. The work of later committees resulted in the publication of biennial updates (*Update 1996*, *Update 1998*, *Update 2000*, *Update 2002*, and *Update 2004*) and of focused reports on the scientific evidence regarding type 2 diabetes, acute myelogenous leukemia in children, and the latent period for respiratory cancer.

Enacted in 2002, PL 107-103, the Veterans Education and Benefits Expansion Act of 2001, mandated that the *VAO* biennial updates continue through 2014. *Update 2006* was the first report published under that legislation. The current update presents this committee's review of peer-reviewed scientific reports concerning associations between health outcomes and exposure to TCDD and other chemicals in the herbicides used in Vietnam that were published in October 2006–September 2008 and the committee's integration of this information with the previously established evidence database.

CHARGE TO THE COMMITTEE

In accordance with PL 102-4 and PL 107-103, the Committee to Review the Health Effects in Vietnam Veterans of Exposure to Herbicides (Seventh Biennial Update) was asked to "determine (to the extent that available scientific data permit meaningful determinations)" the following regarding associations between specific health outcomes and exposure to TCDD and other chemicals in herbicides used by the military in Vietnam:

A) whether a statistical association with herbicide exposure exists, taking into account the strength of the scientific evidence and the appropriateness of the statistical and epidemiological methods used to detect the association;

B) the increased risk of disease among those exposed to herbicides during service in the Republic of Vietnam during the Vietnam era; and

C) whether there exists a plausible biological mechanism or other evidence of a causal relationship between herbicide exposure and the disease.

The committee notes that, as a consequence of congressional and judicial history, both its congressional mandate and the statement of task are phrased with the target of evaluation being "association" between exposure and health outcomes. The rigor of the evidentiary database needed to support a finding of statistical association is weaker than that needed to establish causality, but positive findings for any of the aspects of scientific evidence supportive of causality enhance conviction that an observed statistical association is reliable. Such scientific evidence, of course, would include any information assembled in relation to plausible biologic mechanisms as directed in Article C. In accord with its charge, the committee examined a variety of indicators appropriate for the task, including factors commonly used to evaluate statistical associations, such as the adequacy of control for bias and confounding and the likelihood that an observed association could be explained by chance. Additionally, the committee assessed evidence concerning biologic plausibility derived from laboratory findings in cell-culture or animal models. In particular, associations with multiple supportive indicators are interpreted as having stronger scientific support.

In conducting its study, the present committee operated independently of the Department of Veterans Affairs (VA) and other government agencies. The committee was not asked to make and did not make judgments regarding specific cases in which individual Vietnam veterans have claimed injury from herbicide exposure. This report provides scientific information for the Secretary of Veterans Affairs to consider as VA exercises its responsibilities to Vietnam veterans. The committee was not charged to focus on broader issues, such as the potential costs of compensation for veterans or policies regarding such compensation.

In addition to the above charge, VA made two specific requests to the current committee. First, the committee was asked to consider whether the occurrence of hairy cell leukemia should be regarded as being associated with exposure to the components of herbicides used by the military in Vietnam. Second, the committee was asked to comment on whether effects of herbicide exposure might be manifested at later stages of a child's development than have systematically been evaluated to date or in later generations and on the feasibility of assessing such effects.

COMMITTEE'S APPROACH TO ITS CHARGE

Following the pattern established by prior VAO committees, the present committee concentrated its review on epidemiologic studies to fulfill its charge of assessing whether specific human health effects are associated with exposure to at least one of the herbicides sprayed in Vietnam or to TCDD. The committee also considered controlled laboratory investigations that provided information on whether association between the chemicals of interest and a given effect is biologically plausible.

The *VAO* committees began their evaluation presuming neither the presence nor the absence of association for any particular health outcome. Over the sequence of reviews, evidence of various degrees of association, lack of association, or persisting indeterminacy with respect to a wide array of disease states has accrued. For many conditions, however, particularly ones that are very uncommon, any association with the chemicals of interest has remained unaddressed in the medical research literature; for these (unless the condition is logically subsumed under a broader disease category that has been evaluated), the committee remains neutral, abiding by the maxim that "absence of evidence is not evidence of absence."

In accord with Congress's mandated presumption of herbicide exposure for all Vietnam veterans, VAO committees have treated Vietnam-veteran status as a proxy for some herbicide exposure when no more specific exposure information is available. To obtain information potentially relevant to the evaluation of health effects related to herbicide exposure in addition to that available from studies of Vietnam veterans, the committee reviewed studies of other groups potentially exposed to the constituents of the herbicide mixtures used in Vietnam (2,4-D, 2,4,5-T, TCDD, cacodylic acid, and picloram). In addition to retrieving articles identified on the basis of keywords specifying the compounds and chemical classes of interest, literature searches for the earliest reports in the *VAO* series had been structured to retrieve all studies of several occupational groups, including chemical, agricultural, pulp and paper, sawmill, and forestry workers. To the extent that studies of those workforces were recovered in new searches directed at particular agents of exposure, they were incorporated into the database. Some occupational and environmental cohorts that received exceptionally high exposures (such as the International Agency for Research on Cancer and Seveso cohorts discussed in this report) are now well characterized and are producing a stream of informative results. A continuing prospective cohort study of agricultural populations with specific information on the chemicals of interest is also steadily contributing new findings to the database. Most important, the Vietnam veterans themselves are advancing in age and, when studied, are capable of providing substantial information on chronic health conditions directly. As the information in the database on populations with established exposures to the chemicals of interest has grown, the committee has come to depend less on data from studies with nonspecific exposure information and has been able to focus more on findings of studies with refined exposure specificity.

The original legislation, PL 102-4, did not provide a list of specific diseases and conditions suspected of being associated with herbicide exposure. Such a list was developed on the basis of diseases and conditions that had been mentioned in the scientific literature or in other documents identified through the original *VAO*'s extensive literature searches. The *VAO* list has been augmented in response to developments in the literature, requests by VA, and concerns of Vietnam veterans.

The information that the present committee reviewed was identified through a comprehensive search of relevant databases, including databases covering biologic, medical, toxicologic, chemical, historical, and regulatory information. The search of literature published through September 30, 2008, identified more than 7,000 potentially relevant citations. Screening of those retained about 850 for closer consideration, and roughly 300 ultimately contributed new information to this review. Additional information came from veterans and other interested people who testified at public hearings and offered written submissions.

To determine whether there is an association between exposure and a health outcome, epidemiologists estimate the magnitude of an appropriate measure (such as the relative risk or the odds ratio) that describes the relationship between exposure and disease in a defined population or group. In evaluating the strength of the evidence linking herbicide exposure with a particular outcome, the committee considered whether such estimates of risk might be incorrect (because of confounding, chance, or bias related to errors in selection and measurement) or might accurately represent true associations; although they are not required, data supporting biologic plausibility serve to strengthen confidence that an association is not spurious. It has been the practice of all VAO committees to evaluate all studies according to the same criteria and then to weight findings of similar strength and validity equivalently, whether or not the study subjects are Vietnam veterans, when drawing conclusions. The committee recognizes that an absolute conclusion about the absence of association might never be attained, because, as is generally the case in science, studies of health outcomes after herbicide exposure cannot demonstrate that a purported effect is impossible, only that it is statistically improbable.

EVIDENCE REVIEWED BY THE COMMITTEE

The sections below summarize new epidemiologic information evaluated in this update and integrated with that previously assembled. The epidemiologic studies have been divided, both here and in the health-outcome chapters, into three categories—Vietnam-veteran, occupational, and environmental—depending on the population addressed.

Vietnam-Veterans Studies

Four studies of Vietnam veterans published since *Update 2006* were reviewed by the committee. The Air Force Health Study produced findings related to cancer incidence, diabetes, serum testosterone concentrations, and benign prostatic hyperplasia. Prostate cancer was studied in Vietnam veterans in the California VA Health System. Mortality from all cancers, occurrences of several individual cancers, and other health outcomes were studied in female Vietnam veterans.

Occupational Studies

Several occupational studies have been published since *Update 2006*. Recent reports from the Agricultural Health Study examined the incidence of respiratory outcomes, neurologic symptoms, Parkinson's disease (PD), diabetes, and cancer in private pesticide applicators (farmers), their spouses, and commercial pesticide applicators. Cancer outcomes were investigated in Danish gardeners exposed to pesticides, including 2,4-D and 2,4,5-T; in German nationals with relevant exposures derived from job–exposure matrices; and in members of the United Farm Workers of America occupationally exposed to 2,4-D. Circulatory diseases and neurologic outcomes were studied in a follow-up of Czech production workers who were exposed to TCDD during the production of 2,4,5-T. New case–control studies have investigated occupational exposures and risk factors for various cancer outcomes and childhood leukemia.

Environmental Studies

Studies of the Seveso cohort that update earlier findings concerning cancer, birth outcomes, diabetes, and circulatory, respiratory, and digestive diseases have been published since *Update 2006*. The continuing Seveso Women's Health Study also published studies of ovarian function and fibroids in Seveso women. Cancer outcomes were evaluated in follow-up studies of residents of Italy, New Zealand, and Besançon, France, and respiratory outcomes in participants of the Ontario Farm Family Health Study were investigated. Data from the National Health and Nutrition Examination Survey were used in several studies of health outcomes, including hypertension, cardiovascular disease, diabetes, and increased concentrations of lipids in relation to serum concentrations of dioxin-like compounds. New case–control studies examined occupational and environmental exposures to the chemicals of interest and other risk factors for various reproductive and cancer outcomes and for PD.

THE COMMITTEE'S CONCLUSIONS

Health Outcomes

The present committee weighed the strengths and limitations of the epidemiologic evidence reviewed in this report and in previous VAO reports. Although the studies published since *Update 2006* are the subject of detailed evaluation in this report, the committee drew its conclusions in the context of the entire body of literature. The contribution of recent publications to the evidence database was substantial, but the committee did not weigh them more heavily merely because they were new. Epidemiologic methods and analytic capabilities have improved, but many of the recent studies were also particularly useful for this committee's purpose because they produced results in terms of serum TCDD concentrations or because their findings consisted of observations on the aging population of primary concern, Vietnam veterans.

Table S-1 defines four categories of association and gives criteria for assigning health outcomes to them. On the basis of its evaluation of veteran, occupational, and environmental studies, the committee allocated particular health outcomes to categories of relative certainty of association with exposure to the herbicides that were used in Vietnam or to any of their components or contaminants (with no intention of specifying particular chemicals). The committee notes that experimental data related to biologic plausibility of conditions statistically associated with exposure to Agent Orange has gradually emerged since the beginning of this series of VAO reports and that these findings can inform the decisions

TABLE S-1 Summary of *Seventh Biennial Update* of Findings of Occupational, Environmental, and Veterans Studies Regarding Associations Between Exposure to Herbicides and Specific Health Outcomes[a]

Sufficient Evidence of an Association

Epidemiologic evidence is sufficient to conclude that there is a positive association. That is, a positive association has been observed between exposure to herbicides and the outcome in studies in which chance, bias, and confounding could be ruled out with reasonable confidence.[b] For example, if several small studies that are free of bias and confounding show an association that is consistent in magnitude and direction, there could be sufficient evidence of an association. There is sufficient evidence of an association between exposure to the chemicals of interest and the following health outcomes:

> Soft-tissue sarcoma (including heart)
> Non-Hodgkin's lymphoma
> Chronic lymphocytic leukemia (including **hairy cell leukemia and other chronic B-cell leukemias) (category clarification since *Update 2006*)**
> Hodgkin's disease
> Chloracne

Limited or Suggestive Evidence of an Association

Epidemiologic evidence suggests an association between exposure to herbicides and the outcome, but a firm conclusion is limited because chance, bias, and confounding could not be ruled out with confidence.[b] For example, a well-conducted study with strong findings in accord with less compelling results from studies of populations with similar exposures could constitute such evidence. There is limited or suggestive evidence of an association between exposure to the chemicals of interest and the following health outcomes:

> Laryngeal cancer
> Cancer of the lung, bronchus, or trachea
> Prostate cancer
> Multiple myeloma
> AL amyloidosis
> Early-onset transient peripheral neuropathy
> **Parkinson's disease (category change from *Update 2006*)**
> Porphyria cutanea tarda
> Hypertension
> **Ischemic heart disease (category change from *Update 2006*)**
> Type 2 diabetes (mellitus)
> Spina bifida in offspring of exposed people

Inadequate or Insufficient Evidence to Determine an Association

The available epidemiologic studies are of insufficient quality, consistency, or statistical power to permit a conclusion regarding the presence or absence of an association. For example, studies fail to control for confounding, have inadequate exposure assessment, or fail to address latency. There is inadequate or insufficient evidence to determine association between exposure to the chemicals of interest and the following health outcomes that were explicitly reviewed:

> Cancers of the oral cavity (including lips and tongue), pharynx (including tonsils), or nasal cavity (including ears and sinuses)
> Cancers of the pleura, mediastinum, and other unspecified sites in the respiratory system and intrathoracic organs

continued

TABLE S-1 Continued

Esophageal cancer
Stomach cancer
Colorectal cancer (including small intestine and anus)
Hepatobiliary cancers (liver, gallbladder, and bile ducts)
Pancreatic cancer
Bone and joint cancer
Melanoma
Nonmelanoma skin cancer (basal cell and squamous cell)
Breast cancer
Cancers of reproductive organs (cervix, uterus, ovary, testes, and penis; excluding prostate)
Urinary bladder cancer
Renal cancer (kidney and renal pelvis)
Cancers of brain and nervous system (including eye)
Endocrine cancers (thyroid, thymus, and other endocrine organs)
Leukemia (**other than all chronic B-cell leukemias**, including chronic lymphocytic leukemia and hairy cell leukemia)
Cancers at other and unspecified sites
Infertility
Spontaneous abortion (other than after paternal exposure to TCDD, which appears *not* to be associated)
Neonatal or infant death and stillbirth in offspring of exposed people
Low birth weight in offspring of exposed people
Birth defects (other than spina bifida) in offspring of exposed people
Childhood cancer (including acute myelogenous leukemia) in offspring of exposed people
Neurobehavioral disorders (cognitive and neuropsychiatric)
Neurodegenerative diseases, excluding Parkinson's disease
Chronic peripheral nervous system disorders
Respiratory disorders (wheeze or asthma, chronic obstructive pulmonary disease, and farmer's lung)
Gastrointestinal, metabolic, and digestive disorders (changes in hepatic enzymes, lipid abnormalities, and ulcers)
Immune system disorders (immune suppression, allergy, and autoimmunity)
Circulatory disorders (other than hypertension and ischemic heart disease)
Endometriosis
Effects on thyroid homeostasis

This committee used a classification that spans the full array of cancers. However, reviews for nonmalignant conditions were conducted only if they were found to have been the subjects of epidemiologic investigation or at the request of the Department of Veterans Affairs. *By default, any health outcome on which no epidemiologic information has been found falls into this category.*

Limited or Suggestive Evidence of *No* Association
Several adequate studies, which cover the full range of human exposure, are consistent in not showing a positive association between any magnitude of exposure to the herbicides of interest and the outcome. A conclusion of "no association" is inevitably limited to the conditions, exposures, and length of observation covered by the available studies. *In addition, the possibility of a very small increase in risk at the exposure studied can never be excluded.* There is limited or suggestive

TABLE S-1 Continued

evidence of *no* association between exposure to the herbicides of interest and the following health outcomes:

      Spontaneous abortion after paternal exposure to TCDD

[a] *Herbicides* indicates the following chemicals of interest: 2,4-dichlorophenoxyacetic acid (2,4-D), 2,4,5-trichlorophenoxyacetic acid (2,4,5-T) and its contaminant 2,3,7,8-tetrachlorodibenzo-*p*-dioxin (TCDD, or dioxin), cacodylic acid, and picloram. The evidence regarding association was drawn from occupational, environmental, and veteran studies in which people were exposed to the herbicides used in Vietnam, to their components, or to their contaminants.

[b] Evidence for an association is strengthened by experimental data supporting biologic plausibility, but its absence would not detract from the epidemiologic evidence.

about how to categorize the degree of association for individual conditions; a footnote to this effect has been added to Table S-1.

After considering information related to VA's question about hairy-cell leukemia, the committee concluded that not just hairy-cell leukemia, like chronic lymphoid leukemia, but all chronic B-cell neoplasms belong in the category of "sufficient evidence of an association" with Hodgkin's disease and non-Hodgkin's lymphoma. The committee concluded that ischemic heart disease should move from the category of "inadequate or insufficient evidence of an association" into the category of "limited or suggestive evidence of an association." Several pieces of new information specifically on exposure to the chemicals of interest led the committee to decide that PD should also be promoted from the "inadequate or insufficient evidence" category into the "limited or suggestive evidence" category. These changes to the classifications made in the previous update are bolded in Table S-1.

As mandated by PL 102-4, the distinctions among categories are based on statistical association, not on strict causality. The committee was directed to review the scientific data, not to recommend VA policy; therefore, conclusions reported in Table S-1 are not intended to imply or suggest policy decisions. The conclusions are related to associations between exposure and outcomes in human populations, not to the likelihood that any individual's health problem is associated with or caused by the herbicides in question.

Risk in Vietnam Veterans

There have been numerous health studies of Vietnam veterans, but most have been hampered by relatively poor measures of exposure to herbicides or TCDD and by other methodologic problems. In light of those problems, many conclusions regarding associations between exposure to the chemicals of interest and disease have been based on studies of people exposed in various occupational and environmental settings rather than on studies of Vietnam veterans, although studies of health consequences in the maturing veterans themselves have now begun to generate more informative findings. The committee believes that there is sufficient evidence to reach general or qualitative conclusions about associations between herbicide exposure and health outcomes, but the lack of adequate exposure data on Vietnam veterans themselves makes it difficult to estimate the degree of increased risk of disease in Vietnam veterans as a group or individually. Without information on the extent of herbicide exposure of Vietnam veterans and quantitative information about the dose–time–response relationship for each health outcome in humans, estimation of the risks experienced by veterans exposed to the chemicals of interest during the Vietnam War is not possible.

Because of those limitations, only general assertions can be made about risks to Vietnam veterans, depending on the category of association into which a given health outcome has been placed. If there were "limited or suggestive evidence of *no* association" between herbicide exposure and a health outcome, the evidence would suggest no increased risk of the outcome in Vietnam veterans attributable to exposure to the chemicals of interest (at least for the conditions, exposures, and lengths of observation covered by the studies reviewed). Even qualitative estimates are not possible when there is "inadequate or insufficient" evidence of an association. For outcomes categorized as having "sufficient" or "limited or suggestive" evidence of an association with herbicide exposure, the lack of exposure information on Vietnam veterans prevents calculation of precise risk estimates.

The information needed for assigning risk estimates continues to be absent despite concerted efforts to model the exposure of the troops in Vietnam, to measure the serum TCDD concentrations of individual veterans, and to model the dynamics of retention and clearance of TCDD in the human body. Accordingly, the committee states as a general conclusion that, at least for the present, it is not possible to derive quantitative estimates of any increased risks of various adverse health effects that Vietnam veterans may have experienced in association with exposure to the herbicides sprayed in Vietnam.

COMMITTEE RECOMMENDATIONS

IOM has been asked to make recommendations concerning the need, if any, for additional scientific studies to resolve continuing scientific uncertainties about the health effects of the herbicides used in Vietnam and their contaminants. Great strides have been made over the past several years in understanding the health effects of exposure to the herbicides used in Vietnam and to TCDD and in elucidating the mechanisms that underlie the effects, but there are still subjects on which increased knowledge could be very useful.

While presenting the charge, VA asked that the committee comment on whether effects of herbicide exposures might be manifested at later stages of a child's development than have systematically been evaluated or in later generations and comment on the feasibility of assessing such effects. The chapter on reproductive effects contains the committee's synopsis of toxicologic and epidemiologic information relevant to the request, little of which to date is directly related to the chemicals of interest to the VAO series. Developing understanding of epigenetic mechanisms leads this committee to conclude that it is considerably more plausible than previously believed that exposure to the herbicides sprayed in Vietnam might have caused paternally-mediated transgenerational effects. Such potential would most likely be attributable to the TCDD contaminant in Agent Orange. Consequently, this committee recommends that laboratory research be conducted to address and characterize TCDD's potential for inducing epigenetic modifications. As the offspring of Vietnam veterans grow older, the possibility of a parental effect on the incidence of adult cancers, cognitive problems, and other diseases of maturity are of increasing interest. While information concerning the applicability of epigenetic mechanism to TCDD is being gathered, the committee further recommends innovative epidemiologic protocols be developed to address the logistically challenging task of determining whether adverse effects are being manifested in the adult children and grandchildren of Vietnam veterans.

This committee recommends the pursuit of additional research in toxicology. The development of animal models of various chronic health conditions and their progression would be useful for understanding the possible contributions of the chemicals of interest to compromise the health of aging Vietnam veterans. Additional health problems, such as metabolic syndrome and male-mediated effects in offspring, merit laboratory investigation and study in human populations.

The committee notes that the earlier investment in studying several exposed populations is now producing useful findings; the National Institute for Occupational Safety and Health, Seveso, Air Force Health Study, and Army Chemical Corps cohorts all merit continuing follow-up or more comprehensive analysis. It is especially important that longitudinal analyses be conducted on cancer and reproductive outcomes represented in the complete database assembled in the course of the Air Force Health Study. Consideration should also be given to restarting the congressionally mandated National Vietnam Veterans Longitudinal Study, derived from the cohort originally studied in the National Vietnam Veterans Readjustment Study. New epidemiologic studies, such as a case–control study of tonsil cancer developed from VA's existing files or a study of reproductive effects in the Vietnamese population, could enable the recovery of valuable information.

The committee notes that its recommendations are similar to those offered in previous updates and that there has been little activity in several critical areas. The fate of the assemblage of data and biologic samples from the Air Force Health Study remains unsettled; in the interim, critical integrative analyses such as longitudinal evaluation of the cancer data have not yet been made public, and the unique potential of this resource languishes. It is the committee's conviction that work needs to be undertaken promptly to resolve questions regarding several health outcomes, most urgently tonsil cancer, melanoma, and paternally transmitted transgenerational effects. Creative analysis of VA's own data resources and further work on cohorts that have already been established may well be the most effective way to address those outcomes and to gain a better understanding of the role of herbicide exposure in development of PD in Vietnam veterans.

1

Introduction

The Agent Orange Act of 1991 (Public Law [PL] 102-4, enacted February 6, 1991, and codified as Section 1116 of Title 38 of the United States Code) directed the Secretary of Veterans Affairs to ask the National Academy of Sciences (NAS) to conduct an independent comprehensive review and evaluation of scientific and medical information regarding the health effects of exposure to herbicides used during military operations in Vietnam. The herbicides picloram and cacodylic acid were to be addressed, as were chemicals in various formulations containing the herbicides 2,4-dichlorophenoxyacetic acid (2,4-D) and 2,4,5-trichlorophenoxyacetic acid (2,4,5-T). The most well known of the formulations, Agent Orange, was a 50:50 mixture of 2,4-D and 2,4,5-T. 2,4,5-T contained the contaminant 2,3,7,8-tetrachlorodibenzo-*p*-dioxin (referred to in this report as TCDD to represent a single, and the most toxic, congener of the tetrachlorodibenzo-*p*-dioxins [tetraCDDs], also commonly referred to as dioxin); it should be noted that TCDD and Agent Orange are not the same. NAS also was asked to recommend, as appropriate, additional studies to resolve continuing scientific uncertainties and to comment on particular programs mandated in the law. In addition, the legislation called for biennial reviews of newly available information for a period of 10 years; the period was extended to 2014 by the Veterans Education and Benefits Expansion Act of 2001 (PL 107-103).

In response to the request from the Department of Veterans Affairs (VA), the Institute of Medicine (IOM) of the National Academies convened the Committee to Review the Health Effects in Vietnam Veterans of Exposure to Herbicides. The results of the original committee's work were published in 1994 as *Veterans and Agent Orange: Health Effects of Herbicides Used in Vietnam*, hereafter referred to as *VAO* (IOM, 1994). Successor committees formed to fulfill the requirement for updated reviews produced *Veterans and Agent Orange: Update 1996* (IOM, 1996), *Update 1998* (IOM, 1999), *Update 2000* (IOM, 2001), *Update 2002* (IOM, 2003), *Update 2004* (IOM, 2005), and *Update 2006* (IOM, 2007).

In 1999, VA asked IOM to convene a committee to conduct an interim review of type 2 diabetes; that effort resulted in the report *Veterans and Agent Orange: Herbicide/Dioxin Exposure and Type 2 Diabetes*, hereafter referred to as *Type 2 Diabetes* (IOM, 2000). In 2001, VA asked IOM to convene a committee to conduct an interim review of childhood acute myelogenous leukemia (AML) associated with parental exposure to any of the chemicals of interest; its review of the literature, including literature available since the review for *Update 2000*, was published in *Veterans and Agent Orange: Herbicide/Dioxin Exposure and Acute Myelogenous Leukemia in the Children of Vietnam Veterans*, hereafter referred to as *Acute Myelogenous Leukemia* (IOM, 2002). In PL 107-103, passed in 2001, Congress directed the Secretary of Veterans Affairs to ask NAS to review "available scientific literature on the effects of exposure to an herbicide agent containing dioxin on the development of respiratory cancers in humans" and to address "whether it is possible to identify a period of time after exposure to herbicides after which a presumption of service-connection" of the disease would not be warranted; the result of that effort was *Veterans and Agent Orange: Length of Presumptive Period for Association Between Exposure and Respiratory Cancer*, hereafter referred to as *Respiratory Cancer* (IOM, 2004).

In conducting their work, the committees responsible for those reports operated independently of VA and other government agencies. They were not asked to and did not make judgments regarding specific cases in which individual Vietnam veterans have claimed injury from herbicide exposure. The reports were intended to provide scientific information for the Secretary of Veterans Affairs to consider as VA exercises its responsibilities to Vietnam veterans. This VAO update, and all previous VAO reports, are freely accessible on line at the National Academies Press' website (www.nap.edu).

CHARGE TO THE COMMITTEE

In accordance with PL 102-4, the committee was asked to "determine (to the extent that available scientific data permit meaningful determinations)" the following regarding associations between specific health outcomes and exposure to TCDD and other chemicals in the herbicides used by the military in Vietnam:

A) whether a statistical association with herbicide exposure exists, taking into account the strength of the scientific evidence and the appropriateness of the statistical and epidemiological methods used to detect the association;

B) the increased risk of the disease among those exposed to herbicides during service in the Republic of Vietnam during the Vietnam era; and

C) whether there exists a plausible biological mechanism or other evidence of a causal relationship between herbicide exposure and the disease.

The committee notes that, as a consequence of congressional and judicial history, both its congressional mandate and the statement of task are phrased with the target of evaluation being "association" between exposure and health outcomes, although biologic mechanism and causal relationship are also mentioned as part of the evaluation in Article C. As used technically and as thoroughly addressed in a recent report on decision making (IOM, 2008), the criteria for causation are somewhat more stringent than those for association. The unique mandate of VAO committees to evaluate association, rather than causation, means that the approach delineated in that report (IOM, 2008) is not entirely applicable here. The rigor of the evidentiary database needed to support a finding of statistical association is weaker than that for causality, however, positive findings for any of the indicators for causality would enhance conviction that an observed statistical association was reliable. In accord with its charge, the committee examined a variety of indicators appropriate for the task, including factors commonly used to evaluate statistical associations, such as the adequacy of control for bias and confounding and the likelihood that an observed association could be explained by chance, and additionally assessed evidence concerning biologic plausibility derived from laboratory findings in cell-culture or animal models. The full array of indicators examined was used to categorize the strength of the evidence, as shown in Table 1-1 below. In particular, associations that manifest multiple indicators were interpreted as having stronger scientific support.

In delivering the charge to the current committee, the VA made two additional requests. First, the committee was asked to consider whether the occurrence of hairy cell leukemia should be regarded as associated with exposure to the components of herbicides used by the military in Vietnam. Second, the committee was asked to comment on whether effects of herbicide exposure might be manifested in veterans' children at later stages of their development than have been systematically evaluated to date or in later generations and on the feasibility of assessing such effects.

When the first Veterans and Agent Orange committee received its charge from VA, service in the Republic of Vietnam was defined in Subsections a and f of Section 1116 of Title 38 of the United States Code as including military personnel who served in "the inland waterways of such Republic, the waters offshore of such Republic, and the airspace above such Republic." Using that definition, the original and later Veterans and Agent Orange committees routinely considered any research material pertaining to veterans from any of the armed forces who served in the Vietnam theater as relevant to its charge.

It has recently come to the committee's attention that the definition of a qualifying exposure in VA's manual for processing veterans' applications was modified in 2002 and now limits presumption of exposure to Vietnam veterans

TABLE 1-1 Summary from *Update 2006* of Findings in Occupational, Environmental, and Veterans Studies Regarding the Association Between Specific Health Outcomes and Exposure to Herbicides[a]

Sufficient Evidence of Association
Epidemiologic evidence is sufficient to conclude that there is a positive association. That is, a positive association has been observed between exposure to herbicides and the outcome in studies in which chance, bias, and confounding could be ruled out with reasonable confidence.[b] For example, if several small studies that are free of bias and confounding show an association that is consistent in magnitude and direction, there could be sufficient evidence of an association. There is sufficient evidence of an association between exposure to the chemicals of interest and the following health outcomes:

> Soft-tissue sarcoma (including heart)
> Non-Hodgkin's lymphoma
> Chronic lymphocytic leukemia (CLL)
> Hodgkin's disease
> Chloracne

Limited or Suggestive Evidence of Association
Epidemiologic evidence suggests an association between exposure to herbicides and the outcome, but a firm conclusion is limited because chance, bias, and confounding could not be ruled out with confidence.[b] For example, a well-conducted study with strong findings in accord with less compelling results from studies of populations with similar exposures could constitute such evidence. There is limited or suggestive evidence of an association between exposure to the chemicals of interest and the following health outcomes:

> Laryngeal cancer
> Cancer of the lung, bronchus, or trachea
> Prostate cancer
> Multiple myeloma
> AL amyloidosis (category change from *Update 2004*)
> Early-onset transient peripheral neuropathy
> Porphyria cutanea tarda
> Hypertension (category change from *Update 2004*)
> Type 2 diabetes (mellitus)
> Spina bifida in offspring of exposed people

Inadequate or Insufficient Evidence to Determine Association
The available epidemiologic studies are of insufficient quality, consistency, or statistical power to permit a conclusion regarding the presence or absence of an association. For example, studies fail to control for confounding, have inadequate exposure assessment, or fail to address latency.[b] There is inadequate or insufficient evidence to determine association between exposure to the chemicals of interest and the following health outcomes *that were explicitly reviewed*:

> Cancers of the oral cavity (including lips and tongue), pharynx (including tonsils), or
>   nasal cavity (including ears and sinuses)
> Cancers of the pleura, mediastinum, and other unspecified sites within the respiratory
>   system and intrathoracic organs
> Esophageal cancer (category change from *Update 2004*)
> Stomach cancer (category change from *Update 2004*)
> Colorectal cancer (including small intestine and anus) (category change from *Update
>   2004*)

TABLE 1-1 Continued

      Hepatobiliary cancers (liver, gallbladder, and bile ducts)
      Pancreatic cancer (category change from *Update 2004*)
      Bone and joint cancer
* Melanoma
      Non-melanoma skin cancer (basal cell and squamous cell)
* Breast cancer
      Cancers of reproductive organs (cervix, uterus, ovary, testes, and penis; excluding
          prostate)
      Urinary bladder cancer
      Renal cancer
      Cancers of brain and nervous system (including eye) (category change from *Update
          2004*)
      Endocrine cancers (thyroid, thymus, and other endocrine)
      Leukemia (other than CLL)
      Cancers at other and unspecified sites
      Infertility
      Spontaneous abortion (other than for paternal exposure to TCDD, which appears *not* to
          be associated)[c]
      Neonatal or infant death and stillbirth in offspring of exposed people
      Low birth weight in offspring of exposed people
      Birth defects (other than spina bifida) in offspring of exposed people
      Childhood cancer (including acute myelogenous leukemia) in offspring of exposed
          people
      Neurobehavioral disorders (cognitive and neuropsychiatric)
      Neurodegenerative diseases, including Parkinson's disease and amyotrophic lateral
          sclerosis (ALS)
      Chronic peripheral nervous system disorders
      Respiratory disorders
      Gastrointestinal, metabolic, and digestive disorders (changes in liver enzymes, lipid
          abnormalities, and ulcers)
      Immune system disorders (immune suppression, allergy, and autoimmunity)
* Ischemic heart disease
      Circulatory disorders (other than hypertension and perhaps ischemic heart disease)
      Endometriosis
      Effects on thyroid homeostasis

This committee used a classification that spans the full array of cancers. However, reviews for nonmalignant conditions were conducted only if they were found to have been the subjects of epidemiologic investigation or at the request of the Department of Veterans Affairs. *By default, any health outcome on which no epidemiologic information has been found falls into this category.*

Limited or Suggestive Evidence of *No* Association
Several adequate studies, which cover the full range of human exposure, are consistent in not showing a positive association between any magnitude of exposure to the herbicides of interest and the outcome. A conclusion of "no association" is inevitably limited to the conditions, exposures, and length of observation covered by the available studies. *In addition, the possibility of a very small increase in risk at the exposure studied can never be excluded.* There is limited or suggestive

continued

TABLE 1-1 Continued

evidence of *no* association between exposure to the herbicides of interest and the following health outcomes:

Spontaneous abortion and paternal exposure to TCDD[c]

---

[a] *Herbicides* indicates the following chemicals of interest: 2,4-dichlorophenoxyacetic acid (2,4-D), 2,4,5-trichlorophenoxyacetic acid (2,4,5-T) and its contaminant 2,3,7,8-tetrachlorodibenzo-*p*-dioxin (TCDD, or dioxin), cacodylic acid, and picloram. The evidence regarding association was drawn from occupational, environmental, and veteran studies in which people were exposed to the herbicides used in Vietnam, to their components, or to their contaminants.

[b] The criteria for these categories of association as stated in the current update have added the phrase "Evidence for an association can be strengthened by experimental data supporting biologic plausibility, but it is not required." to clarify the role toxiciologic information has played throughout the history of the VAO series.

[c] This conclusion appropriately constrained by specific chemical and exposed parent was drawn in *Update 2002*, but was not carried into the summary table.

* The committee responsible for *Update 2006* was unable to reach consensus as to whether these health outcomes had **Limited or Suggestive Evidence of an Association** or had **Inadequate or Insufficient Evidence to Determine an Association**, and so left them in the lower category.

whose service involved duty or visitation on land in the Republic of Vietnam. That motivated the legal challenge in *Haas v. Nicholson* and appeals by VA. For consistency, the committee has chosen to maintain the original definition of exposure for its determinations and to consider any veterans who served in the Vietnam theater as included in populations of interest for the committee's findings. This statement is not a change in the committee's procedures but rather is intended to clarify its characterization of populations that it deems relevant for making determinations about possible health effects related to exposure to herbicides during the Vietnam conflict; adopting VA's new definition would have entailed eliminating some data points on naval subpopulations from the evidence database, such as some of the strongest findings on an association with non-Hodgkin's lymphoma. Thus, the Veterans and Agent Orange committee continues to consider studies of and research on all populations that served in the Vietnam theater—the Air Force, the Army, and the Blue Water Navy—to be germane to its work.

Chapter 2 provides details of the committee's approach to its charge and the methods it used in reaching conclusions.

CONCLUSIONS OF PREVIOUS VETERANS AND AGENT ORANGE REPORTS

Health Outcomes

VAO, Update 1996, Update 1998, Update 2000, Update 2002, Update 2004, Type 2 Diabetes, Acute Myelogenous Leukemia, Respiratory Cancer, and *Update*

2006 contain detailed reviews of the scientific studies evaluated by the committees and their implications for cancer, reproductive and developmental effects, neurologic disorders, and other health effects.

The original Veterans and Agent Orange committee addressed the statutory mandate to evaluate the association between herbicide exposure and a given health effect by assigning each of the health outcomes under study to one of four categories on the basis of the epidemiologic evidence reviewed. The categories were adapted from the ones used by the International Agency for Research on Cancer in evaluating evidence of the carcinogenicity of various substances (IARC, 1977). Successor Veterans and Agent Orange committees adopted the same categories.

The question as to whether the committee should be considering "statistical association" rather than "causality," has been controversial. In legal proceedings that predate passage of the legislation mandating this Veterans and Agent Orange (VAO) series of reviews, *Nehmer v. United States Veterans Administration* (712 F. Supp. 1404, 1989) found that

> The legislative history, and prior VA and congressional practice, support our finding that Congress intended that the Administrator predicate service connection upon a finding of a significant statistical association between dioxin exposure and various diseases. We hold that the VA erred by requiring proof of a causal relationship.

The committee believes that the categorization of strength of evidence as shown in Table 1-1 is consistent with that court ruling. In particular, the ruling does not preclude the consideration of the factors usually assessed in determining whether a causal relationship exists (Hill, 1965; IOM, 2008) as indicators of the strength of scientific evidence for an association. In accord with the court ruling, the committee was not seeking proof of a causal relationship, but any information that supports a causal relationship, such as a plausible biologic mechanism as specified in Article C of the charge to the committee, would also lend credence to the reliability of an observed association. Science is principally concerned with causal relationships, and the committee's objective of statistical association is an intermediate (less well-defined) point along a continuum culminating in causality.

The categories, the criteria for assigning a particular health outcome to a category, and the health outcomes that have been assigned to the categories in past updates are discussed below. Table 1-1 summarizes the conclusions of *Update 2006* regarding associations between health outcomes and exposure to the herbicides used in Vietnam or to any of their components or contaminants. That integration of the literature through September 2006 served as the starting point for the current committee's deliberations. It should be noted that the categories of association concern the occurrence of health outcomes in human *populations* in relation to chemical exposure; they do not address the likelihood that any *individual's* health problem is associated with or caused by the chemicals in question.

Health Outcomes with Sufficient Evidence of an Association

In this category, a positive association between herbicides and the outcome must be observed in epidemiologic studies in which chance, bias, and confounding can be ruled out with reasonable confidence. The committee regarded evidence from several studies that have satisfactorily addressed bias and confounding and that show an association that is consistent in magnitude and direction as sufficient evidence of an association. Experimental data supporting biologic plausibility strengthens evidence for an association, but is not a prerequisite.

The original committee found sufficient evidence of an association between exposure to herbicides and three cancers—soft-tissue sarcoma, non-Hodgkin's lymphoma, and Hodgkin's disease—and two other health outcomes, chloracne and porphyria cutanea tarda (PCT). After reviewing all the literature available in 1995, the committee responsible for *Update 1996* concluded that the statistical evidence still supported that classification for the three cancers and chloracne but that the evidence of an association with PCT warranted its being placed in the category of limited or suggestive evidence of an association with exposure. No changes were made in this category in *Update 1998* or *Update 2000*.

As the committee responsible for *Update 2002* began its work, VA requested that it evaluate whether chronic lymphocytic leukemia (CLL) should be considered separately from other leukemias. The committee concluded that CLL could be considered separately and, on the basis of the epidemiologic literature and the etiology of the disease, placed CLL in the "sufficient" category. No additional changes to this category have been made since *Update 2002*.

Health Outcomes with Limited or Suggestive Evidence of an Association

In this category, the evidence must suggest an association between exposure to herbicides and the outcome considered, but the evidence can be limited by the inability to rule out chance, bias, or confounding confidently. The coherence of the full body of epidemiologic information, in light of biologic plausibility, is considered when the committee reaches a judgment about association for a given outcome. Because the VAO series has four herbicides and TCDD as agents of concern whose profiles of toxicity are not expected to be uniform, apparent inconsistencies can be expected among study populations that have experienced different exposures. Even for a single exposure, a spectrum of results would be expected, depending on the power of the studies and other design factors.

The committee responsible for *VAO* found limited or suggestive evidence of an association between exposure to herbicides and three categories of cancer: respiratory cancer (after individual evaluations of laryngeal cancer and of cancers of the trachea, lung, or bronchus), prostate cancer, and multiple myeloma. The *Update 1996* committee added three health outcomes to the list: PCT, acute and subacute transient peripheral neuropathy (hereafter called early-onset transient peripheral neuropathy), and spina bifida in children of veterans. Transient peripheral neuropathies had not been addressed in *VAO*, because they are not amenable to epidemiologic study. In response to a VA request, however, the *Update 1996* committee reviewed those neuropathies and based its determination on case histories. A 1995 analysis of birth defects among the offspring of veterans who served in Operation Ranch Hand, combined with earlier studies of neural-tube defects in the children of Vietnam veterans (published by the Centers for Disease Control and Prevention), led the *Update 1996* committee to distinguish spina bifida from other reproductive outcomes and to classify it in the "limited or suggestive evidence" category. No changes were made in this category in *Update 1998*.

After the publication of *Update 1998*, the committee responsible for type 2 diabetes, on the basis of its evaluation of newly available scientific evidence and the cumulative findings of research reviewed in previous VAO reports, concluded that there was limited or suggestive evidence of an association between exposure to the herbicides used in Vietnam or the contaminant TCDD and type 2 diabetes (mellitus). The evidence reviewed in *Update 2000* supported that finding.

The committee responsible for *Update 2000* reviewed the material in earlier reports and the newly published literature and determined that there was limited or suggestive evidence of an association between exposure to herbicides used in Vietnam or the contaminant TCDD and AML in the children of Vietnam veterans. After release of *Update 2000*, researchers on one of the studies reviewed in it discovered an error in the published data. The committee for *Update 2000* was reconvened to re-evaluate the previously reviewed and new literature regarding AML, and it produced *Acute Myelogenous Leukemia*, which reclassified AML in children from "limited or suggestive evidence of an association" to "inadequate or insufficient evidence to determine an association."

After reviewing the data reviewed in previous VAO reports and recently published scientific literature, the committee responsible for *Update 2006* determined that there was limited or suggestive evidence of an association between exposure to the herbicides used in Vietnam or the contaminant TCDD and hypertension. AL amyloidosis was also moved to the category of "limited or suggestive evidence of an association" primarily on the basis of its close biologic relationship with multiple myeloma.

Health Outcomes with Inadequate or Insufficient Evidence to Determine an Association

By default, any health outcome is in this category before enough reliable scientific data accumulate to promote it to the category of sufficient evidence or limited or suggestive evidence of an association or to move it to the category of limited or suggestive evidence of *no* association. In this category, available studies may have inconsistent findings or be of insufficient quality or statistical power to support a conclusion regarding the presence of an association. Such studies might have failed to control for confounding or might have had inadequate assessment of exposure.

The cancers and other health effects so categorized in *Update 2004* are listed in Table 1-1, but several health effects have been moved into or out of this category since the original Veterans and Agent Orange committee reviewed the evidence then available. Skin cancer was moved into this category in *Update 1996* when inclusion of new evidence no longer supported its classification as a condition with limited or suggestive evidence of *no* association. Similarly, the *Update 1998* committee moved urinary-bladder cancer from the category of limited or suggestive evidence of *no* association to this category; although there was no evidence that exposure to herbicides or TCDD is related to urinary-bladder cancer, newly available evidence weakened the evidence of *no* association. The committee for *Update 2000* had partitioned AML in the offspring of Vietnam veterans from other childhood cancers and put it into the category of suggestive evidence; but a separate review, as reported in *Acute Myelogenous Leukemia*, found errors in the published information and returned it to this category with other childhood cancers. In *Update 2002*, CLL was moved from this category to join Hodgkin's and non-Hodgkin's lymphomas in the category of sufficient evidence of an association.

The committee responsible for *Update 2006* moved several cancers (of the brain, stomach, colon, rectum, and pancreas) from the category of limited or suggestive evidence of *no* association into this category because of changes in evidence since they were originally placed in the "*no* association" category and because that committee had concerns about the lack of information on all five chemicals of interest and each of these cancers.

Health Outcomes with Limited or Suggestive Evidence of *No* Association

The original Veterans and Agent Orange committee defined this category for health outcomes on which several adequate studies covering the "full range of human exposure" were consistent in showing *no* association with exposure to herbicides at any level and had relatively narrow confidence intervals. A conclusion of "no association" is inevitably limited to the conditions, exposures, and observation periods covered by the available studies, and the possibility of a small increase in risk at the levels of exposure studied can never be excluded. However, a change in classification from inadequate or insufficient evidence of an association to limited or suggestive evidence of *no* association would require new studies that correct for the methodologic problems of previous studies and that have samples large enough to limit the possible study results attributable to chance.

The original Veterans and Agent Orange committee found a sufficient number and variety of well-designed studies to conclude that there was limited or suggestive evidence of *no* association between the exposures of interest and a small group of cancers: gastrointestinal tumors (colon, rectum, stomach, and pancreas), skin cancers, brain tumors, and urinary bladder cancer. The *Update 1996* committee removed skin cancers and the *Update 1998* committee removed urinary bladder cancer from this category because the evidence no longer supported a conclusion of *no* association. The *Update 2002* committee concluded that there was adequate evidence to determine that spontaneous abortion is *not* associated with paternal exposure specifically to TCDD; the evidence on this outcome was deemed inadequate for drawing a conclusion about an association with maternal exposure to any of the chemicals of interest or with paternal exposure to any of the chemicals of interest other than TCDD. No changes in this category were made in *Update 2000* or *Update 2004*. The *Update 2006* committee removed brain cancer and several digestive cancers from this category because they were concerned that the overall paucity of information on picloram and cacodylic acid made it inappropriate for those outcomes to remain in this category.

Determining Increased Risk in Vietnam Veterans

The second part of the committee's charge is to determine, to the extent permitted by available scientific data, the increased risk of disease among people exposed to herbicides, or the contaminant TCDD, during service in Vietnam. Previous reports point out that most of the many health studies of Vietnam veterans are hampered by relatively poor measures of exposure to herbicides or TCDD and by other methodologic problems. Most of the evidence on which the findings regarding associations are based, therefore, comes from studies of people exposed to TCDD or herbicides in occupational and environmental settings rather than from studies of Vietnam veterans. The committees that produced *VAO* and the updates found that the body of evidence was sufficient for reaching conclusions about statistical associations between herbicide exposures and health outcomes but that the lack of adequate data on Vietnam veterans themselves complicated consideration of the second part of the charge.

The evidence of herbicide exposure among various groups studied suggests that although some had documented high exposures (such as participants in Operation Ranch Hand or the Army Chemical Corps personnel), most Vietnam veterans had lower exposures to herbicides and TCDD than did the subjects of many occupational and environmental studies. Individual veterans who had very high exposures to herbicides, however, could have risks approaching those described in the occupational and environmental studies.

Estimating the magnitude of risk of each particular health outcome among herbicide-exposed Vietnam veterans requires quantitative information about the dose–time–response relationship for the health outcome in humans, information on the extent of herbicide exposure among Vietnam veterans, and estimates of individual exposure. Committees responsible for *VAO* and the updates have concluded that in general it is impossible to quantify the risk to veterans posed by their exposure to herbicides in Vietnam. Statements to that effect were made for each health outcome in *VAO* (IOM, 1994) and in every update through *Update 2004*. The committee responsible for *Update 2006* chose to eliminate the repetitive restatements in favor of the following general conclusion: "At least for the present, it is not possible to derive quantitative estimates of the increase in risk of various adverse health effects that Vietnam veterans may have experienced in association with exposure to the herbicides sprayed in Vietnam." The current committee retains that approach.

After decades of research, the challenge of estimating the magnitude of potential risk posed by exposure to the compounds of interest remains intractable. The requisite information is still absent despite concerted efforts to reconstruct likely exposure by modeling on the basis of records of troop movements and spraying missions (Stellman and Stellman, 2003, 2004; Stellman et al., 2003a,b), to measure serum TCDD in individual veterans (Kang et al., 2006; Michalek et al., 1995), and to model the pharmacokinetics of TCDD clearance (Aylward et al., 2005a,b; Cheng et al., 2006b; Emond et al., 2004, 2005, 2006). There is still uncertainty about the specific agents that may be responsible for a particular health effect. Even if one accepts an individual veteran's serum TCDD concentration as the optimal surrogate for overall exposure to Agent Orange and the other herbicide mixtures sprayed in Vietnam, not only is the measurement nontrivial but the hurdle of accounting for biologic clearance and extrapolating to the proper timeframe remains. The committee therefore believes that it cannot accurately estimate the risk to Vietnam veterans that is attributable to exposure to the compounds associated with herbicide spraying in Vietnam.

Existence of a Plausible Biologic Mechanism or Other Evidence of a Causal Relationship

Toxicologic data form the basis of the committee's response to the third part of its charge—to determine whether there is a plausible biologic mechanism or other evidence of a causal relationship between herbicide exposure and a health effect. A separate chapter summarizes toxicologic findings on the chemicals of concern. In previous updates, a considerable amount of detail had been provided about individual newly published toxicology studies; the current committee decided it would be more informative for the general reader to provide an integrated profile by interpreting the underlying experimental findings. Specific toxicologic findings pertinent to each health outcome are given in the chapters that review the epidemiologic literature.

In *VAO* and updates before *Update 2006*, this topic has been discussed in the conclusions section for each health outcome after a statement of the committee's judgment about the adequacy of the epidemiologic evidence of an association of that outcome with exposure to the chemicals of interest. As *Update 2006* noted, the degree of biologic plausibility itself influences whether the committee perceives positive findings to be indicative of a pattern or the product of statistical fluctuations. To provide the reader with a more logical sequence, the committee responsible for *Update 2006* placed the biologic-plausibility sections between the presentation of new epidemiologic evidence and the synthesis of all the evidence, which in turn leads to the ultimate statement of the committee's conclusion. The current committee supports that change and has continued to group the sections that way.

ORGANIZATION OF THIS REPORT

The remainder of this report is organized in nine chapters. Chapter 2 briefly describes the considerations that guided the committee's review and evaluation of the scientific evidence. Chapter 3 addresses exposure-assessment issues. Chapter 4 summarizes the toxicology data on the effects of 2,4-D, 2,4,5-T and its contaminant TCDD, cacodylic acid, and picloram; the data contribute to the biologic plausibility of health effects in human populations. Chapter 5 presents the relevant new epidemiologic literature identified in this update period, an overview of populations repeatedly studied by publications reviewed in the series of VAO reports with discussion of the exposure assessments conducted on the major cohorts, and design information on the epidemiologic studies that are newly covered in this update and investigated those populations or that report multiple health outcomes. The committee's evaluation of the epidemiologic literature and its conclusions regarding associations between the exposures of interest and cancer, reproductive and developmental effects, neurologic disorders, and other health effects are discussed in Chapters 6, 7, 8, and 9, respectively. The committee's research recommendations are presented in Chapter 10.

REFERENCES[1]

Aylward LL, Brunet RC, Carrier G, Hays SM, Cushing CA, Needham LL, Patterson DG Jr, Gerthoux PM, Brambilla P, Mocarelli P. 2005a. Concentration-dependent TCDD elimination kinetics in humans: Toxicokinetic modeling for moderately to highly exposed adults from Seveso, Italy, and Vienna, Austria, and impact on dose estimates for the NIOSH cohort. *Journal of Exposure Analysis and Environmental Epidemiology* 15(1):51–65.

Aylward LL, Brunet RC, Starr TB, Carrier G, Delzell E, Cheng H, Beall C. 2005b. Exposure reconstruction for the TCDD-exposed NIOSH cohort using a concentration- and age-dependent model of elimination. *Risk Analysis* 25(4):945–956.

Cheng H, Aylward L, Beall C, Starr TB, Brunet RC, Carrier G, Delzell E. 2006b. TCDD exposure-response analysis and risk assessment. *Risk Analysis* 26(4):1059–1071.

Emond C, Birnbaum LS, DeVito MJ. 2004. Physiologically based pharmacokinetic model for developmental exposures to TCDD in the rat. *Toxicological Sciences* 80(1):115–133.

---

[1]Throughout the report the same alphabetic indicator following year of publication is used consistently for the same article when there were multiple citations by the same first author in a given year. The convention of assigning the alphabetic indicator in order of citation in a given chapter is not followed.

Emond C, Michalek JE, Birnbaum LS, DeVito MJ. 2005. Comparison of the use of physiologically based pharmacokinetic model and a classical pharmacokinetic model for dioxin exposure assessments. *Environmental Health Perspectives* 113(12):1666–1668.

Emond C, Birnbaum LS, DeVito MJ. 2006. Use of a physiologically based pharmacokinetic model for rats to study the influence of body fat mass and induction of CYP1A2 on the pharmacokinetics of TCDD. *Environmental Health Perspectives* 114(9):1394–1400.

Hill AB. 1965. The environment and disease: Association or causation? *Proceedings of the Royal Society of Medicine* 58:295–300.

IARC (International Agency for Research on Cancer). 1977. *Some Fumigants, the Herbicides 2,4-D and 2,4,5-T, Chlorinated Dibenzodioxins and Miscellaneous Industrial Chemicals.* IARC Monographs on the Evaluation of the Carcinogenic Risk of Chemicals to Man, Vol. 15. Lyon, France: World Health Organization, IARC.

IOM (Institute of Medicine). 1994. *Veterans and Agent Orange: Health Effects of Herbicides Used in Vietnam.* Washington, DC: National Academy Press.

IOM. 1996. *Veterans and Agent Orange: Update 1996.* Washington, DC: National Academy Press.

IOM. 1999. *Veterans and Agent Orange: Update 1998.* Washington, DC: National Academy Press.

IOM. 2000. *Veterans and Agent Orange: Herbicide/Dioxin Exposure and Type 2 Diabetes.* Washington, DC: National Academy Press.

IOM. 2001. *Veterans and Agent Orange: Update 2000.* Washington, DC: National Academy Press.

IOM. 2002. *Veterans and Agent Orange: Herbicide/Dioxin Exposure and Acute Myelogenous Leukemia in the Children of Vietnam Veterans.* Washington, DC: The National Academies Press.

IOM. 2003. *Veterans and Agent Orange: Update 2002.* Washington, DC: The National Academies Press.

IOM. 2004. *Veterans and Agent Orange: Length of Presumptive Period for Association Between Exposure and Respiratory Cancer.* Washington, DC: The National Academies Press.

IOM. 2005. *Veterans and Agent Orange: Update 2004.* Washington, DC: The National Academies Press.

IOM. 2007. *Veterans and Agent Orange: Update 2006.* Washington, DC: The National Academies Press.

IOM. 2008. *Improving the Presumptive Disability Decision-making Process for Veterans.* Washington, DC: The National Academies Press.

Kang HK, Dalager NA, Needham LL, Patterson DG, Lees PSJ, Yates K, Matanoski GM. 2006. Health status of Army Chemical Corps Vietnam veterans who sprayed defoliant in Vietnam. *American Journal of Industrial Medicine* 49(11):875–884.

Michalek J, Wolfe W, Miner J, Papa T, Pirkle J. 1995. Indices of TCDD exposure and TCDD body burden in veterans of Operation Ranch Hand. *Journal of Exposure Analysis and Environmental Epidemiology* 5(2):209–223.

Stellman JM, Stellman SD. 2003. *Contractor's Final Report: Characterizing Exposure of Veterans to Agent Orange and Other Herbicides in Vietnam.* Submitted to the National Academy of Sciences, Institute of Medicine in fulfillment of Subcontract VA-5124-98-0019, June 30, 2003.

Stellman SD, Stellman JM. 2004. Exposure opportunity models for Agent Orange, dioxin, and other military herbicides used in Vietnam, 1961–1971. *Journal of Exposure Analysis and Environmental Epidemiology* 14(4):354–362.

Stellman J, Stellman S, Christians R, Weber T, Tomasallo C. 2003a. The extent and patterns of usage of Agent Orange and other herbicides in Vietnam. *Nature* 422:681–687.

Stellman J, Stellman S, Weber T, Tomasallo C, Stellman A, Christian R Jr. 2003b. A geographic information system for characterizing exposure to Agent Orange and other herbicides in Vietnam. *Environmental Health Perspectives* 111(3):321–328.

2

Evaluating the Evidence

This chapter outlines the approach used by the Committee to Review the Health Effects in Vietnam Veterans of Exposure to Herbicides: Seventh Biennial Update and its predecessors to evaluate the available scientific evidence. A more complete description is found in Chapter 5 of *Veterans and Agent Orange: Health Effects of Herbicides Used in Vietnam*, hereafter referred to as *VAO* (IOM, 1994).

CHOICE OF HEALTH OUTCOMES

As discussed in Chapter 1, the committee was charged with summarizing the strength of the scientific evidence of associations between exposure to various herbicides and contaminants during service in the Vietnam War and individual diseases or other health outcomes. Public Law 102-4, which mandated the committee's work, however, did not specify particular health outcomes suspected of being associated with herbicide exposure. Such a list was developed on the basis of diseases and conditions addressed in the scientific literature identified through the original *VAO*'s extensive literature searches. The list has been amended in the VAO updates in response to new publications, to requests from the Department of Veterans Affairs (VA) and various veterans service organizations, and to concerns of Vietnam veterans and their families. Comments received at public hearings and in written submissions from veterans and other interested persons have been valuable in identifying issues to be pursued in greater depth in the scientific literature.

The Veterans and Agent Orange committees began their evaluation by presuming neither the presence nor the absence of an association between exposure and any particular health outcome. Over the series of reviews, evidence of various degrees of association, lack of association, or persistent indeterminacy with respect to a wide array of disease states has accrued. For many conditions, however, particularly ones that are very uncommon, associations with the chemicals of interest have remained unaddressed in the medical research literature; for these, the committee remains neutral based on the understanding that "absence of evidence is not evidence of absence."

IDENTIFICATION OF RELEVANT LITERATURE

Mixtures of 2,4-dichlorophenoxyacetic acid (2,4-D), 2,4,5-trichlorophenoxy-acetic acid (2,4,5-T), picloram, and cacodylic acid made up the bulk of the herbicides sprayed in Vietnam. At the time of the spraying, 2,3,7,8-tetrachloro-dibenzo-p-dioxin (TCDD, one form of dioxin) was an unintended contaminant from the production of 2,4,5-T and was present in Agent Orange and some other herbicide formulations sprayed in Vietnam; it is important to note that TCDD and Agent Orange are not the same. Databases have been searched for the names of those compounds, their synonyms and abbreviations, and their Chemical Abstracts Service (CAS) numbers. The evidence indicates that a tissue protein, the aryl hydrocarbon receptor, mediates most of the toxicity of TCDD, so *aryl hydrocarbon receptor* also was used as a keyword, as were *dioxin*, *Agent Orange*, and *Vietnam veteran*.

One of the herbicides used in Vietnam, cacodylic acid, is dimethyl arsenic acid (DMA), an organic form of arsenic. In addition to being synthesized as a herbicide, DMA is a metabolite of inorganic arsenic in humans. It was long thought to be a biologically inactive metabolite, but recent evidence suggests that one form—DMA[III]—might be responsible for some of the adverse effects of inorganic arsenic. The committee carefully reconsidered that evidence but again determined that it does not support a conclusion that exposure to cacodylic acid would be expected to result in the same adverse health effects as would exposure to toxic concentrations of inorganic arsenic. Therefore, as in prior VAO reports, the literature on the health effects of inorganic arsenic was not considered here. Further details on the effects of inorganic arsenic can be found in *Arsenic in Drinking Water* (NRC, 1999) and *Arsenic in Drinking Water: 2001 Update* (NRC, 2001). For cacodylic acid and picloram, the search terms were the chemical names, synonyms, and CAS numbers of the herbicides.

This report concentrates on the evidence published after the completion of work on *Veterans and Agent Orange: Update 2006* (IOM, 2007). Relevant new contributions to the literature made during the period October 1, 2006–September 30, 2008, were sought. The information that the committee used was compiled from a comprehensive electronic search of public and commercial databases—biologic, medical, toxicologic, chemical, historical, and regulatory—that provide citations of the scientific literature. In addition, the reference lists of some review and research articles, books, and reports were examined for potentially relevant articles. As noted above, the terms used in the search strategy included the chemical names, synonyms, and CAS numbers of the specific chemicals of interest—2,4-D, 2,4,5-T, TCDD, cacocylic acid, and picloram—see Figure 2-1 for chemical structures and CAS numbers—and the more generic terms involved with this project (*Vietnam veteran*, *Agent Orange*, *aryl hydrocarbon receptor*, *dioxin*, *herbicide*, and *phenoxy*). By analogy, results on other specific phenoxy herbicides are also of interest: 2-methyl-4-chlorophenoxyacetic acid (MCPA) and 2-(2-methyl-4-chlorophenoxy) propionic acid (MCPP or Mecoprop) for 2,4-D and 2-(2,4,5-trichlorophenoxy) propionic acid (2,4,5-TP or Silvex) for 2,4,5-T (see Figure 2-1 for chemical structures and CAS numbers); although the ben- zoate herbicide dicamba (2-methoxy-3,6-dichlororbenzoic acid) is not always categorized with the phenoxy herbicides, it shares structural similarities with this class, and measures of its association with various adverse health outcomes have been factored into the evidence. Because some polychlorinated biphenyls (PCBs) and polychlorodibenzofurans (PCDFs) have dioxin-like biologic activity, studies of populations exposed to PCBs or PCDFs were reviewed when results were presented in terms of toxicity equivalent quotients (TEQs). Findings related only to exposure to the diverse chemical families of pesticides were considered too nonspecific for inclusion in the evidence database used to draw conclusions about associations. However, *pesticide* was included among the search terms for VAO updates to ensure that all possible articles on herbicides (the specific tar- gets were only the phenoxy herbicides, cacodylic acid, and picloram) would be identified and subjected to the next phase of screening. (An ancillary analysis of the search results by this committee determined that the term "pesticide" did not identify any relevant citation that was not picked up by more specific terms, and so it will be eliminated from searches in future VAO updates, thereby reducing the number of extraneous hits to be culled.)

Because they are the target population of the charge to the VAO commit- tees, studies of Vietnam veterans (serving in any of the armed forces, American or otherwise) have always been accorded considerable weight in the commit- tees' deliberations, whether or not estimation of exposure to herbicide-related substances has been attempted. Characterization of exposure in studies of the veterans was extremely uncommon at the time of the original *VAO* report, and the Vietnam veterans' own ages were still below the ages at which many chronic illnesses are manifested. Consequently, the original committee made extensive efforts to consider several groups known or thought to have potentially higher and better-characterized exposure to TCDD or phenoxy herbicides than Vietnam veterans themselves—both occupational exposure (as of chemical-production, paper and pulp, sawmill, tannery, waste-incinerator, railroad, agricultural, and forestry workers) and environmental exposure (as of residents of Seveso, Times Beach, Quail Run, and Vietnam).

Successive committees have been able to concentrate more on studies that explicitly addressed the exposures specified in the charge. Some occupational and environmental cohorts that received exceptionally high exposures (such as the

Phenoxy Herbicides

2,4-D [94-75-7]

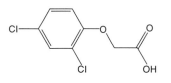

2,4,5-T [93-76-5]

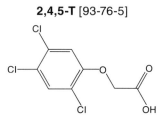

MCPA [94-74-6]

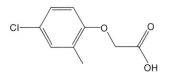

Silvex [93-72-1]

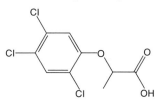

MCPP [93-65-2]

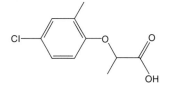

Dicamba [1918-00-9]

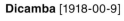
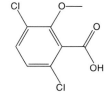

2,3,7,8-TCDD [1746-01-6]

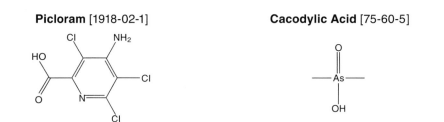

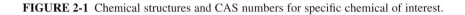

Picloram [1918-02-1]

Cacodylic Acid [75-60-5]

FIGURE 2-1 Chemical structures and CAS numbers for specific chemical of interest.

International Agency for Research on Cancer and Seveso cohorts) are now well characterized and producing a stream of informative results. The Agricultural Health Study, a continuing prospective cohort study of agricultural populations with specific information on the chemicals of interest, is also now contributing a steady stream of information to the database. Most important, the Vietnam veterans themselves are advancing in age and, when studied, capable of directly providing substantial information on chronic health conditions, often as related to serum TCDD concentrations. The committee for *Update 2006* decided that exhaustive searches on job titles, occupations, or industries to identify additional study populations with possible, but not specifically characterized, exposure to the chemicals of interest were no longer an efficient means of augmenting the evidence database, because they are more likely to retrieve citations with information about a health outcome at the expense of considerable uncertainty about exposure.

The current committee adopted the *Update 2006* committee's practice of more circumscribed searching. As the information in the database on populations with established exposure to the chemicals of interest has grown, VAO committees have become less dependent on data from studies with nonspecific exposure information and have been able to focus more on findings of studies with refined exposure specificity. In recognition of the more pivotal role that findings drawn directly from Vietnam veterans are now able to play in its decisions, this committee has reordered its consideration of populations. For each health outcome in this update, studies of Vietnam veterans are now addressed first followed by occupational and environmental studies, rather than last as was the practice established when the information from studies on veterans was quite sparse.

It is well accepted that any TCDD or herbicide effect may be diluted somewhat in studies of Vietnam veterans because some of the veterans may not have been exposed or may have been exposed only at low concentrations. The problem is exacerbated in studies in which exposure is defined in terms of occupation (even on the basis of a full job history). Exploratory studies based on linking to a one-time statement of occupation (for example, on a death certificate or in a census) are thought to be of little usefulness even when a job–exposure matrix is used to "convert" standardized job codes to specific exposures. Not only is there uncertainty about whether all members of the sample have been exposed to one of the chemicals of interest unless detailed personal monitoring and industrial-hygiene work have been performed, but for most occupational categories there is considerable certainty that the workers have been exposed to many other potentially toxic agents. Thus, such studies may well minimize the effects of exposure to dioxin or the herbicides of interest while yielding misleading indications of health problems resulting from other exposures.

The search strategy was devised to ensure that abstracts of all potentially relevant articles were subjected to closer screening, but it also resulted in the identification of a large number of nonrelevant studies. The searches produced 7,000 "hits," including some studies that were identified more than once. It was evident from the abstracts of most of the cited articles that they did not address health effects in association with exposure to the chemicals of interest; for example, many of the cited studies investigated the efficacy of herbicides in killing weeds. All studies that discussed health effects were considered if the search-related information (title, abstract, and keywords) indicated that any of the herbicides of interest (or any of their components) may have been investigated. For each of the more than 850 potentially relevant citations ultimately identified, a copy of the entire article was obtained online or retrieved from library sources and reviewed more thoroughly by the committee for inclusion in its report.

In large part, included reports are peer-reviewed journal articles, but generally available and formally published government studies (particularly those investigating health effects in Vietnam veterans) are also included under the presumption that they have been carefully reviewed. In practice, the articles are generally in English, but the committee would obtain translations for crucial ones that were not in English, as was done for reports of a study of Korean veterans of the Vietnam War (Kim HA et al., 2003; Kim JS et al., 2003) when *Update 2004* was produced.

TCDD, the 2,3,7,8-chlorinated congener of dioxin, is the most potent of the polychlorinated dibenzo-*p*-dioxins, dibenzofurans, and PCBs, so it is presumed to be most problematic. However, our concern is not limited to this single congener. In non-laboratory settings—for example, epidemiologic studies—exposures occur not only to TCDD, but to mixtures of dioxins, dibenzofurans, and PCBs, which vary in their degree of chlorination. A toxicity equivalency factor (TEF) is an estimate of the dioxin-like potency of an individual congener relative to the toxicity of TCDD, as measured in assays of its AH receptor (AHR) activity. TEQs are often used to estimate the cumulative toxic potency of mixtures as the sum of TEFs weighted by the concentration of the corresponding congener in the mixture; this total is denoted as the mixture's TEQ or toxicity equivalent quotient in terms of dioxin-like activity. That approach is often taken in epidemiologic studies focusing on PCBs. Many epidemiologic studies of PCBs were recovered in the literature search although they were not specifically sought. Because dioxin-like and non–dioxin-like PCB congeners are found together in environmental mixtures and are known to mediate toxicity by unique mechanisms, the relative contribution of dioxin-like PCBs to an individual health outcome can be difficult to determine. Therefore, evidence from epidemiologic studies of PCB exposure was retained only for results reported for specific dioxin-like congeners or in terms of TEQs.

Investigation of the pesticides used in greenhouses determined that greenhouse workers are not likely to be exposed to herbicides, particularly those of interest for VAO committee deliberations (Czarnota, 2004; Neal, 2006; University of Connecticut, 2006), so new citations for studies of such workers were not retained and previous results on such populations (Abell et al., 2000, on fertility;

Hansen et al., 1992, on cancer in female workers) were retroactively excluded from the evidence database.

Roughly 300 citations contributed new information to this update. New evidence on each health outcome was reviewed in detail. The conclusions, however, are based on the accumulated evidence, not just on recently published studies. If statistics have been generated on the same study population over time (as noted in Chapter 5), multiple entries for a given health outcome in the summary results tables of Chapters 6–9 correspond to successive updates, but only the most comprehensive version of the information on a given population is factored into the committee's conclusion on that outcome. Primary findings are the components of the evidence that the committee endeavors to integrate in drawing its conclusions; reanalyses, pooled analyses, reviews, and so on may be discussed in conjunction with primary results or in synthesis sections for a given health outcome, but they are not themselves part of the evidence dataset.

COMMITTEE'S APPROACH

The committee's general approach to the evaluation of scientific evidence is presented here. It corresponds very closely with the approach developed by the original committee as delineated in detail in Chapter 5 of *VAO*. The committee had three specific tasks: to determine whether there is a statistical association between exposure to the herbicides used in Vietnam and health outcomes, to determine the increase in risk of effects among Vietnam veterans, and to determine whether plausible biologic mechanisms provide support for a causal relationship with a given health outcome. This section discusses the committee's approach to each task.

Statistical Association

The issues in determining whether a statistical association exists are detailed in Chapter 5 of *VAO*. The committee found that the most relevant evidence came from epidemiologic studies—investigations in which large groups of people are studied to identify an association between exposure to a chemical of interest and the occurrence of particular health outcomes.

Epidemiologists estimate associations between exposure and outcome in a specific population or group by using such measures as relative risk, standardized mortality ratio, and odds ratio. Those measures indicate the magnitude of a difference in the rate of an outcome between two populations. For example, if the rate in an exposed population is twice the rate in a nonexposed population, the relative risk, or rate ratio, is 2. Similarly, if the odds of a health outcome are 1:20 in an exposed population but 1:100 in a nonexposed population, the odds ratio is 5. In this report, *relative risk* refers to the results of cohort studies, and *odds ratio* (an estimate of relative risk) usually refers to the results of case–control studies. (The results of cohort studies sometimes are reported with odds ratios, again to

estimate relative risk.) An estimated relative risk greater than 1 indicates a positive association (that is, it is more likely that the outcome will be seen in exposed
people than in nonexposed people), whereas a relative risk between zero and 1
indicates a negative or inverse association (that is, the outcome is less likely in
exposed people). A ratio of 1 suggests the absence of association. A statistically
significant association is one that would be unlikely to occur by chance (that is,
if the null hypothesis is true).

Determining whether an estimated association between an exposure and an
outcome represents a real relationship requires careful scrutiny because there can
be more than one explanation for an estimate. *Bias* is a distortion of the measure
of association that results from flawed selection in the assembly of the study population or from error in measurement of studied characteristics. *Confounding* is a
distortion of the measure of association that results from failure to recognize or
account for some other factor related both to exposure and to outcome. *Chance* is
the degree to which an estimated association might vary randomly among different samples of the population studied. The width of a *confidence interval* is used
to quantify the likely variability of an exposure–disease association; even when
a relative risk or standardized mortality ratio exceeds 1, a conclusion regarding
increased risk must be qualified when the confidence interval is wide. In drawing
its conclusions, the committee examined the quantitative estimates of association and evaluated the potential influences of bias, confounding, and chance. In
integrating the findings of various studies, the committee considered the degree
of statistical significance associated with every estimated risk (a reflection of the
magnitude of the observed effect and the power of the study designs) rather than
simply tallying the "significant" and "nonsignificant" outcomes as dichotomous
items of evidence. The committee also considered whether controlled laboratory
investigations provide information consistent with the compounds of interest being associated with a given effect and perhaps causally linked to it.

In pursuing the question of statistical association, the committee recognized
that an absolute conclusion about the absence of association is unattainable. As
in science generally, studies of health effects associated with herbicide exposure
cannot demonstrate that a purported effect is impossible or could never occur,
only that it is statistically improbable. Any instrument of observation, even
the most excellent epidemiologic study, is limited in its resolving power. In a
strict technical sense, therefore, the absence of an association between even one
chemical and a health outcome cannot be proven. Convincingly demonstrating
the lack of a particular effect for all five of the compounds of interest simultaneously would be a daunting effort, especially in light of the paucity of information
concerning picloram and cacodylic acid. This committee, therefore, endorses the
decision by the committee for *Update 2006* to reclassify several types of cancer
that had been classified since *VAO* (1994) as having "suggestive evidence of *no*
association" with "exposure to herbicides."

Interaction or synergism among the chemicals of interest or with other agents is another theoretical concern. The committee was not charged with attributing effects to specific chemicals of interest, and joint effects among them should be adequately identified by the committee's approach. The number of combinations of these chemicals with other agents that might be problematic is virtually infinite. Real-life experience, as investigated with epidemiologic studies, effectively integrates any results of exposure to a target substance over all other possibly detrimental or mitigating exposures that a population might have. It may not be possible to partition contributions of the chemicals of interest from those of all other factors quantitatively, but, to the extent that the possibility of confounding influences can be appraised, the committee will have achieved its objective.

Increased Risk in Vietnam Veterans

When all the available epidemiologic evidence has been evaluated, it is presumed that Vietnam veterans are at increased risk for a specific health outcome if there is evidence of a positive association between one or more of the chemicals of interest and the outcome. The best measure of potency for the quantification of risk to veterans would be the rate of the outcome in exposed Vietnam veterans compared with the rate in nonexposed veterans, adjusted for the degree to which any other factors that differ between exposed and nonexposed veterans might influence those rates. A dose–response relationship established in another human population suitably adjusted for such factors would be similarly suitable.

It is difficult to quantify risk when exposures of a population have not been measured accurately. Recent serum TCDD concentrations are available only on subgroups enrolled in the Air Force Health Study (AFHS) (the Ranch Hand and Southeast Asia comparison subjects) and from VA's study of deployed and nondeployed members of the Army Chemical Corps. Pharmacokinetic models, with their own set of assumptions, must then be used to extrapolate back to obtain the most accurate estimates of original exposure available on Vietnam-era veterans. The absence of reliable measures of exposure to the chemicals of interest among Vietnam veterans limits the committee's ability to quantify risks of specific diseases in this population.

Although serum TCDD measurements are available for only a small portion of Vietnam-era veterans, the observed distributions of these most reliable measures of exposure make it clear that they cannot be used as a standard to partition veterans into discrete exposure groups, such as service on Vietnamese soil, service in the Blue Water Navy, and service elsewhere in Southeast Asia. For example, many TCDD values observed in the comparison group from the AFHS exceeded US background levels and overlapped considerably with those of the Ranch Hand subjects.

As explained in Chapter 1, the committee for *Update 2006* decided to make a general statement about its continuing inability to address that aspect of its charge quantitatively rather than reiterate a disclaimer in the concluding section for every health outcome, and this committee has retained that approach.

Plausible Biologic Mechanisms

Chapter 4 details the experimental basis of assessment of biologic plausibility or the extent to which an observed statistical association in epidemiologic studies is consistent with other biologic or medical knowledge. In other words, does the observation of a particular health effect make sense on the basis of what is known about how the chemicals in question act at the tissue, cellular, or molecular level? The relationship between a particular exposure and a specific human health outcome is addressed in the context of research on the effects of the chemicals on biologic systems and of evidence from animal studies.

For this report, the committee reviewed toxicology studies that were published after *Update 2006* (IOM, 2007) and considered them in combination with earlier studies in commenting on the biologic plausibility of individual health outcomes. In the current update, the practice of earlier reports in presenting the toxicologic evidence has been modified. Chapter 4 presents a more streamlined toxicity profile of each of the chemicals of interest without providing commentary on each possibly relevant article published in the update period. Experimental information pertinent to a particular health outcome is now presented immediately after the epidemiologic evidence on that outcome in the "Biologic Plausibility" sections of the individual health outcomes (Chapters 6–9).

A positive statistical association between an exposure and an outcome does not necessarily mean that the exposure is the cause of the outcome. Data from toxicology studies may support or conflict with a hypothesis that a specific compound can contribute to the occurrence of a particular disease. Many toxicology studies are conducted with laboratory animals so that variables, including the amount and duration of exposure, can be controlled precisely. Studies that use isolated cells in culture also can elucidate how a compound alters cellular processes. The objectives of those toxicology studies are to determine what toxic effects are observed at different exposure concentrations and to identify the mechanisms by which the effects are produced. Ultimately, the results of the toxicology studies should be consistent with what is known about the human disease process to support a conclusion that the development of the disease was influenced by an exposure.

That approach is not without shortcomings; for example, the dose of a chemical required to produce an effect in experimental animals is often many times higher than human exposures. (For TCDD, however, effects have been observed in animals whose body burdens are no more than 10-fold higher than the high end of those in the general population in the industrialized world [EPA, 2001].) Furthermore, animal and cell-culture models do not always accurately mimic human responses. The absence of evidence of biologic plausibility from toxicology studies, however, does not rule out the possibility that a biologic relationship exists. In fact, cases in which the epidemiologic evidence is strong, but toxicologic support is lacking, often drive new toxicology research.

As noted in *VAO*, not only is information on biologic plausibility one of the primary elements in the widely accepted Bradford Hill (1965) criteria for causality but insights about biologic processes inform whether an observed pattern of statistical association might be interpreted as the product of more than error, bias, confounding, and chance. The committee used toxicologic information in that fashion and placed the information before its synthesis and conclusion to provide readers with a more coherent argument for its ultimate conclusion about the adequacy of the available evidence to support the existence of a particular association.

EVALUATION OF THE EVIDENCE

Associations between exposures to the chemicals of interest and specific health outcomes are determined through an analysis of available epidemiologic studies that is informed by an understanding of the toxicology of the chemicals and their exposure pathways. In reaching conclusions, Veterans and Agent Orange committees consider the nature of the exposures, the nature of the health outcomes, the populations exposed, and the quality of the evidence examined. Some specific issues that this and prior committees have considered are addressed below.

Human Studies

The committee reviewed studies of Vietnam veterans and of other populations that might have been exposed to the chemicals of interest. In light of the dispute regarding whether veterans who served in the "Blue Water Navy" during the Vietnam War should be presumed to have been exposed to the herbicides sprayed in Vietnam, the committee notes that, like prior VAO committees, it has considered data on such individuals to be a part of the evidentiary database on Vietnam veterans. The other populations factored into the committee's evaluation included cohorts of workers in chemical production and agriculture, populations that reside near sites of environmental contamination, and residents of Vietnam. The committee believes that studies of such nonveteran subjects can help in the assessment of whether the chemicals of interest are associated with particular health outcomes. As noted above in describing the literature search, studies of nonveteran subjects were identified because one of the chemicals of interest was specified by the original researchers as a possible toxic exposure, rather than on the basis of occupational definitions. Some of the studies, especially those of workers in chemical-production plants, provide stronger evidence about health outcomes than do studies of veterans because the industrial exposures were measured sooner after occurrence and were more thoroughly characterized than has been the case in most studies of veterans. Furthermore, in the studies of workers at chemical-production plants, the magnitude and duration of exposure to the chemicals were generally greater, so the likelihood that any possible health consequence would be manifested was greater. The studies were often large enough to examine health risks among groups of people with different levels of exposure, so dose–response relationships could be investigated. The general practice of VAO committees has been to evaluate all studies, whether or not their subjects were Vietnam veterans, according to the same criteria in determining the strength and validity of findings. Because the subjects of studies of Vietnam veterans are the concern of the legislation that mandated the present review, however, demonstrations of increased incidence of particular health outcomes among them are of unquestionable pertinence in drawing conclusions.

The committee has concluded that it would be inappropriate to use quantitative techniques, such as meta-analysis, to combine individual study results into a single summary measure of statistical association. The committee reached that conclusion because of the many differences among studies in definitions of exposure, health outcomes considered, criteria for defining study populations, correction for confounding factors, and degree of detail in reporting results. The appropriate use of meta-analysis requires more methodologic consistency among studies, especially in the definition of exposure, than is present in the literature reviewed by the committee (Egger et al., 2002; Petitti, 2000). A detailed discussion of the results of individual studies in appropriate categories (Vietnam veterans, occupational, or environmental; exposure to Agent Orange or equivalent dioxin-contaminated phenoxy herbicides, to dioxin, to phenoxy herbicides without dioxin contamination, to cacodylic acid, or to picloram) with a thorough examination of each study's strengths and weaknesses is fully informative without making unfounded assumptions of homogeneity.

In general, the committee did not consider case reports, case series, or other published studies that lacked control or comparison groups. An exception was made, however, for early-onset transient peripheral neuropathy. Individual case reports were reviewed because the rapid appearance and transient nature of the condition impose methodologic constraints that might have precluded the application of standard epidemiologic techniques.

Because any effect of Agent Orange in individuals or groups of veterans is evaluated in terms of disease or medical outcome, attention to disease classification was important to the committee in assembling pertinent data related to a particular outcome from various investigations before integrating the information. The researchers who conducted the studies reviewed by the committee faced the same challenge in interpreting the available documentation when assigning diagnostic labels to given subjects and then grouping the labels for analysis.

Pathologists, clinicians, and epidemiologists use several classification systems, including the *International Classification of Diseases* (ICD), the *Interna-*

tional Classification of Diseases, 9th Revision (ICD-9), *Clinical Modification*, and the *International Classification of Diseases for Oncology*. The 10th revision of ICD (ICD-10) is currently used to classify mortality information. Most of the subjects investigated in the studies cited in this update were diagnosed under earlier systems, and most of the articles report results in accordance with ICD-9 if they use ICD codes at all, so the committee has also used ICD-9. ICD codes are a hierarchic system for indicating type of disease and site. For example, ICD-9 162 specifies cancers of the lung, trachea, or bronchus; 162.2 specifies cancer of the main bronchus; 162.3, cancer of the upper lobe of the lung; and 162.4, cancer of the middle lobe of the lung.

For a patient to receive a correct diagnosis, careful staging of the extent of disease is necessary, and a biopsy of the tissue must be analyzed with microscopy, often with special immunohistochemical stains, to confirm a clinical impression. Many of the epidemiologic studies reviewed by this committee did not use the ICD approach to classification of disease and relied instead on clinical impression alone. Death-certificate diagnoses are notoriously inaccurate if the certificates are completed by medical officers who are not familiar with the decedents' medical history (Smith Sehdev and Hutchins, 2001). Self-reported diagnoses, which are obtained from survey questionnaires, often are partially or completely inaccurate; for instance, a patient may report having been treated for stomach cancer although the correct diagnosis was gastric adenocarcinoma, gastric lymphoma, pancreatic cancer, large bowel cancer, or peritoneal cancer.

Many epidemiologic studies report disease outcome by organ system. For instance, the term *digestive system* may be used for conditions that are benign or malignant and that affect the esophagus, stomach, liver, pancreas, small bowel, large bowel, or rectum. Therefore, if a report indicated that a cohort has an increased incidence of digestive system cancer, it would be unclear whether the association was attributable to excess cases of esophageal, gastric, hepatic, pancreatic, or intestinal cancers or to some combination. Such generalization is complicated by the fact that the cause of cancer may differ at various anatomic sites. For instance, there are strong associations between gastric cancer and *Helicobacter pylori* infection, between smoking and squamous cell carcinoma of the esophagus, and between chronic hepatitis B infection and hepatic cancer. Furthermore, a single site may experience a carcinogenic response to multiple agents.

The committee recognizes that outcome misclassification is a possibility when recording of a diagnosis with a specific ICD code is used as the means of entering an observation into an analysis, but this system has been refined over many decades and is virtually universally used and understood, in addition to being exhaustive and explicit. Therefore, this and previous VAO committees have opted to use the ICD system as an organizing tool. Although the groupings of cancer sites for which conclusions about association have been presented may correspond more closely to National Institute for Occupational Safety and Health or National Cancer Institute Surveillance Epidemiology and End Results categories (see Appendix B), the underlying ICD codes provide the most exactitude. In this report, ICD codes appear almost exclusively in the introductory sections of health-outcome discussions (particularly for cancers) to specify precisely what outcome the committee is addressing and, when possible, in the results table to indicate exactly what the primary researchers believed they were investigating. (See Appendix B for cancer groupings with corresponding ICD-9 and ICD-10 codes.)

For *Update 2006*, VA made two specific requests. First, the committee was asked to consider whether the occurrence of hairy cell leukemia should be regarded as associated with exposure to the herbicides used by the military in Vietnam. Second, the committee was asked to comment on whether effects of veterans' herbicide exposures might be manifested at later stages of their children's development than have been systematically evaluated to date or in later generations and on the feasibility of assessing such effects. Those requests are addressed in Chapters 6 and 7, respectively.

Rare diseases, such as hairy cell leukemia and tonsil cancer, are difficult to study because it is hard to accumulate enough cases to permit analysis. Often, the result is that observed cases are included in a broader, less specific category. Thus, epidemiologic data may not be available for assessing whether a particular rare disease is associated with Agent Orange exposure. In some instances, as for chronic lymphocytic leukemia and AL amyloidosis, VAO committees have reached conclusions on the basis of the data available and the etiology of the disease. Through systematic application of the hierarchic nature of the ICD coding system, committees intend to draw an explicit conclusion for every type of cancer about the adequacy of available evidence to support an association between herbicide exposure and each type of cancer. For nonmalignant conditions, however, the diversity of disease processes involved makes the use of broad ICD ranges less useful, but, because VAO committees could not possibly address every rare nonmalignant disease, they do not draw explicit conclusions about diseases that are not discussed. Thus, the category of "inadequate or insufficient evidence to determine an association" is the default or starting point for any health outcome; if a condition or outcome is not addressed specifically, it will be in this category.

The committee is aware of the concerns of some veterans about the role of herbicide exposure in the occurrence of multiple health outcomes, such as multiple cancers, in a given person. Little research has been done to address whether the rate of concurrence is greater than would be expected by chance. Simultaneous analysis of multiple health outcomes could potentially provide more insight into whether the chemicals of interest cause multiple health effects, into competing risks between various health outcomes, and into the interactive effects of some health outcomes on others; but addressing health conditions individually has remained challenging.

VAO committees wanted to be clear in indicating what evidence is factored into their conclusions. The practice in the VAO reports has been to augment the results table for a given health outcome with any additional publications considered in the current update in the categories of Vietnam-veteran, occupational, or environmental studies. Inclusion of sequential sets of results from follow-ups of a study population has the potential to create the appearance of a greater weight of evidence than is warranted, so since *Update 2006* an italicized citation in a table indicates that its results have been superseded.

An issue related to evidence evaluation that was of concern for the *Update 2006* committee was the evidence category of "*no* association." That committee determined that a conclusion of *no* association would require substantive evidence of such a lack of effect of each of the chemicals of interest. Given the paucity of information that has ever been found on cacodylic acid and picloram, that conclusion would seem suspect even if substantial evidence uniformly supported a finding of *no* association both with exposure to the phenoxy herbicides and with exposure to TCDD. The current committee concurs with that determination and has adopted a similar approach to the placement of health outcomes in this category.

Exposure Assessment

Much of the evidence that VAO committees have considered has been drawn from studies of populations that were not in Vietnam during the period when Agent Orange and other herbicides were used as defoliants. The most informative of those studies were well-documented investigations of occupational exposures to TCDD or specific herbicides, such as 2,4-D or 2,4,5-T. In many other studies, TCDD exposure was combined with exposures to an array of "dioxin-like" compounds, and the herbicides were often analyzed as members of a functional class; this is less informative for the committee's purpose than individual results on each specific compound. In the real-world situations investigated in epidemiologic studies, exposure to multiple possibly toxic chemicals is the rule rather than the exception; for example, farmers or other agricultural populations are likely to be exposed to insecticides and fungicides and to herbicides. In such studies, the committee looked for evidence of health effects that are associated with the specific compounds in the defoliants used in Vietnam and also sought consideration of and adjustment for other possibly confounding exposures.

The quality of exposure information in the scientific literature reviewed by this and previous committees spans a broad range. Some studies relied on interviews or questionnaires to determine the extent and frequency of exposure. Such self-reported information generally carries less weight than would more objective measures of exposure. To the extent that questionnaire-based information can be corroborated or validated by other sources, its strength as evidence of exposure is enhanced. Written records of chemical purchase or production can provide one type of objective information. Even more useful are scientific measurements of exposure. In some occupational studies, for example, workers wear air-sampling instruments that measure the concentration of a contaminant in each worker's breathing zone. Measurement of chemicals or their products in biologic specimens, such as blood and urine, also can provide reliable indications of exposure for specific periods. Studies that categorize exposure from well-documented environmental sources of contaminants can be useful in the identification of exposed populations, but their results may be inaccurate if people with different levels of exposure are assigned to the same general category of exposure. Studies that explore environmental exposure and disease frequency in regional populations (such as states and counties) are known as ecologic studies. Most ecologic studies are considered preliminary or "hypothesis-generating" studies because they lack information on exposure and disease on an individual basis and are unable to address potential confounding factors.

Chapter 3 of this update addresses issues of exposure estimation in more detail. The agent of interest may be assessed with various degrees of specificity. For instance, any of the four herbicides in question could be individually measured, and phenoxy herbicides would be a useful broader category for 2,4,5-T and 2,4-D; but a report of findings in terms simply of "herbicides" is on the margin of being informative, whereas results stated in terms of "pesticides" are too vague to be useful. For a given chemical of interest, the measure of exposure may be increasingly imprecise—for example, concentrations in target tissue, serum concentrations, cumulative exposure, possible exposure, and so on down to merely a report of service in a job or industry category. Those approaches can address complexities in specificity, duration, and intensity of exposure with various degrees of success. All may provide some information about association with a chemical of interest, but this committee has determined that investigation of associations between the exposure of concern and most health outcomes has advanced to the stage where some characterizations of exposure are too nonspecific to promote insight. For health outcomes with very little evidence, a somewhat looser criterion would apply so that no possible signal of an association would be overlooked.

Animal and Mechanistic Studies

Animal models used as surrogates for the study of a human disease must reproduce, with some degree of fidelity, the manifestations of the disease in humans. However, a given effect of herbicide exposure in an animal species does not necessarily establish its occurrence in humans. In addition to possible species differences, many factors affect the ability to extrapolate from results of animal studies to health effects in humans. Animals used in experimental studies are most often exposed to purified chemicals, not to mixtures. Even if herbicide formulations or mixtures are used, the conditions of exposure might not realistically reproduce exposures that occur in the field. Furthermore, Vietnam veterans were probably exposed to other agents—such as tobacco smoke, insecticides, therapeutics, drugs, diesel fumes, and alcohol—that may increase or decrease the ability of chemicals in herbicides to produce a particular adverse health outcome. Few, if any, studies either in humans or in experimental animals have examined those interactions.

As discussed in Chapter 4, TCDD, a contaminant of 2,4,5-T, is thought to be responsible for many of the toxic effects of the herbicides used in Vietnam. Attempts to establish correlations in the effects of TCDD between experimental systems and humans are particularly problematic because of known species-, sex-, and outcome-specific differences in susceptibility to TCDD toxicity. Some data indicate that humans might be more resistant than are other species to TCDD's toxic effects (Ema et al., 1994; Moriguchi et al., 2003); other data suggest that, for some outcomes, human sensitivity could be the same as or greater than that of some experimental animals (DeVito et al., 1995). Differences in susceptibility may also be affected by variations in the rate at which TCDD is eliminated from the body (see Chapter 4 for details on the toxicokinetics of TCDD).

It also is important to account for TCDD's mode of action in considering species and strain differences. There is a consensus that most of or all the toxic effects of TCDD involve interaction with the aryl hydrocarbon receptor (AHR), a protein that binds TCDD and other aromatic hydrocarbons with high affinity. Formation of an active complex involving the intracellular receptor, the ligand (the TCDD molecule), and other proteins is followed by interaction of the activated complex with specific sites on DNA. That interaction can alter the expression of genes involved in the regulation of cellular processes. The development of mice that lack the AHR has helped to establish a definitive association between the AHR and TCDD-mediated toxicity. The affinity of TCDD for the AHR is species- and strain-specific, and responses to binding of the receptor vary among cell types and developmental stages. In addition, genetic differences in the properties of the AHR are known in human populations, as they are in laboratory animals, so some people are at intrinsically greater or less risk for the toxic effects of TCDD.

Although studying AHR biology in transformed human cell lines minimizes the inherent error associated with species extrapolations, caution must be exercised because it is still not clear to what extent toxicity is affected by the transformation itself or by the conditions under which cell lines are cultured in vitro.

Publication Bias

Some studies are more likely to be published than others. That is the concept of publication bias, which has been documented in biomedical research (Song et al., 2000; Stern and Simes, 1997). Most commonly, bias can be introduced when studies whose hypotheses are supported by statistically significant results or that are otherwise deemed favorable by their authors are selectively submitted for publication. Conversely, "negative" studies, in which the hypotheses being tested are not supported by the study findings, often go unpublished. Therefore, conclusions about associations between exposure and outcome that are based solely on published results could be subject to bias. Despite that, the committee does not believe that its conclusions have been unduly affected by publication bias, for two reasons: the extensive publicity surrounding the possibility of health effects associated with the herbicides used in Vietnam has created considerable pressure to publish all findings on the subject, and the many published studies assembled and reviewed contain among their results the full range of possible statistical associations, from convincingly negative through indeterminate to strongly positive.

Role of Judgment

This committee's process of reaching conclusions about statistical associations involved more than a formulaic application of quantitative procedures to the assembled evidence. First, the committee had to assess the relevance and validity of individual reports. Then, it had to evaluate the possible influences of measurement error, selection bias, confounding, and chance on the reported results. Next, the committee integrated all the evidence within and among diverse fields of research. Finally, the conclusions drawn were based on consensus within the committee. Those aspects of the committee's review required thoughtful consideration of alternative approaches at several points and could not be accomplished by adherence to a narrowly prescribed formula.

The realized approach, as described here, has been determined to a large extent by the nature of the exposures, of the health outcomes, and of the resulting evidence available for examination; therefore, it has evolved in the course of the work of this and previous VAO committees. The quantitative and qualitative procedures underlying this review have been made as explicit as possible, but ultimately the conclusions about association expressed in this report are based on the committee's collective judgment. The committee has endeavored to express its judgments as clearly and precisely as the data allowed.

REFERENCES[1]

Abell A, Juul S, Bonde JP. 2000. Time to pregnancy among female greenhouse workers. *Scandinavian Journal of Work, Environment and Health* 26(2):131–136.
Czarnota MA. 2004. *Weed Control in Greenhouses: Bulletin 1246*. University of Georgia, College of Agricultural and Environmental Sciences, Cooperative Extension.

---

[1]Throughout the report the same alphabetic indicator following year of publication is used consistently for the same article when there were multiple citations by the same first author in a given year. The convention of assigning the alphabetic indicator in order of citation in a given chapter is not followed.

DeVito MJ, Birnbaum LS, Farland WH, Gasiewicz TA. 1995. Comparisons of estimated human body burdens of dioxin-like chemicals and TCDD body burdens in experimentally exposed animals. *Environmental Health Perspectives* 103(9):820–831.

Egger M, Ebrahim S, Smith GD. 2002. Where now for meta-analysis? *International Journal of Epidemiology* 31(1):1–5.

Ema M, Ohe N, Suzuki M, Mimura J, Sogawa K, Ikawa S, Fujii-Kuriyama Y. 1994. Dioxin binding activities of polymorphic forms of mouse and human arylhydrocarbon receptors. *Journal of Biological Chemistry* 269(44):27337–27343.

EPA (US Environmental Protection Agency). 2001. *Dioxin: Summary of the Dioxin Reassessment Science* (Information Sheet 1). Washington, DC: EPA, Office of Research and Development.

Hansen ES, Hasle H, Lander F. 1992. A cohort study on cancer incidence among Danish gardeners. *American Journal of Industrial Medicine* 21(5):651–660.

Hill AB. 1965. The environment and disease: Association or causation? *Proceedings of the Royal Society of Medicine* 58:295–300.

IOM (Institute of Medicine). 1994. *Veterans and Agent Orange: Health Effects of Herbicides Used in Vietnam.* Washington, DC: National Academy Press.

IOM. 2007. *Veterans and Agent Orange: Update 2006.* Washington, DC: The National Academies Press.

Kim HA, Kim EM, Park YC, Yu JY, Hong SK, Jeon SH, Park KL, Hur SJ, Heo Y. 2003a. Immunotoxicological effects of Agent Orange exposure to the Vietnam War Korean veterans. *Industrial Health* 41(3):158–166.

Kim JS, Lim HS, Cho SI, Cheong HK, Lim MK. 2003b. Impact of Agent Orange exposure among Korean Vietnam veterans. *Industrial Health* 41(3):149–157.

Moriguchi T, Motohashi H, Hosoya T, Nakajima O, Takahashi S, Ohsako S, Aoki Y, Nishimura N, Tohyama C, Fujii-Kuriyama Y, Yamamoto M. 2003. Distinct response to dioxin in an arylhydrocarbon receptor (AHR)-humanized mouse. *Proceedings of the National Academy of Sciences of the United States of America* 100(10):5652–5657.

Neal NC. 2006. *Greenhouse Weed Control: Horticultural Information Leaflet 570.* North Carolina State University.

NRC (National Research Council). 1999. *Arsenic in Drinking Water.* Washington, DC: National Academy Press.

NRC. 2001. *Arsenic in Drinking Water: 2001 Update.* Washington, DC: National Academy Press.

Petitti DB. 2000. *Meta-Analysis, Decision Analysis, and Cost-Effectiveness Analysis: Methods for Quantitative Synthesis in Medicine.* New York: Oxford Press.

Smith Sehdev AE, Hutchins GM. 2001. Problems with proper completion and accuracy of the cause-of-death statement. *Archives of Internal Medicine* 161(2):277–284.

Song F, Eastwood AJ, Gilbody S, Duley L, Sutton AJ. 2000. Publication and related biases. *Health Technology Assessment* 4(10):1–115.

Stern JM, Simes RJ. 1997. Publication bias: Evidence of delayed publication in a cohort study of clinical research projects. *British Medical Journal* 315(7109):640–645.

University of Connecticut. 2006. *Greenhouse Weed Control.* University of Connecticut, Storrs, Cooperative Extension System.

3

Exposure to the Herbicides Used in Vietnam

Assessment of human exposure is a key element in addressing two of the charges that guide the work of this committee. This chapter first presents background information on the military use of herbicides in Vietnam from 1961 to 1971 with a review of our knowledge of exposures of those who served in Vietnam and of the Vietnamese population to the herbicides and to the contaminant 2,3,7,8-tetrachlorodibenzo-p-dioxin (referred to in this report as TCDD, the most toxic congener of the tetrachlorodibenzo-p-dioxins [tetraCDDs], also commonly referred to as dioxin). It then reviews several key methodologic issues in human population studies, namely, disease latency, possible misclassification based on exposure, and exposure specificity required for scientific evaluation of studies.

Exposure of human populations can be assessed in a number of ways, including use of historical information, questionnaires and interviews, measurements in environmental media, and measurements in biologic specimens. Researchers often rely on a mixture of qualitative and quantitative information to derive estimates (Armstrong et al., 1994; Checkoway et al., 2004). The most basic approach compares members of a presumably exposed group with the general population or with a nonexposed group. That method of classification offers simplicity and ease of interpretation. A more refined method assigns each study subject to an exposure category, such as high, medium, or low exposure. Disease risk for each group is calculated separately and compared with a reference or nonexposed group. That method can identify the presence or absence of an exposure–response trend. In some cases, more detailed information is available for quantitative exposure estimates, and these can be used to construct what are sometimes called exposure metrics. The metrics integrate quantitative estimates of exposure intensity (such as chemical concentration in air or extent of skin contact) with exposure duration to produce an estimate of cumulative exposure. Exposure also can be assessed by measuring chemicals and their metabolites in human tissues. Such biologic markers of exposure integrate absorption from all routes, and their interpretation requires knowledge of pharmacokinetic processes. All those approaches have been used in studies of Vietnam veterans.

MILITARY USE OF HERBICIDES IN VIETNAM

Military use of herbicides in Vietnam took place from 1962 through 1971. Selection of the specific herbicides to be used was based on tests conducted in the United States and elsewhere that were designed to evaluate their defoliation efficacy (IOM, 1994; Young and Newton, 2004). Four compounds were used in the herbicide formulations in Vietnam: 2,4-dichlorophenoxyacetic acid (2,4-D), 2,4,5-trichlorophenoxyacetic acid (2,4,5-T), 4-amino-3,5,6-trichloropicolinic acid (picloram), and dimethylarsinic acid (cacodylic acid). The chemical structures of those compounds are presented in Chapter 2 (Figure 2-1). The herbicides were used to defoliate inland hardwood forests, coastal mangrove forests, cultivated land, and zones around military bases. In 1974, a National Academy of Sciences committee estimated the amount of herbicides sprayed from helicopters and other aircraft by using records gathered from August 1965 through February 1971 (NAS, 1974). That committee calculated that about 18 million gallons (about 68 million liters) of herbicide were sprayed over about 3.6 million acres (about 1.5 million hectares) in Vietnam in that period. The amount of herbicides sprayed on the ground to defoliate the perimeters of base camps and fire bases and the amount sprayed by Navy boats along river banks were not estimated.

A new analysis of spray activities and exposure potential of troops emerged from a recent study overseen by a committee of the Institute of Medicine (IOM) (IOM, 1997, 2003a,b). That work yielded new estimates of the use of military herbicides in Vietnam from 1961 through 1971 (Stellman et al., 2003a). The investigators reanalyzed the original data sources that were used to develop herbicide-use estimates in the 1970s and identified errors that inappropriately removed spraying missions from the dataset. They also added new data on spraying missions that took place before 1965. Finally, a comparison of procurement records with spraying records indicated errors in both types and suggested that additional spraying had taken place but gone unrecorded at the time.

The new analyses led to a revision in estimates of the amounts of the agents applied, as indicated in Table 3-1. The new research effort estimated that about 77 million liters were applied, about 9 million liters more than the previous estimate.

Herbicides were identified by the color of a band on 55-gal containers and were called Agents Pink, Green, Purple, Orange, White, and Blue. Agent Green and Agent Pink were used in 1961 and 1965, and Agent Purple in 1962–1965. Agent Orange was used in 1965–1970, and a slightly different formulation (Agent

TABLE 3-1 Military Use of Herbicides in Vietnam (1961–1971)

Code Name	Chemical Constituents[a]	Concentration of Active Ingredient[a]	Years Used[a]	Amount Sprayed	
				VAO Estimate[b]	Revised Estimate[a]
Pink	60% n-butyl: 40% isobutyl ester of 2,4,5-T	961–1,081 g/L acid equivalent	1961, 1965	464,817 L (122,792 gal)	50,312 L sprayed; 413,852 L additional on procurement records
Green	n-butyl ester of 2,4,5-T	—	1961, 1965	31,071 L (8,208 gal)	31,026 L on procurement records
Purple	50% n-butyl ester of 2,4-D, 30% n-butyl ester of 2,4,5-T, 20% isobutyl ester of 2,4,5-T	1,033 g/L acid equivalent	1962–1965	548,883 L (145,000 gal)	1,892,733 L
Orange	50% n-butyl ester of 2,4-D, 50% n-butyl ester of 2,4,5-T	1,033 g/L acid equivalent	1965–1970	42,629,013 L (11,261,429 gal)	45,677,937 L (could include Agent Orange II)
Orange II	50% n-butyl ester of 2,4-D, 50% isooctyl ester of 2,4,5-T	910 g/L acid equivalent	After 1968	—	Unknown; at least 3,591,000 L shipped
White	Acid weight basis: 21.2% triisopropanolamine salts of 2,4-D, 5.7% picloram	By acid weight, 240 g/L 2,4-D, 65 g/L picloram	1966–1971	19,860,108 L (5,246,502 gal)	20,556,525 L
Blue powder	Cacodylic acid (dimethylarsinic acid) sodium cacodylate	Acid, 65% active ingredient; salt, 70% active ingredient	1962–1964	—	25,650 L
Blue aqueous solution	21% sodium cacodylate + cacodylic acid to yield at least 26% total acid equivalent by weight	Acid weight, 360 g/L	1964–1971	4,255,952 L (1,124,307 gal)	4,715,731 L
Total, all formulations				67,789,844 L (17,908,238 gal)	76,954,766 L (including procured)

[a] Based on Stellman et al. (2003a).
[b] Based on data from MRI (1967), NAS (1974), and Young and Reggiani (1988).

Orange II) probably was used after 1968. Agent White was used in 1966–1971. Agent Blue was used in powder form in 1962–1964 and as a liquid in 1964–1971. Agents Pink, Green, Purple, Orange, and Orange II all contained 2,4,5-T and were contaminated to some extent with TCDD. Agent White contained 2,4-D and picloram. Agent Blue (powder and liquid) contained cacodylic acid. The chlorinated phenoxy acids 2,4-D and 2,4,5-T persist in soil for only a few weeks; picloram is much more stable, persisting in soil for years; and cacodylic acid is nonvolatile and stable in sunlight (NAS, 1974). More details on the herbicides used are presented in the initial National Academy of Sciences report (NAS, 1974) and the initial *VAO* report (IOM, 1994).

TCDD IN HERBICIDES USED IN VIETNAM

TCDD is formed during the manufacture of 2,4,5-T in the following manner: trichlorophenol (2,4,5-TCP), the precursor for the synthesis of 2,4,5-T, is formed by the reaction of tetrachlorobenzene and sodium hydroxide (Figure 3-1a); 2,4,5-T is formed when 2,4,5-TCP reacts with chloroacetic acid (Figure 3-1b); small amounts of TCDD are formed as a byproduct of the intended main reaction (Figure 3-1b) when a molecule of 2,4,5-TCP reacts with the tetrachlorobenzene stock (Figure 3-1c) instead of with chloroacetic acid. For each step in the reaction, a chlorine atom is replaced with an oxygen atom, and this leads to the final TCDD molecule (NAS, 1974). In the class of compounds known as polychlorinated dibenzo-*p*-dioxins (PCDDs), 75 congeners can occur, depending on the number and placement of the chlorines. Cochrane et al. (1982) noted that TCDD had been found in pre-1970 samples of 2,4,5-TCP. Other PCDDs—2,7-dichloro-dibenzo-*p*-dioxin and 1,3,6,8-tetrachloro-dibenzo-*p*-dioxin—were measured in the same samples. The concentration of TCDD in any given lot of 2,4,5-T depended on the manufacturing process (FAO/UNEP, 2009; Young et al., 1976).

The manufacture of 2,4-D is based on a different process. Its synthesis is based on dichlorophenol, a molecule formed from the reaction of phenol with chlorine (NZIC, 2009). Neither tetrachlorobenzene nor trichlorophenol is formed during this reaction, so TCDD is not normally a byproduct of the synthetic process. However, other, less toxic PCDDs have been detected in pre-1970 commercial-grade 2,4-D (Cochrane et al., 1982; Rappe et al., 1978; Tosine, 1983). Cochrane et al. (1982) found multiple PCDDs in isooctyl ester, mixed butyl ester, and dimethylamine salt samples of 2,4-D. It has also been noted that cross-contamination of 2,4-D by 2,3,7,8-TCDD occurred in the operations of at least one major manufacturer (Lilienfeld and Gallo, 1989).

TCDD concentrations in individual herbicide shipments were not recorded but were known to vary from batch to batch and between manufacturers. TCDD concentrations in stocks of Agent Orange remaining after the conflict, which either had been returned from South Vietnam or had been procured but not shipped, ranged from less than 0.05 ppm to almost 50 ppm and averaged 2–3 ppm in two

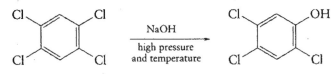

a. Trichlorophenol, the precursor for the synthesis of 2,4,5-T, is formed by the reaction of tetrachlorobenzene and sodium hydroxide (NaOH).

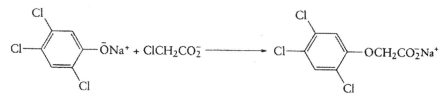

b. The herbicide 2,4,5-T is formed when a reactive form of trichlorophenol (2,4,5-trichlorophenoxide) reacts with chloroacetic acid.

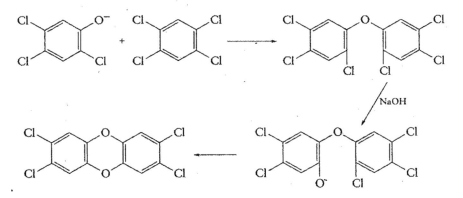

c. TCDD is formed when a molecule of trichlorophenol reacts with its own precursor, tetrachlorobenzene. Two intermediate steps are shown in this diagram. At each step, an oxygen–carbon bond forms as a chlorine atom is released. This reaction does not occur in the synthesis of 2,4-D, because these precursors with adjacent chlorines are not used in its production.

FIGURE 3-1 TCDD formation during 2,4,5-T production.

sets of samples (NAS, 1974; Young et al., 1978). Comparable manufacturing standards for the domestic use of 2,4,5-T in 1974 required that TCDD not be present at over 0.05 ppm (NAS, 1974).

    Until recently, data from Young and Gough have been used to estimate the amount of TCDD in the various herbicide formulations (Gough, 1986; Young,

1992; Young et al., 1978). Young et al. (1978) estimated that Agents Green, Pink, and Purple—used early in the program (through 1965)—contained 16 times the mean TCDD content of the formulations used in 1965–1970, whereas mean TCDD concentrations in Agents Pink and Green were estimated at 66 ppm. Gough (1986) estimated that about 167 kg of TCDD was sprayed in Vietnam over a 6-year period.

A new analysis by researchers at Columbia University benefited from access to military spray records that had not been available earlier and has resulted in substantial revisions of the estimates (Stellman et al., 2003a). The investigators were able to incorporate newly found data on spraying in the early period of the war (1961–1965) and to document that larger volumes of TCDD-containing herbicides were used in Vietnam than had been estimated previously. They also found that the earlier estimates of TCDD contamination in the herbicide formulations were too low, noting that the original estimates were based on samples at the lower end of the distribution of concentration values. They concluded that mean TCDD concentrations in Agent Orange were closer to 13 ppm than to the earlier estimates of 3 ppm. They therefore proposed 366 kg of TCDD as a plausible estimate of the total amount of TCDD applied in Vietnam during 1961–1971.

EXPOSURE OF VIETNAM VETERANS

Determination of exposure among US military personnel who served in Vietnam has been a great challenge in the study of health effects associated with herbicides and TCDD. Some military personnel stationed in cities or on large bases may have received little or no herbicide exposures, whereas troops who moved through defoliated areas soon after treatment may have been exposed through soil contact, drinking water, or bathing. Reliable estimates of the magnitude and duration of such exposures are not possible in most cases, given the lack of contemporaneous chemical measurements and the lack of records of individual behaviors. In accord with Congress's mandated presumption of herbicide exposure for all Vietnam veterans, VAO committees have treated Vietnam-veteran status as a proxy for some herbicide exposure when no more specific exposure information is available.

Exposure of Herbicide Handlers

Military personnel who came into direct contact with the herbicidal compounds through mixing, loading, spraying, and clean-up activities had relatively high exposures to herbicides. The US Environmental Protection Agency refers to such personnel as pesticide handlers and provides special guidance for preventing or minimizing their exposure during those activities in its worker protection standard for pesticides (EPA, 1992). The number of US military personnel who handled herbicides directly is not known precisely, but two groups have been identified as high-risk subpopulations among veterans: Air Force personnel involved in fixed-wing aircraft spraying activities (often referred to as Operation Ranch Hand), and members of the US Army Chemical Corps (ACC) who used hand-operated equipment and helicopters to conduct smaller-scale operations, including defoliation around special-forces camps; clearing of the perimeters of airfields, depots, and other bases; and small-scale crop destruction (NRC, 1980; Thomas and Kang, 1990; Warren, 1968). Additional units and individuals handled or sprayed herbicides around bases or lines of communication; for example, Navy river patrols were reported to have used herbicides to clear inland waterways, and engineering personnel used herbicides to remove underbrush and dense growth in constructing fire-support bases. However, they have not been the subject of epidemiologic studies. The herbicides used in Vietnam were not considered to present an important human health hazard at that time, so few precautions were taken to prevent exposure of personnel (GAO, 1978, 1979); that is, military personnel did not typically use chemical-protective gloves, coveralls, or protective aprons, so substantial skin exposure almost certainly occurred in these populations in addition to exposure by inhalation and incidental ingestion (such as by hand-to-mouth contact).

The Air Force personnel who participated in Operation Ranch Hand were the first Vietnam-veteran subpopulation to receive special attention with regard to herbicide exposure. In the Air Force Health Study (AFHS), the members of this Ranch Hand cohort were contrasted with Air Force personnel who had served elsewhere in Southeast Asia during the Vietnam era. The AFHS began in 1979 (IOM, 2006). The exposure index initially proposed in it relied on military spray records for the TCDD-containing herbicides (Agents Orange, Purple, Pink, Green) and helped to identify the members of the cohort. The subjects were further characterized by military occupation, and exposure in the cohort and comparison group was evaluated through measurement of TCDD in blood (serum) samples drawn in 1987 or later. A general increase in serum TCDD was detected in people whose jobs involved more frequent handling of herbicides, but there was no clear demarcation between the distributions of serum concentrations in the Ranch Hand subjects and in the comparison group (AFHS, 1991). Several methods for estimating herbicide exposure of members of the cohort were developed on the basis of questionnaires and focused on such factors as number of days of skin exposure, percentage of skin area exposed, and the concentration of TCDD in the different herbicidal formulations (Michalek et al., 1995). Most recent analyses of the AFHS data have relied on serum TCDD concentration as the primary exposure metric for epidemiologic classification (Kern et al., 2004; Michalek et al., 2001, 2003; Pavuk et al., 2003). The IOM has issued a comprehensive review of the AFHS with recommendations for the use of the extensive data collected in the project (IOM, 2006).

Members of the ACC performed chemical operations on the ground and by helicopter and were thereby involved in the direct handling and distribution of herbicides in Vietnam. They were identified for detailed study of health effects related to herbicide exposure only in the late 1980s (Thomas and Kang, 1990). An initial feasibility study recruited Vietnam veterans and nondeployed Vietnam-era veterans from within the ACC (Kang et al., 2001). Blood samples collected in 1996 from 50 Vietnam veterans showed an association between those who reported spraying herbicides and higher TCDD concentrations; this finding was confirmed in a follow-up study of a larger fraction of the cohort (Kang et al., 2006).

Exposure of Ground Troops

In light of the widespread use of herbicides in Vietnam for many years, it is reasonable to assume that many military personnel were inadvertently exposed to the chemicals of concern. Surveys of Vietnam veterans who were not part of the Ranch Hand or ACC groups have indicated that 25–55% believe that they were exposed to herbicides (CDC, 1989a). That view has been supported by government reports (GAO, 1979) and reiterated by veterans and their representatives in testimony to the VAO committees over the last several years.

Numerous attempts were made in the 1980s to characterize herbicide exposures of people who served as ground troops in Vietnam (CDC, 1988; Erickson et al., 1984; NRC, 1982; Stellman and Stellman, 1986; Stellman et al., 1988). The efforts combined self-reported contact with herbicides or military service records with aerial-spray data to produce an "exposure opportunity" index. For example, Erickson et al. (1984) created five exposure categories based on military records to examine the risks of birth defects among the offspring of veterans. Those studies were conducted carefully and provided reasonable estimates based on available data, but no means of testing the validity of the estimates were available at the time.

The search for a validation method led to the development of exposure biomarkers in veterans. Initial studies measured concentrations of dioxin in adipose tissue of veterans (Gross et al., 1984; Schecter et al., 1987). A study sponsored by the New Jersey Agent Orange Commission was the first to link dioxin concentrations in adipose tissue to dioxin concentrations in blood (Kahn et al., 1988). At the same time, the Center for Disease Control undertook what came to be called the Agent Orange Validation Study, measuring TCDD in the serum portion of blood from a relatively large sample of Vietnam veterans and veterans who served elsewhere during the Vietnam era (CDC, 1989b). The study did not find a significant difference in TCDD serum concentrations among the groups. A review of a preliminary report of the work by an advisory panel established through the IOM concluded that the long lag between exposure and the serum measurements (about 20 years) called into question the accuracy of exposure classification based on serum concentrations. The panel concluded that estimates based on troop locations and herbicide-spraying activities might be more reliable indicators of exposure serum measurements (IOM, 1987).

The report of the *VAO* committee (IOM, 1994) proposed further work on exposure reconstruction and development of a model that could be used to categorize exposures of ground troops. The committee cautioned that serum TCDD measurements not be regarded as a "gold standard" for exposure, that is, as a fully accurate measure of herbicide exposure. Recent efforts to develop exposure-reconstruction models for US Vietnam veterans are discussed later in this chapter.

One other effort to reconstruct exposure has been reported by researchers in the Republic of Korea (Kim et al., 2001, 2003). They developed an exposure index for Korean military personnel who served in Vietnam. The exposure index was based on herbicide-spray patterns in military regions in which Korean personnel served during 1964–1973, time–location data on the military units stationed in Vietnam, and an exposure score derived from self-reported activities during service. The researchers were not successful in an attempt to validate their exposure index with serum dioxin measurements.

Exposure of Personnel Who Had Offshore Vietnam Service

US Navy riverine units are known to have used herbicides while patrolling inland waterways (IOM, 1994; Zumwalt, 1993), and it is generally acknowledged that estuarine waters became contaminated with herbicides and dioxin as a result of shoreline spraying and runoff from spraying on land. Thus, military personnel who did not serve on land were among those exposed to the chemicals during the Vietnam conflict. A particular concern for the personnel has been possible contamination of drinking water. Most vessels serving offshore but within the territorial limits of the Republic of Vietnam converted seawater to drinking water through distillation.

Higher than expected mortality among Royal Australian Navy Vietnam veterans prompted a study of potable-water contamination on ships offshore during the Vietnam conflict (Mueller et al., 2001, 2002). Specifically, the study investigated the potential for naval personnel to ingest TCDD and cacodylic acid in drinking water. The study focused on the evaporative distillation process that was used to produce potable water from surrounding estuarine waters. The study found that codistillation of dioxins was observable in all experiments conducted and that distillation increased the concentration of dioxins in the distillate compared with the concentration in the source water. The study also found that dimethylarsenic acid did not codistill to a great extent during evaporation and concluded that drinking water on ships was unlikely to have been contaminated with this herbicide. In a follow-up discussion of the study with its authors, it was noted that vessels would take up water for distillation as close to shore as possible to minimize salt content (Wells, 2006). On the basis of that study and other evidence, the Australian Department of Veterans Affairs determined that Royal Australian Navy personnel who served offshore were exposed to dioxins that resulted from herbicide spraying in Vietnam even if they did not go ashore during their tour of duty (ADVA, 2005).

The current committee engaged Steven Hawthorne as a consultant to review the Mueller et al. (2002) publication and to comment generally on the ability of organic compounds to codistill during the production of potable water. Hawthorne is an environmental chemist at the University of North Dakota's Energy and Environmental Research Center and has specific expertise in the study of organic emissions from water (Hawthorne et al., 1985). He affirmed the findings of the Australian study, citing Henry's law for an explanation of how contaminants with low water solubility would evaporate from water and noting that the distillation process would enhance the process by adding heat and reducing pressure (SB Hawthorne, University of North Dakota Energy Research Center, personal communication on October 23, 2008). No measurements of dioxin concentrations in seawater were collected during the Vietnam conflict, so it is not possible to ascertain the extent to which drinking water on US vessels may have been contaminated through distillation processes. However, it seems likely that vessels with such distillation processes that traveled near land or even at some distance from river deltas would periodically collect water that contained dioxin. Thus, a presumption of exposure of military personnel serving on those vessels is not unreasonable.

In its charge to the original *VAO* committee, the Department of Veterans Affairs asked the committee to include military personnel who served in inland waterways, offshore of the Republic of Vietnam, and in the airspace above the Republic of Vietnam. A presumption of exposure to Agent Orange and other herbicides used as defoliants applied to each of those groups as well as to those who served on land. In light of the findings of the Australian study regarding potential drinking-water contamination and those serving offshore, the presumption seems well founded.

EXPOSURE OF THE VIETNAMESE POPULATION

Studies of exposure to herbicides among the residents of South Vietnam have compared nonexposed residents of the South with residents of the North (Constable and Hatch, 1985). Other studies have attempted to identify wives of veterans of North Vietnam who served in South Vietnam. Records of herbicide spraying have been used to refine exposure measurements, comparing people who lived in sprayed villages in the South with those living in unsprayed villages. In some studies, village residents were considered exposed if a herbicide mission had passed within 10 km of the village center (Dai et al., 1990). Other criteria for classifying exposure included length of residence in a sprayed area and the number of times the area reportedly had been sprayed.

A small number of studies have provided information on TCDD concentrations in Vietnamese civilians exposed during the war (Schecter et al., 1986, 2002,

2006). Dwernychuk et al. (2002) have emphasized the need to evaluate dioxin contamination around former air bases in Vietnam. They collected environmental and food samples, human blood, and breast milk from residents of the Aluoi Valley of central Vietnam. The investigators identified locations where relatively high dioxin concentrations remained in soil or water systems. Soil dioxin concentrations were particularly high around former air fields and military bases where herbicides were handled. Fish harvested from ponds in those areas were found to contain high dioxin concentrations. More recently, Dwernychuk (2005) elaborated on the importance of "hot spots" as important locations for future studies and argued that herbicide use at former US military installations was the most likely cause of the hot spots. The above studies are not directly relevant to this committee's task, but they may prove useful in future epidemiologic studies of the Vietnamese population and in the development of risk-mitigation policies.

The only new study of dioxin in Vietnam reviewed by the committee examined dioxin contamination in soils (Mai et al., 2007). The study focused on the Bien Hoa Air Base, considered a hot spot because of the use of chemical defoliants around the base, and found high dioxin concentrations. The study did not involve estimates of exposure of the population living in the vicinity of the bases.

NEW MODELS FOR CHARACTERIZING HERBICIDE EXPOSURE

IOM, following up on the recommendations contained in the original *VAO* report (IOM, 1994), issued a request for proposals seeking individuals and organizations to develop historical exposure-reconstruction approaches suitable for epidemiologic studies of herbicide exposure among US veterans during the Vietnam War (IOM, 1997). The request resulted in the project Characterizing Exposure of Veterans to Agent Orange and Other Herbicides in Vietnam. The project was carried out under contract by a team of researchers in Columbia University's Mailman School of Public Health. The Columbia University project integrated various sources of information concerning spray activities to generate individualized estimates of the exposure potential of troops serving in Vietnam (Stellman and Stellman, 2003). Location data on military units assigned to Vietnam were compiled into a database.

"Mobility-factor" analysis, a new concept for studying troop movement, was developed for use in reconstructing herbicide-exposure histories. The analysis is a three-part classification system for characterizing the location and movement of military units in Vietnam. It comprises a mobility designation (stable or mobile), a distance designation (usually in a range of kilometers) to indicate how far a unit might travel in a day, and a notation of the modes of travel available to the unit (air; ground by truck, tank, or armored personnel carrier; or water). A mobility factor was assigned to every unit that served in Vietnam.

The data were combined into a geographic information system (GIS) for Vietnam. Herbicide-spraying records were integrated into the GIS and linked with data on military-unit locations to permit estimation of individual exposure-opportunity scores. The results are the subject of reports by the contractor (Stellman and Stellman, 2003) and the Committee on the Assessment of Wartime Exposure to Herbicides in Vietnam (IOM, 2003a,b). A summary of the findings regarding the extent and pattern of herbicide spraying (Stellman et al., 2003a), a description of the GIS for characterizing exposure to Agent Orange and other herbicides in Vietnam (Stellman et al., 2003b), and an explanation of the exposure-opportunity models based on that work (Stellman and Stellman, 2004) have been published in peer-reviewed journals. The publications have argued that it is now feasible to conduct epidemiologic investigations of veterans who served as ground troops during the Vietnam War.

A different perspective has been put forth by Young and colleagues in a series of papers (Young et al., 2004a,b). They have argued that ground troops had little direct contact with herbicide sprays and that TCDD residues in Vietnam had low bioavailability. Those conclusions were based on analyses of previously unpublished military records and environmental-fate studies. They have also argued that ground-troop exposures were relatively low because herbicide-spraying missions were carefully planned, and spraying occurred only when friendly forces were not in the target area.

Since *Update 2006*, IOM has issued a report that examined the feasibility of using the Agent Orange Reconstruction Model developed by Columbia University (IOM, 2008). The report concluded that "despite the shortcomings of the exposure assessment model in its current form and the inherent limitations in the approach, the committee agreed that the model holds promise for supporting informative epidemiologic studies of herbicides and health among Vietnam veterans and that it should be used to conduct studies."

METHODOLOGIC ISSUES IN EXPOSURE ASSESSMENT

Analyses of Vietnam-veteran studies have been an important source of information for understanding associations between the herbicides used in Vietnam and specific health outcomes, but, as discussed in Chapter 2, the committee has extended its review of the scientific literature to other populations in which exposure could be estimated with greater accuracy. Those populations are discussed in detail in Chapter 5. We focus here on several key methodologic issues that complicate development of accurate exposure estimates in the Vietnam-veteran population and in the other study populations discussed in this report: the latent period between exposure and disease, exposure misclassification, and exposure specificity.

Latency

The temporal relationship between exposure and disease is complex and often difficult to define in studies of human populations. Many diseases do not appear immediately after exposure. In the case of cancer, for example, the disease may not appear for many years after exposure. The time between a defined exposure period and the occurrence of disease is often referred to as a latency period (IOM, 2004). Exposures can be brief (sometimes referred to as acute exposures) or protracted (sometimes referred to as chronic exposures). At one extreme, an exposure can be the result of a single event, as in an accidental poisoning. At the other extreme, a person exposed to a chemical that is stored in the body may continue to experience "internal exposure" for years even if exposure from the environment has ceased. The definition of the proper timeframe for duration of exposure constitutes a challenge to exposure scientists.

Misclassification

Exposure misclassification in epidemiologic studies can affect estimates of risk. A typical situation is in a case–control study in which the reported measurement of exposure of either group or both groups can be misclassified. The simplest situation to consider is one in which the exposure is classified into just two levels, for example, ever vs never exposed. If the probability of exposure misclassification is the same in cases and controls (that is, non-differential), then it can be shown that the estimated association between disease and exposure is biased toward the null value; in other words, one would expect the true association to be stronger than the association observed. However, if the probability of misclassification is different between cases and controls, bias in the estimated association can occur in either direction; in this case, the true association might be stronger or weaker than the association observed.

The situation in which exposure is classified into more than two levels is somewhat more complicated. Dosemeci et al. (1990) have demonstrated that in that situation the slope of a dose–response trend is not necessarily attenuated toward the null value even if the probability of misclassification is the same in the two groups of subjects being compared; in other words, the observed trend in disease risk across the several levels of exposure may be either an overestimate or an underestimate of the true trend in risk. Greenland and Gustafson (2006) have discussed the effect of exposure misclassification on the statistical significance of the result, demonstrating that if one adjusts for exposure misclassification when the exposure is represented as binary (for example, ever vs never exposed), the resulting association is not necessarily more significant than in the unadjusted estimate. That result remains true even though the observed magnitude of the association (for example, the relative risk) might be increased.

Specificity

Only a few herbicidal compounds were used as defoliants during the Vietnam conflict: esters and salts of 2,4-D and 2,4,5-T, cacodylic acid, and picloram in various formulations. Many scientific studies reviewed by the committee have reported exposures to broad categories of chemicals rather than to those specific compounds. The categories are presented in Table 3-2, with their relevance to the committee's charge. The information in Table 3-2 represents the current committee's thinking and has helped to guide our evaluation of epidemiologic studies. Previous VAO committees did not necessarily address the issue of exposure specificity in this manner.

Many studies have examined the relationship between exposure to "pesticides" and adverse health outcomes, and others have used the category of "herbicides" without identifying specific compounds. A careful reading of a scientific report often reveals that none of the compounds of interest (those used in Vietnam, as delineated above) contributed to the exposures of the study population, so such studies could be excluded from consideration. But in many cases, the situation is more ambiguous. For example, reports that define exposure in the broad category of "pesticides" with no further information have little relevance to the committee's charge to determine associations between exposures to herbicides used in Vietnam and adverse health outcomes. Reports that define exposure in the more restricted category of "herbicides" are of greater relevance but are of little value unless it is clear from additional information that exposure to one or more of the herbicides used in Vietnam occurred in the study population, for example,

TABLE 3-2 Current Committee Guidance for the Classification of Exposure Information in Epidemiologic Studies That Focus on the Use of Pesticides or Herbicides, and Relevance of the Information to the Committee's Charge to Evaluate Exposures to 2,4-D and 2,4,5-T (phenoxy herbicides), Cacodylic Acid, and Picloram

Specificity of Exposure Reported in Study	Additional Information	Relevance to Committee's Charge
Pesticides	Chemicals of interest were not used or no additional information	Not relevant
	Chemicals of interest were used	Limited relevance
Herbicides	Chemicals of interest were not used	Not relevant
	No additional information	Limited relevance
	Chemicals of interest were used	Relevant
Phenoxy herbicides		Highly relevant
2,4-D or 2,4,5-T		Highly relevant
Cacodylic acid[a]		Highly relevant
Picloram		Highly relevant

[a] None of the epidemiologic studies reviewed by the committee to date have specified exposure to cacodylic acid.

if the published report indicates that the chemicals of interest were among the pesticides or herbicides used by the study population, the lead author of a published report has been contacted and has indicated that the chemicals of interest were among the chemicals used, the chemicals of interest are used commonly for the crops identified in the study, or the chemicals of interest are used commonly for a specific purpose, such as removal of weeds and shrubs along highways.

Among the various chemical classes of herbicides that have been identified in published studies reviewed by the committee, phenoxy herbicides, particularly 2,4-D and 2,4,5-T, are directly relevant to the exposures experienced by US military forces in Vietnam. On the basis of the assumption that compounds with similar chemical structure may have analogous biologic activity, information on the effects of other chemicals in the phenoxy herbicide class—such as Silvex, 2-methyl-4-chlorophenoxyacetic acid (MCPA), 2-(2-methyl-4-chlorophenoxy) propionic acid (MCPP, Mecoprop), and dicamba—has been factored into the committee's deliberations with somewhat less weight. The very few epidemiologic findings on exposure to picloram or cacodylic acid have been regarded as highly relevant. The committee has decided to include many studies that report on unspecified herbicides in the discussions in the health-effects sections, and their results have been entered into the health-outcome–specific tables. However, these studies tend to contribute little to the evidence considered by the committee. The many studies that provide chemical-specific exposure information are believed to be far more informative for the committee's purposes.

A similar issue arises in the evaluation of studies that document exposure to dioxin-like compounds. Most "dioxin" studies reviewed by the committee have focused on TCDD, but TCDD is only one of a number of PCDDs. The committee recognizes that in real-world conditions exposure to TCDD virtually never occurs in isolation and that there are hundreds of similar compounds to which humans might be exposed, including other PCDDs, polychlorinated dibenzofurans, and polychlorinated biphenyls (PCBs). Exposure to TCDD is almost always accompanied by exposure to one or more of the other compounds. The literature on the other compounds, particularly PCBs, was not reviewed systematically by the committee unless TCDD was identified as an important component of the exposure or the risks of health effects were expressed in terms of toxicity equivalent quotients, which are the sums of toxicity equivalency factors for individual dioxin-like compounds as measured by activity with the aryl hydrocarbon receptor (AHR). We took that approach for two reasons. First, exposure of Vietnam veterans to substantial amounts of the other compounds, relative to exposure to TCDD, has not been documented. Second, the most important mechanism for TCDD toxicity involves its ability to bind to and activate the AHR. Many of the other compounds act by different or multiple mechanisms, so it is difficult to attribute toxic effects after such exposures to TCDD.

REFERENCES[1]

ADVA (Australian Department of Veterans' Affairs). 2005. *The Third Australian Vietnam Veterans Mortality Study 2005.* Canberra: Australian Department of Veterans' Affairs.

AFHS (Air Force Health Study). 1991. *An Epidemiologic Investigation of Health Effects in Air Force Personnel Following Exposure to Herbicides. Serum Dioxin Analysis of 1987 Examination Results.* Air Force Health Study. Brooks AFB, TX: USAF School of Aerospace Medicine. 9 vols.

Armstrong BK, White E, Saracci R. 1994. *Principles of Exposure Assessment in Epidemiology.* New York: Oxford University Press.

CDC (Center for Diseases Control). 1988. Serum 2,3,7,8-tetrachlorodibenzo-*p*-dioxin levels in US Army Vietnam era veterans. *Journal of the American Medical Association* 260:1249–1254.

CDC. 1989a. *Health Status of Vietnam Veterans.* Vietnam Experience Study. Atlanta: US Department of Health and Human Services. Vols. I–V, Supplements A–C.

CDC. 1989b. *Comparison of Serum Levels of 2,3,7,8-Tetrachlorodibenzo-p-Dioxin with Indirect Estimates of Agent Orange Exposure Among Vietnam Veterans: Final Report.* Centers for Disease Control. Atlanta: US Department of Health and Human Services.

Checkoway H, Pearce NE, Kriebel D. 2004. *Research Methods in Occupational Epidemiology.* Second Edition. New York: Oxford University Press.

Cochrane WP, Sirgh J, Miles W, Wakeford B, Scott J. 1982. Analysis of technical and formulated products of 2,4-dichlorophenoxyacetic acid for the presence of chlorinated dibenzo-*p*-dioxins. In: Hutzinger O, Frei RW, Merian E, Pocchiari F, eds. *Chlorinated Dioxins and Related Compounds: Impact on the Environment.* Oxford: Pergamon Press, pp. 209–213.

Constable JD, Hatch MC. 1985. Reproductive effects of herbicide exposure in Vietnam: Recent studies by the Vietnamese and others. *Teratogenesis, Carcinogenesis, and Mutagenesis* 5:231–250.

Dai LC, Phuong NTN, Thom LH, Thuy TT, Van NTT, Cam LH, Chi HTK, Thuy LB. 1990. A comparison of infant mortality rates between two Vietnamese villages sprayed by defoliants in wartime and one unsprayed village. *Chemosphere* 20:1005–1012.

Dosemeci M, Wacholder S, Lubin JH. 1990. Does nondifferential misclassification of exposure always bias a true effect toward the null value? *American Journal of Epidemiology* 132(4):746–748.

Dwernychuk LW. 2005. Dioxin hot spots in Vietnam. *Chemosphere* 60(7):998–999.

Dwernychuk LW, Cau HD, Hatfield CT, Boivin TG, Hung TM, Dung PT, Thai ND. 2002. Dioxin reservoirs in southern Viet Nam—A legacy of Agent Orange. *Chemosphere* 47(2):117–137.

EPA (US Environmental Protection Agency). 1992. *Worker Protection Standard.* Washington, DC: US Environmental Protection Agency.

Erickson JD, Mulinare J, Mcclain PW. 1984. Vietnam veterans' risks for fathering babies with birth defects. *Journal of the American Medical Association* 252:903–912.

FAO/UNEP (Food and Agriculture Organization, United Nations Environment Programme). 2009. *2,4,5-T and its salts and esters. Decision Guidance Documents.* Secretariat for the Rotterdam Convention on the Prior Informed Consent Procedure for Certain Hazardous Chemicals and Pesticides in International Trade. Joint FAO/UNEP Programme for the Operation of the Prior Informed Consent. Accessed March 9, 2009, at http://www.pic.int/en/DGDs/2,4,5-TEN.doc.

GAO (General Accounting Office). 1978. *Use of Agent Orange in Vietnam.* Washington, DC: GAO. CED-78-158.

GAO. 1979. *US Ground Troops in South Vietnam Were in Areas Sprayed with Herbicide Orange.* Report by the Comptroller General of the United States. Washington, DC: GAO. FPCD 80-23.

---

[1]Throughout the report the same alphabetic indicator following year of publication is used consistently for the same article when there were multiple citations by the same first author in a given year. The convention of assigning the alphabetic indicator in order of citation in a given chapter is not followed.

Gough M. 1986. *Dioxin, Agent Orange: The Facts.* New York: Plenum Press.

Greenland P, Gustafson S. 2006. The performance of random coefficient regression in accounting for residual confounding. *Biometrics* 62(3):760–768.

Gross ML, Lay JO, Lippstreu D, Lyon PA, Kangas N, Harless RL, Taylor SE. 1984. 2,3,7,8-tetra-chlorodibenzo-*p*-dioxin levels in adipose tissue of Vietnam veterans. *Environmental Research* 33:261.

Hawthorne SB. 2008. *Review of Mueller et al., 2002.* October 23, 2008 e-mail from Steven Hawthorne to Mary Paxton. Dr. Hawthorne's evaluation of this study was requested by the VAO committee.

Hawthorne SB, Sievers RE, Barkley RM. 1985. Organic emissions from shale oil wastewater and their implications for air quality. *Environment and Science Technology* 19:992–997.

IOM (Institute of Medicine). 1987. *Review of Comparison of Serum Levels of 2,3,7,8-TCDD with Indirect Estimates of Agent Orange Exposure in Vietnam Veterans.* Fifth Letter Report. Washington, DC: National Academy Press.

IOM. 1994. *Veterans and Agent Orange: Health Effects of Herbicides Used in Vietnam.* Washington, DC: National Academy Press.

IOM. 1997. *Characterizing Exposure of Veterans to Agent Orange and Other Herbicides Used in Vietnam: Scientific Considerations Regarding a Request for Proposals for Research.* Washington, DC: National Academy Press.

IOM. 2003a. *Characterizing Exposure of Veterans to Agent Orange and Other Herbicides Used in Vietnam: Interim Findings and Recommendations.* Washington, DC: The National Academies Press.

IOM. 2003b. *Characterizing Exposure of Veterans to Agent Orange and Other Herbicides Used in Vietnam: Final Report.* Washington, DC: The National Academies Press.

IOM. 2004. *Veterans and Agent Orange: Length of Presumptive Period for Association Between Exposure and Respiratory Cancer.* Washington, DC: The National Academies Press.

IOM. 2006. *Disposition of the Air Force Health Study.* Washington, DC: The National Academies Press.

IOM. 2008. *The Utility of Proximity-Based Herbicide Exposure Assessment in Epidemiologic Studies of Vietnam Veterans.* Washington DC: The National Academies Press.

Kahn PC, Gochfeld M, Nygren M, Hansson M, Rappe C, Velez H, Ghent-Guenther T, Wilson WP. 1988. Dioxins and dibenzofurans in blood and adipose tissue of Agent Orange-exposed Vietnam veterans and matched controls. *Journal of the American Medical Association* 259:1661–1667.

Kang HK, Dalager NA, Needham LL, Patterson DG, Matanoski GM, Kanchanaraksa S, Lees PSJ. 2001. US Army Chemical Corps Vietnam Veterans Health Study: Preliminary results. *Chemosphere* 43:943–949.

Kang HK, Dalager NA, Needham LL, Patterson DG, Lees PSJ, Yates K, Matanoski GM. 2006. Health status of Army Chemical Corps Vietnam veterans who sprayed defoliant in Vietnam. *American Journal of Industrial Medicine* 49(11):875–884.

Kern PA, Said S, Jackson WG Jr, Michalek JE. 2004. Insulin sensitivity following agent orange exposure in Vietnam veterans with high blood levels of 2,3,7,8-tetrachlorodibenzo-*p*-dioxin. *Journal of Clinical Endocrinology and Metabolism* 89(9):4665–4672.

Kim JS, Kang HK, Lim HS, Cheong HK, Lim MK. 2001. A study on the correlation between categorizations of the individual exposure levels to Agent Orange and serum dioxin levels among the Korean Vietnam veterans. *Korean Journal of Preventive Medicine* 34(1):80–88.

Kim JS, Lim HS, Cho SI, Cheong HK, Lim MK. 2003. Impact of Agent Orange exposure among Korean Vietnam veterans. *Industrial Health* 41:149–157.

Lilienfeld DE, Gallo MA. 1989. 2,4-D, 2,4,5-T and 2,3,7,8-TCDD: An overview. *Epidemiological Review* 11:28–58.

Mai TA, Doan TV, Tarradellas J, de Alencastro LF, Granjean D. 2007. Dioxin contamination in soils in Southern Vietnam. *Chemosphere* 67(9):1802–1807.

Michalek JE, Wolfe WH, Miner JC, Papa TM, Pirkle JL. 1995. Indices of TCDD exposure and TCDD body burden in veterans of Operation Ranch Hand. *Journal of Exposure Analysis and Environmental Epidemiology* 5(2):209–223.

Michalek JE, Akhtar FZ, Longnecker MP, Burton JE. 2001. Relation of serum 2,3,7,8-tetrachlorodibenzo-*p*-dioxin (TCDD) level to hematological examination results in veterans of Operation Ranch Hand. *Archives of Environmental Health* 56(5):396–405.

Michalek JE, Ketchum NS, Tripathi RC. 2003. Diabetes mellitus and 2,3,7,8-tetrachlorodibenzo-*p*-dioxin elimination in veterans of Operation Ranch Hand. *Journal of Toxicology and Environmental Health, Part A* 66(3):211–221.

MRI (Midwest Research Institute). 1967. *Assessment of Ecological Effects of Extensive or Repeated Use of Herbicides.* MRI Project No. 3103-B. Kansas City, MO: MRI. NTIS AD-824-314.

Mueller J, Gaus C, Bundred K, Alberts V, Moore MR, Horsley K. 2001. Co-distillation of TCDD and other POPs during distillation of water: A potential source for exposure. *Organohalogen Compounds* 52:243–246.

Mueller J, Gaus C, Alberts V, Moore M. 2002. *Examination of the Potential Exposure of Royal Australian Navy (RAN) Personnel to Polychlorinated Dibenzodioxins and Polychlorinated Dibenzofurans via Drinking Water.* Brisbane, Queensland, Australia: National Research Centre for Environmental Toxicology and the Queensland Health Services.

NAS (National Academy of Sciences). 1974. *The Effects of Herbicides in South Vietnam.* National Research Council, Washington, DC: National Academy Press.

NRC (National Research Council). 1980. *Review of U.S. Air Force Protocol: Epidemiological Investigation of Health Effects in Air Force Personnel Following Exposure to Herbicide Orange.* National Research Council, Washington, DC: National Academy Press.

NRC. 1982. *The Effects of Exposure to Agent Orange on Ground Troops in Vietnam: A Report of the Subcommittee Appointed to Review a Protocol.* National Research Council, Washington, DC: National Academy Press.

NZIC (New Zealand Institute of Chemistry). 2009. *The production of phenoxy herbicides.* New Zealand Institute of Chemistry. Accessed March 9, 2009 at http://nzic.org.nz/ChemProcesses/production/index.html

Pavuk M, Schecter AJ, Akhtar FZ, Michalek JE. 2003. Serum 2,3,7,8-tetrachlorodibenzo-*p*-dioxin (TCDD) levels and thyroid function in Air Force veterans of the Vietnam War. *Annals of Epidemiology* 13(5):335–343.

Rappe C, Buser HR, Bosshardt HP. 1978. Identification and quantitation of polychlorinated dibenzo-*p*-dioxins (PCDDs) and dibenzofurans (PCDFs in 2,4,5-T ester formulations and herbicide orange. *Chemosphere* 5:431–438.

Schecter A, Ryan JJ, Constable JD. 1986. Chlorinated dibenzo-*p*-dioxin and dibenzofuran levels in human adipose tissue and milk samples from the north and south of Vietnam. *Chemosphere* 15:1613–1620.

Schecter A, Constable JD, Arghestani S, Tong H, Gross ML. 1987. Elevated levels 2,3,7,8-tetrachlorodibenzodioxin in adipose tissue of certain US veterans of the Vietnam war. *Chemosphere* 16:1997–2002.

Schecter A, Pavuk M, Constable JD, Dai LC, Papke O. 2002. A follow-up: High level of dioxin contamination in Vietnamese from Agent Orange, three decades after the end of spraying [letter]. *Journal of Occupational and Environmental Medicine* 44(3):218–220.

Schecter A, Quynh HT, Papke O, Tung KC, Constable JD. 2006. Agent Orange, dioxins, and other chemicals of concern in Vietnam: Update 2006. *Journal of Occupational and Environmental Medicine* 48(4):408–413.

Stellman SD, Stellman JM. 1986. Estimation of exposure to Agent Orange and other defoliants among American troops in Vietnam: A methodological approach. *American Journal of Industrial Medicine* 9:305–321.

Stellman JM, Stellman SD. 2003. *Contractor's Final Report: Characterizing Exposure of Veterans to Agent Orange and Other Herbicides in Vietnam.* Submitted to the National Academy of Sciences, Institute of Medicine in fulfillment of Subcontract VA-5124-98-0019, June 30, 2003.

Stellman SD, Stellman JM. 2004. Exposure opportunity models for Agent Orange, dioxin, and other military herbicides used in Vietnam, 1961–1971. *Journal of Exposure Analysis and Environmental Epidemiology* 14:354–362.

Stellman SD, Mager-Stellman J, Sommer JF Jr. 1988. Combat and herbicide exposures in Vietnam among a sample of American Legionnaires. *Environmental Research* 47:112–128.

Stellman JM, Stellman SD, Christian R, Weber T, Tomasallo C. 2003a. The extent and patterns of usage of Agent Orange and other herbicides in Vietnam. *Nature* 422:681–687.

Stellman JM, Stellman SD, Weber T, Tomasallo C, Stellman AB, Christian R. 2003b. A geographic information system for characterizing exposure to Agent Orange and other herbicides in Vietnam. *Environmental Health Perspectives* 111:321–328.

Thomas TL, Kang HK. 1990. Mortality and morbidity among Army Chemical Corps Vietnam veterans: A preliminary report. *American Journal of Industrial Medicine* 18:665–673.

Tosine H. 1983. Dioxins: A Canadian perspective. In *Chlorinated Dioxins and Dibenzofurans in the Total Environment*, Choudhary G, Keith LH, Rappe C, eds. Woburn, MA: Butterworth Publishers, pp. 3–14.

Warren WF. 1968. *A Review of the Herbicide Program in South Vietnam.* San Francisco: Scientific Advisory Group. Working Paper No. 10-68. NTIS AD-779-797.

Wells J. 2006. *Report on a meeting by Janice Wells with Professor Michael Moore and Research Fellow Ms. Carol Gaus.* Brisbane, Australia, July 3.

Young AL. 1992. *The Military Use of Herbicides in Vietnam.* Presentation to the Institute of Medicine Committee to Review the Health Effects in Vietnam Veterans of Exposure to Herbicides. December 8, 1992. Washington, DC.

Young AL, Reggiani GM, eds. 1988. *Agent Orange and Its Associated Dioxin: Assessment of a Controversy.* Amsterdam: Elsevier.

Young AL, Newton M. 2004. Long overlooked historical information on Agent Orange and TCDD following massive applications of 2,4,5-T-containing herbicides, Eglin Air Force Base, Florida. *Environmental Science and Pollution Research* 11(4):209–221.

Young AL, Thalken CE, Arnold EL, Cupello JM, Cockerham LG. 1976. *Fate of 2,3,7,8 tetrachlorodibenzo-p-dioxin (TCDD) in the Environment: Summary and Decontamination Recommendations.* Colorado Springs: US Air Force Academy. USAFA TR 76 18.

Young AL, Calcagni JA, Thalken CE, Tremblay JW. 1978. *The Toxicology, Environmental Fate, and Human Risk of Herbicide Orange and Its Associated Dioxin.* Brooks AFB, TX: Air Force Occupational and Environmental Health Lab. USAF OEHL TR 78 92.

Young AL, Cecil PF Sr, Guilmartin JF Jr. 2004a. Assessing possible exposures of ground troops to Agent Orange during the Vietnam War: The use of contemporary military records. *Environmental Science and Pollution Research* 11(6):349–358.

Young AL, Giesy JP, Jones P, Newton M, Guilmartin JF Jr, Cecil PF Sr. 2004b. Assessment of potential exposure to Agent Orange and its associated TCDD. *Environmental Science and Pollution Research* 11(6):347–348.

Zumwalt ER Jr. 1993. Letter to the Institute of Medicine Committee to Review the Health Effects in Vietnam Veterans of Exposure to Herbicides regarding draft version of the IOM chapter on the US military and the herbicide program in Vietnam, May 20.

4

Information Related to Biologic Plausibility

The committee reviewed all relevant experimental studies of 2,4-dichlorophenoxyacetic acid (2,4-D), 2,4,5-trichlorophenoxyacetic acid (2,4,5-T), picloram, cacodylic acid, and 2,3,7,8-tetrachlorodibenzo-*p*-dioxin (TCDD) that have been published since *Update 2006* (IOM, 2007) and has incorporated the findings, when it was appropriate, into this chapter or into the biologic-plausibility sections of Chapters 6–9 when they are of consequence for particular health outcomes. For each substance, this chapter includes a review of toxicokinetic properties, a brief summary of the toxic outcomes investigated in animal experiments, and a discussion of underlying mechanisms of action as illuminated by in vitro studies.

To achieve the goals of this chapter more effectively, the current committee has slightly modified the presentation of toxicologic information used by previous Veterans and Agent Orange (VAO) committees. The toxicology chapter of each earlier update presented information about each of the several hundred potentially relevant toxicologic articles published in the preceding 2 years. In contrast with the committee's responsibility to evaluate each potentially relevant epidemiologic study of the chemicals of interest published in the preceding 2 years, its charge with respect to the toxicologic literature is to distill experimental toxicologic findings to judge whether it is biologically plausible to attribute adverse health outcomes reported in epidemiologic investigations to the chemicals. The current committee recognized that for most readers of the VAO series the implications of most toxicologic results reported are not immediately obvious. Therefore, starting with this update, the committee will focus on integrating and interpreting the toxicologic evidence rather than delineating the entire body of new experimental findings.

Establishment of biologic plausibility through laboratory studies strengthens the evidence of a cause–effect relationship between herbicide exposure and health effects reported in epidemiologic studies and thus supports the existence of the less stringent relationship of association, which is the target of this committee's charge. Experimental studies of laboratory animals or cultured cells allow observation of effects of herbicide exposure under highly controlled conditions that are difficult or impossible to control in epidemiologic studies. Such conditions include frequency and magnitude of exposure, exposure to other chemicals, preexisting health conditions, and genetic differences between people, all of which can be controlled in a laboratory animal study.

Once a chemical contacts the body, it begins to interact through the processes of absorption, distribution, metabolism, and excretion. Those four biologic processes characterize the disposition of a foreign substance that enters the organism. Their combination determines the concentration of the compound in the body and how long each organ is exposed to it and thus influences its toxic or pharmacologic activity.

Absorption is the entry of the substance into the organism, normally by uptake into the bloodstream via mucous surfaces, such as the intestinal walls of the digestive tract during ingestion. Low solubility, chemical instability in the stomach, and inability to permeate the intestinal wall can all reduce the extent to which a substance is absorbed after being ingested. The solubility of a chemical in fat and its hydrophobicity influence the pathways by which it is metabolized (structurally transformed) and whether it persists in the body or is excreted. Absorption is a critical determinant of the chemical's bioavailability, that is, the fraction of it that reaches the systemic circulation. Other routes of absorption experienced by free-ranging humans are inhalation (entry via the airways) and dermal exposure (entry via the skin). Animal studies may involve additional routes of exposure that are not ordinarily encountered by humans, such as intravenous or intraperitoneal injection, in which the chemical is injected into the bloodstream or abdominal cavity, respectively.

Distribution refers to the travel of a substance from the site of entry to the tissues and organs where they will have their ultimate effect or be sequestered. Distribution takes place most commonly via the bloodstream. The term *metabolism* is used to describe the breaking down that all substances begin to experience as soon as they enter the body. Metabolism of most foreign substances takes place in the liver by the action of oxidative enzymes collectively termed cytochrome P450. As metabolism occurs, the initial (parent) chemical is converted to new chemicals called metabolites. When metabolites are pharmacologically or toxicologically inert, metabolism deactivates the administered dose of the parent chemical reducing its effects on the body. Sometimes metabolism may activate the compound to a metabolite more potent or more toxic than the parent compound.

Excretion, also referred to as elimination, is the removal of substances or their metabolites from the body, most commonly in urine or feces. Excretion is often incomplete, and incomplete excretion results in the accumulation of foreign substances that can adversely affect function.

The routes and rates of absorption, distribution, metabolism, and excretion of a toxic substance collectively are termed toxicokinetics (or pharmacokinetics). Those processes determine the amount of a particular substance or metabolite that reaches specific organs or cells and that persists in the body. Understanding the toxicokinetics of a chemical is important for valid reconstruction of exposure of humans and for assessing the risk of effects of a chemical. The principles involved in toxicokinetics are similar among chemicals, although the degree to which different processes influence the distribution depends on the structure and other inherent properties of the chemicals. Thus, the lipophilicity or hydrophobicity of a chemical and its structure influence the pathways by which it is metabolized and whether it persists in the body or is excreted. The degree to which different toxicokinetic processes influence the toxic potential of a chemical depends on metabolic pathways, which often differ among species. For that reason, attempts at extrapolation from experimental animal studies to human exposures must be done with extreme care.

Many chemicals were used by the US armed forces in Vietnam. The nature of the substances themselves was discussed in more detail in Chapter 6 of the original *VAO* report (IOM, 1994). Four herbicides documented in military records were of particular concern and are examined here: 2,4-D, 2,4,5-T, 4-amino-3,5,6-trichloropicolinic acid (picloram), and cacodylic acid (dimethyl arsenic acid, DMA). This chapter also examines 2,3,7,8-tetrachlorodibenzo-*p*-dioxin (referred to in this report as TCDD to represent a single, and the most toxic, congener of the tetrachlorodibenzo-*p*-dioxins [tetraCDDs], also commonly referred to as dioxin), a contaminant of 2,4,5-T, because its potential toxicity is of concern; considerably more information is available on TCDD than on the herbicides. Other contaminants present in 2,4-D and 2,4,5-T are of less concern. Except as noted, the laboratory studies of the chemicals of concern used pure compounds or formulations; the epidemiologic studies discussed in later chapters often tracked exposures to mixtures.

TCDD

Chemistry

TCDD is a polychlorinated dibenzo-*p*-dioxin that has a triple-ring structure consisting of two benzene rings connected by an oxygenated ring (Figure 4-1); chlorine atoms are attached at the 2, 3, 7, and 8 positions of the benzene rings. The chemical properties of TCDD include a molecular weight of 322, a melting point of 305–306°C, a boiling point of 445.5°C, and a log octanol–water partition coefficient of 6.8 (NTP substance profile). It is virtually insoluble in water

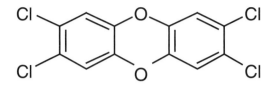

2,3,7,8-tetrachlorodibenzo-*p*-dioxin

FIGURE 4-1 Chemical structure of TCDD.

(19.3 ng/L), but is soluble in organic solvents, such as benzene and acetone. It has been suggested (EPA 2004 Draft Document) that volatilization of dioxin from water may be an important mechanism of transfer from the aqueous to the atmospheric phase.

Absorption, Distribution, Metabolism, and Elimination

The absorption, distribution, metabolism, and elimination of TCDD have been extensively studied in a number of animal models in the last 25 years. Given the plethora of data, this section only highlights and summarizes key findings. A more exhaustive review may be found at http://www.epa.gov/ncea/pdfs/dioxin/nas-review.

TCDD is absorbed into the body rapidly but is eliminated slowly. Because of the slow elimination, the concentration of TCDD in lipid or blood is thought to be in dynamic equilibrium with that in other tissue compartments and is thus considered to be reasonable for use in estimating total body burdens. Exposure of humans to TCDD is thought to occur primarily via the mouth, skin, and lungs. In laboratory animals, oral administration of TCDD has been shown to result in absorption of 50–93% of the administered dose (Nolan et al., 1979; Rose et al., 1976). Similarly, a study performed in a 42-year-old man found that 87% of the oral dose was absorbed. Dermal absorption appears to be dose-dependent, with lower absorption occurring at higher doses (Banks and Birnbaum, 1991). Studies performed in humans indicate that human skin may be more resistant to absorption (Weber, 1991).

After ingestion and gastrointestinal absorption, TCDD associates primarily with the lipoprotein fraction of the blood and later partitions into the cellular membranes and tissues (Henderson and Patterson, 1988). TCDD is distributed to all compartments of the body; the amounts differ from organ to organ, but most studies indicate that the primary disposition of TCDD is in the liver and adipose tissues. For example, in a human volunteer, it was found that at 135 days after ingestion, 90% of TCDD was in fat (Poiger and Schlatter, 1986); in the rhesus monkey, TCDD is very persistent in adipose tissue (Bowman et al., 1989). The disposition and elimination of TCDD depend on the tissue examined, the time that has elapsed since exposure, total exposure, and other factors. For example, the concentration of cytochrome P450 1A2 (CYP1A2) (Poland et al., 1989) in the liver is increased by TCDD. Direct binding of TCDD to the CYP1A2 is thought to result in sequestration of TCDD in the liver and to inhibit its distribution to other tissues. The importance of CYP1A2 concentrations for the toxic actions of TCDD has also been shown in studies performed in laboratory animals in which maternal hepatic CYP1A2 was found to sequester TCDD and protect the fetus against TCDD-induced teratogenesis (Dragin et al., 2006). In addition, distribution of TCDD is age-dependent, as shown by studies in which young animals displayed the highest concentration of TCDD in the liver and older animals the highest concentrations in kidney, skin, and muscle (Pegram et al., 1995). Finally, the elimination rate of TCDD, in particular after low exposures, depends heavily on the amount of adipose tissue mass (Aylward et al., 2005; Emond et al., 2005, 2006).

In laboratory animals and humans, metabolism of TCDD occurs slowly. It is eliminated primarily in feces as both the parent compound and its more polar metabolites. However, elimination appears to be dose-dependent; at low doses, about 35% of the administered dose of TCDD was detected in the feces; at higher doses, about 46% was observed (Diliberto et al., 2001). The dose-dependent occurrence of TCDD metabolites in the feces is thought to be due to increased expression of metabolizing enzymes at higher doses. A measure of elimination is half-life, which is defined as the time required for the plasma concentration or the amount of a chemical in the body to be reduced by one-half. The half-life of TCDD in humans varies with body mass index, age, sex, and concentration and has been found to vary from 0.4 to over 10 years (Table 4-1).

In light of the variables discussed above and the effect of differences in physiologic states and metabolic processes, which can affect the mobilization of lipids and possibly of compounds stored in them, complex models known as physiologically based pharmacokinetic models have been developed to integrate exposure dose with organ mass, blood flow, metabolism, and lipid content to predict the movement of toxicants into and out of each organ. A number of recent modeling studies have been performed in an effort to understand the relevance of animal experimental studies to exposures that occur in human populations (Aylward et al., 2005a,b; Emond et al., 2005).

Toxicity Profile

The administration of TCDD to laboratory animals affects many tissues and organs. The effects of TCDD in laboratory animals have been observed in a number of species (rats, mice, guinea pigs, hamsters, monkeys, cows, and rabbits) after the administration of a variety of doses and after periods that represent acute (less than 24 hr), subchronic (more than 1 day up to 3 months), and chronic (more

TABLE 4-1 Estimates of TCDD Half-Life in Humans and Animals

Reference	Half-Life[a]	Confidence Interval	Comment
Human studies:			
Leung et al., 2006	0.4 year		Breast-fed infants, 0–1 year after exposure
Kumagai and Koda, 2005	1.1–2.3 years		Adult male, incinerator workers, 0–1.3 years after exposure
Aylward et al., 2005a	< 3 years		Calculated for exposures > 10,000 pg/g of serum lipid
	> 10 years		Calculated for exposures < 50 pg/g of serum lipid
Flesch-Janys et al., 1996	7.2 years		Adult males, Boehringer cohort
Geusau et al., 2002	1.5 years[b]		Adult female, severe exposure, 0–3 years after exposure
	2.9 years[b]		Adult female, severe exposure, 0–3 years after exposure
Michalek et al., 2002	0.34 year[b]		Adult males, Seveso cohort, 0–3 months after exposure
	6.9 years		Adult males, Seveso cohort, 3–16 years after exposure
	9.8 years		Adult females, Seveso cohort, 3–16 years after exposure
	7.5 years		Adult males, Ranch Hands, 9–33 years after exposure
Needham et al., 1994	7.8 years	7.2–9.7 years	Adults, Seveso cohort
Pirkle et al., 1989	7.1 years	5.8–9.6 years	Adult males, Ranch Hands, 9–23 years after exposure
Animal studies:			
Neubert et al., 1990	73.7 days	60.9–93.8 days	Monkeys, marmoset, single injection
DeVito and Birnbaum, 1995	15 days		Mice, female B6C3F1
Gasiewicz et al., 1983	11.0 days[c]		Mice, C5BL/6J
	24.4 days[c]		Mice, DBA/2J
	12.6 days[c]		Mice, B6D2F1/J
Koshakji et al., 1984	20 days		Mice, male ICR/Ha Swiss
Hurst et al., 1998	8 days		Rats, Long-Evans, excretion from liver
Pohjanvirta and Tuomisto, 1990	21.9 days		Rats, male Han/Wistar, resistant strain
Viluksela et al., 1996	20.2 days		Rats, Long-Evans, TurkuAB strain
	28.9 days[d]		Rats, Long-Evans, Charles River strain
Weber et al., 1993	16.3 ± 3.0 days		Rats, male Sprague-Dawley

[a] Half-lives of TCDD in humans based on measurement of TCDD in serum samples.
[b] Shorter half-lives measured in humans during first months after exposure or in severely contaminated persons consistent with nonlinear elimination predicted by physiologically based pharmacokinetic modeling (for example, by Carrier et al., 1995). Greater half-life in females attributed to greater body-mass index.
[c] Total cumulative excretion of ^{3}H-TCDD-derived radioactivity.

than 3 months) exposures. Some differences are observed in the different species, particularly with respect to their degree of sensitivity, but in general the effects observed are qualitatively similar. Relatively high exposures of TCDD affect a variety of organs and result in organ dysfunction and death. The specific organ dysfunction that constitutes the lethal event, however, is not known. A characteristic of TCDD exposure is a wasting syndrome with loss of adipose and muscle tissues and severe weight loss. In most rodents, exposure to TCDD affects the liver, as indicated by hepatic enlargement, the presence of hepatic lesions, and impaired hepatic function. The thymus is also sensitive. Finally, in both humans and nonhuman primates, TCDD exposure results in chloracne and associated dermatologic changes. As will be discussed in more detail in Chapters 6–9, studies performed in animal models have indicated that exposure to TCDD adversely affects the heart, the skin, and the immune, endocrine, and reproductive systems, and increases the incidence of cancers of the liver, skin, thyroid, adrenal cortex, hard palate, nasal turbinates, tongue, and respiratory and lymphatic systems (Huff et al., 1994). When TCDD has been administered to pregnant animals, such birth defects as cleft palate, malformations of the reproductive organs of the male and female progeny, and abnormalities in the cardiovascular system have been observed.

The administration of TCDD to laboratory animals and cultured cells affects enzymes, hormones, and receptors. In addition to adversely affecting the ability of specific organs to fulfill their normal physiologic roles, TCDD has been found to alter the function and expression of essential proteins. Some of the proteins are enzymes, specialized proteins that increase the rates of chemical reactions and aid in the body's ability to convert chemicals into different molecules. The metabolism of foreign chemicals often changes their biologic properties and in some cases increases the body's ability to eliminate them in urine. The enzymes that are most affected by TCDD are ones that act on or metabolize xenobiotics and hormones. Xenobiotics are chemicals that are not expected to be present in the body, and hormones are made by the body and serve as chemical messengers that transport a signal from one cell to another. Among the enzymes affected by TCDD, the best studied is CYP1A1, which metabolizes xenobiotics. In laboratory animals, exposure to TCDD commonly results in an increase in the CYP1A1 present in most tissues; CYP1A1 therefore is often used as a marker of TCDD exposure.

Other enzymes that are affected by TCDD are ones that metabolize hormones such as thyroid hormones, retinoic acid, testosterone, estrogens, and adrenal steroids. Those hormones transmit their signals by interacting with specific proteins called receptors and in this manner initiate a chain of events in many tissues of the body. For example, binding of the primary female sex hormone, estrogen, to the estrogen receptor promotes the formation of breasts and the thickening of the endometrium and regulates the menstrual cycle. Exposure to TCDD can increase the metabolism of estrogen, and this leads to a decrease in the amount of estrogen available for binding and activating the estrogen receptor. The ultimate effect of TCDD is an interference with all the bodily functions that are regulated by estrogens. Similarly, the actions of TCDD on the adrenal steroids can adversely affect their ability to regulate glucose tolerance, insulin sensitivity, lipid metabolism, obesity, vascular function, and cardiac remodeling. In addition to changing the amount of hormone present, TCDD has been found to interfere with the ability of receptors to fulfill their role in transmitting hormone signals. Animal models have shown that exposure to TCDD can increase the amounts of enzymes in the body and interfere with the ability of hormones to activate their specific hormone receptors. Those actions of TCDD on enzymes and hormone receptors are thought to underlie, in part, observed developmental and reproductive effects and cancers that are hormone-responsive.

TCDD alters the paths of cellular differentiation. Research performed primarily in cultured cells has shown that TCDD can affect the ability of cells to undergo such processes as proliferation, differentiation, and apoptosis. During the proliferative process, cells grow and divide. When cells are differentiating, they are undergoing a change from less specialized to more specialized. Cellular differentiation is essential for an organism to mature from a fetal to an adult state. In the adult, proper differentiation is required for normal functions of the body, for example, in maintaining a normally responsive immune system. Processes of controlled cell death, such as apoptosis, are similarly important during development of the fetus and are necessary for normal physiologic functions in the adult. Apoptosis is a way for the body to eliminate damaged or unnecessary cells. The ability of a cell to undergo proliferation, differentiation, and apoptosis is tightly controlled by an intricate network of signaling molecules that allows the body to maintain the appropriate size and number of all the specialized cells that form the fabric of complex tissues and organs. Disruption of that network that alters the delicate balance of cell fate can have severe consequences, including impairment of the function of the organ because of the absence of specialized cells. Alternatively, the presence of an excess of some kinds of cells can result in the formation and development of tumors. Thus, the ability of TCDD to disrupt the normal course of a specific cell to proliferate, differentiate, or undergo apoptosis is thought to underlie (at least in part) its adverse effects on the immune system and the developing fetus and its ability to promote the formation of certain cancers.

Definition of Dioxin-like Compounds and TEF and TEQ Terminology

Many compounds have dioxin-like properties: they have similar chemical structure, have similar physiochemical properties, and cause a common battery of toxic responses. Because of their hydrophobic nature and resistance to metabolism, these chemicals persist and bioaccumulate in fatty tissues of animals and humans. Several hundred chemicals—such as the polychlorinated dibenzo-*p*-dioxins, polychlorinated dibenzofurans, polybrominated dibenzo-*p*-dioxins, polybrominated dibenzofurans, and polychlorinated biphenyls—are described as dioxin-like compounds (DLCs), although only a few of them are thought to display dioxin-like toxicity. For most purposes, only 17 polychlorinated dibenzo-*p*-dioxins and polychlorinated dibenxofurans and a few of the coplanar polychlorinated biphenyls that are often encountered in environmental samples are recognized as being true DLCs. In the context of risk assessment, these polychlorinated dibenzo-*p*-dioxins, polychlorinated dibenxofurans, and polychlorinated biphenyls are commonly found as complex mixtures when detected in environmental media and biologic tissues or when measured as environmental releases from specific sources. That complicates the human health risk assessment that may be associated with exposures to varied mixtures of DLCs. To address the problem, the concept of toxic equivalency has been elaborated by the scientific community, and the toxic equivalency factor (TEF) has been developed and introduced to facilitate risk assessment of exposure to those chemical mixtures. On the most basic level, TEFs compare the potential toxicity of each DLC found in a mixture with the toxicity of TCDD, the most toxic member of the group. The procedure involves assigning individual TEFs to the DLCs with consideration of chemical structure, persistence, and resistance to metabolism. TEF ascribe specific order-of-magnitude toxicity to each DLC relative to that of TCDD, which is assigned a TEF of 1.0. The DLCs have TEFs ranging from 0.00001 to 1.0. When several compounds are present in a mixture, the toxicity of the mixture is estimated by multiplying the TEF of each DLC in the mixture by its mass concentration and summing the products to yield the TCDD toxicity equivalent quotient (TEQ) of the mixture.

Mechanism of Action

TCDD binds and activates the aryl hydrocarbon receptor (AHR). The AHR is a member of a family of basic-helix-loop-helix (bHLH) transcription factors, that is, one of many proteins in the cell that controls the transfer (or transcription) of genetic information from DNA to RNA. bHLH proteins are characterized by the presence of a string of basic amino acid residues followed by two alpha helices joined by a loop. Generally, the larger of the two helices participates in binding to DNA in a specific sequence motif; the specificity is determined largely by the amino acid sequence of the helix. bHLH transcription factors are dimeric, forming functional heterodimers with other members of the family. By mechanisms that are poorly understood, binding of the heterodimeric complex to DNA recruits the transcriptional machinery needed to activate gene expression and results in a large increase in the rate of synthesis of mRNA molecules for the genes regulated by the complex and ultimately in a large increase in the corresponding protein.

The best known AHR target is the expression of a mixed-function oxidase enzyme that was termed aryl hydrocarbon hydroxylase (AHH) in the 1960s and is now better known as the CYP1A1 enzyme. Expression of this protein is an acute outcome of AHR activation and may not faithfully represent the consequences of chronic exposure to AHR ligands.

In its inactive state, the AHR is found in the cytosol of the cell, where it is protected from proteolytic degradation by several chaperones and cochaperones. As a receptor, the AHR is a protein capable of receiving and forming a complex with specific substances, termed ligands, which confer on it the ability to perform a biologic function. In the case of the AHR, the function is to induce the transcription of specific target genes. Hence, the AHR belongs to a class of ligand-activated transcription factors. If the ligand is a chemical, such as TCDD, the AHR dissociates from the chaperones and translocates into the nucleus of the cell, where it forms a heterodimer with another bHLH protein, the AHR nuclear translocator (ARNT). This heterodimer binds to its cognate DNA motifs and recruits the macromolecular complexes needed to initiate gene transcription.

AHR Functional Domains

The AHR contains several regions, or domains, that perform distinct functions. The receptor is a member of the Per-Arnt-Sim (PAS) bHLH subfamily (Burbach et al., 1992; Fukunaga et al., 1995). The bHLH motif is found in the amino terminus of the protein and is common to all transcription factors in this subfamily (Jones, 2004). The members of the bHLH family also have several highly conserved domains with functionally distinctive biochemical roles. One of the domains is the basic region, described earlier, which is involved in the binding of AHR/ARNT complexes to DNA. Another domain is the HLH region, which facilitates the stable interaction between AHR and ARNT. A third domain is termed the PAS domain and consists of a stretch of 200–350 amino acids with high sequence relatedness to protein domains that were originally found in the *Drosophila melanogaster* genes *period* (Per) and *single minded* (Sim) and in the AHR's dimerization partner ARNT; hence the name PAS. The AHR contains two PAS domains, PAS-A and PAS-B (Ema et al., 1992). The PAS domains support secondary interactions with other PAS-domain–containing proteins, with the chaperones and cochaperones, and with many other transcription factors, coactivators and corepressors. The ligand-binding site of AHR is in the PAS-B domain (Coumailleau et al., 1995) and contains several conserved residues critical for ligand binding (Goryo et al., 2007). A fourth important domain in the carboxyl terminus of the protein, is rich in glutamine and is involved in coregulator recruitment and transactivation (Kumar et al., 2001).

AHR Ligands

From an environmental point of view, there are two classes of AHR ligands—synthetic and naturally occurring—that total more than 400 known ligands. Many of the first ligands to be discovered were synthetic polycyclic aromatic hydrocarbons (PAHs), such as 3-methylcholanthrene, benzo[a]pyrene (B[a]P), benzanthracene, and naphthoflavone. The biologic consequences of experimental exposure of mice to those chemicals led to the prediction of a receptor-dependent mechanism long before the existence of the AHR was directly demonstrated. Comparison of the effects of 3-methylcholanthrene treatment in two inbred mouse strains revealed a major difference in PAH responsiveness. Hepatic CYP1A1 enzyme increased more than 6-fold after 3-methylcholanthrene treatment in C57BL/6 mice but not in DB/2 mice. Appropriate genetic crosses between responsive C57BL/6 mice but in non-responsive DB/2 mice indicated that responsiveness in these prototype strains was inherited as a simple autosomal dominant trait. The genetic locus defined in the crosses was termed the *aromatic hydrocarbon responsiveness (Ahr) locus* (Nebert et al., 1982). Molecular biologic studies during the next decade showed that responsive and nonresponsive mice had equally functional CYP1A1 enzymes and that the *Ahr* locus encoded a regulatory gene responsible for induction of the *Cyp1a1* gene. The members of the polyhalogenated aromatic hydrocarbons—such as the dibenzodioxins, dibenzofurans, and polychlorinated and polybrominated biphenyls—were recognized as AHR ligands much later, after the discovery by Poland and co-workers that dioxin was a potent inducer of hepatic AHH in the rat. At that time, it was found that high concentrations of TCDD could induce AHH activity in the nonresponsive DB/2 mouse to levels as high as those in the responsive C57BL/6 mouse. The difference between responsive and nonresponsive strains was in sensitivity to the inducer: DB/2 mice required 18 times more TCDD than C57BL/6 mice for 50% of the maximal response. Later, a receptor protein for TCDD, 3-methylcholanthrene and other PAHs, was identified, characterized in the hepatic cytosol of C57BL/6 mice, and termed Ah receptor (Poland et al., 1976). The available evidence indicated that the protein was the product of the *Ahr* locus, which was localized to mouse chromosome 12 and human chromosome 7, and later cloned (Burbach et al., 1992; Ema et al., 1992).

Recent work has focused on naturally occurring compounds in hopes of identifying an endogenous ligand (Denison and Nagy, 2003). Several such naturally occurring compounds have been identified as AHR ligands, including the tryptophan derivatives indigo and indirubin (Adachhi et al., 2001), the tetrapyrroles bilirubin (Sinal and Bend, 1997), the arachidonic acid metabolites lipoxin A4 and prostaglandin G (Seidel et al., 2001), modified low-density lipoprotein (McMillan and Bradfield, 2007), several dietary carotenoids (Denison and Negy, 2003; Probst et al., 1993), and cAMP (Oesch-Bartlomowicz et al., 2005). One assumption made in the search for an endogenous ligand is that the ligand will be a receptor agonist, that is, that it will activate the receptor. However, recent work has shown that may not be the case inasmuch as one such natural ligand, 7-ketocholesterol, competitively inhibits AHR-dependent signal transduction (Savouret et al., 2001).

AHR Signaling Pathway

In the absence of bound ligand, the inactive AHR is retained in the cytoplasm of the cell in a complex consisting of two molecules of the heat shock protein hsp90, one molecule of prostaglandin E synthase 3 (p23) (Kazlauskas et al., 1999), and one molecule of the immunophilin-like protein hepatitis B virus X-associated protein 2 (XAP2) (Petrulis et al., 2003), previously identified as AHR-interacting protein (Ma and Whitlock, 1997) and AHR-activated 9 (Carver and Bradfield, 1997). The hsp90 dimer–p23 complex plays multiple roles in the protection of the AHR from proteolysis, maintaining it in a conformation that makes the receptor accessible to ligand binding at the same time that it prevents the premature binding of ARNT (Carver and Bradfield, 1994; Pongratz et al., 1992; Whitelaw et al., 1993). XAP2 interacts with the carboxyl terminus of hsp90 and with the AHR nuclear-localization signal (NLS), a short amino acid domain in the bHLH region that targets the receptor for interaction with nuclear-transport proteins. Binding of XAP2 blocks such interaction, preventing the inappropriate trafficking of the receptor into the nucleus (Petrulis et al., 2003).

Binding of ligand induces the release of XAP2 and the exposure of the NLS and leads to the binding of nuclear-import proteins and translocation of the cytosolic complex into the nucleus (Davarinos and Pollenz, 1999; Song and Pollenz, 2002). Once in the nucleus, chaperones and cochaperones dissociate from the AHR, exposing the two PAS domains and allowing the binding of ARNT (Hoffman et al., 1991; Probst et al., 1993). The activated AHR/ARNT heterodimeric complex is then capable of directly or indirectly interacting with DNA by binding to recognition sequences in the regulatory region of responsive genes (Dolwick et al., 1993; Probst et al., 1993).

The canonical DNA recognition motif of the AHR/ARNT complex is referred to as the AHR-responsive element (AHRE, also referred to as the dioxin-responsive element [DRE] or the xenobiotic-responsive element [XRE]). This element is found in the promoter region of AHR-responsive genes and contains the core sequence 5'-GCGTG-3' (Shen and Whitlock, 1992), which is part of a more extensive consensus binding sequence, 5'-T/GNGCGTGA/CG/CA-3' (Lusska et al., 1993; Yao and Denison, 1992). The AHR/ARNT complex binds to the AHRE core sequence in such a manner that ARNT binds to the 5'-GTG-3' and AHR binds to 5'-TC/TGC-3' (Bacsi et al., 1995; Swanson et al., 1995). A second type of element, termed AHRE-II, 5'-CATG(N6)C[T/A]TG-3', has recently been shown to be capable of acting indirectly with the AHR/ARNT complex (Boutros et al., 2004; Sogawa et al., 2004). The end result of the process is the recruitment of the transcriptional machinery associated with RNA polymerase II and the initiation of differential changes in the expression of the genes bearing the AHR/ ARNT recognition motif. Many of the genes code for proteins responsible for detoxification reactions directed at the elimination of the ligand. Recent research suggests that posttranslational modifications in histone proteins may modify the response (Hestermann and Brown, 2003; Schnekenburger et al., 2007).

AHR Physiology

The vertebrate AHR is presumed to have evolved from its counterpart in invertebrates, in which it serves a ligand-independent role in normal development processes. The ancestral function of the AHR appears to be the regulation of specific aspects of embryonic development, it having acquired the ability to bind xenobiotic compounds only during vertebrate evolution (Hahn, 2001). The invertebrate AHR also functions as a transcription factor and binds to the same dimerization partner (ARNT) and DNA response elements as the vertebrate protein, but it does not respond to any of the environmental ligands recognized by the vertebrate receptor. Instead, it regulates diverse developmental processes that are independent of exogenous ligand exposure, such as neuronal differentiation during worm development in *Caenorhabditis elegans* (Huang et al., 2004; Qin and Powell-Coffman, 2004) or normal morphogenesis of legs, antennae, and bristles in *Drosophila melanogaster* (Adachi-Yamada et al., 2005). In developing vertebrates, the AHR seems to play a role in cellular proliferation and differentiation and, in keeping with this role in invertebrates, also possesses a developmental role in craniofacial, renal, and cardiovascular morphogenesis (Birnbaum et al., 1989; Fernandez-Salguero et al., 1997; Lahvis et al., 2005).

The clearest adaptive physiologic response of AHR activation is the induction of xenobiotic-metabolizing enzymes involved in detoxification of toxic ligands. Evidence of that response, which was described above, was first observed from the induction of *Cyp1a1*, resulting from exposure to PAHs or TCDD, and directly related to activation of the AHR signaling pathway (Israel and Whitlock, 1983, 1984). Because of the presence of AHRE motif in their gene promoters, other metabolizing genes were tested and found to be induced by AHR ligands, and this led to the identification of a so-called AHR gene battery of phase I and phase II detoxification genes that code for the drug-metabolizing enzymes CYP1A1, CYP1A2, CYP1B1, NQO1, ALHD3A1, UGT1A2, and GSTA1 (Nebert et al., 2000). Presumably, vertebrates have evolved those enzymes to detect a wide array of foreign, potentially toxic chemicals, represented in the wide variety of substrates that AHR is able to bind whose biotransformation and elimination it is able to facilitate.

A potential complication of the adaptive responses elicited by AHR activation is the induction of a toxic response. Toxicity may result from the adaptive response itself if the induction of metabolizing enzymes results in the production of toxic metabolites. For example, the PAH B[a]P, an AHR ligand, induces its own metabolism and detoxification by the AHR-dependent signaling mechanism described earlier but paradoxically becomes bioactivated to a toxic metabolite in several tissues by metabolism that depends on CYP1A1 and CYP1B1 enzymatic activity (Harrigan et al., 2004). A second potential source of AHR-mediated toxicity may be aberrant changes in global gene expression beyond those observed in the AHR gene battery. The global changes in gene expression may lead to deleterious changes in cellular processes and physiology. Microarray analysis has proved invaluable in understanding and characterizing that response (Martinez et al., 2002; Puga et al., 2000, 2004; Vezina et al., 2004).

It is clear that the AHR is an essential component of the toxicity of dioxin and of DLCs. Homozygous deletion of the AHR in mice leads to a phenotype that is resistant to the toxic effects of TCDD and to the carcinogenic effects of B[a]P (Fernandez-Salguero et al., 1996; Lahvis and Bradfield, 1998; Schmidt et al., 1996). AHR knockout mice, however, have other phenotypic effects, including reduced liver size and hepatic fibrosis and cardiovascular abnormalities. Hence, it is likely that dioxin has effects due to gratuitous deregulation of endogenous AHR functions, unrelated to the intrinsic toxicity of some of its ligands.

Carcinogenic Classification of TCDD

The US Environmental Protection Agency (EPA) and the International Agency for Research on Cancer (IARC), a branch of the World Health Organization, have defined criteria to classify the potential carcinogenicity of chemicals on the basis of the weight of scientific evidence from animal, human, epidemiologic, mechanistic, and mode-of-action studies. EPA classified TCDD as a "probable human carcinogen" in 1985 and as "carcinogenic to humans" in a 2003 reassessment. In 1998, the IARC panel of experts concluded that the weight of scientific evidence supported the classification of dioxin as a class I carcinogen, that is, as "carcinogenic to humans." Four years later, the US National Toxicology Program upgraded its classification to "known to be a human carcinogen." In 2006, a panel of experts convened by the National Research Council to evaluate the EPA reassessment concluded that TCDD was "likely to be carcinogenic to humans." That designation reflected the revised EPA *Guidelines for Carcinogen Risk Assessment* made public in 2005.

Other Toxic Health Outcomes of Dioxin

There is an extensive body of evidence from experimental studies in animal model systems that TCDD, other dioxins, and several DLCs are immunotoxic. Although the available evidence on humans is scant, mechanistic considerations support the notion that chemical alterations to immune function would cause adverse health outcomes because of the critical role that the immune system plays in general protection, fighting off infection and eliminating cancer cells at early stages. Because of those considerations, these compounds are potential immunotoxicants.

Similarly, reproduction and embryonic development clearly are targets of TCDD, other dioxins, and DLCs; it is found consistently that the adverse effects are more prevalent during fetal development than in the adult. However, data on those effects in humans are practically nonexistent.

TCDD, other dioxins, and DLCs are also recognized as potentially capable of causing birth defects, reproductive disorders, immunotoxicity, and chloracne. Human and animal studies have revealed other potential health outcomes including cardiovascular disease, hepatic disease, thyroid dysfunction, lipid disorders, neurotoxicity, and metabolic disorders, such as diabetes.

A number of effects of TCDD exposure in vitro appear to be independent of AHR-mediated mechanisms. The salient ones are induction of transforming growth factor-α and other genes involved in extracellular matrix deposition in cells from mice with homozygous ablation of the *Ahr* gene (Guo et al., 2004); mobilization of calcium from intracellular sources and imported from the culture medium (Puga et al., 1995); and related to calcium mobilization, the induction of mitochondria oxidative stress (Senft et al., 2002). Calcium mobilization by TCDD may have an important effect on signal-transduction mechanisms that control gene expression, inasmuch as several proto-oncogenes, such as *c-fos,* are activated by calcium changes.

Recent Findings from Mechanistic Studies That May Be Relevant to Health Outcomes

Several reports published since *Update 2006* (IOM, 2007) have contributed to the understanding of how TCDD exposure may have contributed to particular health outcomes, as follows:

- Insight into the role of the AHR repressor protein in mediating cell-type–specific responsiveness to TCDD (Evans et al., 2008; Haarmann-Stemmann et al., 2007).
- Identification of genes that may be regulated by TCDD through activation of AHR that are involved in cholesterol biosynthesis, lipogenesis, and glucose metabolism (Sato et al., 2008; Zarzour et al., 2008); development of thymocytes (the KLF2 regulon) (McMillian et al., 2007); glucose uptake (the glucose transporter) (Tonack et al., 2007); and metabolism of the steroid hydroxysteroid 17-beta dehydrogenase; plus a novel gene (*Hectd2*) with poorly defined function (Hayes et al., 2007).
- Examination of the effect of TCDD on signaling pathways, such as that of protein kinase C (Lee et al., 2007) and integrin signaling (Liu and

Jefcoate, 2006) that may underlie TCDD's adverse effects on neurons in cell culture and cell adhesion, respectively.

- Elucidation of crosstalk between the AHR and receptors involved in regulation of cellular responses to stress (Burchiel et al., 2008; Dvorak et al., 2008; Sonneveld et al., 2007) and estrogen (Boverhof et al., 2008; Marquez-Bravo and Gierthy, 2008; Tanaka et al., 2007).
- Progress pertaining to TCDD's effects on oxidative stress and DNA damage (Lin et al., 2007; Lu et al., 2007) and events in the mitochondria (Biswas et al., 2008; Shertzer et al., 2006).
- Study of TCDD's effects on determination of cell-fate. Mechanisms by which TCDD induces G1 arrest in hepatic cells (Mitchell et al., 2006; Weiss et al., 2008) and decreases viability of endometrial endothelial cells (Bredhult et al., 2007), insulin-secreting beta cells (Piaggi et al., 2007), peripheral T cells (Singh et al., 2008), and neuronal cells (Bredhult et al., 2007) were identified. The findings may be relevant to cancer, reproductive health, diabetes, immune function, and neurotoxicity. Insights were also gained into TCDD's effects on maturation and differentiation of adipocytes (Arsenescu et al., 2008), granule neuron precursors (Collins et al., 2008), dendritic cells (Lee et al., 2007), and how TCDD induces the differentiation of regulatory T cells (Funatake et al., 2008; Gill et al., 2008; Hollingshead et al., 2008; Kimura et al., 2008; Quintana et al., 2008; Veldhoen et al., 2008; Vogel et al., 2008).
- Increased evidence that the TCDD–AHR pathway may impinge on the cytokine-inflammatory response (Chiaro et al., 2008; Dong and Matsumura, 2008; Hollingshead et al., 2008; Ito et al., 2008; Li et al., 2007; Vogel et al., 2007a,b).

Those publications collectively have added to what was already strong support of an association of TCDD exposure with adverse health effects in laboratory animals and, by extension, in humans.

Summary on Biologic Plausibility of TCDD Inducing Adverse Effects in Humans

Mechanistic studies in vitro and in laboratory animals have characterized the biochemical pathways and types of biologic events that contribute to adverse effects of exposure to TCDD. For example, much evidence indicates that TCDD acting via the AHR in partnership with ARNT alters gene expression. Receptor binding may result in release of other cytoplasmic proteins that alter the expression or activity of other cell-regulatory proteins. Mechanistic studies also indicate that many other cellular component proteins contribute to the gene-regulatoring effect and that the response to TCDD exposure involves a complex interplay between genetic and environmental factors. Comparative data from animal and human cells in vitro and from tissues suggest a strong qualitative similarity among species in response to TCDD, and this further supports the applicability to humans of the generalized model of initial events in response to dioxin exposure. Biochemical and biologic responses to TCDD exposure are considered adaptive or simply reflective of exposure and not adverse in themselves if they take place within the normal homeostatic parameters of an organism. However, they may exceed physiologic parameters or constitute an early event in a pathway leading to damage to sensitive members of the population. In the latter case, the response is toxic and would be expected to cause an adverse health effect. From a mechanistic standpoint, adverse effects identified in vitro are expected to occur in all the cells of an organism and to all the organisms that express these proteins. That generalization sets the ground rules for the concept of *biologic plausibility*, which relies on extrapolation from laboratory tests to human risks, and on the *precautionary principle*, which bases decision-making on precaution if the precise nature or magnitude of the potential damage that a substance may cause in humans is uncertain.

When deemed useful, the findings from individual publications are presented in the biologic-plausibility sections associated with specific health outcomes.

PHENOXY HERBICIDES: 2,4-D AND 2,4,5-T

Chemistry

2,4-D (Chemical Abstracts Service [CAS] No. 94-75-7) is an odorless and, when pure, white crystalline powder (Figure 4-2); it may appear yellow when phenolic impurities are present. The melting point of 2,4-D is 138°C, and the free acid is corrosive to metals. It is soluble in water and in a variety of organic solvents (such as acetone, alcohols, ketones, ether, and toluene). 2,4,5-T (CAS No. 93-76-5) is an odorless, white to light-tan solid with a melting point of 158°C.

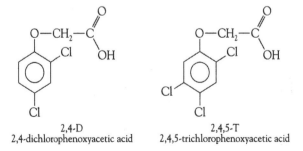

2,4-D
2,4-dichlorophenoxyacetic acid

2,4,5-T
2,4,5-trichlorophenoxyacetic acid

FIGURE 4-2 Structure of selected phenoxy herbicides.

2,4,5-T is noncorrosive and is soluble in alcohol and water. It reacts with organic and inorganic bases to form salts and with alcohols to form esters.

Uses of 2,4-D and 2,4,5-T

2,4-D has been used commercially in the United States since World War II to control the growth of broadleaf plants and weeds on range lands, lawns, golf courses, forests, roadways, parks, and agricultural land and remains today a widely used herbicide approved for use by the European Union and the US EPA. Formulations include 2,4-D amine and alkali salts and esters, which are mobile in soil and easily absorbed through the leaves and roots of many plants. Like 2,4-D, 2,4,5-T was developed and marketed as a herbicide during World War II. However, the registration for 2,4,5-T was canceled by EPA in 1978 when it became clear that it was contaminated with TCDD during the manufacturing process.

The herbicidal properties of 2,4-D and 2,4,5-T are related to their ability to mimic the plant growth hormone indole acetic acid. They are selective herbicides in that they affect the growth of only broadleaf dicots (which include most weeds) and do not affect monocots, such as wheat, corn, and rice.

Absorption, Distribution, Metabolism, and Elimination

Several studies have examined the absorption, distribution, metabolism, and excretion of 2,4-D and 2,4,5-T in animals and humans. Data on both compounds are consistent among species and support the conclusion that absorption of oral or inhaled doses is rapid and complete. Absorption through the skin is much lower but may be increased with the use of sunscreens or alcohol (Brand et al., 2002; Pont et al., 2004). After absorption, 2,4-D and 2,4,5-T are distributed widely in the body but are eliminated quickly, predominantly in unmetabolized form in urine (Sauerhoff et al., 1977). Neither 2,4-D nor 2,4,5-T is metabolized to a great extent in the body although 2,4,5-trichlorophenol and 2,4-dichlorophenol have been identified as trace metabolites in urine. The half-life in humans after single doses of 2,4-D or 2,4,5-T has been estimated to be about 18–23 hours (Gehring et al., 1973; Kohli et al., 1974; Sauerhoff et al., 1977; WHO, 1984). Results of a recent study that examined concentrations of 2,4-D and its metabolites in the urine of herbicide applicators was consistent with 2,4-D urinary half-life estimates of 13–40 hours in humans (Hines et al., 2003).

Toxicity Profile

The toxicity data base on 2,4-D is extensive (http://www.epa.gov/ttn/atw/hlthef/di-oxyac.html: accessed January 21, 2009), whereas the data available on the toxicity of purified 2,4,5-T, independent of its contamination by TCDD, are sparse. TCDD is much more toxic than 2,4,5-T, and much of the toxicity attributed to 2,4,5-T in early studies was later shown to be caused by the TCDD contaminant. The following summary therefore focuses on 2,4-D toxicity, and information on pure 2,4,5-T is added when it is available.

After a single oral dose, 2,4-D is considered to produce moderate acute toxicity with an LD_{50} (dose lethal to 50% of exposed animals) of 375 mg/kg in rats, 370 mg/kg in mice, and from less than 320 to 1,000 mg/kg in guinea pigs. Rats and rabbits have dermal LD_{50}s of 1,500 mg/kg and 1,400 mg/kg, respectively. 2,4,5-T itself also produces moderate acute toxicity, with oral LD_{50}s of 389 mg/kg in mice and 500 mg/kg in rats. Death from acute poisoning with 2,4-D or 2,4,5-T has been attributed to the ability of the chemicals to uncouple oxidative phosphorylation, a vital process used by almost all cells in the body as the primary means of generating energy. After exposure to high doses, death can occur rapidly from multiple organ failure. Studies in rats, cats, and dogs indicate that the central nervous system is the principal target organ for acute 2,4-D toxicity in mammals and suggest that the primary site of action is the cerebral cortex or the reticular formation (Arnold et al., 1991; Dési et al., 1962a,b). Neurotoxicity in humans is the predominant effect of acute inhalation and oral exposure to 2,4-D; symptoms include stiffness of arms and legs, incoordination, lethargy, anorexia, stupor, and coma. 2,4-D is also an irritant of the gastrointestinal tract, causing nausea, vomiting, and diarrhea.

Chronic exposure to 2,4-D at relatively high concentrations has been shown to produce a variety of toxic effects, including hepatic and renal toxicity, neurotoxicity, and hematologic changes. A no-observed-effect level (NOEL) of 2,4-D of 1 mg/kg was identified for renal toxicity in rats (Hazleton Laboratories America, 1987). The reproductive toxicity of 2,4-D is limited to reduced survival and decreased growth rates of offspring of mothers fed high doses during pregnancy and was associated with maternal toxicity. However, even at high exposures, 2,4-D did not affect fertility and did not produce teratogenic effects in the offspring. The purity of 2,4,5-T has been shown to influence its reproductive toxicity; TCDD contamination increases its fetotoxic effects and induces teratogenic effects. Immunotoxicity of 2,4-D has been reported in a small number of studies. At high doses that produced clinical toxicity, suppression of the antibody response was observed, whereas other measures of immune function were normal. The immunotoxicity of 2,4,5-T has not been evaluated in laboratory animals.

Carcinogenicity

The carcinogenicity of 2,4-D or 2,4,5-T has been studied in rats, mice, and dogs after exposure in their food, direct placement in their stomachs, or exposure of their skin. All the studies had negative results except one that found an increased incidence of brain tumors in male rats, but not female rats, that received the highest dose of 2,4-D. The occurrence of malignant lymphoma in dogs kept as pets was reported to be higher when owners reported that they used 2,4-D on their lawns than when they did not (Hayes et al., 1991, 1995), but detailed reanalysis did not confirm this finding (Kaneene and Miller, 1999). A controlled study using dogs exposed to 2,4-D in the laboratory had negative results. Timchalk (2004) suggested that dogs are not relevant for comparative evaluation of human health risk attributable to 2,4-D exposure, because they excrete 2,4-D less efficiently than rats or humans. 2,4-D is not metabolized to reactive intermediates capable of interacting with DNA, and the evidence supports the conclusion that 2,4-D is not a carcinogen.

CACODYLIC ACID

Chemistry

Arsenic (As) is a naturally occurring element that exists in trivalent form (As^{+3} or As^{III}) and pentavalent form (As^{+5} or As^V). The As^{III} in sodium arsenite is generally considered to be the most toxic—see Figure 4-3 for chemical struc-

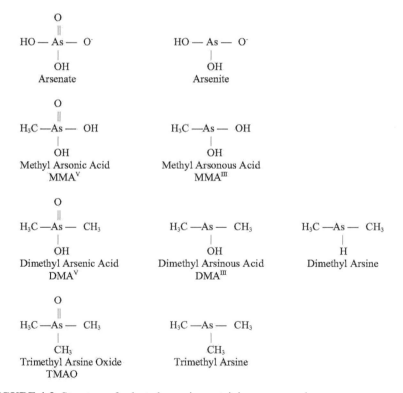

FIGURE 4-3 Structure of selected arsenic-containing compounds.

tures of selected arsenic-containing compounds. Arsenic is commonly present in drinking-water sources associated with volcanic soils and can reach high concentrations (over 50 ppb). Numerous human health effects have been attributed to drinking-water exposure, particularly bladder, skin, and lung cancers and vascular diseases.

Arsenic exists in both inorganic and organic (methylated) forms and is readily metabolized in humans and other species. Inorganic arsenic can be converted to organic forms, but organic forms cannot be converted into inorganic forms (Cohen et al., 2006). Cacodylic acid has a valence of +5 and is commonly referred to as dimethylarsinic acid (DMA^V). Cacodylic acid, disodium methanearsonate, and monosodium methanearsonate are herbicides that EPA-approved for use in the United States, where they are occasionally applied on golf courses and large open spaces. Cacodylic acid was the form of arsenic used in Agent Blue; DMA^V made up about 30% of Agent Blue, one of the mixtures used for defoliation in Vietnam. Agent Blue was chemically and toxicologically unrelated to Agent Orange, which consisted of phenoxy herbicides contaminated with DLCs. As shown in Figure 4-4, DMA and monomethyl arsonic acid (MMA) are metabolic products of exposure to inorganic arsenic. Methylation of inorganic arsenic used to be considered a detoxification process associated with increased excretion (Vahter and Concha, 2001). More recently, however, some of the methylated metabolic intermediates have been thought to be more toxic than the parent compound. The

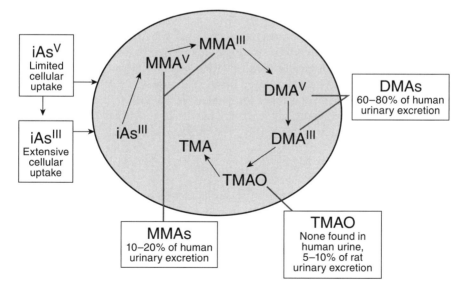

FIGURE 4-4 General pathways of arsenic metabolism after exposure to inorganic arsenic (iAs).
SOURCE: Adapted with permission from Cohen et al., 2006.

methylation pathway of inorganic arsenic results in the formation of pentavalent DMA (DMA^V) and trivalent DMA (DMA^{III}). The committee contemplated the relevance to DMA of data on exposure to inorganic arsenic. Although inorganic arsenic is a human carcinogen, there is no evidence that direct exposure to DMA produces cancer in humans. DMA also is not demethylated to inorganic arsenic (Vahter et al., 1984). It has not been established, nor can it be inferred, that the observed effects of exposure to inorganic arsenic are also caused by exposure to DMA. Therefore, the literature on inorganic arsenic is not considered in this report. The reader is referred to *Arsenic in Drinking Water* (NRC, 1999a) and *Arsenic in Drinking Water: 2001 Update* (NRC, 2001).

Toxicokinetics

The metabolism and disposition of DMA^V has recently been reviewed (Cohen et al., 2006). In general, DMA^V is rapidly excreted mostly unchanged in the urine of most animal species after systemic exposure. However, rats are unique in that a small percentage (10%) of DMA^V binds to hemoglobin in red blood cells and leads to a longer half-life in blood (Cui et al., 2004; Suzuki et al., 2004). Rat hemoglobin is unique in its binding of DMA^V in that its binding affinity to DMA^V is 10 times higher than that of human hemoglobin (Lu et al., 2004). Chronic exposure of normal rat hepatocytes to DMA^V resulted in reduced uptake over time and in acquired cytotoxic tolerance (Kojima et al., 2006); the tolerance was mediated by induction of glutathione-*S*-transferase activity and of multiple-drug–resistant protein expression. Adair et al. (2007) recently examined the tissue distribution of DMA in rats after dietary exposures for 14 days; they found that it was extensively metabolized to trimethylated forms that may play a role in toxicity.

Recently, a physiologically based pharmacokinetic model for intravenous and ingested DMA^V has been developed based on mouse data (Evans et al., 2008). Similar models have been developed for humans on the basis of exposure to inorganic arsenic (El-Masri and Kenyon, 2008), but these models have limited utility in considering the toxicity of DMA^V exposures that are relevant to veterans.

Toxicity Profile

This section discusses the toxicity associated with organic forms of arsenic, most notably DMA^V because this is the active ingredient in Agent Blue. The toxicity of inorganic arsenic is not considered relevant to veteran exposures to Agent Blue.

Neurotoxicity

Kruger et al. (2006) found that DMA^{III} and DMA^V significantly attenuated neuronal ion currents through *N*-methyl-D-aspartate receptor ion channels whereas only DMA^V inhibited ion currents through α-amino-3-hydroxy-5-methylisoxazole-4-propionic acid receptors. The data suggest that those methylated forms of arsenic may have neurotoxic potential.

Immunotoxicity

Previous studies have shown that a low concentration of DMA^V (10^{-7} M) could increase proliferation of human peripheral blood monocytes after their stimulation with phytohemagglutinin whereas it took a high concentration (10^{-4} M) to inhibit release of interferon-γ; this suggested that immunomodulatory effects of DMA^V are concentration-specific (Di Giampaolo et al., 2004).

Genotoxicity and Carcinogenicity

Cancer has been induced in the urinary bladder, kidneys, liver, thyroid glands, and lungs of laboratory animals exposed to high concentrations of DMA (Wei et al., 2002). Exposure to DMA^V resulted in necrosis of the urinary bladder epithelium followed by regenerative hyperplasia (Cohen et al., 2002).

DMA^{III} was considerably more potent than DMA^V in inducing DNA damage in Chinese hamster ovary cells (Dopp et al., 2004), and this was associated with a 10% uptake of DMA^{III} into the cells compared with 0.03% uptake of DMA^V. An additional study showed that DMA^V is poorly membrane-permeable, but when forced into cells by electroporation it can induce DNA damage (Dopp et al., 2005). Furthermore, DMA^V induced protein-DNA adducts in lung fibroblast cells (MRC-5) (Mouron et al., 2005) and transformation loci in 3T3 fibroblasts following subsequent treatment with the tumor promoter 12-*O*-tetradecanoylphorbol-13-acetate (TPA) (Tsuchiya et al., 2005). However, DMA^V was devoid of promotion activity in 3T3 fibroblasts when cells were pretreated with 3-methylcholanthrene or sodium arsenite.

DMA^V, but not inorganic arsenic species, exhibited genotoxicity in *Drosophila* as assessed with the somatic mutation and recombination test (Rizki et al., 2006). *Drosophila* lacks the ability to methylate arsenic, so the data suggest that arsenic biomethylation is a key determinant of arsenic genotoxicity.

DMA^{III} and DMA^V have been shown to induce DNA damage by increasing oxidative stress. Chronic exposure of ddY mice to DMA^V at 400 ppm in drinking water increased staining for 4-hydroxy-2-nonenal adducts, which are indicative of oxidative stress, and for 8-oxo-2′-deoxyguanosine (8-oxodG), reactive oxygen-species–induced DNA damage, in Clara cells of the lung (An et al., 2005). Gomez et al. (2005) demonstrated that DMA^{III} induced a dose-related increase in DNA damage and oxidative stress in Jurkat cells.

Two studies investigated the degree to which oxidative stress may mediate DMA^V cytotoxicity. In one study, an antioxidant (*N*-acetylcysteine, vitamin C, or melatonin) and DMA^V at 100 ppm were coadministered to F344 rats for 10 weeks

(Wei et al., 2005). *N*-Acetylcysteine inhibited DMA^V-induced proliferation of the urinary bladder epithelium whereas neither vitamin C nor melatonin had an effect; this suggested that oxidative stress may mediate the cytotoxic process in the urothelium. In the second, metallothionein wild-type and null mice were exposed to a single oral dose of DMA^V at 0, 188, 375, or 750 mg/kg (Jia et al., 2004). DMA^V induced a dose-dependent increase in metallothionein in the livers of wild-type mice, but metallothionein was undetectable and uninducible in the null mice. At 24 hours after exposure, DMA^V induced dose-dependent DNA adducts, DNA strand breaks, and pulmonary and bladder apoptosis in both genotypes, but the incidence of damage was significantly higher in the null mice. Those results suggest that metallothionein may play a protective role against DMA^V-induced DNA damage.

Gene-expression profiling of bladder urothelium after chronic exposure to DMA^V in drinking water showed significant increases in genes that regulate apoptosis, the cell cycle, and oxidative stress (Sen et al., 2005). Furthermore, doses that were nontoxic, according to a lack of histologic and ultrastructural changes, could be distinguished from toxic doses on the basis of the expression of a subset of genes involved in control of cell signaling and the stress response, such as thioredoxin E-cadherin. Xie et al. (2004) administered DMA^V at 1,000 ppm in drinking water to v-Ha-*ras* transgenic mice for 17 weeks and after 4 weeks of treatment applied TPA to the skin twice a week. The results were an initial 10% body-weight loss, a cumulative mortality of 20%, hepatic arsenic accumulation, hepatocellular degeneration and foci of inflammation without evidence of hepatic tumors, and hepatic DNA hypomethylation. Hepatic gene-expression profiling showed that DMA^V exposure induced changes consistent with oxidative stress, including induction of heme oxygenase, NAD(P)H:quinone oxidoreductase, and glutathione-*S*-transferase.

Mizoi et al. (2005) found that chronic administration of DMA^V at 400 ppm to mice after their initiation with 4-nitroquinolone 1-oxide (4NQO) significantly increased the number of lung tumors and the percentage of mice that had lung tumors. DMA^V also significantly increased pulmonary 8-oxodG adducts regardless of whether the mice had been treated with 4NQO. Hairless mice treated with DMA^{III} on the skin after initiation with dimethylbenz[*a*]anthracene exhibited a significant increase in epidermal 8-oxodG adducts and skin tumors.

In a 2-year bioassay, F344 rats were exposed to DMA^V at 0, 2, 10, 40, or 100 ppm in drinking water, and C57BL/6 mice were exposed at 0, 8, 40, 200, or 500 ppm (Arnold et al., 2006). The rats developed epithelial carcinomas and papillomas in the urinary bladder and nonneoplastic changes in the kidneys. The mice failed to develop any tumors but exhibited glomerular nephropathy, nephrocalcinosis, and vacuolation of the urinary epithelium. The murine NOEL based on nonneoplastic changes was 40 ppm in males and 8 ppm in females; the rat NOEL based on neoplastic and nonneoplastic changes was 10 ppm in both sexes. In a recent study, Cohen et al. (2007) exposed F344 rats to DMA^V at

2–100 ppm in the diet for 2 years and found an increase in bladder tumors; they postulated that trimethylated forms of arsenic may be responsible for bladder cancer in rats. Similar findings have not been reported in other species. In light of the significant differences in metabolism of arsenic by different species and the lack of supportive data in humans, it cannot be concluded that DMA^V leads to an increase in cancer risk in humans.

Mechanisms

Oxidative stress is a common theme that runs through the literature on the mechanisms of action of arsenic, particularly with regard to cancer in animals, although some studies have suggested that methylated arsenicals (MMA^{III} and DMA^{III}) can induce mutations in mammalian cells at concentrations below those required to produce oxidative stress after in vitro exposures (Klein et al., 2008). Recent studies have shown that mice deficient in DNA-repair enzymes associated with oxidative stress are highly susceptible to formation of tumors, particularly lung tumors, induced by DMA^V (Kinoshita et al., 2007). The chemical reaction of arsenicals with thiol groups in sensitive target tissues, such as red blood cells and kidneys, may also be a mechanism of action of organic arsenicals (Naranmandura and Suzuki, 2008).

The variation in the susceptibility of various animal species to tumor formation caused by inorganic and organic arsenic is thought to depend heavily on differences in metabolism and distribution. Thus, genetic differences may play an important role. Numerous investigators are examining potential human susceptibility factors and gene polymorphisms that may increase a person's risk of cancer and other diseases induced by arsenicals. Several such studies were reported during the update period covered by this update (Hernandez et al., 2008; Huang SK et al., 2008; Huang YK et al., 2008; McCarty et al., 2007; Meza et al., 2007; Steinmaus et al., 2007). However, the studies are in early stages, and it is not possible to identify polymorphisms that may contribute to a person's susceptibility to DMA-induced cancer or tissue injury.

PICLORAM

Chemistry

Picloram (4-amino-3,5,6-trichloropyridine-2-carboxylic acid or 4-amino-3,5,6-trichloropicolinic acid; see chemical structure in Figure 4-5) was used with 2,4-D in the herbicide formulation Agent White, which was sprayed in Vietnam. Picloram is also used commonly in Australia in a formulation with the trade name Tordon 75D®. Tordon 75D contains several chemicals, including 2,4-D, picloram, a surfactant diethyleneglycolmonoethyl ether, and a silicone defoamer. A number

Picloram [1918-02-1]

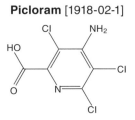

FIGURE 4-5 Structure of picloram.

of studies of picloram used such mixtures as Tordon or other mixtures of 2,4-D and picloram that are similar to Agent White.

Toxicokinetics

The original *VAO* committee reviewed studies of the toxicokinetics of picloram. Studies of animals showed rapid absorption through the gastrointestinal tract and rapid elimination of picloram as the unaltered parent compound in urine. Nolan et al. (1984) examined the toxicokinetics of picloram in six healthy male volunteers who were given single oral doses of 0.5 or 5.0 mg/kg and a dermal dose of 2.0 mg/kg. Picloram was rapidly absorbed in the gavage study and rapidly excreted as unchanged compound in urine. More than 75% of the dose was excreted within 6 hours, and the remainder with an average half-life of 27 hours. On the basis of the quantity of picloram excreted in urine in the skin study, the authors noted that only 0.2% of the picloram applied to the skin was absorbed. Because of its rapid excretion, picloram has low potential to accumulate in humans.

In general, the literature on picloram toxicity continues to be sparse. Studies of humans and animals indicate that picloram is rapidly eliminated as the parent compound. Studies of animals have indicated that picloram is sparingly toxic at high doses.

Toxicity Profile

The original *VAO* committee reviewed studies of the carcinogenicity, genotoxicity, acute toxicity, chronic systemic toxicity, reproductive and developmental toxicity, and immunotoxicity of picloram. In general, there is limited evidence for cancer in some rodent models but not in other species (NCI, 1978). In those studies, there was some concern that contaminants in the picloram (in particular, hexachlorobenzene) might be responsible for the carcinogenicity. Therefore, picloram has not been established as a chemical carcinogen.

There is also no evidence that picloram is a genotoxic agent on the basis of studies conducted by EPA (1988c). Picloram is considered a mild irritant; erythema is seen in rabbits only at high doses. The available information on the acute toxicity of picloram is also paltry. Some neurologic effects—including hyperactivity, ataxia, and tremors—were reported in pregnant rats exposed to picloram at 750 or 1,000 mg/kg (Thompson et al., 1972).

Chronic Systemic Toxicity

Several studies have reported various effects of technical-grade picloram on the livers of rats. In the carcinogenicity bioassay conducted by Stott and colleagues (1990) described above, treatment-related hepatomegaly, hepatocellular swelling, and altered tinctorial properties in the central regions of the liver lobules were noted in the groups exposed at 60 and 200 mg/kg per day. In addition, males and females exposed at the high dose had higher liver weights than controls. The NOEL was 20 mg/kg per day, and the lowest effect level was 60 mg/kg per day for histologic changes in centrilobular hepatocellular tissues. According to EPA, hexachlorobenzene (at 197 ppm) was probably not responsible for the hepatic effects (EPA, 1988c). Gorzinski and colleagues (1987) also reported a dose-related increase in liver weights, hepatocellular hypertrophy, and changes in centrilobular tinctorial properties in male and female F344 rats exposed to picloram at 150 mg/kg per day and higher in the diet for 13 weeks. In a 90-day study, cloudy swelling in the liver cells and bile duct epithelium occurred in male and female F344 rats given 0.3% or 1% technical picloram in the diet (EPA, 1988c). Hepatic effects have also been reported in dogs exposed to picloram: increased liver weights were reported in beagles that received 35 mg/kg per day or more in the diet for 6 months (EPA, 1988c). No other effects of chronic exposure to picloram have been reported.

Reproductive and Developmental Toxicity

The reproductive toxicity of picloram was evaluated in a two-generation study; however, too few animals were evaluated, and no toxicity was detected at the highest dose tested, 150 mg/kg per day (EPA, 1988c). Some developmental toxicity was produced in rabbits exposed to picloram by gavage at 400 mg/kg per day on days 6–18 of gestation. Fetal abnormalities included single-litter incidences of forelimb flexure, fused ribs, hypoplastic tail, and omphalocele (John-Greene et al., 1985). Some maternal toxicity was observed at that dose, however, and EPA concluded on the basis of the low-litter incidence of the findings, that the malformations were not treatment-related (EPA, 1988c). No teratogenic effects were produced in the offspring of rats given picloram by gavage at up to 1,000 mg/kg per day on days 6–15 of gestation, although the occurrence of bilateral accessory ribs was significantly increased (Thompson et al., 1972).

Immunotoxicity

Studies of the potential immunotoxicity of picloram included dermal sensitization and rodent immunoassays. In one study, 53 volunteers received nine 24-hour applications of 0.5 mL of a 2% potassium picloram solution on the skin of both upper arms. Each volunteer received challenge doses 17–24 days later. The formulation of picloram (its potassium salt) was not a skin sensitizer or an irritant (EPA, 1988c). In a similar study, a 5% solution of picloram (M-2439, Tordon 101 formulation) produced slight dermal irritation and a sensitization response in 6 of the 69 volunteers exposed. When the individual components of M-2439—picloram, triisopropanolamine (TIPA) salt, and 2,4-D TIPA salt—were tested separately, no sensitization reaction occurred (EPA, 1988c). Tordon K+, but not technical-grade picloram, was also found to be a skin sensitizer in guinea pigs (EPA, 1988c). CD1 mice exposed to Tordon 202C (94% 2,4-D and 6% picloram) had no consistent adverse effects on antibody responses (Blakley, 1997).

Mechanisms

There are no well-characterized mechanisms of toxicity known for picloram, and therefore they are not discussed here.

REFERENCES[1]

Adachi J, Mori Y, Matsui S, Takigami H, Fujino J, Kitagawa H, Miller C III, Kato T, Saeki K, Matsuda T. 2001. Indirubin and indigo are potent aryl hydrocarbon receptor ligands present in human urine. *Journal of Biological Chemistry* 276:31475–31478.

Adachi-Yamada T, Harumoto T, Sakurai K, Ueda R, Saigo K, O'Connor MB, Nakato H. 2005. Wing-to-leg homeosis by spineless causes apoptosis regulated by fish-lips, a novel leucine-rich repeat transmembrane protein. *Molecular & Cellular Biology* 25(8):3140–3150.

Adair BM, Moore T, Conklin SD, Creed JT, Wolf DC, Thomas DJ. 2007. Tissue distribution and urinary excretion of dimethylated arsenic and its metabolites in dimethylarsinic acid- or arsenate-treated rats. *Toxicology and Applied Pharmacology* 222(2):235–242.

An Y, Kato K, Nakano M, Otsu H, Okada S, Yamanaka K. 2005. Specific induction of oxidative stress in terminal bronchiolar Clara cells during dimethylarsenic-induced lung tumor promoting process in mice. *Cancer Letters* 230(1):57–64.

Arnold EK, Beasley VR, Parker AJ, Stedelin JR. 1991. 2,4-D toxicosis II: A pilot study of clinical pathologic and electroencephalographic effects and residues of 2,4-D in orally dosed dogs. *Veterinary and Human Toxicology* 33:446–449.

Arnold LL, Eldan M, Nyska A, van Gemert M, Cohen SM. 2006. Dimethylarsinic acid: Results of chronic toxicity/oncogenicity studies in F344 rats and in B6C3F1 mice. *Toxicology* 223(1-2): 82–100.

---

[1]Throughout the report the same alphabetic indicator following year of publication is used consistently for the same article when there were multiple citations by the same first author in a given year. The convention of assigning the alphabetic indicator in order of citation in a given chapter is not followed.

Arsenescu V, Arsenescu RI, King V, Swanson H, Cassis LA. 2008. Polychlorinated biphenyl–77 induces adipocyte differentiation and proinflammatory adipokines and promotes obesity and atherosclerosis. *Environmental Health Perspectives* 116(6):761–768.

Aylward LL, Brunet RC, Carrier G, Hays SM, Cushing CA, Needham LL, Patterson DG Jr, Gerthoux PM, Brambilla P, Mocarelli P. 2005a. Concentration-dependent TCDD elimination kinetics in humans: Toxicokinetic modeling for moderately to highly exposed adults from Seveso, Italy, and Vienna, Austria, and impact on dose estimates for the NIOSH cohort. *Journal of Exposure Analysis and Environment Epidemiology* 15(1):51–65.

Aylward LL, Brunet RC, Starr TB, Carrier G, Delzell E, Cheng H, Beall C. 2005b. Exposure reconstruction for the TCDD-exposed NIOSH cohort using a concentration- and age-dependent model of elimination. *Risk Analysis* 25(4):945–956.

Bacsi SG, Reisz-Porszasz S, Hankinson O. 1995. Orientation of the heterodimeric aryl hydrocarbon (dioxin) receptor complex on its asymmetric DNA recognition sequence. *Molecular Pharmacology* 47(3):432–438.

Banks YB, Birnbaum LS. 1991. Absorption of 2,3,7,8-tetrachlorodibenzo-*p*-dioxin (TCDD) after low dose dermal exposure. *Toxicology and Applied Pharmacology* 107(2):302–310.

Birnbaum L, Harris M, Stocking L, Clark A, Morrissey R. 1989. Retinoic acid and 2,3,7,8-tetrachlorodibenzo-*p*-dioxin selectively enhance teratogenesis in C57BL/6N mice. *Toxicology and Applied Pharmacology* 98:487–500.

Biswas G, Srinivasan S, Anandatheerthavarada HK, Avadhani NG. 2008. Dioxin-mediated tumor progression through activation of mitochondria-to-nucleus stress signaling. *Proceedings of the National Academy of Sciences of the United States of America* 105(1):186–191.

Blakley BR. 1997. Effect of Roundup and Tordon 202C herbicides on antibody production in mice. *Veterinary and Human Toxicology* 39(4):204–206.

Boutros PC, Moffat ID, Franc MA, Tijet N, Tuomisto J, Pohjanvirta R, Okey AB. 2004. Dioxin-responsive AHRE–II gene battery: Identification by phylogenetic footprinting. *Biochemical and Biophysical Research Communications* 321(3):707–715.

Boverhof DR, Burgoon LD, Williams KJ, Zacharewski TR. 2008. Inhibition of estrogen-mediated uterine gene expression responses by dioxin. *Molecular Pharmacology* 73(1):82–93.

Bowman RE, Schantz SL, Weerasinghe NCA, Gross ML, Barsotti DA. 1989. Chronic dietary intake of 2,3,7,8-tetrachlorodibenzo-*p*-dioxin (TCDD) at 5 and 25 parts per trillion in the monkey: TCDD kinetics and dose–effect estimate of reproductive toxicity. *Chemosphere* 18:243–252.

Brand RM, Spalding M, Mueller C. 2002. Sunscreens can increase dermal penetration of 2,4-dichlorophenoxyacetic acid. *Journal of Toxicology–Clinical Toxicology* 40(7):827–832.

Bredhult C, Backlin BM, Olovsson M. 2007. Effects of some endocrine disruptors on the proliferation and viability of human endometrial endothelial cells in vitro. *Reproductive Toxicology* 23(4):550–559.

Burbach KM, Poland A, Bradfield CA. 1992. Cloning of the Ah–receptor cDNA reveals a distinctive ligand-activated transcription factor. *Proceedings of the National Academy of Sciences of the United States of America* 89:8185–8189.

Burchiel SW, Thompson TA, Lauer FT, Oprea TI. 2008. Corrigendum to "Activation of dioxin response element (DRE)–associated genes by benzo(a)pyrene 3,6-quinone and benzo(a)pyrene 1,6-quinone in MCF-10A human mammary epithelial cells." *Toxicology and Applied Pharmacology* 226(3):345–346.

Carrier G, Brunet RC, Brodeur J. 1995. Modeling of the toxicokinetics of polychlorinated dibenzo-*p*-dioxins and dibenzofurans in mammalians, including humans. II. Kinetics of absorption and disposition of PCDDs/PCDFs. *Toxicology and Applied Pharmacology* 131(2):267–276.

Carver L, Bradfield C. 1997. Ligand-dependent interaction of the aryl hydrocarbon receptor with a novel immunophilin homolog in vivo. *Journal of Biological Chemistry* 272:11452–11456.

Carver L, Jackiw V, Bradfield C. 1994. The 90-kDa heat shock protein is essential for Ah receptor signaling in a yeast expression system. *Journal of Biological Chemistry* 269:30109–30112.

Chiaro CR, Morales JL, Prabhu KS, Perdew GH. 2008. Leukotriene A4 metabolites are endogenous ligands for the Ah receptor. *Biochemistry* 47(32):8445–8455.

Cohen SM, Arnold LL, Uzvolgyi E, Cano M, St John M, Yamamoto S, Lu X, Le XC. 2002. Possible role of dimethylarsinous acid in dimethylarsinic acid–induced urothelial toxicity and regeneration in the rat. *Chemical Research in Toxicology* 15(9):1150–1157.

Cohen SM, Arnold LL, Eldan M, Lewis AS, Beck BD. 2006. Methylated arsenicals: The implications of metabolism and carcinogenicity studies in rodents to human risk assessment. *Critical Reviews in Toxicology* 36(2):99–133.

Cohen SM, Ohnishi T, Arnold LL, Le XC. 2007. Arsenic-induced bladder cancer in an animal model. *Toxicology and Applied Pharmacology* 222(3):258–263.

Collins LL, Williamson MA, Thompson BD, Dever DP, Gasiewicz TA, Opanashuk LA. 2008. 2,3,7,8-tetracholorodibenzo-*p*-dioxin exposure disrupts granule neuron precursor maturation in the developing mouse cerebellum. *Toxicological Sciences* 103(1):125–136.

Coumailleau P, Poellinger L, Gustafsson J, Whitelaw M. 1995. Definition of a minimal domain of the dioxin receptor that is associated with hsp90 and maintains wild type ligand binding affinity and specificity. *Journal of Biological Chemistry* 270:25291–25300.

Cui X, Kobayashi Y, Hayakawa T, Hirano S. 2004. Arsenic speciation in bile and urine following oral and intravenous exposure to inorganic and organic arsenics in rats. *Toxicological Sciences* 82(2):478–487.

Davarinos N, Pollenz R. 1999. Aryl hydrocarbon receptor imported into the nucleus following ligand binding is rapidly degraded via the cytosplasmic proteasome following nuclear export. *Journal of Biological Chemistry* 274:28708–28715.

Denison M, Nagy S. 2003. Activation of the aryl hydrocarbon receptor by structurally diverse exogenous and endogenous chemicals. *Annual Review of Pharmacology Toxicology* 43:309–334.

Dési I, Sos J, Nikolits I. 1962a. New evidence concerning the nervous site of action of a chemical herbicide causing professional intoxication. *Acta Physiologica Academiae Scientiarum Hungaricae* 22:73–80.

Dési I, Sos J, Olasz J, Sule F, Markus V. 1962b. Nervous system effects of a chemical herbicide. *Archives of Environmental Health* 4:95–102.

DeVito M, Birnbaum L. 1995. The importance of pharmacokinetics in determining the relative potency of 2,3,7,8-tetrachlorodibenzo-*p*-dioxin and 2,3,7,8-tetrachlorodibenzofuran. *Fundamental and Applied Toxicology* 24:145–148.

Di Giampaolo L, Di Gioacchino M, Qiao N, Travaglini P, D'Intino A, Kouri M, Ponti J, Castellani ML, Reale M, Gabriele E, Boscolo P. 2004. "In vitro" effects of different arsenic compounds on PBMC (preliminary study). *Giornale Italiano di Medicina del Lavoro Ed Ergonomia* 26(3): 183–186.

Diliberto JJ, Devito MJ, Ross DG, Birnbaum LS. 2001. Subchronic exposure of [3H]-2,3,7,8-tetrachlorodibenzo-*p*-dioxin (TCDD) in female B6C3F1 mice: Relationship of steady-state levels to disposition and metabolism. *Toxicological Sciences* 61:241–255.

Dolwick KM, Swanson HI, Bradfield CA. 1993. In vitro analysis of Ah receptor domains involved in ligand-activated DNA recognition. *Proceedings of the National Academy of Sciences (USA)* 90:8566–8570.

Dong B, Matsumura F. 2008. Roles of cytosolic phospholipase A2 and Src kinase in the early action of 2,3,7,8-tetrachlorodibenzo-*p*-dioxin through a nongenomic pathway in MCF10A cells. *Molecular Pharmacology* 74(1):255–263.

Dopp E, Hartmann LM, Florea AM, von Recklinghausen U, Pieper R, Shokouhi B, Rettenmeier AW, Hirner AV, Obe G. 2004. Uptake of inorganic and organic derivatives of arsenic associated with induced cytotoxic and genotoxic effects in Chinese hamster ovary (CHO) cells. *Toxicology and Applied Pharmacology* 201(2):156–165.

Dopp E, Hartmann LM, von Recklinghausen U, Florea AM, Rabieh S, Zimmermann U, Shokouhi B, Yadav S, Hirner AV, Rettenmeier AW. 2005. Forced uptake of trivalent and pentavalent methylated and inorganic arsenic and its cyto-/genotoxicity in fibroblasts and hepatoma cells. *Toxicological Sciences* 87(1):46–56.

Dragin N, Dalton TP, Miller ML, Shertzer HG, Nebert DW. 2006. For dioxin-induced birth defects, mouse or human CYP1A2 in maternal liver protects whereas mouse CYP1A1 and CYP1B1 are inconsequential. *Journal of Biological Chemistry* 281(27):18591–18600.

Dvorak Z, Vrzal R, Pavek P, Ulrichova J. 2008. An evidence for regulatory cross-talk between aryl hydrocarbon receptor and glucocorticoid receptor in HepG2 cells. *Physiological Research* 57(3):427–435.

El-Masri HA, Kenyon EM. 2008. Development of a human physiologically based pharmacokinetic (PBPK) model for inorganic arsenic and its mono- and di-methylated metabolites. *Journal of Pharmacokinetics and Pharmacodynamics* 35(1):31–68.

Ema M, Sogawa K, Watanabe N, Chujoh Y, Matsushita N, Gotoh O, Funae Y, Fujii-Kuriyama Y. 1992. cDNA cloning and structure of mouse putative Ah receptor. *Biochemical and Biophysical Research Communications* 184:246–253.

Emond C, Michalek JE, Birnbaum LS, DeVito MJ. 2005. Comparison of the use of physiologically based pharmacokinetic model and a classical pharmacokinetic model for dioxin exposure assessments. *Environmental Health Perspectives* 113(12):1666–1668.

Emond C, Birnbaum LS, DeVito MJ. 2006. Use of a physiologically based pharmacokinetic model for rats to study the influence of body fat mass and induction of CYP1A2 on the pharmacokinetics of TCDD. *Environmental Health Perspectives* 114(9):1394–1400.

EPA (US Environmental Protection Agency). 1988c. *Guidance for the Reregistration of Pesticide Products Containing Picloram as the Active Ingredient.* Washington, DC: EPA, Office of Pesticide Programs.

Evans BR, Karchner SI, Allan LL, Pollenz RS, Tanguay RL, Jenny MJ, Sherr DH, Hahn ME. 2008. Repression of aryl hydrocarbon receptor (AHR) signaling by AHR repressor: Role of DNA binding and competition for AHR nuclear translocator. *Molecular Pharmacology* 73(2):387–398.

Fernandez-Salguero PM, Hilbert DM, Rudikoff S, Ward JM, Gonzalez FJ. 1996. Aryl-hydrocarbon receptor-deficient mice are resistant to 2,3,7,8-tetrachlorodibenzo-*p*-dioxin-induced toxicity. *Toxicology and Applied Pharmacology* 140:173–179.

Fernandez-Salguero PM, Ward JM, Sundberg JP, Gonzalez FJ. 1997. Lesions of aryl-hydrocarbon receptor-deficient mice. *Veterinary Pathology* 34(6):605–614.

Flesch-Janys D, Becher H, Gurn D, Jung D, Konietzko J, Manz A, Papke O. 1996. Elimination of polychlorinated dibenzo-*p*-dioxins and dibenzofurans in occupationally exposed persons. *Journal of Toxicology and Environmental Health* 47(4):363–378.

Fukunaga BN, Probst MR, Reisz-Porszasz S, Hankinson O. 1995. Identification of functional domains of the aryl hydrocarbon receptor. *Journal of Biology and Chemistry* 270:29270–29278.

Funatake CJ, Marshall NB, Kerkvliet NI. 2008. 2,3,7,8-tetrachlorodibenzo-*p*-dioxin alters the differentiation of alloreactive CD8+ T cells toward a regulatory T cell phenotype by a mechanism that is dependent on aryl hydrocarbon receptor in CD4+ T cells. *Journal of Immunotoxicology* 5(1):81–91.

Gasiewicz T, Geiger L, Rucci G, Neal R. 1983. Distribution, excretion, and metabolism of 2,3,7,8-tetrachlorodibenzo-*p*-dioxin in C57BL/6J, DBA/2J, and B6D2F1/J mice. *Drug Metabolism and Disposition* 11:397–403.

Gehring PJ, Kramer CG, Schwetz BA, Rose JQ, Rowe VK. 1973. The fate of 2,4,5-trichlorophenoxyacetic acid (2,4,5-T) following oral administration to man. *Toxicology and Applied Pharmacology* 26:352–361.

Geusau A, Schmaldienst S, Derfler K, Päpke O, Abraham K. 2002. Severe 2,3,7,8-tetrachlorodibenzo-*p*-dioxin (TCDD) intoxication: Kinetics and trials to enhance elimination in two patients. *Archives of Toxicology* 76:316–325.

Gill BC, Jeon CH, Sung HN, Kim HL, Jin DW, Park JH. 2008. 2,3,7,8-tetrachlorodibenzo-*p*-dioxin modulates the expression of cKrox and Runx3, transcription regulatory factors controlling the lineage commitment of $CD4^+CD8^+$ into CD4 and CD8 thymocytes, respectively. *Toxicology Letters* 180(3):189–195.

Gómez SE, Del Razo LM, Muñoz Sanchez JL. 2005. Induction of DNA damage by free radicals generated either by organic or inorganic arsenic (As^{III}, MMA^{III}, and DMA^{III}) in cultures of B and T lymphocytes. *Biological Trace Element Research* 108(1-3):115–126.

Goryo K, Suzuki A, Del Carpio CA, Siizaki K, Kuriyama E, Mikami Y, Kinoshita K, Yasumoto K, Rannug A, Miyamoto A, Fujii-Kuriyama Y, Sogawa K. 2007. Identification of amino acid residues in the Ah receptor involved in ligand binding. *Biochemical and Biophysical Research Communications* 354:396–402.

Gorzinski SJ, Johnson KA, Campbell RA, Landry TD. 1987. Dietary toxicity of picloram herbicide in rats. *Journal of Toxicology and Environmental Health* 20:367–377.

Guo SW. 2004. The link between exposure to dioxin and endometriosis: A critical reappraisal of primate data. *Gynecologic and Obstetric Investigation* 57(3):157–173.

Haarmann-Stemmann T, Bothe H, Kohli A, Sydlik U, Abel J, Fritsche E. 2007. Analysis of the transcriptional regulation and molecular function of the aryl hydrocarbon receptor repressor in human cell lines. *Drug Metabolism and Disposition* 35(12):2262–2269.

Hahn ME. 2001. Dioxin toxicology and the aryl hydrocarbon receptor: Insights from fish and other non-traditional models. *Marine Biotechnology (New York, NY)* 3(Supplement 1):S224–S238.

Harrigan JA, Vezina CM, McGarrigle BP, Ersing N, Box HC, Maccubbin AE, Olson JR. 2004. DNA adduct formation in precision-cut rat liver and lung slices exposed to benzo[a]pyrene. *Toxicological Sciences* 77(2):307–314.

Hayes HM, Tarone RE, Cantor KP, Jessen CR, McCurnin DM, Richardson RC. 1991. Case–control study of canine malignant lymphoma: Positive association with dog owner's use of 2,4-D herbicides. *Journal of the National Cancer Institute* 83(17):1226–1231.

Hayes HM, Tarone RE, Cantor KP. 1995. On the association between canine malignant lymphoma and opportunity for exposure to 2,4-dichlorophenoxyacetic acid. *Environmental Research* 70(2): 119–125.

Hayes KR, Zastrow GM, Nukaya M, Pande K, Glover E, Maufort JP, Liss AL, Liu Y, Moran SM, Vollrath AL, Bradfield CA. 2007. Hepatic transcriptional networks induced by exposure to 2,3,7,8-tetrachlorodibenzo-*p*-dioxin. *Chemical Research in Toxicology* 20(11):1573–1581.

Hazleton Laboratories America. 1987. Oncogenicity Study in Mice with 2,4-Dichlorophenoxyacetic Acid (2,4-D). Final Report. Prepared for the Industry Task Force on 2,4-D Research Data.

Henderson L, Patterson DJ. 1988. Distribution of 2,3,7,8-tetrachlorodibenzo-*p*-dioxin in human whole blood and its association with, and extractability from, lipoproteins. *Bulletin of Environmental Contamination and Toxicology* 40(4):604–611.

Hernandez A, Xamena N, Surralles J, Sekaran C, Tokunaga H, Quinteros D, Creus A, Marcos R. 2008. Role of the Met(287)Thr polymorphism in the AS3MT gene on the metabolic arsenic profile. *Mutation Research* 637(1-2):80–92.

Hestermann E, Brown M. 2003. Agonist and chemopreventative ligands induce differential transcriptional cofactor recruitment by aryl hydrocarbon receptor. *Molecular and Cellular Biology* 7920–7925.

Hines CJ, Deddens JA, Striley CA, Biagini RE, Shoemaker DA, Brown KK, Mackenzie BA, Hull RD. 2003. Biological monitoring for selected herbicide biomarkers in the urine of exposed custom applicators: Application of mixed-effect models. *Annals of Occupational Hygiene* 47(6): 503–517.

Hoffman EC, Reyes H, Chu FF, Sander F, Conley LH, Brooks BA, Hankinson O. 1991. Cloning of a factor required for activity of the Ah (dioxin) receptor. *Science* 252:954–958.

Hollingshead BD, Beischlag TV, Dinatale BC, Ramadoss P, Perdew GH. 2008. Inflammatory signaling and aryl hydrocarbon receptor mediate synergistic induction of interleukin 6 in MCF-7 cells. *Cancer Research* 68(10):3609–3617.

Huang SK, Chiu AW-H, Pu Y-S, Huang Y-K, Chung C-J, Tsai H-J, Yang M-H, Chen C-J, Hsueh Y-M. 2008. Arsenic methylation capability, heme oxygenase-1 and NADPH quinone oxidoreductase-1 genetic polymorphisms and the stage and grade of urothelial carcinomas. *Urologia Internationalis* 80(4):405–412.

Huang X, Powell-Coffman JA, Jin Y. 2004. The AHR-1 aryl hydrocarbon receptor and its co-factor the AHA-1 aryl hydrocarbon receptor nuclear translocator specify GABAergic neuron cell fate in C. elegans. *Development* 131(4):819–828.

Huang YK, Pu YS, Chung CJ, Shiue HS, Yang MH, Chen CJ, Hsueh YM. 2008. Plasma folate level, urinary arsenic methylation profiles, and urothelial carcinoma susceptibility. *Food and Chemical Toxicology* 46(3):929–938.

Huff J, Lucier G, Tritscher A. 1994. Carcinogenicity of TCDD: Experimental, mechanistic, and epidemiologic evidence. *Annual Review of Pharmacology and Toxicology* 34:343–372.

Hurst CH, Abbott BD, DeVito MJ, Birnbaum LS. 1998. 2,3,7,8-Tetrachlorodibenzo-*p*-dioxin in pregnant Long Evans rats: Disposition to maternal and embryo/fetal tissues. *Toxicological Sciences* 45(2):129–136.

IOM (Institute of Medicine). 1994. *Veterans and Agent Orange: Health Effects of Herbicides Used in Vietnam*. Washington, DC: National Academy Press.

IOM. 1996. *Veterans and Agent Orange: Update 1996*. Washington, DC: National Academy Press.

IOM. 1999. *Veterans and Agent Orange: Update 1998*. Washington, DC: National Academy Press.

IOM. 2001. *Veterans and Agent Orange: Update 2000*. Washington, DC: National Academy Press.

IOM. 2003. *Veterans and Agent Orange: Update 2002*. Washington, DC: The National Academies Press.

IOM. 2005. *Veterans and Agent Orange: Update 2004*. Washington, DC: The National Academies Press.

IOM. 2006. *Health Risks from Dioxin and Related Compounds: Evaluation of the EPA Reassessment*. Washington, DC: The National Academies Press.

IOM. 2007. *Veterans and Agent Orange: Update 2006*. Washington, DC: The National Academies Press.

Israel DI, Whitlock JP Jr. 1983. Induction of mRNA specific for cytochrome P1-450 in wild type and variant mouse hepatoma cells. *Journal of Biological Chemistry* 258:10390–10394.

Israel DI, Whitlock JP Jr. 1984. Regulation of cytochrome P1-450 gene transcription by 2,3,7,8-tetrachlorodibenzo-*p*-dioxin in wild type and variant mouse hepatoma cells. *Journal of Biological Chemistry* 259:5400–5402.

Ito T, Inouye K, Nohara K, Tohyama C, Fujimaki H. 2008. TCDD exposure exacerbates atopic dermatitis-related inflammation in NC/Nga mice. *Toxicology Letters* 177(1):31–37.

Jia G, Sone H, Nishimura N, Satoh M, Tohyama C. 2004. Metallothionein (I/II) suppresses genotoxicity caused by dimethylarsinic acid. *International Journal of Oncology* 25(2):325–333.

John-Greene JA, Ouellette JH, Jeffries TK, Johnson KA, Rao KS. 1985. Teratological evaluation of picloram potassium salt in rabbits. *Journal of Food and Chemical Toxicology* 23:753–756.

Jones S. 2004. An overview of the basic helix–loop–helix proteins. *Genome Biology* 5:226.

Kaneene JB, Miller R. 1999. Re-analysis of 2,4-D use and the occurrence of canine malignant lymphoma. *Veterinary and Human Toxicology* 41(3):164–170.

Kazlauskas A, Poellinger L, Pongratz I. 1999. Evidence that the Co-chaperone p23 regulates ligand responsiveness of the dioxin (Aryl hydrocarbon) receptor. *Journal of Biological Chemistry* 274:13519–13524.

Kimura A, Naka T, Nohara K, Fujii–Kuriyama Y, Kishimoto T. 2008. Aryl hydrocarbon receptor regulates Stat1 activation and participates in the development of Th17 cells. *Proceedings of the National Academy of Sciences of the United States of America* 105(28):9721–9726.

Kinoshita A, Wanibuchi H, Wei M, Yunoki T, Fukushima S. 2007. Elevation of 8-hydroxydeoxy-guanosine and cell proliferation via generation of oxidative stress by organic arsenicals contributes to their carcinogenicity in the rat liver and bladder. *Toxicology and Applied Pharmacology* 221(3):295–305.

Klein OD, Kostiner DR, Weisiger K, Moffatt E, Lindeman N, Goodman S, Tuchman M, Packman S. 2008. Acute fatal presentation of ornithine transcarbamylase deficiency in a previously healthy male. *Hepatology International* 2(3):390–394.

Kohli JD, Khanna RN, Gupta BN, Dhar MM, Tandon JS, Sircar KP. 1974. Absorption and excretion of 2,4,5-trichlorophenoxy acetic acid in man. *Archives Internationales de Pharmacodynamie et de Therapie* 210:250–255.

Kojima C, Qu W, Waalkes MP, Himeno S, Sakurai T. 2006. Chronic exposure to methylated arsenicals stimulates arsenic excretion pathways and induces arsenic tolerance in rat liver cells. *Toxicological Sciences* 91(1):70–81.

Koshakji RP, Harbison RD, Bush MT. 1984. Studies on the merabolic fate of [14C] 2,3,7,8-tetrachlorodibenzo-*p*-dioxin (TCDD) in the mouse. *Toxicology and Applied Pharmacology* 73:69–77.

Kruger K, Gruner J, Madeja M, Hartmann LM, Hirner AV, Binding N, Muhoff U. 2006. Blockade and enhancement of glutamate receptor responses in Xenopus oocytes by methylated arsenicals. *Archives of Toxicology* 80(8):492–501.

Kumagai S, Koda S. 2005. Polychlorinated dibenzo-*p*-dioxin and dibenzofuran concentrations in serum samples of workers at an infectious waste incineration plant in Japan. *Journal of Occupational and Environmental Hygiene* 2(2):120–125.

Kumar M, Ramadoss P, Reen R, Vanden Heuvel J, Perdew G. 2001. The Q-rich sub-domain of the human Ah receptor transactivation domain is required for dioxin-mediated transcriptional activity. *Journal of Biology and Chemistry* 276(45):42302–42310.

Lahvis G, Bradfield C. 1998. Ahr null alleles: Distinctive or different? *Biochemical Pharmacology* 56(7):781–787.

Lahvis GP, Pyzalski RW, Glover E, Pitot HC, McElwee MK, Bradfield CA. 2005. The aryl hydrocarbon receptor is required for developmental closure of the ductus venosus in the neonatal mouse. *Molecular Pharmacology* 67(3):714–720.

Lee JA, Hwang JA, Sung HN, Jeon CH, Gill BC, Youn HJ, Park JH. 2007. 2,3,7,8-tetrachlorodibenzo-*p*-dioxin modulates functional differentiation of mouse bone marrow-derived dendritic cells downregulation of RelB by 2,3,7,8-tetrachlorodibenzo-*p*-dioxin. *Toxicology Letters* 173(1):31–40.

Leung HW, Kerger BD, Paustenbach DJ. 2006. Elimination half-lives of selected polychlorinated dibenzodioxins and dibenzofurans in breast-fed human infants. *Journal of Toxicology and Environmental Health, Part A* 69(6):437–443.

Li W, Vogel CFA, Matsumura F. 2007. Studies on the cell treatment conditions to elicit lipolytic responses from 3T3-L1 adipocytes to TCDD, 2,3,7,8-tetrachlorodibenzo-*p*-dioxin. *Journal of Cellular Biochemistry* 102(2):389–402.

Lin PH, Lin CH, Huang CC, Chuang MC, Lin P. 2007. 2,3,7,8-tetrachlorodibenzo-*p*-dioxin (TCDD) induces oxidative stress, DNA strand breaks, and poly(ADP-ribose) polymerase-1 activation in human breast carcinoma cell lines. *Toxicology Letters* 172(3):146–158.

Liu X, Jefcoate C. 2006. 2,3,7,8-tetrachlorodibenzo-*p*-dioxin and epidermal growth factor cooperatively suppress peroxisome proliferator-activated receptor-gamma1 stimulation and restore focal adhesion complexes during adipogenesis: Selective contributions of Src, Rho, and Erk distinguish these overlapping processes in C3H10T1/2 cells. *Molecular Pharmacology* 70(6):1902–1915.

Lu F, Zahid M, Saeed M, Cavalieri EL, Rogan EG. 2007. Estrogen metabolism and formation of estrogen-DNA adducts in estradiol-treated MCF-10F cells. The effects of 2,3,7,8-tetrachlorodibenzo-*p*-dioxin induction and catechol-O-methyltransferase inhibition. *Journal of Steroid Biochemistry and Molecular Biology* 105(1–5):150–158.

Lu M, Wang H, Li XF, Lu X, Cullen WR, Arnold LL, Cohen SM, Le XC. 2004. Evidence of hemoglobin binding to arsenic as a basis for the accumulation of arsenic in rat blood. *Chemical Research in Toxicology* 17(12):1733–1742.

Lusska A, Shen E, Whitlock JP Jr. 1993. Protein-DNA interactions at a dioxin-responsive enhancer. *Journal of Biological Chemistry* 268:6575–6580.

Ma Q, Whitlock J Jr. 1997. A novel cytoplasmic protein that interacts with the Ah receptor, contains tetratricopeptide repeat motifs, and augments the transcriptional response to 2,3,7,8-tetrachlorodibenzo-*p*-dioxin. *Journal of Biological Chemistry* 272(14):8878–8884.

Marquez-Bravo LG, Gierthy JF. 2008. Differential expression of estrogen receptor alpha (ERalpha) protein in MCF-7 breast cancer cells chronically exposed to TCDD. *Journal of Cellular Biochemistry* 103(2):636–647.

Martinez JM, Afshari CA, Bushel PR, Masuda A, Takahashi T, Walker NJ. 2002. Differential toxicogenomic responses to 2,3,7,8-tetrachlorodibenzo-*p*-dioxin in malignant and nonmalignant human airway epithelial cells. *Toxicological Sciences* 69(2):409–423.

McCarty KM, Chen YC, Quamruzzaman Q, Rahman M, Mahiuddin G, Hsueh YM, Su L, Smith T, Ryan L, Christiani DC. 2007. Arsenic methylation, GSTT1, GSTM1, GSTP1 polymorphisms, and skin lesions. *Environmental Health Perspectives* 115(3):341–345.

McMillan BJ, Bradfield CA. 2007. The aryl hydrocarbon receptor is activated by modified low-density lipoprotein. *Proceedings of the National Academy of Sciences of the United States of America* 104(4):1412–1417.

Meza M, Gandolfi AJ, Klimecki WT. 2007. Developmental and genetic modulation of arsenic biotransformation: A gene by environment interaction? *Toxicology and Applied Pharmacology* 222(3):381–387.

Michalek JE, Pirkle JL, Needham LL, Patterson DG Jr, Caudill SP, Tripathi RC, Mocarelli P. 2002. Pharmacokinetics of 2,3,7,8-tetrachlorodibenzo-*p*-dioxin in Seveso adults and veterans of Operation Ranch Hand. *Journal of Exposure Analysis and Environmental Epidemiology* 12(1):44–53.

Mitchell KA, Lockhart CA, Huang G, Elferink CJ. 2006. Sustained aryl hydrocarbon receptor activity attenuates liver regeneration. *Molecular Pharmacology* 70(1):163–170.

Mizoi M, Takabayashi F, Nakano M, An Y, Sagesaka Y, Kato K, Okada S, Yamanaka K. 2005. The role of trivalent dimethylated arsenic in dimethylarsinic acid-promoted skin and lung tumorigenesis in mice: Tumor-promoting action through the induction of oxidative stress. *Toxicology Letters* 158(2):87–94.

Mouron SA, Grillo CA, Dulout FN, Golijow CD. 2005. DNA-protein cross-links and sister chromatid exchanges induced by dimethylarsinic acid in human fibroblasts cells. *Mutation Research* 581(1-2):83–90.

Naranmandura H, Suzuki KT. 2008. Formation of dimethylthioarsenicals in red blood cells. *Toxicology and Applied Pharmacology* 227(3):390–399.

NCI (National Cancer Institute). 1978. *Bioassay of Picloram for Possible Carcinogenicity. Report Series No. 23*. Bethesda, MD: NCI.

Nebert DW, Negishi M, Lang M, Hjelmeland L, Eisen H. 1982. The Ah locus, a multigene family necessary for survival in a chemically adverse environment: Comparison with the immune system. *Advances in Genetics* 21:1–52.

Nebert DW, Roe AL, Dieter MZ, Solis WA, Yang Y, Dalton TP. 2000. Role of the aromatic hydrocarbon receptor and [Ah] gene battery in the oxidative stress response, cell cycle control, and apoptosis. *Biochemical Pharmacology* 59(1):65–85.

Needham L, Gerthoux P, Patterson D, Brambilla P, Pirkle J, Tramacere P, Turner W, Beretta C, Sampson E, Mocarelli P. 1994. Half-life of 2,3,7,8-tetrachlorodibenzo-*p*-dioxin in serum of Seveso adults: Interim report. *Organohalogen Compounds* 21:81–85.

Neubert D, Wiesmuller T, Abraham K, Krowke R, Hagenmaier H. 1990. Persistence of various polychlorinated dibenzo-*p*-dioxins and dibenzofurans (PCDDs and PCDFs) in hepatic and adipose tissue of marmoset monkeys. *Archives of Toxicology* 64:431–442.

Nolan R, Smith F, Hefner J. 1979. Elimination and tissue distribution of 2,3,7,8-tetrachlorodibenzo-para-dixion (TCDD) in female guinea-pigs following a single oral dose. *Toxicology and Applied Pharmacology* 48(1):A162.

Nolan RJ, Freshour NL, Kastl PE, Saunders JH. 1984. Pharmacokinetics of picloram in male volunteers. *Toxicology and Applied Pharmacology* 76:264–269.

NRC (National Research Council). 1999a. *Arsenic in Drinking Water.* Washington, DC: National Academy Press.

NRC. 2001. *Arsenic in Drinking Water: Update 2001.* Washington, DC: National Academy Press.

Oesch-Bartlomowicz B, Huelster A, Wiss O, Antoniou-Lipfert P, Dietrich C, Arand M, Weiss C, Bockamp E, Oesch F. 2005. Aryl hydrocarbon receptor activation by cAMP vs. dioxin: Divergent signaling pathways. *Proceedings of the National Academy Sciences of the United States of America* 102:9218–9223.

Pegram RA, Diliberto JJ, Moore TC, Gao P, Birnbaum LS. 1995. 2,3,7,8-tetrachlorodibenzo-*p*-dioxin (TCDD) distribution and cytochrome P4501A induction in young adult and senescent male mice. *Toxicology Letters* 76:119–126.

Petrulis J, Kusnadi A, Ramadoss P, Hollingshead B, Perdew G. 2003. The hsp90 co-chaperone XAP2 alters importin beta recognition of the bipartite nuclear localization signal of the Ah receptor and represses transcriptional activity. *Journal of Biological Chemistry* 278:2677–2685.

Piaggi S, Novelli M, Martino L, Masini M, Raggi C, Orciuolo E, Masiello P, Casini A, De Tata V. 2007. Cell death and impairment of glucose-stimulated insulin secretion induced by 2,3,7,8-tetrachlorodibenzo-*p*-dioxin (TCDD) in the beta-cell line INS-1E. *Toxicology and Applied Pharmacology* 220(3):333–340.

Pirkle J, Wolfe W, Patterson D, Needham L, Michalek J, Miner J, Peterson M, Phillips D. 1989. Estimates of the half-life of 2,3,7,8-tetrachlorodibenzo-*p*-dioxin in Vietnam veterans of Operation Ranch Hand. *Journal of Toxicology and Environmental Health* 27:165–171.

Pohjanvirta R, Tuomisto J. 1990. Remarkable residual alterations in responses to feeding regulatory challenges in Han/Wistar rats after recovery from the acute toxicity of 2,3,7,8-tetrachlorodibenzo-*p*-dioxin (TCDD). *Food and Chemical Toxicology* 28:677–686.

Poiger H, Schlatter C. 1986. Pharmacokinetics of 2,3,7,8-TCDD in man. *Chemosphere* 15:1489–1494.

Poland A, Glover E, Kende A. 1976. Stereospecific, high affinity binding of 2,3,7,8-tetrachlorodibenzo-*p*-dioxin by hepatic cytosol. Evidence that the binding species is receptor for induction of aryl hydrocarbon hydroxylase. *Journal of Biological Chemistry* 251:4936–4946.

Poland A, Teitelbaum P, Glover E. 1989. [125I]2-iodo-3,7,8-trichlorodibenzo-*p*-dioxin-binding species in mouse liver induced by agonists for the Ah receptor: Characterization and identification. *Molecular Pharmacology* 36(1):113–120.

Pongratz I, Mason GGF, Poellinger L. 1992. Dual roles of the 90-kDa heat shock protein hsp90 in modulating functional activities of the dioxin receptor. *Journal of Biological Chemistry* 267:13728–13734.

Pont AR, Charron AR, Brand RM. 2004. Active ingredients in sunscreens act as topical penetration enhancers for the herbicide 2,4-dichlorophenoxyacetic acid. *Toxicology and Applied Pharmacology* 195:348–354.

Probst MR, Reisz-Porszasz S, Agbunag RV, Ong MS, Hankinson O. 1993. Role of the aryl hydrocarbon receptor nuclear translocator protein in aryl hydrocarbon (dioxin) receptor action. *Molecular Pharmacology* 44:511–518.

Puga A, Bohm J, Hoffer A, Leikauf G, Shertzer H, Zhou S. 1995. Dioxin alters calcium homeostasis and the regulation of arachidonate metabolism in mouse hepatoma cells. *Proceeding of the 15th International Symposium on Chlorinated Dioxins and Related Compounds* 25:381–386.

Puga A, Maier A, Medvedovic M. 2000. The transcriptional signature of dioxin in human hepatoma hepg2 cells. *Biochemical Pharmacology* 60(8):1129–1142.

Puga A, Sartor MA, Huang MY, Kerzee JK, Wei YD, Tomlinson CR, Baxter CS, Medvedovic M. 2004. Gene expression profiles of mouse aorta and cultured vascular smooth muscle cells differ widely, yet show common responses to dioxin exposure. *Cardiovascular Toxicology* 4(4):385–404.

Qin H, Powell-Coffman JA. 2004. The Caenorhabditis elegans aryl hydrocarbon receptor, AHR-1, regulates neuronal development. *Developmental Biology* 270(1):64–75.

Quintana FJ, Basso AS, Iglesias AH, Korn T, Farez MF, Bettelli E, Caccamo M, Oukka M, Weiner HL. 2008. Control of T(reg) and T(H)17 cell differentiation by the aryl hydrocarbon receptor. *Nature* 453(7191):65–71.

Rizki M, Kossatz E, Velazquez A, Creus A, Farina M, Fortaner S, Sabbioni E, Marcos R. 2006. Metabolism of arsenic in Drosophila melanogaster and the genotoxicity of dimethylarsinic acid in the Drosophila wing spot test. *Environmental and Molecular Mutagenesis* 47(3):162–168.

Rose JQ, Ransy JC, Wentzler TH, Hummel RA, Gehring PJ. 1976. The fate of 2,3,7,8-tetrachlorodibenzo-*p*-dioxin following single and repeated oral doses to the rat. *Toxicology and Applied Pharmacology* 36:209–226.

Sato S, Shirakawa H, Tomita S, Ohsaki Y, Haketa K, Tooi O, Santo N, Tohkin M, Furukawa Y, Gonzalez FJ, Komai M. 2008. Low-dose dioxins alter gene expression related to cholesterol biosynthesis, lipogenesis, and glucose metabolism through the aryl hydrocarbon receptor-mediated pathway in mouse liver. *Toxicology and Applied Pharmacology* 229(1):10–19.

Sauerhoff MW, Braun WH, Blau GE, Gehring PJ. 1977. The fate of 2,4-dichlorophenoxyacetic acid (2,4-D) following oral administration to man. *Toxicology* 8:3–11.

Savouret J, Antenos M, Quesne M, Xu J, Milgrom E, Casper R. 2001. 7-ketocholesterol is an endogenous modulator for the arylhydrocarbon receptor. *Journal of Biological Chemistry* (276): 3054–3059.

Schmidt JV, Su GH, Reddy JK, Simon MC, Bradfield CA. 1996. Characterization of a murine Ahr null allele: Involvement of the Ah receptor in hepatic growth and development. *Proceedings of the National Academy of Sciences of the United States of America* 93(13):6731–6736.

Schnekenburger M, Peng L, Puga A. 2007. HDAC1 bound to the Cyp1a1 promoter blocks histone acetylation associated with Ah receptor-mediated trans-activation. *Biochimica et Biophysica ACTA/General Subjects* 1769:569–578.

Seidel S, Winters G, Rogers W, Ziccardi M, Li V, Keser B, Denison MS. 2001. Activation of the Ah receptor signaling pathway by prostaglandins. *Journal of Biochemistry and Molecular Toxicology* 15:187–196.

Sen B, Wang A, Hester SD, Robertson JL, Wolf DC. 2005. Gene expression profiling of responses to dimethylarsinic acid in female F344 rat urothelium. *Toxicology* 215(3):214–226.

Senft AP, Dalton TP, Nebert DW, Genter MB, Puga A, Hutchinson RJ, Kerzee JK, Uno S, Shertzer HG. 2002. Mitochondrial reactive oxygen production is dependent on the aromatic hydrocarbon receptor. *Free Radical Biology and Medicine* 33(9):1268–1278.

Shen ES, Whitlock JP. 1992. Protein–DNA interactions at a dioxin responsive enhancer: Mutational analysis of the DNA binding site for the liganded Ah receptor. *Journal of Biological Chemistry* 267:6815–6819.

Shertzer HG, Genter MB, Shen D, Nebert DW, Chen Y, Dalton TP. 2006. TCDD decreases ATP levels and increases reactive oxygen production through changes in mitochondrial F(0)F(1)-ATP synthase and ubiquinone. *Toxicology and Applied Pharmacology* 217(3):363–374.

Sinal C, Bend J. 1997. Aryl hydrocarbon receptor–dependent induction of cyp1a1 by bilirubin in mouse hepatoma hepa 1c1c7 cells. *Molecular Pharmacology* 52:590–599.

Singh NP, Nagarkatti M, Nagarkatti P. 2008. Primary peripheral T cells become susceptible to 2,3,7,8-tetrachlorodibenzo-*p*-dioxin–mediated apoptosis in vitro upon activation and in the presence of dendritic cells. *Molecular Pharmacology* 73(6):1722–1735.

Sogawa K, Numayama-Tsuruta K, Takahashi T, Matsushita N, Miura C, Nikawa J, Gotoh O, Kikuchi Y, Fujii-Kuriyama Y. 2004. A novel induction mechanism of the rat CYP1A2 gene mediated by Ah receptor–Arnt heterodimer. *Biochemical and Biophysical Research Communications* 318(3):746–755.

Song Z, Pollenz RS. 2002. Ligand-dependent and independent modulation of aryl hydrocarbon receptor localization, degradation, and gene regulation. *Molecular Pharmacology* 62(4):806–816.

Sonneveld E, Jonas A, Meijer OC, Brouwer A, van der Burg B. 2007. Glucocorticoid-enhanced expression of dioxin target genes through regulation of the rat aryl hydrocarbon receptor. *Toxicological Sciences* 99(2):455–469.

Steinmaus C, Moore LE, Shipp M, Kalman D, Rey OA, Biggs ML, Hopenhayn C, Bates MN, Zheng S, Wiencke JK, Smith AH. 2007. Genetic polymorphisms in MTHFR 677 and 1298, GSTM1 and T1, and metabolism of arsenic. *Journal of Toxicology and Environmental Health, Part A* 70(2):159–170.

Stott WT, Johnson KA, Landry TD, Gorzinski SJ, Cieszlak FS. 1990. Chronic toxicity and oncogenicity of picloram in Fischer 344 rats. *Journal of Toxicology and Environmental Health* 30:91–104.

Suzuki KT, Katagiri A, Sakuma Y, Ogra Y, Ohmichi M. 2004. Distributions and chemical forms of arsenic after intravenous administration of dimethylarsinic and monomethylarsonic acids to rats. *Toxicology and Applied Pharmacology* 198(3):336–344.

Swanson HI, Chan WK, Bradfield CA. 1995. DNA binding specificities and pairing rules of the Ah receptor, ARNT, and SIM proteins. *Journal of Biological Chemistry* 270(44):26292–26302.

Tanaka J, Yonemoto J, Zaha H, Kiyama R, Sone H. 2007. Estrogen-responsive genes newly found to be modified by TCDD exposure in human cell lines and mouse systems. *Molecular and Cellular Endocrinology* 272(1-2):38–49.

Thompson DJ, Emerson JL, Strebing RJ, Gerbig CG, Robinson VB. 1972. Teratology and postnatal studies on 4-amino-3,5,6-trichloropicolinic acid (picloram) in the rat. *Food and Cosmetics Toxicology* 10:797–803.

Timchalk C. 2004. Comparative inter-species pharmacokinetics of phenoxyacetic acid herbicides and related organic acids. Evidence that the dog is not a relevant species for evaluation of human health risk. *Toxicology* 200(1):1–19.

Tonack S, Kind K, Thompson JG, Wobus AM, Fischer B, Santos AN. 2007. Dioxin affects glucose transport via the arylhydrocarbon receptor signal cascade in pluripotent embryonic carcinoma cells. *Endocrinology* 148(12):5902–5912.

Tsuchiya M, Katoh T, Motoyama H, Sasaki H, Tsugane S, Ikenoue T. 2005. Analysis of the AhR, ARNT, and AhRR gene polymorphisms: Genetic contribution to endometriosis susceptibility and severity. *Fertility and Sterility* 84(2):454–458.

Vahter M, Concha G. 2001. Role of metabolism in arsenic toxicity. *Pharmacology and Toxicology* 89(1):1–5.

Vahter M, Marafante E, Dencker L. 1984. Tissue distribution and retention of 74As-dimethylarsinic acid in mice and rats. *Archives of Environmental Contamination and Toxicology* 13:259–264.

Veldhoen M, Hirota K, Westendorf AM, Buer J, Dumoutier L, Renauld JC, Stockinger B. 2008. The aryl hydrocarbon receptor links TH17-cell-mediated autoimmunity to environmental toxins. *Nature* 453(7191):106–109.

Vezina CM, Walker NJ, Olson JR. 2004. Subchronic exposure to TCDD, PeCDF, PCB126, and PCB153: Effect on hepatic gene expression. *Environmental Health Perspectives* 112(16):1636–1644.

Viluksela M, Duong TV, Stahl BU, Li X, Tuomisto J, Rozman KK. 1996. Toxicokinetics of 2,3,7,8-tetrachlorodibenzo-*p*-dioxin (TCDD) in two substrains of male Long-Evans rats after intravenous injection. *Fundamental and Applied Toxicology* 31:184–191.

Vogel CF, Sciullo E, Li W, Wong P, Lazennec G, Matsumura F. 2007a. RelB, a new partner of aryl hydrocarbon receptor–mediated transcription. *Molecular Endocrinology* 21(12):2941–2955.

Vogel CF, Sciullo E, Matsumura F. 2007b. Involvement of RelB in aryl hydrocarbon receptor-mediated induction of chemokines. *Biochemical and Biophysical Research Communications* 363(3):722–726.

Vogel CF, Goth SR, Dong B, Pessah IN, Matsumura F. 2008. Aryl hydrocarbon receptor signaling mediates expression of indoleamine 2,3-dioxygenase. *Biochemical and Biophysical Research Communications* 375(3):331–335.

Weber LW, Zesch A, Rozman K. 1991. Penetration, distribution and kinetics of 2,3,7,8-tetrachlorodibenzo-*p*-dioxin in human skin in vitro. *Archives of Toxicology* 65:421–428.

Weber LW, Ernst SW, Stahl BU, Rozman K. 1993. Tissue distribution and toxicokinetics of 2,3,7,8-tetrachlorodibenzo-*p*-dioxin in rats after intravenous injection. *Fundamental and Applied Toxicology* 21:523–534.

Wei M, Wanibuchi H, Morimura K, Iwai S, Yoshida K, Endo G, Nakae D, Fukushima S. 2002. Carcinogenicity of dimethylarsinic acid in male F344 rats and genetic alterations in induced urinary bladder tumors. *Carcinogenesis* 23(8):1387–1397.

Wei M, Arnold L, Cano M, Cohen SM. 2005. Effects of co-administration of antioxidants and arsenicals on the rat urinary bladder epithelium. *Toxicological Sciences* 83(2):237–245.

Weiss C, Faust D, Schreck I, Ruff A, Farwerck T, Melenberg A, Schneider S, Oesch-Bartlomowicz B, Zatloukalova J, Vondracek J, Oesch F, Dietrich C. 2008. TCDD deregulates contact inhibition in rat liver oval cells via Ah receptor, JunD and cyclin A. *Oncogene* 27(15):2198–2207.

Whitelaw M, Pongratz I, Wilhelmsson A, Gustafsson JA, Poellinger L. 1993. Ligand-dependent recruitment of the ARNT coregulatory determines DNA recognition by the dioxin receptor. *Molecular and Cellular Biology* 13:2504–2514.

WHO (World Health Organization). 1984. 2,4-Dichlorophenoxyacetic Acid (2,4-D). *Environmental Health Criteria* 29. Geneva: WHO.

Xie Y, Trouba KJ, Liu J, Waalkes MP, Germolec DR. 2004. Biokinetics and subchronic toxic effects of oral arsenite, arsenate, monomethylarsonic acid, and dimethylarsinic acid in v-Ha-ras transgenic (Tg.AC) mice. *Environmental Health Perspectives* 112(12):1255–1263.

Yao E, Denison M. 1992. DNA sequence determinants for binding of transformed Ah receptor to a dioxin-responsive enhancer. *Biochemistry* 31:5060–5067.

Zarzour AH, Selim M, Abd-Elsayed AA, Hameed DA, AbdelAziz MA. 2008. Muscle invasive bladder cancer in Upper Egypt: The shift in risk factors and tumor characteristics. *BMC Cancer* 8(250).

5

Epidemiologic Studies—New Citations and Background on Repeatedly Studied Populations

The continuing effort to evaluate and integrate all results of human studies pertinent to possible health effects of exposure to any of the chemicals of interest—2,4-dichlorophenoxyacetic acid (2,4-D), 2,4,5-trichlorophenoxyacetic acid (2,4,5-T) and its contaminant 2,3,7,8-tetrachlorodibenzo-p-dioxin (TCDD), 4-amino-3,5,6-trichloropicolinic acid (picloram), and cacodylic acid (dimethyl arsenic acid or DMA)—has involved the consideration of thousands of citations over the successive updates. Results of a study of a single population may be reported in connection with a multiplicity of health outcomes and more than one publication, particularly if a study is of the cohort design with repeated follow-ups.

The major purpose of the chapters on epidemiology or epidemiologic studies in the original *Veterans and Agent Orange: Health Effects of Herbicides Used in Vietnam (VAO)* report and its updates has always been to reduce repetition of design information in the health-outcomes chapters from outcome to outcome and from update to update. Deviating somewhat from the format of previous *Veterans and Agent Orange* (VAO) reports, this chapter first provides tables listing the epidemiologic citations that are new, which represent a compendium of the sources of new information on health outcomes in humans considered by this committee. The citations correspond to publications that appeared from October 1, 2006 (the closing date for inclusion in *Veterans and Agent Orange: Update 2006* [*Update 2006*; IOM, 2007]) through September 30, 2008.

For this chapter, for discussions of health outcomes, and for results tables in earlier reports in the VAO series, an organizational framework was used that categorized each publication containing primary epidemiologic findings as an occupational study, an environmental study, or a study of Vietnam veterans.

Those categories were not intended to imply that any of the populations is intrinsically more valuable for the committee's purpose. Various study designs (most importantly, cohort, case–control, and cross-sectional) have strengths and weaknesses (see Chapter 2) that influence their potential to contribute evidence of an association with the health outcomes considered in Chapters 6–9. This update retains the categorization scheme. The second part of this chapter discusses the design details of new reports on populations already under study and on multiple outcomes in new populations. The occupational-studies section covers studies of production workers, agriculture and forestry workers (including herbicide and pesticide applicators), and paper and pulp workers. The environmental-studies section covers studies of populations unintentionally exposed to unusually high concentrations of herbicides or dioxins as a result of where they lived, such as Seveso, Italy; Times Beach, Missouri; and the southern portion of Vietnam. The section on Vietnam–veteran studies covers studies of US veterans conducted by the Air Force, the Centers for Disease Control and Prevention (CDC), the Department of Veterans Affairs (VA), the American Legion, and individual states; it also discusses studies of veterans from other nations (such as Australia and Korea) that fought in Vietnam.

In addition to reviewing studies involving exposures to the chemicals of interest (2,4-D, 2,4,5-T and its contaminant TCDD, cacodylic acid, and picloram), this and earlier VAO committees have examined any available studies that address compounds chemically related to the herbicides used in Vietnam, such as 2-(2-methyl-4-chlorophenoxy) propionic acid, hexachlorophene, and chlorophenols, particularly 2,4,5-trichlorophenol. Some study investigators did not indicate in their published reports the specific herbicides to which study participants were exposed or the magnitude of exposure; those complicating factors were considered when the committee weighed the relevance of a study, as detailed in Chapter 2. Available details of exposure assessment and use of the resulting data in analyses are discussed in Chapter 3, which follows the same sequence to categorize study populations.

NEW CITATIONS

To elucidate further the new epidemiologic data reviewed by the committee for this update, three tables that list new citations are included.

Citations Reporting on a Single Health Outcome in New Populations

New studies reporting on only a single health outcome in previously unstudied populations are listed in Table 5-1 with an indication of the outcome. Descriptions and critiques of the studies will appear only in the sections of the report that discuss the results on the particular health outcomes.

TABLE 5-1 Citations on Study Populations New in *Update 2008* with Results on a Single Health Outcome

Author	Study Design	Exposure Measure(s) Having Results	Health Outcome Reported	Study Population
Studies of Vietnam Veterans				
Chamie et al., 2008	Case–control	Self-reported exposure to Agent Orange	Prostate cancer	Vietnam veterans who registered with Northern California VA Health System and were followed in 1998–2006
Occupational Studies				
Monge et al., 2007	Population-based case–control	Pesticides, including picloram, 2,4-D	Childhood leukemia	Costa Rican parents of children with childhood leukemia
Samanic et al., 2008	Case–control	Herbicides (unspecified) from JEM, self-reported occupational history	Adult brain tumors	Patients with new diagnosis of glioma or meningioma
Solomon et al., 2007	Cross-sectional	Pesticides; herbicide users were 40% of "other pesticides" users	Neurologic symptoms	Men born between 1933–1977 identified in 1991 census in rural areas of England and Wales
Environmental Studies				
Abdelouahab et al., 2008	Cross-sectional	Serum concentrations of POPs, including dl PCBs 105, 118, 156	Thyroid homeostasis	Men and women who consume freshwater fish from Canadian lakes
Brighina et al., 2008	Case–control	Herbicides, discussion of 2,4-D	PD	PD patients from Wisconsin, Iowa, South Dakota, North Dakota
Chao et al., 2007	Cross-sectional	Serum concentrations of PCDDs, PCDFs, PCBs	Menstrual-cycle characteristics	Healthy Taiwanese mothers (18–40 years old)
Chevrier et al., 2008	Birth cohort	34 PCBs, including dl PCBs 118, 156	Thyroid levels during pregnancy	Pregnant women in Salinas Valley, CA
Cok et al., 2008	Case–control	Serum concentrations of PCDDs, PCDFs, dl PCBs	Male infertility	Surgical patients from Ankara University, School of Medicine, Turkey

TABLE 5-1 Continued

Author	Study Design	Exposure Measure(s) Having Results	Health Outcome Reported	Study Population
Cooney et al., 2007	Case–control	Pesticides, herbicides	Wilm's tumor (childhood cancer)	523 case mothers and 517 controls from US and Canada
Dhooge et al., 2006	Cross-sectional	Serum concentrations of TCDD (5 months after PCB, dioxin food-contamination episode in Belgium)	Reproductive parameters	101 Flemish men 20–40 years old
Eriksson et al., 2008	Population-based case–control	Herbicides; specific phenoxy herbicides, including 2,4,5-T; 2,4-D; MCPA	NHL	Swedish patients with diagnosis of NHL December 1, 1999–April 30, 2002
Hancock et al., 2008	Family-based case–control	Self-reported herbicide or chlorophenoxy acid or ester use	PD	PD patients, family members (with, without PD)
Heilier et al., 2006	Cross-sectional	Serum concentrations of dl compounds	PE, DEN	47 patients with endometriosis, DEN
Heilier et al., 2007	Matched case–control	Serum concentrations of PCDDs, PCDFs, PCBs	PE, DEN	88 matched triads: women with DEN, women with PE, controls
Hertz-Picciotto et al., 2008	Cohort	Serum concentrations of PCBs, including dl PCBs 105, 118, 170, 180	Sex ratio	Cord blood extracted from pregnant women in San Francisco Bay area
Meyer et al., 2006	Case–control	Agricultural pesticides including 2,4-D and dicamba. Pounds of pesticides applied or persisting within 600 m of subject's home during gestational weeks 6–16	Hypospadias	Cases and controls born 1998–2002 in eastern Arkansas
Nishijo et al., 2008	Cross-sectional	Serum TEQs, seven pesticides	Birth weight	Japanese women, their newborn infants
Polsky et al., 2007	Case–control	Serum concentrations of PCBs, including dl PCBs 118, 156; total PCBs, chlorinated pesticides	Erectile dysfunction	Ontario men

continued

TABLE 5-1 Continued

Author	Study Design	Exposure Measure(s) Having Results	Health Outcome Reported	Study Population
Rudant et al., 2007	Case–control	Maternal household herbicide use during pregnancy	Childhood hematopoietic malignancies	Residents of France
Sagiv et al., 2007	Cohort	Serum concentrations of PCBs, including dl PCBs 118, 180; non-dl PCBs 138, 153	Infant size at birth (weight, length, head circumference)	Four towns near PCB-contaminated harbor in Massachusetts
Spinelli et al., 2007	Population-based case–control	Serum concentrations of dl PCBs 105, 118, 156; non-dl PCBs	NHL	Residents of British Columbia, Canada
Teitelbaum et al., 2007	Population-based case–control	Self-reported lifetime residential use of lawn and garden pesticides (unspecified)	Breast cancer	Women living on Long Island, New York
Toft et al., 2007	Cross-sectional	Endocrine-disrupting compounds; dl activity by CALUX, AHR competitive activity	Semen quality	Inuits, three European populations
Tsuchiya et al., 2007	Case–control	Serum TEQ of dioxin (sum of dl compounds); TEQ of PCBs (sum of mono-ortho PCBs)	Endometriosis, polymorphisms	Infertile Japanese women
Tsukimori et al., 2008	Retrospective survey	Serum concentrations of PeCDF; dl PCBs 126, 169	Pregnancy outcomes (loss, preterm)	Yusho subjects 36 years after 1968 incident
Xu et al., 2007	Case–control	Herbicides (unspecified)	Nasal NK/T-cell lymphoma	Patients in East Asia
Zambon et al., 2007	Population-based, case–control	Residential duration and distance from 33 industrial sources	Sarcoma	Residents of Province of Venice, Italy

ABBREVIATIONS: 2,4-D, 2,4-dichlorophenoxyacetic acid; 2,4,5-T, 2,4,5-trichlorophenoxyacetic acid; AHR, aryl hydrocarbon receptor; CALUX, chemically activated luciferase gene expression; DEN, deep endometriotic nodules; dl, dioxin-like; JEM, job–exposure matrix; MCPA, 2-methyl-4-chlorophenoxyacetic acid; NK/T-cell, natural killer T-cell; NHL, non-Hodgkin's lymphoma; PCB, polychlorinated biphenyl; PCDD, polychlorinated dibenzo-*p*-dioxin; PCDF, polychlorinated dibenzofuran; PD, Parkinson's disease; PE, peritoneal endometriosis; PeCDF, 2,3,4,7,8-pentachlorodibenzofuran; POP, persistent organic pollutants; TCDD, 2,3,7,8-tetrachlorodibenzo-*p*-dioxin; TEQ, toxicity equivalent quotient; TSH, thyroid-stimulating hormone; VA, Department of Veterans Affairs.

Citations Reporting on Multiple Health Outcomes in New Populations

Newly accessed citations reporting on multiple health outcomes in populations that have not been studied before are listed in Table 5-2, which indicates which outcomes were investigated. Single comprehensive discussions of the studies are presented in this chapter, organized according to the type of study population. The results, with comments related to their reliability or limitations, appear in the appropriate outcome-specific sections of Chapters 6–9.

TABLE 5-2 Citations on Study Populations New in *Update 2008* with Results on Multiple Health Outcomes

Author	Study Design	Exposure Measures(s) Having Results	Health Outcome(s) Reported	Study Population
Occupational Studies				
Richardson et al., 2008	Population-based case–control	Exposure estimates derived from JEM for chlorophenols, herbicides, others	NHL, CLL	German nationals, 15–75 years of age, newly diagnosed NHL cases that occurred between 1986 and 1998
Environmental Studies				
Karouna-Renier et al., 2007	Cross-sectional	Serum concentrations of 17 PCDD and PCDF congeners	Hypertension, diabetes, liver function	Former employees, their families, residents living near Pensacola, Florida, wood treatment plant
Read et al., 2007	Ecologic	2,4,5-T	All cancers, STS, HD, NHL, CLL	Residence near 2,4,5-T manufacturing plant in New Zealand
Ueruma et al., 2008a,b	Cross-sectional	Serum concentrations of PCDD/Fs, dl PCBs, total TEQ	Diabetes, lipid levels	Stratified sample of Japanese men and women aged 15–73 years old
	The remainder of these citations report on a variety of individual outcomes addressed in the NHANES surveys conducted in 1999–2002 and 2003–2004.			
Everett et al., 2007	Cross-sectional	Serum concentrations of HxCDD, dl PCB-126, DDT	Diabetes	NHANES-IV

continued

TABLE 5-2 Continued

Author	Study Design	Exposure Measures(s) Having Results	Health Outcome(s) Reported	Study Population
Everett et al., 2008a,b	Cross-sectional	Serum concentrations of PCBs, including dl PCBs 118 and 126	Hypertension	NHANES (1999–2002, 1999–2004)
Ha et al., 2007	Cross-sectional	Serum concentrations of PCDDs, PCDFs, dl and non-dl PCBs, including dl PCBs 118, 126, 156, 169, 170, 180	Cardiovascular disease	NHANES (1999–2002) (1/3 subsample)
Lee DH et al., 2006	Cross-sectional	Serum concentrations of 6 POPs, including HpCDD, OCDD	Diabetes	NHANES (1999–2002)
Lee DH et al., 2007a	Cross-sectional	Serum concentrations of 19 POPs, including PCDDs; PCDFs; dl PCBs 118, 126, 169	Arthritis, rheumatoid arthritis	NHANES (1999–2002)
Lee DH et al., 2007b	Cross-sectional	Serum concentrations of 19 POPs, including PCDDs; PCDFs; dl PCBs 118, 126, 169	Insulin resistance in nondiabetic adults	NHANES (1999–2002)
Lee DH et al., 2007c	Cross-sectional	Serum concentrations of 19 POPs, including PCDDs; PCDFs; dl PCBs 118, 126, 169	Lipid levels, hypertension	NHANES (1999–2002)
Turyk et al., 2007	Cross-sectional	Serum concentrations of total PCBs, total TEQs (dioxin, furans, coplanar mono-ortho-substituted PCBs)	Thyroid hormones	NHANES (1999–2000, 2001–2002)

ABBREVIATIONS: 2,4,5-T, 2,4,5-trichlorophenoxyacetic acid; CLL, chronic lymphocytic leu-kemia; DDT, dichlorodiphenyltrichloroethane; dl, dioxin-like; HD, Hodgkin's disease; HpCDD, 1,2,3,4,6,7,8-heptachlorodibenzo-*p*-dioxin; HxCDD, 1,2,3,6,7,8-hexachlorodibenzo-*p*-furan; JEM, job–exposure matrix; NHANES, National Health and Nutritional Examination Survey; NHL, non-Hodgkin's lymphoma; OCDD, 1,2,3,4,6,7,8,9-octachlorodibenzo-*p*-dioxin; PCB, polychlorinated biphenyl; PCDD, polychlorinated dibenzo-*p*-dioxin; PCDD/Fs, dioxins and furans combined; PCDF, polychlorinated dibenzofuran; POP, persistent organic pollutants; STS, soft-tissue sarcoma; TEQ, toxicity equivalent quotient.

New Citations on Previously Studied Populations

A number of long-term studies of populations exposed to the herbicides sprayed in Vietnam or to their components are of particular importance to the VAO project. Placing each new publication in historical context helps the com-mittee to avoid factoring into its deliberations repeatedly what is actually a single observation. Such clusters of studies are useful in describing the course of a population's response to an exposure, and joint consideration of an entire body of research on a population may yield insight into relationships with potential confounding factors. Many of the cohorts that have contributed to the cumulative findings of the VAO committees are no longer being followed; however, the cohorts' histories are briefly recapitulated in the body of this report. Additional background information can be found in earlier reports in this series.

Many cohorts potentially exposed to any of the chemicals of interest are monitored periodically, including the cohorts of the National Institute for Occupational Safety and Health (NIOSH), the International Agency for Research on Cancer (IARC), and the National Cancer Institute (NCI); residents of Seveso; and Ranch Hand personnel. For the sake of thoroughness, the discussions of specific health outcomes and the associated cumulative-results tables in Chapters 6–9 include references to studies discussed in previous VAO reports and to new studies. However, in drawing its conclusions, the committee focused on the most recent update (*Update 2006*) when multiple reports on the same cohorts and health outcomes were available. Individual researchers who belong to research consortia evaluating cohorts in large multicenter studies (such as the IARC and NCI cohort studies) sometimes publish reports based solely on the subset of subjects they themselves are monitoring. All the studies are noted in the present report, but in drawing its conclusions the committee focused on the studies of the larger, multicenter cohorts.

The new citations on previously studied populations are listed in Table 5-3. For citations listed there, the current citation is discussed in the context of the history of publications on the population with an explanation of how the new work meshes with earlier efforts.

TABLE 5-3 Citations on Previously Studied Populations[a]

Author	Study Design	Exposure Measure(s) Having Results	Health Outcome(s) Reported	Study Population
Studies of Vietnam Veterans				
Cypel and Kang, 2008	Retrospective cohort	Service in Vietnam during Vietnam War	Mortality from all causes; all cancers; cancers of large intestine, pancreas, lung, breast, uterus, CNS, lymphopoietic system; circulatory system diseases	VA Environmental Epidemiology Service cohort of female Vietnam, Vietnam-era veterans

continued

TABLE 5-3 Continued

Author	Study Design	Exposure Measure(s) Having Results	Health Outcome(s) Reported	Study Population
Gupta et al., 2006	Longitudinal prospective cohort	Serum concentrations of TCDD	Serum testosterone, benign prostatic hyperplasia	AFHS (sprayers vs nonsprayers)
Michalek and Pavuk, 2008	Prospective cohort	Serum concentrations of TCDD	Diabetes, cancer	AFHS (calendar period of service, days spraying, years in SEA)

Occupational Studies

Author	Study Design	Exposure Measure(s) Having Results	Health Outcome(s) Reported	Study Population
Hansen et al., 2007	Cohort	Pesticides, including 2,4-D; 2,4,5-T	Cancer: buccal cavity and pharynx, digestive organs and peritoneum, respiratory system, male genital organs, urinary system, skin, STS, lymphatic and hematopoietic tissue	Danish male gardeners
Hoppin et al., 2006c	Cohort	Pesticides, including 2,4-D; 2,4,5-T	Respiratory outcomes (wheeze)	AHS
Hoppin et al., 2007a	Cohort (cross-sectional analysis)	Pesticides, including 2,4-D; 2,4,5-T	Farmer's lung	AHS
Hoppin et al., 2007b	Cohort	Pesticides, including 2,4-D; 2,4,5-T	Chronic bronchitis	AHS
Hoppin et al., 2008c	Cohort (cross-sectional analysis)	Pesticides, including 2,4-D	Atopic and nonatopic asthma	AHS (women only)
Kamel et al., 2007a	Cross-sectional	Pesticides, including 2,4-D; 2,4,5-T	Neurologic symptoms	AHS
Kamel et al., 2007b	Case–control	Pesticides, including 2,4-D; 2,4,5-T	PD	AHS
Lee WJ et al., 2007	Cohort	Pesticides, including 2,4-D; 2,4,5-T	Colorectal cancer	AHS

TABLE 5-3 Continued

Author	Study Design	Exposure Measure(s) Having Results	Health Outcome(s) Reported	Study Population
Mills and Yang, 2007	Nested case–control	Pesticides, including 2,4-D	Gastric cancer	California Cancer Registry; United Farm Workers roster (1973–1996), California Department of Pesticide Regulation
Montgomery et al., 2008	Cohort	Pesticides, including 2,4-D; 2,4,5-T; 2,4,5-TP; dicamba	Diabetes	AHS (5-year follow-up of licensed pesticide applicators)
Pelclová et al., 2007	Case–control	Serum concentrations of TCDD	Endothelial dysfunction, impaired microvascular reactivity	Poisoned Czech production workers
Saldana et al., 2007	Cohort	Pesticides, including 2,4-D; 2,4,5-T; 2,4,5-TP; dicamba	Gestational diabetes	AHS
Samanic et al., 2006	Cohort	Dicamba	Cancer incidence	AHS
Urban et al., 2007	Case series	Serum concentrations of TCDD	Polyneuropathy, other neurologic effects	Poisoned Czech production workers
Valcin et al., 2007	Cohort	Herbicides	Chronic bronchitis	AHS (nonsmoking women)
Weselak et al., 2007	Cohort	In utero exposure to phenoxy herbicides, including 2,4-D; 2,4-DB; MCPA; dicamba	Cough, asthma, allergy	Ontario Farm Family Health Study

Environmental Studies

Author	Study Design	Exposure Measure(s) Having Results	Health Outcome(s) Reported	Study Population
Baccarelli et al., 2008	Cohort (residential-based population)	Serum concentrations of TCDD; maternal exposure to TCDD	Neonatal thyroid function (TSH), birth weight, sex ratio	Seveso births 1994–2005

continued

TABLE 5-3 Continued

Author	Study Design	Exposure Measure(s) Having Results	Health Outcome(s) Reported	Study Population
Consonni et al., 2008	Cohort	Serum concentrations of TCDD	Mortality—all cancers; specific cancers: diabetes, circulatory, respiratory, digestive disease	Seveso population by zone
Eskenazi et al., 2007	Cohort	Serum concentrations of TCDD	Fibroids	Seveso Women's Health Study
Miligi et al., 2006	Case–control	Herbicides including phenoxy herbicides, 2,4-D, MCPA	Cancers of hematolymphopoietic system (NHL, CLL, HD, leukemia, multiple myeloma)	Italian multicenter case–control study
Mocarelli et al., 2008	Cohort	Serum concentrations of TCDD	Male fertility	Seveso Zone A men vs age-matched men residing outside contamination zone
Viel et al., 2008	Population-based case–control	Residential proximity to municipal solid-waste incinerator (GIS-derived dioxin exposure)	Breast cancer	Residents of Besancon, France
Warner et al., 2007	Cohort	Serum concentrations of TCDD	Ovarian function	Seveso Women's Health Study

ABBREVIATIONS: 2,4-D, 2,4-dichlorophenoxyacetic acid; 2,4-DB, 2-(2,4-diichlorophenoxy) butyric acid; 2,4,5-T, 2,4,5-trichlorophenoxyacetic acid; 2,4,5-TP, 2-(2,4,5-trichlorophenoxy) propionic acid; AFHS, Air Force Health Study; AHS, Agricultural Health Study; ALL, acute lymphocytic leukemia; CLL, chronic lymphocytic leukemia; CNS, central nervous system; GIS, geographic information system; HD, Hodgkin's disease; MCPA, 2-methyl-4-chlorophenoxyacetic acid; NHL, non-Hodgkin's lymphoma; PCB, polychlorinated biphenyl; PD, Parkinson's disease; SEA, Southeast Asia; STS, soft-tissue sarcoma; TCDD, 2,3,7,8-tetrachlorodibenzo-*p*-dioxin; THS, thyroid-stimulating hormone; VA, Department of Veterans Affairs.

*a*Throughout the report the same alphabetic indicator following year of publication is used consistently for the same article when there were multiple citations by the same first author in a given year. The convention of assigning the alphabetic indicator in order of citation in a given chapter is not followed.

RELEVANT POPULATIONS: NEW REPORTS WITH MULTIPLE HEALTH OUTCOMES OR WITH RESULTS ON PREVIOUSLY STUDIED GROUPS

One-time reports on given study populations that addressed only single health outcomes are not discussed in the rest of the chapter.

Of particular importance to the VAO project are a number of continuing studies of populations that have been exposed to the herbicides sprayed in Vietnam or to their components. Properly integrating new information into the existing database can enhance its usefulness. If new results are updatings on or concern a subset of previously considered study populations, "double-counting" resulting from ignoring this can bias overall findings, but separately reported information can impart new relevance to other data on a study population.

To avoid repetition in the health-outcome chapters (Chapters 6–9), this section summarizes the design characteristics of studies involving multiple health outcomes even if the study populations have not been addressed in other VAO publications. Detailed descriptions of many of the study populations can be found in Chapter 2 of the original *VAO* report, and the criteria for inclusion were discussed in Appendix A of that report. Available details of exposure assessment and use of exposure data are discussed in Chapter 3 of the present report.

The section below on Vietnam veterans covers studies conducted in the United States by the Air Force, CDC, VA, the American Legion, and the state of Michigan; it also discusses studies of Australian and South Korean Vietnam veterans. The section "Occupational Studies" covers studies of production workers, agriculture and forestry workers (including herbicide and pesticide applicators), and paper and pulp workers; case–control studies are of interest primarily for their evaluation of occupational exposures, so ones that address multiple outcomes or that are represented by several citations considered in VAO reports are presented at the end of the section. The section "Environmental Studies" covers studies of populations unintentionally exposed to unusually high concentrations of herbicides or dioxins as a result of where they lived, such as Seveso, Italy; Times Beach, Missouri; and the southern portion of Vietnam.

VIETNAM-VETERAN STUDIES

Studies of Vietnam veterans who might have been exposed to herbicides, including Agent Orange, have been conducted in the United States at the national and state levels and in Australia, Korea, and Vietnam. Exposures have been estimated by various means, and health outcomes have been evaluated with reference to various comparison or control groups. This section is organized primarily by research sponsor because it is more conducive to a methodologic presentation of the articles. Exposure measures fall on a crude scale from individual exposures of Ranch Hand personnel, as reflected in serum TCDD measurements, to some statewide studies' use of service in Vietnam as a surrogate for TCDD exposure.

Several comparison groups have been used for veteran cohort studies: Vietnam veterans who were stationed in areas where herbicide-spraying missions were unlikely to have taken place and who therefore were unlikely to have been in areas sprayed with herbicides; Vietnam-era veterans who were in the military at the time of the conflict but did not serve in Vietnam; non-Vietnam veterans who served in other wars or conflicts, such as the Korean War or World War II; and various US male populations (either state or national).

In all studies of Vietnam veterans (whether or not the subjects are American), the study subjects are in fact the target population of our charge, and they are assumed to have a higher probability of having received exposures of concern than people who did not serve in Vietnam, whether or not their individual exposures are characterized beyond the mere fact that they were deployed.

United States

Air Force Health Study of Operation Ranch Hand Subjects

Major defoliation activities in Vietnam were conducted by Air Force personnel as part of Operation Ranch Hand. Veterans who took place in the defoliation activities became the first subpopulation of Vietnam veterans to receive special attention with regard to Agent Orange and have become known as the Ranch Hand cohort within the Air Force Health Study (AFHS). To determine whether exposure to herbicides, including Agent Orange, had adverse health effects, the Air Force made a commitment to Congress and the White House in 1979 to conduct an epidemiologic study of Ranch Hand personnel (AFHS, 1982). Results of biologic-marker studies of Ranch Hand personnel have been consistent with their being exposed, as a group, to TCDD. When the Ranch Hand cohort was classified by military occupation, a general increase in serum TCDD was detected in people whose jobs involved more frequent handling of herbicides (AFHS, 1991a).

The exposure index initially proposed in the AFHS relied on military records of TCDD-containing herbicides (Agents Orange, Purple, Pink, Green) sprayed as reported in the HERBS tapes for the period starting in July 1965 and on military procurement records and dissemination information for the period before July 1965. In 1991, the exposure index was compared with the results of the Ranch Hand serum-TCDD analysis. The exposure index and the TCDD body burden correlated weakly.

Michalek et al. (1995) developed several indexes of herbicide exposure of members of the Ranch Hand cohort and tried to relate them to the measurements of serum TCDD from 1987 to 1992. Self-administered questionnaires completed by veterans of Operation Ranch Hand were used to develop three indexes of herbicide or TCDD exposure: number of days of skin exposure, percentage of skin area exposed, and the product of the number of days of skin exposure, percentage of skin exposed, and a factor for the concentration of TCDD in the herbicide. A fourth index, which used no information gathered from individual subjects, was calculated by multiplying the volume of herbicide sprayed during a person's tour of duty by the concentration of TCDD in herbicides sprayed in that period and then dividing the product by the number of crew members in each job specialty at the time.

Each of the four indexes tested was significantly related to serum TCDD although the models explained only 19–27% of the variability in serum TCDD concentrations. Days of skin exposure had the highest correlation. Military job classification (non–Ranch Hand combat troops, Ranch Hand administrators, Ranch Hand flight engineers, and Ranch Hand ground crew), which is separate from the four indexes, explained 60% of the variability in serum TCDD. When the questionnaire-derived indexes were applied within each job classification, days of skin exposure added statistical significance, but not substantially, to the variability explained by job alone.

A retrospective matched-cohort study design was used to examine morbidity and mortality; follow-up was scheduled to continue until 2002. Records from the National Personnel Records Center and the US Air Force Human Resources Laboratory were searched and cross-referenced to identify all Ranch Hand personnel (AFHS, 1982; Michalek et al., 1990). A total of 1,269 participants were originally identified (AFHS, 1983). A control population of 24,971 C-130 crew members and support personnel assigned to duty in Southeast Asia (SEA) but not occupationally exposed to herbicides (AFHS, 1983) was selected from the same data sources. Control subjects were individually matched for age, type of job (based on Air Force specialty code), and race (white or not white) to control for age-related, educational, socioeconomic-status, and race-related differences in development of chronic disease. To control for many potential confounders related to the physical and psychophysiologic effects of combat stress and the SEA environment, Ranch Hands were matched to control subjects who performed similar combat or combat-related jobs (AFHS, 1982). Rank also was used as a surrogate of exposure. Alcohol use and smoking were included in the analysis when they were known risk factors for the outcome of interest.

Ten matches formed a control set for each exposed subject. For the mortality study, the intent was to follow each exposed subject and a random sample of half of each subject's control set for 20 years in a 1:5 matched design. The morbidity component of follow-up consisted of a 1:1 matched design; the first control was randomized to the mortality-ascertainment component of the study. If a control was noncompliant, another control from the matched "pool" was selected; controls who died were not replaced.

The baseline physical examination occurred in 1982 and examinations took place in 1985, 1987, 1992, 1997, and 2002. Morbidity was ascertained through questionnaires and physical examination, which emphasized dermatologic, neurobehavioral, hepatic, immunologic, reproductive, and neoplastic conditions. Some 1,208 Ranch Hands and 1,668 comparison subjects were eligible for baseline examination. Initial questionnaire response rates were 97% for the exposed cohort and 93% for the nonexposed; baseline physical-examination responses were 87% and 76%, respectively (Wolfe et al., 1990). Deaths were identified and reviewed by using US Air Force Military Personnel Center records, the VA Beneficiary Identification Record Locator Subsystem (BIRLS), and the Internal Revenue Service (IRS) database of active Social Security numbers. Death certificates were obtained from the appropriate health departments (Michalek et al., 1990).

Ranch Hands were divided into three categories on the basis of their potential exposure:

- *Low potential.* Pilots, copilots, and navigators. Exposure was primarily through preflight checks and spraying.
- *Moderate potential.* Crew chiefs, aircraft mechanics, and support personnel. Exposure could occur by contact during dedrumming and aircraft loading operations, onsite repair of aircraft, and repair of spray equipment.
- *High potential.* Spray-console operators and flight engineers. Exposure could occur during operation of spray equipment and through contact with herbicides in the aircraft.

Ostensibly, the AFHS was designed to answer exactly the question that the VAO project is asking, but the realized nature of the "exposed" (Ranch Hand veterans) and "comparison" (SEA veterans) groups and the evolving practices of VAO committees endeavoring to fulfill the intention of their congressional mandate make interpretation less straightforward.

Results have been published for baseline morbidity (AFHS, 1984a) and baseline mortality (AFHS, 1983) studies; the first (1984), second (1987), third (1992), fourth (1997), and fifth (2002) follow-up examinations (AFHS, 1987, 1990, 1995, 2000, 2005); and the reproductive-outcomes study (AFHS, 1992; Michalek et al., 1998a; Wolfe et al., 1995). Mortality updates have been published for 1984–1986, 1989, and 1991 (AFHS, 1984b, 1985, 1986, 1989, 1991a). An interim technical report updated cause-specific mortality in Ranch Hands through 1993 (AFHS, 1996). Michalek et al. (1998b) and Ketchum and Michalek (2005) reported on 15-year and 20-year follow-up of postservice mortality, respectively, in veterans of Operation Ranch Hand, updating an earlier cause-specific mortality study by Michalek et al. (1990).

Blood samples for determination of serum TCDD concentrations were drawn at the cycle examinations in 1982 from 36 Ranch Hands (Pirkle et al., 1989), in 1987 from 866 Ranch Hands (AFHS, 1991b), in 1992 from 455 Ranch Hands (AFHS, 1995), and in 1997 from 443 Ranch Hands (AFHS, 2000). Analyses of the serum TCDD readings were included in the report on the 1987 follow-up examination (AFHS, 1991b), and other Ranch Hand publications have addressed the relationship between serum TCDD and reproductive hormones (Henriksen et al., 1996); diabetes mellitus, glucose, and insulin (Henriksen et al., 1997); skin disorders (Burton et al., 1998); infant death (Michalek et al., 1998a); sex ratios (Michalek et al., 1998c); skin cancer (Ketchum et al., 1999); insulin, fasting glucose, and sex-hormone–binding globulin (Michalek et al., 1999a); immunologic responses (Michalek et al., 1999b); diabetes mellitus (Longnecker and Michalek, 2000; Steenland et al., 2001a); cognitive function (Barrett et al., 2001); hepatic abnormalities (Michalek et al., 2001a); peripheral neuropathy (Michalek et al., 2001b); hematologic results (Michalek et al., 2001c); psychologic functioning (Barrett et al., 2003); correlations between diabetes and TCDD elimination (Michalek et al., 2003); thyroid function (Pavuk et al., 2003); cancer incidence (Akhtar et al., 2004; Pavuk et al., 2005); insulin sensitivity (Kern et al., 2004), and prostate cancer (Pavuk et al., 2006). All of the VAO updates, *Veterans and Agent Orange: Herbicide/Dioxin Exposure and Type 2 Diabetes* (IOM, 2000) and *Veterans and Agent Orange: Length of Presumptive Period for Association Between Exposure and Respiratory Cancer* (IOM, 2004), have discussed reports and papers addressing the cohort in more detail.

In a recent study, Gupta et al. (2006) examined associations between TCDD exposure, serum testosterone, and risk of benign prostate hyperplasia in the AFHS cohort. The investigation included 971 Ranch Hands and 1,266 Air Force veterans who flew non–herbicide-related aircraft missions in SEA during the Vietnam War.

Another recent study by Michalek and Pavuk (2008) investigated diabetes and cancer incidence in Vietnam veterans and Vietnam-era veterans. The study population consisted of Air Force veterans who served in Operation Ranch Hand and in SEA during the period 1962–1971 and participated in at least one physical examination in 1982, 1985, 1987, 1992, 1997, or 2002. For veterans whose TCDD was not measured in 1987 but was measured later, the later measurement was extrapolated to 1987 by using a first-order kinetics model with a constant half-life of 7.6 years. For diabetes, the study period began with a veteran's departure from Vietnam or SEA and extended through December 2004. From an initial sample size of 1,196 subjects, 1,020 Ranch Hand veterans were included in the diabetes analyses after exclusion for pre-existing conditions, noncompliance, and absent TCDD measurements. Comparison veterans served in SEA during the same period but were not involved in spraying herbicides. The final comparison group included 1,449 people in the diabetes analyses. Diabetes diagnoses were determined during one of the physical examinations or verified from medical records; veterans were excluded if they had a history of diabetes before service in SEA or if they had no TCDD measurements. Time to onset was defined as the number of years between the end of the tour of duty and the date of first diagnosis of diabetes. For cancer incidence, the study period was January 1983–September 2004. The final analyses for cancer incidence included 986 Ranch Hand veterans and 1,597 comparison people that met the inclusion criteria. Cancer incidence was obtained from medical records and coded according to *International Clas-*

sification of Diseases, revision 9 (ICD-9). Malignancies discovered at death were coded from the causes of death on death certificates. Study results were correlated by body mass index (BMI), tour dates, number of days spent in Vietnam, number of days spent in SEA; for Ranch Hand veterans, the last day of service in the Ranch Hand unit and number of days of spraying; and for comparison veterans, the last day of service in SEA.

The tendency of the AFHS researchers to use differing cutpoints and population definitions for analogous analyses suggests their a-posteriori selection in a fashion that influences the results. For example, Michalek and Pavuk (2008) allude to the commonly held assumption that Agent Orange was more heavily contaminated earlier in the war as the motivation for making various temporal partitions in their analyses, but the choices were not consistent. For cancer, 1968 or before was the cutpoint for the "date of service" variable, while "days of spraying" were counted through 1967 and the distribution was partitioned at 30 days. For diabetes, however, "date of service" was divided at 1969 or before and "number of days of spraying" was split at 90 days or more, with no specification of the time period over which the counting was done.

In trying to harvest evidence from a fairly broad spectrum of populations targeted in epidemiologic studies, the VAO committees have factored in results on Vietnam veterans in general on the grounds that they are representative of all subjects who might have had increased exposure to herbicide components (as surrogates for VA's clientele). With respect to the Blue Water Navy issue, the AFHS data document that herbicide spraying did not occur solely in Vietnam and did not affect only those deployed to Vietnam. Serum TCDD results from the AFHS demonstrate that the Ranch Hands in general were, indeed, more highly exposed than the SEA veterans, but the SEA veterans had serum TCDD concentrations that tended to exceed background values in the US population.

The AFHS is perceived by many to be the central piece of research for decision making by the committees preparing the VAO reports. However, it represents an unwieldy body of information that was gathered in evolving accord with a protocol that was intended to address specific questions but in practice generated data that have proved far more challenging to interpret than expected. It took the committee that produced *Disposition of the Air Force Health Study* (IOM, 2006) much effort to sort out which data were sought and which data were actually assembled in the course of an enterprise that went on for more than 20 years. The report's conclusions (IOM, 2006, pp. 80–81) about the limitations of the AFHS were as follows:

Limitations Related to the Design and Execution of the Study

The AFHS—like all epidemiologic studies—suffers from limitations related to factors intrinsic to its design and resulting from implementation decisions made by the investigators. Many of these are specific to the study of the health effects of wartime exposure to herbicides and would carry into future research on this topic, although some of the limitations can be addressed by making different assumptions in analyses. However, the limitations would not necessarily extend to more general studies using the data assets.

Study limitations were a central topic of the 1999 GAO report on the AFHS . . . The GAO study director, Kwai-Cheung Chan . . . , summarized that report's findings as follows:

The [AFHS] has two major limitations: it has difficulty in detecting low to moderate increases in risks of rare diseases because of the relatively small size of the Ranch Hand population, and its findings cannot be generalized to all Vietnam veterans because Ranch Hands and ground troops were exposed to different levels of herbicides in different ways. Blood measurements of dioxin . . . suggest that the Ranch Hands' exposure levels were significantly higher than those of many ground troops. But ground troops may have been exposed in ways (such as through contaminated food and water) that Ranch Hands were not, and little is known about the potential effects of such differences.

GAO asserted that "the Air Force has not clearly or effectively communicated these limitations to the public" . . . and suggested that lack of knowledge of these issues was leading to misunderstanding of the study's results.

In congressional testimony concerning the GAO report in 2000, Dr. Linda Spoonster Schwartz—a Yale University researcher and retired Major USAF nurse—offered additional observations. . . . Among her comments were that the AFHS protocol (AFHS, 1982) stated that data collected from active duty personnel[17] were not confidential because information that indicated a risk to "public safety or national defense" would be made known to the USAF. The fact that a subject's information could affect his career could, she said, have had an influence on the subject's responses and willingness to submit to certain tests. Dr. Schwartz also indicated that, since all of the AFHS participants were in Vietnam at one time, it could not be assumed that the comparison subjects had no significant exposure to herbicides,[18] and that this called into question the validity of the comparison group for studies of the health effects of herbicides.

Dr. Joel Michalek, then principal investigator of the AFHS, spoke in a January 2005 presentation before the committee about how the study had dealt with obstacles. . . . He noted four limitations of the study related to herbicide health effects research: the inherently small size of the cohort; lack of any biomarkers of herbicide exposure other than dioxin; little information on participants' locations in the theater of operations; and unavailability of a detailed exposure history. Michalek also indicated that AFHS investigators had confronted several exposure-related design and analysis issues. Lack of a good herbicide exposure metric led to concerns over exposure misclassification and bias that were recognized in the study's original protocol (AFHS, 1982).[19] After CDC developed an assay for measuring serum TCDD levels in the late 1980s that AFHS adopted as a proxy, more issues arose. One of these was the effect of measurement error in the estimation of TCDD half-life, an issue because this value was used to estimate a common baseline serum dioxin level for each study participant. Papers by Caudill et al. . . . and Michalek et al. . . . discuss this in greater detail. Later papers addressed the validity of dioxin body burden as an exposure index . . . , reliability of the dioxin assay. . . , and the correction of bias in half-life calculations. . . . The AFHS web site notes a weakness specific to the examination of questions outside of the study's stated mission to evaluate the health effects of wartime exposure to herbicides: "[b]ecause all of our study subjects served in Vietnam or Southeast Asia, contrasting Ranch Hands with comparisons may not fully reveal health differences associated with service in Vietnam". . . .

An additional obstacle identified by this committee is related to study design. As described above, the design allowed the addition of replacement comparisons at each cycle. The integration of replacements in statistical analyses cannot be handled using standard statistical techniques.

Subjects who were found to have been misclassified (designated as a comparison subject when in fact they were a Ranch Hand subject and vice versa) were in turn reassigned to the other group and followed under this new group assignment. Such a design, coupled with the usual issues of missing data and losses to followup, complicates the reanalysis of results presented in AFHS reports and papers.

---

[17]At the time of the Cycle 1 exam, 185 Ranch Hands and 184 comparison subjects were on active duty; in addition, 210 Ranch Hand subjects and 234 comparison subjects held current military or civilian flying certificates, which have rigorous physical and mental fitness requirements (AFHS, 1984a).

[18]Serum dioxin levels in study subjects are not a reliable proxy for exposure because these levels decrease over time in the absence of exposure, blood draws were not taken until several years after the end of US military involvement in Vietnam, and not all herbicides were contaminated with dioxin.

[19]The protocol also addresses a number of other recognized study difficulties and planned correction measures.

In the preface of the report on the 2002 physical examinations (AFHS, 2005, p. ii), the AFHS researchers themselves warned against considering the contents (and those of the five earlier sets of examinations) as the most definitive presentations of the assembled information on the Ranch Hand subjects and the comparison veterans:

This report is comprehensive and detailed, but limited in that (a) it included only those veterans who attended the final physical examination, (b) it addressed only those risk factors that were thought to be important when the study was designed, and (c) it did not account for potentially important risk factors that were discovered after the analytical plan was set. In addition to these six reports, study results have been summarized in articles published in peer-reviewed scientific journals. Such articles differ from the reports in that they (a) incorporate all participants who attended at least one physical examination, (b) use different methods of analysis, (c) focus on particular health endpoints, and (d) include recently discovered risk factors. The results in the journal articles are often consistent, but sometimes lead to conclusions that differ from the six reports. For example, published articles on diabetes in Ranch Hand veterans revealed an association with dioxin exposure consistent with the current report. Published articles on peripheral neuropathy, memory loss, and cancer, however, revealed associations not discussed in this report.

As the preface notes, the conclusions of the examination reports and of the journal articles are not always in obvious accord.

The methods sections of the AFHS report (2005; for example, p. 10-7 for neoplasia) state that cumulative individual histories were compiled on men who participated in the 2002 cycle (giving something akin to cumulative prevalence for 1987–2002 among participating survivors) for the neoplastic, neurologic, pychologic, gastrointestinal, dermatologic, cardiovascular, renal, endocrinologic, and pulmonary variables. For general health, hematologic, and immunologic variables, however, the analyses in the 2002 examination report were apparently only of information gathered in that cycle.

The multiple analysis models, changing inclusion criteria, different exposure groupings, and so on applied to the evolving dataset make it challenging to track the findings on an outcome through the course of the study. For example, noting the number of various types of cancer cases reported to have been analyzed in various documents produced during the final stages of the AFHS gives a confusing picture (see Table 5-4). The discrepancies in the table are large enough to require explanation:

- The paucity of prostate-cancer cases in the Ranch Hand subjects as analyzed in Akhtar et al. (2004) compared with the number in Pavuk et al. (2006).
- The 15 melanoma cases and 54 prostate-cancer cases in the comparison group (Akhtar et al., 2004) are far fewer than the corresponding numbers that had ever been diagnosed before the 2002 examinations.

It is unclear whether the large differences in the numbers of melanoma and prostate-cancer cases analyzed in the comparison subjects between Akhtar et al. (2004) and Pavuk et al. (2005, 2006) are entirely accounted for by the fact that the Akhtar dataset did not include subjects who received diagnoses during the 2002 examination cycle (melanoma and prostate cancer are among the cancers likely to be detected during a thorough physical examination). If so, especially given the asymmetric nature of the changes in the numbers of Ranch Hand and comparison subjects, would it imply that the results reported by Akhtar et al. could not be considered representative of the final AFHS sample? The AFHS researchers remarked in the preface to the final report on the final physical-examination cycle:

TABLE 5-4 Numbers of Ranch Hand and SEA Comparison Subjects with Particular Types of Cancer Included in Various Analyses Based on AFHS Data

Tumor type	Cases Among Ranch Handers			Cases Among SEA Comparisons			
	AFHS (2005)	Akhtar et al. (2004) Table 4 (Table 7)	Pavuk et al. (2006) Table 1	AFHS (2005)	Akhtar et al. (2004) Table 4 (Table 7)	Pavuk et al. (2005) Table 4	Pavuk et al. (2006) Table 1
Digestive system (not clear whether SEER system used)		16 (6 dead)			31 (14 dead)	24	
Respiratory system (not clear whether SEER system used)	13	33 (21 dead)		7	48 (38 dead)	36	
Melanoma	19	17 (< 4 dead)		31	15 (< 2 dead)	25	
Basal cell or squamous cell	175	nr		213	nr	253	
Basal cell	154			183			
Squamous cell	45			61			
Prostate	53	36 (2 dead)	62 total 59 TCDD	67	54 (3 dead)	83	89 total 81 TCDD

ABBREVIATIONS: nr, not reported; SEA, Southeast Asia; SEER, Surveillance, Epidemiology, and End Results program; TCDD, 2,3,7,8-tetrachlorodibenzo-p-dioxin (measurements available).

NOTES: Case counts from AFHS (2005) are cumulative for cases diagnosed from the end of service in SEA through 2003 for those who participated in the 2002 examination cycle (that is, deceased excluded). A person was counted only once for having any tumor in a given analysis. The analyses for melanoma and nonmelanoma skin cancers only excluded black veterans.

Case counts from Akhtar et al. (2004) are cumulative for whites from the end of service in SEA through 1999, so did not include any cancers found in the 2002 examination cycle. The analyses for all sites excluded veterans whose race was black or "other."

Case counts from Pavuk et al. (2005) are cumulative for first cancers diagnosed from 1982 to 2003 for SEA comparison subjects with TCDD readings. The analyses for melanoma and nonmelanoma skin cancers only excluded black veterans.

Case counts from Pavuk et al. (2006) are cumulative for first prostate cancers diagnosed from 1982 to 2003 for those with TCDD readings.

The lack of a particular finding does not prove that no association exists and should not lead the reader to conclude that there is no association between herbicide exposure and adverse health. In particular, a recently published analysis showed an increase in cancer risk with increased dioxin body burden in Ranch Hand veterans who spent less than 2 years in Southeast Asia; a stratified analysis was performed because years of service in Southeast Asia was identified as a risk factor for cancer in Comparison veterans. These patterns require that more sophisticated statistical models be used to study cancer in Ranch Hand veterans. Consistent with the protocol, study investigators continue to question the underlying assumptions of all analyses, explore new ways to analyze data, and collaborate with specialists to determine whether exposure to Agent Orange adversely affected the health of Ranch Hand veterans.

Not only have the "exposed" subjects (Ranch Hand veterans) been compared with the "comparison" subjects (SEA veterans), but both groups have been contrasted with nonveteran US men, and various subsets (some seemingly arcane) of the entire sample have been analyzed on the basis of serum TCDD concentrations. For purposes of the VAO project, all that actually represents a unitary observation on each of a multitude of health outcomes, which it would be desirable to distill as concisely as possible. In seeking a consistent approach to incorporating the AFHS data for a variety of outcomes, the current committee adopts the decisions of the committee for *Update 2006* that:

- The limitations of the AFHS are such that it was under-powered for detecting actual effects, so indications of positivity, especially if they are repeated over examination cycles, are likely to be a real signal. The findings in the examination-cycle reports are not much more than a large data dump with analyses dictated by the original protocol; they have not really been scientifically processed and interpreted.
- The examination-cycle reports are not useful for assessing **cancer endpoints** (they are only "sort of cumulative" for incidence; people who have died are excluded from the cycle sample); the committee worked from the more fully cumulative and thoughtfully analyzed findings in the published peer-reviewed articles.
- For assessing **some** of the **non-cancer endpoints**, the findings seem to be useful, but they would need to be combined with other findings to support a conclusion other than "inadequate."

Centers for Disease Control and Prevention

Surveys of US Vietnam veterans who were not part of the Ranch Hand or Army Chemical Corps (ACC) groups indicate that 25–55% believe that they were exposed to herbicides (CDC, 1989; Erickson et al., 1984a,b; Stellman and Stellman, 1986). Several attempts have been made to estimate exposure of

Vietnam veterans who were not part of the Ranch Hand or ACC groups. CDC has undertaken a series of studies to examine various health outcomes in Vietnam veterans as directed by Congress in the Veterans Health Programs Extension and Improvement Act of 1979 (Public Law [PL] 96-151) and the Veterans' Health Care, Training, and Small Business Loan Act of 1981 (PL 97-72). *VAO* and *Veterans and Agent Orange: Update 1996*, referred to as *Update 1996* (IOM, 1996) describe those studies in detail. The first was a case–control interview study of birth defects in offspring of men who served in Vietnam (Erickson et al., 1984a,b). In 1983, the US government asked CDC to conduct a study of possible long-term health effects in Vietnam veterans exposed to Agent Orange. The CDC Agent Orange study (CDC, 1985) attempted to classify veterans' service-related exposures to herbicides. That involved determining the proximity of troops to Agent Orange spraying by using military records to track troop movement and the HERBS tapes to locate herbicide-spraying patterns. The CDC birth-defects study developed an exposure-opportunity index to score Agent Orange exposure (Erickson et al., 1984a,b).

In 1987, CDC conducted the Agent Orange Validation Study to test the validity of the various indirect methods used to estimate exposure of ground troops to Agent Orange in Vietnam. The study measured serum TCDD in a nonrandom sample of Vietnam veterans and in Vietnam-era veterans who did not serve in Vietnam (CDC, 1988b). Vietnam veterans were selected for study on the basis of the number of Agent Orange hits that they were thought to have experienced, as derived from the number of days on which their company was within 2 km and 6 days of a recorded Agent Orange spraying event. Blood samples were obtained from 66% of Vietnam veterans (n = 646) and from 49% of the eligible comparison group of veterans (n = 97). More than 94% of those whose serum was obtained had served in one of five battalions.

The median serum TCDD in Vietnam veterans in 1987 was 4 ppt (range, under 1 to 45 ppt). Only two veterans had concentrations above 20 ppt. The "low" exposure group consisted of 298 Vietnam veterans, the "medium" exposure group 157 veterans, and the "high" exposure group 191 veterans. The distribution of TCDD measurements was nearly identical with that in the control group of 97 non-Vietnam veterans. The CDC validation study concluded that study subjects could not be distinguished from controls on the basis of serum TCDD. In addition, neither record-derived estimates of exposure nor self-reported exposure to herbicides could predict Vietnam veterans with currently high serum TCDD (CDC, 1988b, 1989a). The report concluded that it was unlikely that military records alone could be used to identify a large number of veterans who might have been heavily exposed to TCDD in Vietnam.

Using those exposure estimates, CDC conducted the Vietnam Experience Study (VES), a historical cohort study of the health experience of Vietnam veterans (CDC, 1989b). The study was divided into three parts: physical health, reproductive outcomes and child health, and psychosocial characteristics (CDC,

1987, 1988a,b,c, 1989b). Using VES data, CDC examined postservice mortality (through 1983) in a cohort of 9,324 US Army veterans who served in Vietnam and in 8,989 Vietnam-era Army veterans who served in Korea, Germany, or the United States (Boyle et al., 1987; CDC, 1987). Another study (O'Brien et al., 1991) combined the mortality and interview data to identify all veterans with non-Hodgkin's lymphoma (NHL). To evaluate whether self-reported assessment of exposure to herbicides influences the reporting of adverse health outcomes, CDC designed a study of VES subjects (Decoufle et al., 1992). In a follow-up of CDC's VES cohort, Boehmer et al. (2004) reported findings on mortality during 1965–2000.

The serum TCDD measurements in Vietnam veterans also suggested that exposure to TCDD in Vietnam was substantially lower, *on the average*, than that of persons exposed as a result of the industrial explosion in Seveso or that of the heavily exposed occupational workers who are the focus of many of the studies evaluated by the committee. The assessment of *average* exposure does not preclude heavy exposure of subgroups of Vietnam veterans.

CDC undertook the Selected Cancers Study (CDC, 1990a) to investigate the effects of military service in Vietnam and of exposure to herbicides on the health of American veterans, specifically NHL (CDC, 1990b), soft-tissue sarcoma (STS) and other sarcomas (CDC, 1990c), Hodgkin's disease (HD; CDC, 1990d), and nasal, nasopharyngeal, and primary liver cancers (CDC, 1990d).

Department of Veterans Affairs

Numerous cohort and case–control studies are discussed in detail in *VAO*, *Update 1996*, *Veterans and Agent Orange: Update 1998* referred to as *Update 1998* (IOM, 1999); *Update 2000* (IOM, 2001); *Update 2002* (IOM, 2003a); *Update 2004* (IOM, 2005); and *Update 2006* (IOM, 2007). Among the earliest was a proportionate-mortality study by Breslin et al. (1988). The subjects were ground troops who served in the US Army or Marine Corps at any time from July 4, 1965, through March 1, 1973, or veterans who were born in 1934–1957. A list of 186,000 Vietnam-era veterans who served in the Army or Marine Corps and were reported deceased as of July 1, 1982, was assembled from VA's BIRLS; 75,617 names were randomly selected from the list for inclusion in the study. Information extracted from the selected military records included the places, dates, and branch of military service; date of birth; sex; race; military occupation specialty codes; education level; type of discharge; and confirmation of service in Vietnam. Additional information was extracted on veterans who served in SEA, including the first and last dates of service in SEA, the military unit, and the country where the veteran served. Of the final sample of 52,253 Army and Marine Corps veterans, cause of death was ascertained from death certificates or Department of Defense Report of Casualty forms for 51,421 men, including 24,235 who served in Vietnam and 26,685 men who did not serve in SEA; 501 deaths were excluded from the final analyses because service in SEA was in a country other than Vietnam or the location of military service was unknown. Each veteran's cause of death was coded by a nosologist who used ICD-8.

On the basis of the proportionate-mortality study (Breslin et al., 1988), Burt et al. (1987) conducted a nested case–control study of NHL with controls selected from among the cardiovascular-disease deaths. In a follow-up of the Breslin et al. study, Bullman et al. (1990) compared cause-specific proportionate mortality of 6,668 Army I Corps Vietnam veterans—veterans who served in the northernmost part of South Vietnam in a combat zone designated as Military Region I by the US military—with that of 27,917 Army Vietnam-era veterans who had not served in Vietnam. The study by Bullman et al. included the study population identified by Breslin et al. and an additional 9,555 Army Vietnam-era veteran deaths that were identified after the BIRLs mortality data were extended through December 31, 1984. Similarly, Watanabe et al. (1991) updated the Vietnam-veteran mortality experience reported by Breslin et al. (1988) by extending the follow-up from January 1, 1982, to December 31, 1984. An additional 11,325 deceased Army and Marine Vietnam-era veterans were identified from the period and included in the study. The study population for Watanabe et al. consisted of 62,068 military veterans, of whom 29,646 served in Vietnam and 32,422 never served in SEA. Proportionate mortality ratios were calculated by three referent groups: branch-specific (Army and Marine Corps) non-Vietnam veterans, all non-Vietnam veterans combined, and, the US male population. A third follow-up proportionate-mortality study using the veterans from Breslin et al. (1988) and Watanabe et al. (1991) also was conducted (Watanabe and Kang, 1996); it included an additional 9,040 randomly selected Vietnam-era veterans who died from July 1, 1984, through June 30, 1988. The final study included 70,630 veterans—33,833 who served in Vietnam and 36,797 who never served in SEA—and the analyses were performed with the same referent groups described previously (Watanabe et al., 1991).

VA also conducted studies focusing on specific health outcomes, using data from VA's Agent Orange Registry (AOR), a computer database containing health information on Vietnam veterans who voluntarily undergo physical examinations at a VA hospital. The AOR was set up in 1978 to monitor Vietnam veterans' health complaints or problems that could be related to Agent Orange exposure during military service in Vietnam. The physical examinations consist of an exposure history, a medical history, laboratory tests, and an examination of body systems most commonly affected by toxic chemicals. As of June 1, 2008, the registry contained information from 506,184 examinations (Agent Orange Review, 2008).

Using early data from the registry, Bullman et al. (1991) examined the risk of post-traumatic stress disorder (PTSD) in a case–control study of veterans who received AOR medical examinations during January 1983–December 1987. The final analyses include 374 PTSD cases and 373 controls for whom military records were used to verify Vietnam service, Military Occupational Specialty Codes (MOSCs), primary duties, military branch, dates of Vietnam service, medals, awards, and disciplinary actions for each veteran. Similarly, Bullman et al. (1994)

studied the risk of testicular cancer by using the AOR health records of veterans who received Agent Orange medical examinations during March 1982–January 1991. The final analyses in that study included 97 testicular-cancer cases and 311 controls. A surrogate metric for Agent Orange exposure was developed by using branch of service, combat MOSCs, geographic area of service in Vietnam, location of military units in relation to herbicide spray missions, and the length of time between spray missions and military operations in sprayed areas.

Watanabe and Kang (1995) compared postservice mortality in Vietnam veterans in the Marine Corps with that in Vietnam-era marines who did not serve in Vietnam. All study participants were on active duty during 1967–1969 and were followed from their discharge date or from the date of the US military withdrawal from Vietnam until their date of death or December 31, 1991, whichever came first. The final study population included 10,716 Vietnam and 9,346 non-Vietnam veteran marines.

Kang et al. (1991) conducted a case–control study that compared dioxin and dibenzofuran concentrations in the adipose tissue of 36 Vietnam veterans with those in 79 non-Vietnam veterans and a sample 80 of US men born in 1936–1954. All tissue samples were archived specimens from the US Environmental Protection Agency (EPA) National Human Adipose Tissue Survey and had been collected by hospitals and medical examiners from men who died from external causes or surgical procedures. Military service—branch of service, MOSC, and geographic service location in Vietnam, if applicable—was researched and verified with military records. Controls were matched by birth year and sample collection year (± 2 years), and the final analyses were adjusted by age and BMI.

Female Veterans   Although estimates vary, 5,000–7,000 women are believed to have served in Vietnam after volunteering for military service in the United States (Thomas et al., 1991). The vast majority of them served as combat nurses—most serving in the Army Nurse Corps—but they also served with the Women's Army Corps and the Air Force, Navy, and Marine Corps (Spoonster-Schwartz, 1987; Thomas et al., 1991).

In 1986, PL 99-972 was enacted, requiring that an epidemiologic study be conducted to examine long-term adverse health effects in female Vietnam veterans as a result of their exposure to traumatic experiences, exposure to such herbicides as Agent Orange or other chemicals or medications, or any other similar experience or exposure during such service. The first study that VA conducted to assess mortality in female Vietnam veterans was by Thomas et al. (1991). No comprehensive record of female personnel who served in Vietnam in 1964–1972 existed, so researchers gathered military service data from each branch of the armed forces to conduct the mortality study through December 31, 1987. Female Army and Navy personnel were identified from morning reports and muster rolls of hospitals and administrative support units where women were likely to have served. Military personnel were identified as female by their names, leaving open the possibility that some women may have been inadvertently excluded from the analysis. Women who served in the Air Force and Marine Corps were identified through military records. The combined roster of all female personnel from the military branches was considered by the researchers to be relatively complete. Comparisons were female veterans identified through the same process as the female Vietnam veterans but who had not served in Vietnam during their military service. Demographic information and information on overseas tours of duty, unit assignments, jobs, and principal duties were abstracted from military records. Mortality information was obtained from VA's beneficiary records, the Social Security Administration, IRS, National Death Index, and military personnel records. When women whose service in the military fell outside the period of interest, whose records were lacking data, or who served in SEA but not Vietnam were excluded, the analysis included 132 deaths in 4,582 female Vietnam veterans and 232 deaths in 5,324 comparison veterans who served in the military in July 4, 1965–March 28, 1973. Cause-specific mortality was derived for Vietam veterans and comparison veterans and compared with mortality in US women, adjusted for race, age, and calendar period. Dalager et al. (1995a) updated mortality in the original cohort until December 31, 1991, using the same study protocol as Thomas et al. (1991). After updating of mortality figures and adjustment of the existing cohort on the basis of new information to the study groups based on the inclusion criteria, 4,586 Vietnam veterans and 5,325 comparison veterans were included in the final analyses.

VA also published studies on pregnancy outcomes and gynecologic cancers—namely, neoplasms of the cervix, uterus, and ovary—in US female Vietnam veterans (Kang et al., 2000a,b). Army veterans were identified from a list obtained by the US Army and Joint Services Environmental Support group; computerized lists were also provided by the Air Force, Navy, and Marine Corps. Military-service data were abstracted from personnel records. Of 5,230 eligible veterans, 4,390 whose permanent tour of duty included service in Vietnam were alive on January 1, 1992. From a pool of 6,657 potential control subjects whose military units did not serve in Vietnam, 4,390 veterans who were alive on January 1, 1992, were randomly selected as controls. After exclusion of 250 veterans and 250 nonveterans who participated in a pilot study, an attempt was made to locate the remaining 4,140 veterans in each group. Various location strategies were used, and fewer than 5% (370) were not located; another 339 were deceased. A full telephone interview was conducted on 6,430; 775 refused (13% of Vietnam veterans and 17% of non-Vietnam veterans), and another 366 completed only a short written questionnaire. A questionnaire was administered on demographic background, general health, lifestyle, menstrual history, pregnancy history, pregnancy outcomes, and military experience, including nursing occupation and combat exposure. Information on pregnancy complications—including smoking, infections, medications, exposure to x rays, occupational history, and exposure to anesthetic gases, ethylene oxide, herbicides, and pesticides—was collected for each pregnancy. In Kang et al. (2000a), the first pregnancy after the beginning of Vietnam service was designated as the index pregnancy for each woman. For the comparison group, the first pregnancy after July 4, 1965, was used as the index pregnancy. Odds ratios were calculated for reproductive history and pregnancy outcomes. The study analyzed data on 3,392 Vietnam and 3,038 non-Vietnam veterans and on 1,665 Vietnam and 1,912 non-Vietnam veteran index pregnancies. In Kang et al. (2000b), a self-reported history of gynecologic cancers (defined by the authors as cancers of the breast, ovary, uterus, and cervix) was collected. The authors attempted to "retrieve hospital records on all reported cancers as far back as 30 years." Of records successfully found, 99% of the breast cancers were confirmed, and 90% of all cancers were confirmed. The authors did not provide data on validation of the three sites other than breast, but stated that Vietnam status was not associated with verification of outcome.

After the publications by Kang et al. (2000a,b), Congress passed PL 106-419, which provides compensation for children of female Vietnam veterans who are born with birth defects unrelated to an existing familial disorder, to a birth-related injury, or to a fetal or neonatal infirmity with a well-established cause. Eighteen birth defects are covered by the legislation, including cleft lip or palate, congenital heart disease, hypospadias, neural-tube defects, and Williams's syndrome. A complete list of covered birth defects can be found in Section 3.815 of the legislation.

Since *Update 2006*, Cypel and Kang (2008) have conducted a mortality study of female Vietnam veterans and compared their mortality with that in a control group of women who were in military service but did not participate in the Vietnam War. For their retrospective cohort study, eligible subjects were on active duty in Vietnam and in other areas in 1964–1972, and researchers considered the study period to extend from the time when each woman separated from active-duty service or the end of the Vietnam War (March 1973), whichever came first, through December 2004. After exclusion for unmet eligibility criteria or lack of evidence of Vietnam service, the Vietnam cohort consisted of 4,586 female veterans, primarily nurses, who served in Vietnam during July 1965–March 1973. Non-Vietnam veterans were selected randomly from among women who never served in Vietnam and were matched (presumably by frequency matching) to the Vietnam veterans according to rank and military occupation; this resulted in a comparison group of 6,575 non-Vietnam veterans. The final sample size for non-Vietnam veterans was 5,325, after exclusions due to unmet eligibility criteria (not specified) and exclusion of about 1,000 nurses who served in Guam, the Phillipines, Japan, Korea, Okinawa, or Thailand, because of concerns about having conditions similar to those of women who served in Vietnam. It is not clear whether veterans other than nurses who served in those locations were also excluded. The exclusion of the nurses led to a difference in the distributions of occupation and broke the matching strategy (formerly 1:4); for example, the proportions of "officer/nurses" in the Vietnam cohort and the non-Vietnam cohorts were 80.5% and 61.7%, respectively. In addition, the non-Vietnam cohort was younger at time of entry than the Vietnam cohort (those less than 25 years old made up 32.4% of the Vietnam cohort and 49.5% of the non-Vietnam cohort), but the crude mortality in the comparison population was 32.3% higher (40.14 vs 53.09 per 10,000). Thus, there was an imbalance in the cohorts in age but also a peculiarity in mortality so the results of the analyses resembled a situation in which the healthy-worker effect was operative. For example, the crude rate ratio for all-causes mortality was 0.76, and the adjusted one was 0.92. The committee was therefore concerned about potential selection biases built into the study that may lead to biased results.

Army Chemical Corps   Members of the US ACC performed chemical operations on the ground and by helicopter and were thereby involved in the direct handling and distribution of herbicides in Vietnam. That population was belatedly identified for the study of health effects related to herbicide exposure (Thomas and Kang, 1990). In an extension, Dalager and Kang (1997) compared mortality in veterans of the ACC specialties, including Vietnam veterans and non-Vietnam veterans. Results of an initial feasibility study were reported by Kang et al. (2001). They recruited 565 veterans: 284 Vietnam veterans and 281 non-Vietnam veteran control subjects. Blood samples were collected in 1996 from 50 Vietnam veterans and 50 control veterans, and 95 of the samples met CDC standards of quality assurance and quality. Comparison of the entire Vietnam cohort with the entire non-Vietnam cohort showed that the geometric mean TCDD concentrations did not differ significantly ($p = 0.6$). Of the 50 Vietnam veterans sampled, analysis of questionnaire responses indicated that those who reported spraying herbicides had higher TCDD concentrations than did those who reported no spraying activities. The authors concluded that Agent Orange exposure was a likely contributor to TCDD concentrations in Vietnam veterans who had a history of spraying herbicides.

Kang et al. (2006) reported findings from the main study. A health survey of 1,499 Vietnam veterans and 1,428 non-Vietnam veterans was administered by telephone. Exposure to herbicides was assessed by analyzing serum specimens from a sample of 897 veterans for dioxin. Veterans who reported spraying herbicides had significantly higher TCDD serum concentrations than did Vietnam veterans and other veterans who did not report herbicide spraying. The final analysis compared Vietnam-veteran sprayers with Vietnam-veteran nonsprayers in the entire study population.

VA has evaluated specific health outcomes, including case–control studies of STS (Kang et al., 1986, 1987), NHL (Dalager et al., 1991), testicular cancer (Bullman et al., 1994), HD (Dalager et al., 1995b), and lung cancer (Mahan et al., 1997). It also has conducted a study of self-reported physical health (Eisen et al., 1991) and PTSD (Goldberg et al., 1990) in monozygotic twins who served during the Vietnam era.

Dalager et al. (1991) examined NHL in male Vietnam veterans in a hospital-based case–control study. Study participants were identified via inpatient discharge records from VA medical centers for fiscal years 1969–1985. Cases were identified as having a malignant lymphoma and a birth date during 1937–1954. Controls were identified from VA medical-center discharge records and were matched by hospital, discharge date, and birth date. The location and dates of each veteran's military service were verified by using military records. A surrogate Agent Orange exposure opportunity was also developed for each Vietnam veteran according to branch of service, combat experience, and geographic location of the military unit assignment. The final analysis included 201 cases and 358 controls. Another study by Dalager et al. (1995b) examined the association between HD and Vietnam service. It used the same method as the 1991 Dalager et al. study; the analysis included 283 HD cases and 404 controls.

VA has examined other outcomes in Vietnam veterans: PTSD (Bullman et al., 1991; True et al., 1988), suicide and motor-vehicle crashes (Bullman and Kang, 1996; Farberow et al., 1990), and tobacco use (McKinney et al., 1997). The studies have been included for completeness, but the outcomes that they address are outside the purview of this committee. *VAO* and *Update 1998* discuss them in detail; most did not discuss exposure to Agent Orange, and exposure to "combat" was evaluated as the risk factor of interest.

American Legion   The American Legion, a voluntary service organization for veterans, conducted a cohort study of the health and well-being of Vietnam veterans who were members. Studies examined physical health and reproductive outcomes, social–behavioral consequences, and PTSD in veterans who had served in SEA and elsewhere (Snow et al., 1988; Stellman JM et al., 1988; Stellman SD et al., 1988). No new studies have been published on the cohort.

State Studies   Several states have conducted studies of Vietnam veterans, most of them unpublished in the scientific literature. *VAO* and *Update 1996* reviewed studies on veterans of Hawaii (Rellahan, 1985), Iowa (Wendt, 1985), Maine (Deprez et al., 1991), Massachusetts (Clapp, 1997; Clapp et al., 1991; Kogan and Clapp, 1985, 1988; Levy, 1988), Michigan (Visintainer et al., 1995), New Jersey (Fiedler and Gochfeld, 1992; Kahn et al., 1988, 1992a,b,c), New Mexico (Pollei et al., 1986), New York (Greenwald et al., 1984; Lawrence et al., 1985), Pennsylvania (Goun and Kuller, 1986), Texas (Newell, 1984), West Virginia (Holmes et al., 1986), and Wisconsin (Anderson et al., 1986a,b).

Other US Vietnam-Veteran Studies   Additional studies have examined health outcomes that included spontaneous abortion (Aschengrau and Monson, 1989) and late adverse pregnancy outcomes in spouses of Vietnam veterans (Aschengrau and Monson, 1990). After a published study indicated a potential association for testicular cancer in dogs that served in Vietnam (Hayes et al., 1990), Tarone et al.

(1991) conducted a case–control study of testicular cancer in male veterans. *VAO* summarized those studies, and no new studies have been published.

The 1997 Institute of Medicine request for proposals for historical-exposure reconstruction has led to the development of new methods for estimating Vietnam veterans' exposures to Agent Orange. The resulting Columbia University project integrated various sources of information on spraying activities to generate individualized estimates of the exposure potential of troops who served in Vietnam (Stellman and Stellman, 2003). Location data on military units assigned to Vietnam were compiled into a database developed from five primary and secondary sources: the Unit Identification Code list (a reference list of units serving in Vietnam created and used by the Army), a command-post list (division-level data on command locations of army personnel), Army Post Office lists (compilations of locations down to and including battalion size and other selected units that were updated on monthly), troop-strength reports (data assembled by the US Military Assistance Command on troop allocations, updated monthly and generally collected on the battalion level), and order-of-battle information (data on command post, arrival and departure dates, and authorized strength of many units). For units that served in the III Corps Tactical Zone during 1966–1969, battalion-tracking data were also available; these are data on the grid coordinate locations of battalion-sized units derived from daily journals, which recorded company locations over 24-hour periods.

Mobility-factor analysis, a new concept for studying troop movement, was developed for use in reconstructing herbicide-exposure histories. The analysis is a three-part classification system for characterizing the location and movement of military units in Vietnam. It comprises a mobility designation (stable, mobile, or elements mobile), a distance designation (usually in a range of kilometers) to indicate how far the unit might travel in a day, and a notation of the modes of travel available to the unit: air, ground (truck, tank, or armored personnel carrier), or water. A mobility factor was assigned to every unit that served in Vietnam.

All those data were combined into a geographic information system (GIS) for Vietnam with a grid resolution of 0.01° latitude and 0.01° longitude. Herbicide-spraying records were integrated into the GIS and linked with data on military-unit locations to permit estimation of exposure-opportunity scores for individuals. The results are the subject of reports by the contractor (Stellman and Stellman, 2003) and the *Update 2002* committee (IOM, 2003a,b). A summary of the findings regarding the extent and pattern of herbicide spraying (Stellman et al., 2003a), a description of the GIS for characterizing exposure to Agent Orange and other herbicides in Vietnam (Stellman et al., 2003b), and an explanation of the exposure-opportunity models based on that work (Stellman and Stellman, 2004) have been published in peer-reviewed journals. The publications argue that it is now feasible to conduct epidemiologic investigations of veterans who served as ground troops during the Vietnam War.

A different perspective has been put forth in a series of papers (Young and

Newton, 2004; Young et al., 2004a,b) that argue that ground troops had little direct contact with herbicide sprays and that TCDD residues in Vietnam had low bioavailability. Those conclusions were based on analyses of previously un-published military records and environmental-fate studies. They also argue that ground-troop exposures were relatively low because herbicide-spraying missions were carefully planned and spraying occurred only when friendly forces were not in the target area. Finally, they note that the GIS-based exposure-opportunity model has not yet been validated through measurement of serum dioxin concentrations in veterans (Young, 2004).

Australia

The Australian government has commissioned studies to investigate health risks to Australian veterans: birth anomalies (Donovan et al., 1983, 1984; Evatt, 1985), death (ADVA, 2005b; CIH, 1984a,b,c; Crane et al., 1997a,b; Evatt, 1985; Fett et al., 1987a,b; Forcier et al., 1987), morbidity (AIHW, 1999, 2000, 2001; CDVA 1998a,b), cancer (ADVA, 2005a; results supersede those in CDVA, 1998a), and death and cancer in Australian National Service veterans (ADVA, 2005c; results supersede those in CIH, 1984a; Crane et al., 1997b; Fett et al., 1984). An independent study in Tasmania evaluated reproductive and child-hood-health problems for associations with paternal service in Vietnam (Field and Kerr, 1988). O'Toole et al. (1996a,b,c) described self-reported health status in a random sample of Australian Army Vietnam veterans. Leavy et al. (2006) reported the results of a case–control study examining prostate cancer incidence that factored in self-reported military-service history. *VAO, Update 1998, Update 2000*, the acute myelogenous leukemia report (IOM, 2001), and *Update 2004* describe the studies.

One of the recent studies of Australian Vietnam veterans did not characterize the veterans' exposure to the herbicides sprayed in Vietnam beyond the fact that they served on land or in Vietnamese waters during May 23, 1962–July 1, 1973. It is the convention of this committee to regard Vietnam veterans in general as being more likely to have received higher exposures to the chemicals of concern than the general public.

Korea

Military personnel of the Republic of Korea served in Vietnam during 1964–1973. Kim et al. (2001) attempted to use serum dioxin concentrations to validate an index for estimating group exposure. The study involved 720 veterans who served in Vietnam and 25 veterans who did not. The exposure index was based on Agent Orange spraying patterns in military regions in which Korean person-nel served, time–location data on the military units stationed in Vietnam, and an exposure score derived from self-reported activities during service. A total of 13 pooled samples were submitted to CDC for serum dioxin analysis. One analytic sample was prepared from the pooled blood of the 25 veterans who did not serve in Vietnam. The remaining 12 samples were intended to correspond to 12 exposure categories; each was created by pooling blood samples from 60 veterans. The 12 exposure categories ultimately were reduced to four exposure groups, each representing a quartile of 180 Vietnam veterans but characterized by only three serum TCDD measurements.

The paper by Kim et al. (2001) reported highly significant Pearson correlation coefficients and multiple-logistic-regression-analysis results. The statistical analyses apparently were based on the assignment of the pooled-serum-dioxin value to each individual in the exposure group, thereby inflating the true sample size. The multiple regression analysis evaluated such variables as age, body mass index (BMI), and consumption of tobacco or alcohol. In a later report on the same exposure groups and serum-dioxin data, the authors corrected their analysis (Kim JS et al., 2003). A correlation was observed between serum-dioxin concentrations and ordinal exposure categories, but the correlation was not statistically significant. The authors attributed the lack of statistical significance to the small sample size, and they noted that the data exhibited a distinct monotonic upward trend (average serum dioxin concentrations 0.3, 0.6, 0.62, 0.78, and 0.87 pg/g [lipid adjusted] for exposure categories 0–4, respectively). The decision to pool blood samples from a large number of persons within each exposure set (Kim et al., 2001) greatly reduced the power of the validation study. Instead of 180 samples in each of the final exposure categories, the pooled analysis produced only three samples in each category. The lipid-adjusted serum TCDD concentrations from the 12 pooled samples from Vietnam veterans ranged from 0.25 to 1.2 pg/g, whereas the single sample from the non-Vietnam veterans contained 0.3 pg/g. The narrow range of results makes the biologic relevance of any differences questionable.

Thus, it appears that there was not a clear separation between Korean Vietnam veterans and non-Vietnam veterans. Furthermore, the range of mean values for the four Vietnam-veteran exposure categories was narrow, and all concentrations were relatively low (less than 1 pg/g). The relatively low serum-dioxin concentrations observed in the 1990s in those people are the residua of substantially higher initial concentrations, as has been seen in other Vietnam-veteran groups. However, the concentrations reported in the Korean veterans study are significantly lower than those reported in American Vietnam veterans in the 1988 CDC Agent Orange Validation Study, which was nonetheless unable to distinguish Vietnam veterans from non-Vietnam veterans on the basis of serum dioxin (CDC, 1988b). The Korean authors were able to construct plausible exposure categories based on military records and self-reporting, but they were unable to validate the categories with serum dioxin measurements.

Epidemioligic studies also looked at immunotoxicologic effects (Kim H-A et al., 2003) and skin and general disease patterns (Mo et al., 2002) in Korean Vietnam veterans who were exposed to Agent Orange during the Vietnam conflict.

No additional reports on Korean Vietnam veterans have been published since *Update 2004*.

Other Vietnam-Veteran Studies

Health effects in Vietnam veterans from countries other than the United States, Austrialia, or Korea who are believed to have been exposed to dioxin have been studied. A study reviewed in an earlier update examined antinuclear and sperm autoantibodies in Vietnamese veterans (Chinh et al., 1996). No new studies of other Vietnam-veteran groups were identified by the present committee.

OCCUPATIONAL STUDIES

Several occupational groups in the United States and elsewhere have been exposed to the chemicals of interest. Exposure characterization varies widely in the metric used, the extent of detail, confounding by other exposures, and whether individual, surrogate, or group (ecologic) measures are used. Some studies use job titles as broad surrogates of exposure; others rely on disease-registry data.

The committee reviewed many epidemiologic studies of occupationally exposed groups for evidence of an association between health risks and exposure to TCDD or to the herbicides used in Vietnam, primarily the phenoxy herbicides 2,4-D and 2,4,5-T. TCDD is an unwanted byproduct of 2,4,5-T production but not of 2,4-D production. Other contaminants, including other dioxins (such as 1,3,6,8-tetrachlorodibenzo-*p*-dioxin) have been reported at low concentrations in 2,4-D, but those identified do not have the toxicity of TCDD (ATSDR, 1998; Huston, 1972; Norström et al., 1979). In reviewing the studies, the committee considered two types of exposure separately: exposure to 2,4-D or 2,4,5-T and exposure to TCDD from 2,4,5-T or other sources. That separation is necessary because some health effects could be associated with exposure to 2,4-D or 2,4,5-T in the absence of substantial TCDD exposure. After recognition of the problem of dioxin contamination in phenoxy herbicides, production conditions were modified to minimize contamination, but use of the products most subject to containing specifically TCDD (2,4,5-T and Silvex) was banned. As a result, study subjects exposed to phenoxy herbicides only after the late 1970s would not be assumed to have been at risk for exposure to TCDD.

The distinction is particularly important for workers in agriculture and forestry, including farmers and herbicide appliers, whose exposure is primarily the result of mixing, loading, and applying herbicides. In addition to those occupational groups, the committee considered studies of occupational exposure to dioxins, focusing on workers in chemical plants that produced phenoxy herbicides or chlorophenols, which tend to be contaminated with polychlorinated dibenzo-*p*-dioxins (PCDDs). Waste-incineration workers were also included in the occupation category because they can come into contact with dioxin-like compounds while handling byproducts of incineration. Other occupationally exposed groups included were pulp and paper workers exposed to dioxins through bleaching processes that use chlorinated compounds and sawmill workers exposed to chlorinated dioxins that can be contaminants of chlorophenates used as wood preservatives.

Production Workers

National Institute for Occupational Safety and Health

Starting in 1978, an extensive set of data on chemical production workers potentially contaminated with TCDD in 1942–1984 has been compiled by NIOSH. More than 5,000 workers who were involved in production or maintenance at any of 12 companies were identified from personnel and payroll records; 172 additional workers identified previously by their employers as being exposed to TCDD were also included in the study cohort. The employees' possible exposure resulted from working with substances of which TCDD was a contaminant: 2,4,5-T; 2,4,5-trichlorophenol (2,4,5-TCP); 2-(2,4,5-trichlorophenoxy) propionic acid (Silvex, 2,4,5-TP); 2-(2,4,5-trichlorophenoxy) ethyl 2,2-dichloropropionate (Erbon); *o,o*-dimethyl *o*-(2,4,5-trichlorophenoxy) phosphorothioate (Ronnel); and hexachlorophene. The 12 plants involved were large manufacturing sites of major chemical companies, so many of the subjects were potentially exposed to many other compounds, some of which could be toxic and carcinogenic. The NIOSH cohort was added to the IARC cohort as of the 1987 publication by Kogenvinas et al.

Exposure status was determined initially through a review of process operating conditions, employee duties, and analytic records of TCDD in industrial-hygiene samples, process streams, products, and waste (Fingerhut et al., 1991). Occupational exposure to TCDD-contaminated processes was confirmed by measuring serum TCDD in 253 cohort members. Duration of exposure was defined as the number of years worked in processes contaminated with TCDD and was used as the primary exposure metric in the study. The use of duration of exposure as a surrogate for cumulative exposure was based on a correlation (Pearson correlation efficient, 0.72) between log-transformed serum TCDD and years worked in TCDD-contaminated processes. Duration of exposure of individual workers was calculated from work records, and exposure-duration categories were created: less than 1 year, 1 to less than 5 years, 5 to less than 15 years, and 15 years and longer. In some cases, information on duration of exposure was not available, so a separate metric, duration of employment, was defined as the total time that each worker was employed at the study plant.

Before the publication of the first study of the main cohort, NIOSH conducted a cross-sectional study that included a comprehensive medical history, medical examination, and measurement of pulmonary function of workers employed in chemical manufacturing at a plant in Newark, New Jersey, during 1951–1969 and at a plant in Verona, Missouri, during 1968–1969 and 1970–1972. Control subjects were recruited from surrounding neighborhoods (Alderfer et al., 1992; Calvert et al., 1991, 1992; Sweeney et al., 1989, 1993). The New Jersey plant manufactured 2,4,5-TCP and 2,4,5-T; the Missouri plant manufactured 2,4,5-TCP, 2,4,5-T, and hexachlorophene.

Later studies examined specific health outcomes in the cohort members, including porphyria cutanea tarda (Calvert et al., 1994) and effects on pulmonary function (Calvert et al., 1991), hepatic and gastrointestinal function (Calvert et al., 1992), mood (Alderfer et al., 1992), the peripheral nervous system (Sweeney et al., 1993), and reproductive hormones (Egeland et al., 1994). Sweeney et al. (1996, 1997/1998) evaluated noncancer outcomes—including hepatic function, gastrointestinal disorders, chloracne, serum glucose concentration, hormone and lipid concentrations, and diabetes—in a subgroup of the original cohort studied by Calvert et al. (1991). More recent studies of the main cohort examined cardiovascular effects (Calvert et al., 1998); diabetes mellitus, thyroid function, and endocrine function (Calvert et al., 1999); immune characteristics (Halperin et al., 1998); and cancer incidence (Kayajanian, 2002). Cross-sectional medical surveys reported serum TCDD concentrations and surrogates of cytochrome P450 induction (Halperin et al., 1995) in that cohort.

A follow-up study (Steenland et al., 1999) examined the association between TCDD exposure and cause of death; it examined specific health outcomes, including cancer (all and site-specific), respiratory disease, cardiovascular disease, and diabetes. The researchers used a more refined exposure assessment than previously; it excluded workers whose records were inadequate to determine duration of exposure, and this reduced the number of study participants to a subcohort of 3,538 workers (69% of the overall cohort). The exposure assessment for the subcohort was based on a job–exposure matrix (JEM) that assigned each remaining worker a quantitative exposure score for each year of work (Piacitelli and Marlow, 1997).

Steenland et al. (2001a) reanalyzed data from two studies of TCDD and diabetes mellitus: one in the US workers of the NIOSH cohort (Calvert et al., 1999) and one in veterans of Operation Ranch Hand in which the herbicides were sprayed from planes in Vietnam (Henriksen et al., 1997). Another study by Steenland et al. (2001b) included a detailed exposure–response analysis of data on workers at one of the original 12 companies in the cohort study. A group of 170 workers who had serum TCDD greater than 10 ppt, as measured in 1988, was identified. The investigators conducted a regression analysis by using the work history of each worker, the exposure score for each job held by each worker, a simple pharmacokinetic model of the storage and excretion of TCDD, and an estimated TCDD half-life of 8.7 years. The pharmacokinetic model allowed calculation of the estimated serum TCDD concentration at the time of last exposure of each worker. Results of the analysis were used to estimate the serum TCDD concentration that was attributable to occupational exposure of all 3,538 workers in the subcohort defined in 1999.

Using exposure data for the NIOSH cohort from Steenland et al. (2001b), Crump et al. (2003) conducted a meta-analysis of dioxin dose–response studies in three occupational cohorts: the NIOSH cohort (Fingerhut et al., 1991), the Hamburg cohort (Flesch-Janys et al., 1998), and the BASF cohort (Ott and Zober, 1996). Bodner et al. (2003) compared mortality in Dow Chemical Company workers with mortality in the NIOSH and IARC cohorts; study details are in the Dow Chemical Company section of this chapter. Lawson et al. (2004) continued the NIOSH cross-sectional medical study reported by Sweeney et al. (1989, 1993) in a study of three birth outcomes—birth weight, preterm delivery, and birth defects—in offspring, by comparing serum TCDD concentrations in the NIOSH cohort with those in a reference population. TCDD exposures at conception were estimated by using physiologically based pharmacokinetic modeling approaches (Dankovic et al., 1995; Thomaseth and Salvan, 1998).

Aylward et al. (2005a) applied a concentration- and age-dependent elimination model to the NIOSH cohort data to determine the impact of these factors on estimates of serum TCDD concentrations. The authors found that their model produced a better fit to serum sampling data than first-order models did. Dose rates varied by a factor of 50 among different combinations of input parameters, elimination models, and regression models. The authors concluded that earlier dose-reconstruction efforts may have underestimated peak exposure levels in these populations. Aylward et al. (2005b) also applied the concentration- and age-dependent elimination model to serial measurements of serum lipid TCDD concentrations in 36 adults from Seveso, Italy, and three adults from Vienna, Austria with documented TCDD exposure. They concluded that a large degree of uncertainty is characteristic of back-calculated dose estimates of peak TCDD exposure and recommended that further analyses explicitly recognize the uncertainty.

VAO, Update 1996, Update 1998, Update 2000, Update 2002, Update 2004, and *Update 2006* describe the details of those studies. No new studies have been published on the NIOSH cohort or the smaller cohorts that make up the NIOSH cohort.

Monsanto

The NIOSH study cohort (Fingerhut et al., 1991) included employees of the Monsanto facility in Nitro, West Virginia, that produced 2,4,5-T in 1948–1969. Zack and Suskind (1980) examined the mortality experience of the 121 men who had chloracne associated with an unintentional release that occurred on March 8, 1949. Other studies considered mortality and other health outcomes in additional workers involved in numerous aspects of 2,4,5-T production at the Monsanto plant (Collins et al., 1993; Moses et al., 1984; Suskind and Hertzberg, 1984; Zack and Gaffey, 1983). The Monsanto studies were discussed in more detail in *VAO*. No additional studies on those subjects alone have been published; they have since been followed as part of the NIOSH and IARC cohorts.

Dow Chemical Company

Workers at Dow Chemical Company facilities where 2,4-D was manufactured, formulated, or packaged have been the focus of a cohort analysis since the 1980s (Bond et al., 1988). Several studies of Dow production workers are summarized in *VAO*, *Update 1996*, *Update 1998*, *Update 2002*, and *Update 2004*. Originally, Dow conducted a study of workers engaged in the production of 2,4,5-T (Ott et al., 1980) and one on TCP-manufacturing workers who had chloracne (Cook et al., 1980). Industrial hygienists developed a JEM that ranked employee exposures as low, moderate, or high on the basis of available air-monitoring data and professional judgment. The matrix was merged with employee work histories to assign an estimate of exposure to each job. A cumulative dose was then developed for each of the 878 employees by multiplying the representative 8-hour time-weighted average (TWA) exposure value for each job by the number of years in the job and then adding the products for all jobs. A 2,4-D TWA of 0.05 mg/m^3 was used for low, 0.5 mg/m^3 for moderate, and 5 mg/m^3 for high exposure. The role of dermal exposure in the facilities does not appear to have been considered in the exposure estimates. It is not clear to what extent the use of air measurements alone can provide accurate classification of workers into low-, moderate-, and high-exposure groups. Biologic monitoring of 2,4-D apparently was not included in the study.

Extension and follow-up studies compared potential exposure to TCDD with morbidity (Bond et al., 1983) and potential paternal TCDD exposure with reproductive outcomes (Townsend et al., 1982). Dow employees who had a diagnosis of chloracne or who were classified as having chloracne on the basis of clinical description were followed prospectively for mortality (Bond et al., 1987). Large-scale cohort mortality studies of workers exposed to herbicides in several of the plants (Bloemen et al., 1993; Bond et al., 1988; Burns et al., 2001) also were conducted with the same exposure-assessment procedures.

Dow assembled a large cohort at the Midland, Michigan, plant (Bond et al., 1989a; Cook et al., 1986, 1987). Exposure to TCDD in the cohort was characterized on the basis of chloracne diagnosis (Bond et al., 1989b). Within the cohort, a cohort study of women (Ott et al., 1987) and a case–control study of STS (Sobel et al., 1987) were conducted. The Dow cohorts have been followed as part of the NIOSH and IARC cohorts since 1991 and 1997, respectively.

Dow also has conducted a cohort study of its manufacturing workers exposed to pentachlorophenol (PCP) (Ramlow et al., 1996). Assessment of exposure of the cohort was based on consideration of the available industrial-hygiene and process data, including process and job-description information obtained from employees, process and engineering-control change information, industrial-hygiene surface-wipe sample data, area exposure monitoring, and personal breathing-zone data. Jobs with higher estimated potential exposure involved primarily dermal exposure to airborne PCP in the flaking–prilling–packaging area; the industrial-hygiene data suggested a difference of about a factor of 3 between the areas of highest and lowest potential exposure. All jobs were therefore assigned an estimated exposure-intensity score of 1–3 (from lowest to highest potential exposure intensity). Reliable information concerning the use of personal protective equipment was not available. Cumulative PCP and TCDD exposure indexes were calculated for each subject by multiplying the duration of each exposed job by its estimated exposure intensity and then summing across all exposed jobs.

Bodner et al. (2003) published a 10-year follow-up of the work of Cook et al. (1986), comparing the mortality experience of 2,187 male Dow workers potentially heavily exposed to dioxin before 1983 with that of the NIOSH and IARC cohorts. Dow researchers have published a study of serum dioxin concentrations measured in 2002 in former chlorophenol workers (Collins et al., 2006). Most of the workers in the study were included in the NIOSH and IARC cohorts. The authors used their data to estimate worker exposures at the time of exposure termination by using several pharmacokinetic models. They concluded that their findings were consistent with those of other studies that reported high serum dioxin concentrations in chlorophenol workers after occupational exposures. No new studies have been published on the Dow Chemical Company cohort.

BASF

An accident on November 17, 1953, during the manufacture of TCP at BASF plant in Germany, resulted in extreme exposure of some workers to TCDD. *VAO, Update 1996, Update 1998*, and *Update 2000* summarized studies of those workers, including a mortality study of persons initially exposed or later involved in cleanup (Thiess et al., 1982), an update and expansion of that study (Zober et al., 1990), and a morbidity follow-up (Zober et al., 1994). In addition, Ott and Zober (1996) and Zober et al. (1997) examined cancer incidence and mortality in workers exposed to TCDD after the accident or during reactor cleanup, maintenance, or demolition.

No new studies have been published on those cohorts since *Update 2000*.

International Agency for Research on Cancer

A multisite study by IARC involved 18,390 production workers and herbicide sprayers working in 10 countries (Saracci et al., 1991). The full cohort was established by using the International Register of Workers Exposed to Phenoxy Herbicides and Their Contaminants. Twenty cohorts were combined for the analysis: one each in Canada, Finland, and Sweden; two each in Australia, Denmark, Italy, the Netherlands, and New Zealand; and seven in the United Kingdom. There were 12,492 production workers and 5,898 sprayers in the full cohort.

Questionnaires were constructed for workers manufacturing chlorophenoxy herbicides or chlorinated phenols and for herbicide sprayers and were completed with the assistance of industrial hygienists. Information from production records and job histories were examined when available. Workers were classified as exposed, probably exposed, with unknown exposure, or nonexposed. The exposed-workers group (n = 13,482) consisted of all those known to have sprayed chlorophenoxy herbicides and all who worked in particular aspects of chemical production. Two subcohorts (n = 416) had no job titles available but worked in chemical-production facilities that were likely to produce TCDD exposure, so they were deemed probably exposed. Workers with no exposure information (n = 541) were classified as "exposure unknown." Nonexposed workers (n = 3,951) were those who had never been employed in parts of factories that produced chlorophenoxy herbicides or chlorinated phenols and had never sprayed chlorophenoxy herbicides.

One study evaluated mortality from STS and malignant lymphoma in people in 10 countries (Kogevinas et al., 1992). A cohort study of cancer incidence and mortality was conducted in 701 women in seven countries who were occupationally exposed to chlorophenoxy herbicides, chlorophenols, and dioxins (Kogevinas et al., 1993). Two nested case–control studies were undertaken with the IARC cohort to evaluate the relationship between STS and NHL (Kogevinas et al., 1995). An expanded and updated analysis of the IARC cohort was published in 1997 (Kogevinas et al., 1997). The researchers added herbicide-production workers in 12 plants in the United States (the NIOSH cohort) and four plants in Germany. The 21,863 workers exposed to phenoxy herbicides or chlorophenols were classified in three categories of exposure to TCDD or higher-chlorinated dioxins: those exposed (n = 13,831), those not exposed (n = 7,553), and those with unknown exposure (n = 479). Several exposure metrics were constructed for the cohort—years since first exposure, duration of exposure (in years), year of first exposure, and job title—but detailed methods were not described. Vena et al. (1998) studied nonneoplasm mortality in the IARC cohorts. *VAO, Update 1996, Update 1998*, and *Update 2000* highlight those studies.

In addition to the NIOSH cohort and its component subcohorts (discussed above), several of the other subcohorts that make up the IARC cohort have been evaluated apart from the IARC-coordinated efforts. They include Danish production workers (Lynge, 1985, 1993), British production workers (Coggon et al., 1986, 1991), Dutch production workers (Bueno de Mesquita et al., 1993; Hooiveld et al., 1998), Austrian production workers (Jäger et al., 1998; Neuberger et al., 1998, 1999), New Zealand production workers (Smith AH et al., 1981, 1982; 't Mannetje et al., 2005), and German production workers (Becher et al., 1996; Flesch-Janys, 1997; Flesch-Janys et al., 1995; Manz et al., 1991).

The study by Flesch-Janys et al. (1995) updated the cohort and added a quantitative exposure assessment based on blood or adipose measurements of PCDDs and polychlorinated dibenzofurans (PCDFs). The authors estimated maximum PCDD and PCDF exposure of 190 workers with a first-order kinetics model, half-lives with an elimination study of 48 workers in the cohort, and background concentrations in the German population. They then regressed the estimated maximum PCDD and PCDF exposures of the workers against the length of time that they worked in each production department in the plant. The working-time weights were then used with work histories of the remainder of the cohort to estimate PCDD and PCDF exposure of each person at the end of that person's exposure. Those values were used to estimate TCDD doses in the population.

Becher et al. (1996) conducted an analysis of several German cohorts, including the Boehringer–Ingelheim cohort described above (Kogevinas et al., 1997), a cohort from the BASF Ludwigshafen plant that did not include those involved in a 1953 accident, and cohorts from a Bayer plant in Uerdingen and a Bayer plant in Dormagen. All the plants were involved in production of phenoxy herbicides or chlorophenols. Exposure assessment involved estimates of duration of employment from the start of work in a department where exposure was possible until the end of employment in the plant. Analysis was based on time since first exposure.

Hooiveld et al. (1998) updated the mortality experience of production workers in two chemical factories in the Netherlands with known exposure to dioxins: workers in herbicide production, nonexposed production workers, and workers known to have been exposed as a result of an accident that occurred in 1963. Assuming first-order TCDD elimination with an estimated half-life of 7.1 years, measured TCDD concentrations were extrapolated to the time of maximum TCDD exposure for a group of 47 workers. A regression model was then used to estimate, for each cohort member, the effect on estimated maximum TCDD exposure attributable to exposure as a result of the accident, duration of employment in the main production department, and time of first exposure before (or after) 1970.

VAO, *Update 1996*, *Update 1998*, *Update 2000*, and *Update 2006* discuss those studies in more detail.

Waste-Incineration Worker Studies

A study of infectious-waste–incineration plant workers in Japan used serum dioxin concentrations to document higher PCDD and PCDF exposures of workers than of controls (Kumagai and Koda, 2005). A second study in Japan examined the association between serum-dioxin concentrations (total value of toxicity equivalent quotient [TEQ]-PCDDs, PCDFs, and coplanar-polychlorinated-biphenyls) and oxidative DNA-damage markers in municipal-waste–incineration workers (Yoshida et al., 2006).

Researchers in South Korea compared plasma protein concentrations in 31 waste-incineration workers with those in 33 nonexposed subjects (Kang et al., 2005). A second Korean study evaluated immunologic and reproductive toxicity (DNA damage and sperm quality) in 31 waste-incineration workers and 84 control subjects (Oh et al., 2005). Rather than measuring serum dioxin, both studies inferred dioxin exposure of individual workers on the basis of dioxin concentrations in air and estimated exposures to polycyclic aromatic hydrocarbons by analyzing two urinary metabolites: 1-hydroxypyrene and 2-naphthol.

No new studies relevant to the chemicals of interest have been published on waste-incineration workers since *Update 2006*.

Czech Worker Studies

Several studies of Czech workers have been reviewed by VAO committees. The original committee reviewed a 10-year follow-up study of 55 men in Czechoslovakia who were exposed to TCDD during the production of 2,4,5-T (Pazderova-Vejlupková et al., 1981). The exposure occurred because of excessive temperature and pressure in the production process over an extended period (1965–1968) rather than as a consequence of a major release at a single time. More than 80 workers were affected, but the researchers provided little information about those who were not included in the study. Researchers observed several disorders in the workers, including chloracne, metabolic disturbances; abnormal results of glucose tolerance tests, evidence of a mild hepatic lesion, nervous system focal damage, and psychologic disorders. In a 30-year follow-up, Pelclová et al. (2001, 2002) examined biochemical, neuropsychologic, neurologic, and lipid-metabolism abnormalities in the surviving Czech cohort. Previous VAO committees concluded that there were methodologic problems of selection bias; lack of control for confounding by educational achievement, tobacco use, or alcohol use; the use of self-reported symptoms; and the lack of an objective measure of exposure. An essential limitation is the lack of a comparison group, which precludes any inference of causality.

Since *Update 2006*, two new studies of the exposed Czech cohort have been published. In 2004, Pelclová and colleagues (2007) compared vascular function in 15 exposed workers with that of 14 healthy male health-care workers who had no history of occupational exposure to TCDD. Urban et al. (2007) evaluated the same set of workers, looking at over-all health effects. In reviewing the study by Pelclová et al. (2007), the committee found that the data were difficult to interpret with respect to the health effects of TCDD. The study authors did not explain how the 15 subjects in the reports were contacted and the extent to which this small sample was biased toward increased symptoms. It is unclear how the case series was selected, so it is unclear to what degree the participants are representative of all still-living workers, especially with respect to chronic-disease burden. Because the exposed group had a large number of metabolic and comorbid conditions of which the control group was largely free, the effects of disease could not be separated from the effects of TCDD. Finally, the relationship between microvascular and thermal reactivity and clinical cardiovascular events is unclear. Flow-mediated reactivity of brachial arteries can predict clinical disease (Yeboah et al., 2007), but the predictive value of the particular measures used in the study has not been demonstrated. The committee was concerned that the study by Urban et al. (2007) lacked a comparison group, and although the study supports the idea that exposure to large amounts of TCDD over a period of years can produce neurologic abnormalities during or shortly after exposure that can continue for more than 30 years, the committee was concerned that some of the testing methods used could not adequately support the assumptions of the researchers, and many other environmental or age-related factors could have affected the results.

Other Chemical Plants

Studies have reviewed health outcomes in UK chemical workers exposed to TCDD as a result of an industrial accident in 1968 (Jennings et al., 1988; May, 1982, 1983), 2,4-D production workers in the former Soviet Union (Bashirov, 1969), 2,4-D and 2,4,5-T production workers in the United States (Poland et al., 1971), white men employed at a US chemical plant that manufactured flavors and fragrances (Thomas, 1987), and US chemical workers engaged in the production of pentachlorophenol, lower-chlorinated phenols, and esters of chlorophenoxy acids (Hryhorczuk et al., 1998). The long-term immunologic effects of TCDD were examined in 11 industrial workers involved in production and maintenance operations at a German chemical factory that produced 2,4,5-T (Tonn et al., 1996), and immunologic effects were studied in a cohort of workers formerly employed at a German pesticide-producing plant (Jung et al., 1998). *VAO, Update 1998*, and *Update 2000* detailed those studies. Garaj-Vrhovac and Zeljezic (2002) conducted a study of workers occupationally exposed to a complex mixture of pesticides (atrazine, alachlor, cyanazine, 2,4-D, and malathion) during their production.

No new studies relevant to the chemicals of interest of cohorts in other chemical plants have been published since *Update 2000*.

Agriculture, Forestry, and Other Outdoor Work

Various methods have been used to estimate occupational exposure of agricultural workers to herbicides or TCDD. The simplest method derives data from death certificates, cancer registries, or hospital records (Burmeister, 1981). Although such information is relatively easy to obtain, it cannot be used to estimate duration or intensity of exposure or to determine whether a worker was exposed to a specific agent. In some studies of agricultural workers, examination of differences in occupational practices has allowed identification of subsets of workers who were likely to have had higher exposures (Hansen et al., 1992; Musicco et al., 1988; Ronco et al., 1992; Vineis et al., 1986; Wiklund and Holm, 1986; Wilklund et al., 1988a). In other studies, county of residence was used as a surrogate for exposure, relying on agricultural censuses of farm production and chemical use to characterize exposure in individual counties (Blair and White, 1985; Cantor, 1982; Gordon and Shy, 1981), or exposure was estimated according to the number of years of employment in a specific occupation as a surrogate for exposure duration, using supplier records of pesticide sales to estimate exposure or estimating acreage sprayed to determine the amount used (Morrison et al., 1992; Wigle et al., 1990). Still other studies used self-reported information on exposure that recounted direct handling of a herbicide, whether it was applied by tractor or hand-held sprayer, and what types of protective equipment or safety precautions were used (Hoar et al., 1986; Zahm et al., 1990). Another set of studies validated self-reported information with written records, signed statements, or telephone interviews with coworkers or former employers (Carmelli et al., 1981; Woods and Polissar, 1989).

Forestry and other outdoor workers, such as highway-maintenance workers, are likely to have been exposed to herbicides and other compounds. Exposure of those groups has been classified by using approaches similar to those noted above for agricultural workers, for example, by using the number of years employed, job category, and occupational title.

Agricultural Health Study

The US Agricultural Health Study (AHS) is a prospective investigation of cohorts of private pesticide applicators (farmers), their spouses, and commercial pesticide applicators—a total of almost 90,000 people. It is sponsored by NCI and the National Institute of Environmental Health Sciences of the National Institutes of Health and by EPA. Enrollment in the study was offered to applicants for applicator certification in Iowa and North Carolina. The project's Web site (www.aghealth.org) provides many details about conduct of the study, including specification of which pesticides had information gathered from the enrollment forms and mailed questionnaires (Alavanja et al., 1994). In phase I (1993–1997), the enrollment form for both commercial and private (largely farmers) applicators asked for the details of use of 22 pesticides (10 herbicides, including 2,4-D; nine insecticides; two fungicides; and one fumigant) and yes–no responses as to whether 28 other pesticides (eight herbicides, including 2,4,5-T and Silvex, 2,4,5-TP; 13 insecticides; four fungicides; and three fumigants) had ever been used. A subset of 24,034 applicators also completed a take-home questionnaire. The mailed questionnaire for this phase asked for details about use of the 28 yes–no pesticides and yes–no as to whether 108 other pesticides (34 herbicides, including organic arsenic, which would cover cacodylic acid; 36 insecticides; 29 fungicides; and nine fumigants) had ever been "frequently" used. Dosemeci et al. (2002) published an algorithm designed to characterize personal exposures of that population. Weighting factors for key exposure variables were developed from the literature on pesticide exposure. This quantitative approach has the potential to improve the accuracy of exposure classification for the cohort but has not yet been used in published epidemiologic studies.

In phase II (a 5-year follow-up of farmers, 1999–2003), computer-assisted telephone interviews specified "pesticides" in general to include herbicides. It asked about specific pesticides on individual crops; for several crops, only if atrazine or 2,4-D was specified was the subject asked whether it had been used alone or as part of the manufacturer's mixture. A full pesticide list was not posted on the Web site with this follow-up questionnaire.

Several reports on the AHS effort have been considered in earlier updates. All have developed pesticide-exposure estimates or exposure categories from self-administered questionnaires. They have addressed a variety of health outcomes: doctor visits resulting from pesticide exposure (Alavanja et al., 1998), chemical predictors of wheeze (Hoppin et al., 2002), prostate-cancer incidence (Alavanja et al., 2003, 2005), lung-cancer incidence (Alavanja et al., 2004), reproductive effects (Farr et al., 2004, 2006), cancer risk in the 21,375 children of pesticide appliers born in 1975 or later (Flower et al., 2004), mortality (Blair, 2005a), morbidity (Blair et al., 2005b), rheumatoid arthritis (DeRoos et al., 2005b), breast-cancer incidence (Engel et al., 2005), neurotoxicity of chronic exposure to modest amounts of pesticides (Kamel et al., 2005), and prevalance of wheeze (Hoppin et al., 2006a). Three additional publications have discussed pesticide-use patterns in the population (Hoppin, 2005, 2006b; Kirrane et al., 2004; Samanic et al., 2005). The AHS questionnaire collected detailed information regarding herbicide use; 2,4-D was the most commonly reported herbicide.

Since *Update 2006*, researchers have published several new studies of the AHS cohort. Kamel et al. (2007a) evaluated questionnaire responses from more than 18,000 AHS subjects, who listed a variety of neurologic symptoms, including memory and concentration problems. Another study by Kamel et al. (2007b) evaluated Parkinson's disease (PD) in participants in the AHS. People were contacted twice within 5 years; those who reported a doctor's diagnosis of PD initially were classified as prevalent cases, and those who reported a diagnosis of PD that occurred in the 5 years preceding the second contact were classified as incident cases. During both telephone contacts, a detailed pesticide-exposure history was collected with information about protective techniques used.

Two studies looked at cancer incidence in the AHS cohort. Lee WJ et al. (2007) analyzed incident colorectal cancers diagnosed in AHS subjects in 1993–2005. Associations with self-reported exposures to 50 pesticides (including 2,4-D, 2,4,5-T, and 2,4,5-TP) were studied. Samanic et al. (2006) reported on the incidence of all cancers combined and selected individual cancers in male pesticide applicators in the AHS particularly with respect to reported exposures to the benzoic acid herbicide Dicamba (3,6-dichloro-2-methoxybenzoic acid). Dicamba was used in combination with other herbicides, such as 2,4-D and Agent Orange.

Montgomery and colleagues (2008), reported on the relationship between self-reported incident diabetes and pesticide and herbicide exposure in 31,787 licensed pesticide applicators and their spouses. Physician-diagnosed incident diabetes was assessed during a follow-up questionnaire. Saldana and colleagues (2007) reported on the cross-sectional relationship between pesticide and herbicide exposure and a history of gestational diabetes in the wives of licensed applicators. Women (n = 11,273) were asked about their pregnancy closest to enrollment, and 506 (4.5%) reported gestational diabetes. Exposure to 2,4,5-T and 2,4-D was assessed by questionnaire.

Several new studies concerning respiratory health problems in the AHS cohort have also been published since *Update 2006*. They used a common method; at the time of enrollment, questionnaires regarding use of pesticides and health outcomes were administered, and subjects who returned both of them (about 40%) were included in the analyses. The new studies evaluated subjects who had experienced different health outcomes: wheeze (Hoppin et al., 2006c), farmer's lung (hypersensitivity pneumonitis) (Hoppin et al., 2007a), chronic bronchitis (Hoppin et al., 2007b; Valcin et al., 2007), and atopic and nonatopic asthma in women (Hoppin et al., 2008). Wheeze was defined as a positive response to the question, How many episodes of wheezing or whistling in your chest have you had in the past 12 months? Farmer's lung and chronic bronchitis were defined if a subject reported having a doctor's diagnosis. Atopic asthma and nonatopic asthma were defined if a woman reported at enrollment that she had received a diagnosis of asthma after the age of 19 years. Use of 40 specific chemicals in the year before enrollment was assessed from the questionnaires.

California United Farm Workers of America Study

Mills et al. (2005a) and Mills and Yang (2005b) analyzed lymphohematopoietic cancer and breast cancer, respectively, in nested case–control studies of Hispanic workers drawn from a cohort of 139,000 Californians who were members of the United Farm Workers of America (UFW). Estimates of exposure to specific pesticides, including 2,4-D, were developed through linkage of the union's job histories with the California Pesticide Use Reporting Database of the state's Department of Pesticide Regulation, which has records of all agricultural applications of pesticides in the state since 1970. Vital status and cancer incidence were ascertained through a probabilistic record linkage to the California Cancer Registry for the period 1988–2001.

Since *Update 2006*, Mills and Yang (2007) have conducted a nested case–control study of gastric cancer embedded in the UFW cohort and identified cases of gastic cancer newly diagnosed in 1988–2003.

Upper Midwest Health Study

The Upper Midwest Health Study (UMHS) has published several studies that have been reviewed in previous updates. Chiu et al. (2004) and Lee WJ et al. (2004b) conducted pooled (combined) analyses of two earlier case–control studies of NHL carried out by the UMHS in Iowa and Minnesota (Cantor et al., 1992) and Nebraska (Zahm et al., 1990). Chiu et al. (2004) examined the association of NHL with agricultural pesticide use and familial cancer, and Lee WJ et al. (2004b, 2006) looked at NHL in asthmatics who reported pesticide exposure. Data from the Nebraska data (Chiu et al., 2006, based on Zahm et al., 1990, 1993) were used to identify whether there were subtypes of NHL that expressed a higher risk. Specifically, tissue samples were analyzed according to the presence of a specific chromosomal translocation (t[14;18][q32;q21]); only 172 of 385 cases were included. Researchers evaluated farm pesticide exposure in men (Ruder et al., 2004) and women (Carreon et al., 2005) in Iowa, Michigan, Minnesota, and Wisconsin in relation to gliomas as part of the UMHS.

Two studies focused on pesticide use and the risk of adenocarcinomas of the stomach and esophagus (Lee WJ et al., 2004a) and the risk of gliomas (Lee WJ et al., 2005). Cases were white Nebraska residents over 21 years old who were identified from the Nebraska Cancer Registry and matched to controls drawn from an earlier study by Zahm et al. (1990).

Since *Update 2006*, Ruder et al. (2006) have published a follow-on study to Ruder et al. (2004) evaluating gliomas in UMHS subjects. The new analyses provided no evidence of greater use of pesticides in cases than in controls, and there was no breakdown of specific agents.

Ontario Farmers

The Ontario Farm Family Health Study (OFFHS) has produced several reports on exposure to phenoxyacetic acid herbicides, including 2,4-D. A study of male pesticide exposure and pregnancy outcome (Savitz et al., 1997) developed an exposure metric based on self-reports of mixing or application of crop herbicides, crop insecticides, and fungicides; livestock chemicals; yard herbicides; and building pesticides. Subjects were asked whether they participated in those activities during each month, and their exposure classifications were based on activities in 3-month periods. Exposure classification was refined with answers to questions about use of protective equipment and specificity of pesticide use.

A related study included analysis of 2,4-D residues in semen as a biologic marker of exposure (Arbuckle et al., 1999a). The study began with 773 potential participants, but only 215 eventually consented to participation. Of the 215, 97 provided semen and urine samples for 2,4-D analysis.

The OFFHS also examined pregnancy outcomes of stillbirth, gestational age, and birth weight (Savitz et al., 1997) and the effect of exposure to pesticides, including 2,4-D, on time to pregnancy (Curtis et al., 1999) and on the risk of spontaneous abortion (Arbuckle et al., 1999b, 2001). About 2,000 farm couples participated in the study. Exposure information was pooled from interviews with husbands and wives to construct a history of monthly agricultural and residential pesticide use. Exposure classification was based on a yes–no response for each month. Data on such variables as acreage sprayed and use of protective equipment were collected but were not available in all cases. Other studies have used herbicide biomonitoring in a subset of the population to evaluate the validity of self-reported predictors of exposure (Arbuckle et al., 2002). Assuming that the presence of 2,4-D in urine was an accurate measure of exposure and that the results of the questionnaire indicating 2,4-D use were more likely to be subject to exposure-classification error (that is, assuming that the questionnaire results were less accurate than the results of urinalysis), the questionnaire's prediction of exposure, compared with the urinary 2,4-D concentrations, had a sensitivity of 57% and a specificity of 86%. In multivariate models, the variables for pesticide formulation, protective clothing and gear, application equipment, handling practice, and personal-hygiene practice were valuable as predictors of urinary herbicide concentrations in the first 24 hours after application was initiated.

Additional publications have reported results from the cohort and were included in previous updates. Urinary concentrations of 2,4-D and 2-methyl-4-chlorophenoxyacetic acid (MCPA) were measured in samples from farm applicators (Arbuckle et al., 2005) and from women who lived on Ontario farms (Arbuckle and Ritter, 2005). Indirect sources of herbicide exposure of farm families were evaluated through wipe sampling of surfaces and drinking-water samples (Arbuckle et al., 2006).

Since *Update 2006*, Weselak et al. (2008) has examined occupational exposures and birth defects in the offspring of OFFHS subjects. Spouses completed questionnaires that requested the history of pesticide use on the farm. Pregnancies resulting in birth defects were reported by the female study participants. All birth defects were combined for study analyses, and exposure was examined by pesticide class, family, and active ingredient for two 3-month periods—before and after conception.

Mortality Study of Male Canadian Farm Operators

The Mortality Study of Canadian Male Farm Operators evaluated the risk to farmers of death and of specific health outcomes: NHL (Morrison et al., 1994; Wigle et al., 1990), prostate cancer (Morrison et al., 1992), brain cancer (Morrison et al., 1993), multiple myeloma (Semenciw et al., 1993), leukemia (Semenciw et al., 1994), and asthma (Senthilselvan et al., 1992).

No new reports on relevant health outcomes have been published on subjects in the study since *Update 1996*.

Swedish Cancer-Environment Registry

The Swedish Cancer-Environment Registry (CER) linked the cancer cases entered in the Swedish Cancer Registry with the records of people who responded to the 1960 and 1970 national censuses, which had obtained data on current occupation. The resulting database has been used in studies that evaluated cancer mortality and farm work (Wiklund, 1983); STS and malignant lymphoma in agricultural and forestry workers (Wiklund and Holm, 1986; Wiklund et al., 1988a); and the risk of NHL, HD, and multiple myeloma in relation to occupational activities (Eriksson et al., 1992).

No new studies using the CER have been published since the original *VAO* report that are relevant to the chemicals of interest for this report.

Farmers of Italian Piedmont

Corrao et al. (1989) evaluated cancer incidence in farmers licensed to spray pesticides in Italy's southern Piedmont region (Corrao et al., 1989). In a continuation of that study, Torchio et al. (1994) reported on the mortality experience of a cohort of 23,401 male farmers in the Piedmont area from the time they registered to use agricultural pesticides (1970–1974) through 1986. That area is characterized by higher use of herbicides, particularly 2,4-D and MCPA, than the rest of the country. The cohort was partitioned into people who lived near arable land, those who lived near woodlands, and those who lived near mixed-use land; separate results were reported for the first two groups.

Other Studies of Agricultural Workers

Studies of proportionate mortality were conducted in Iowa farmers (Burmeister, 1981) and male and female farmers in 23 states (Blair et al., 1993). Cancer mortality in a cohort of rice growers in the Novara Province of northern Italy was investigated (Gambini et al., 1997), and cancer incidence in Danish gardeners was studied (Hansen et al., 1992). Lerda and Rizzi (1991) studied the incidence of sperm abnormalities in Argentinian farmers. Ronco et al. (1992) studied mortality in Danish farmers and the incidence of specific types of cancer in Italian farmers. The utility of the findings was limited by their being the largely unanalyzed products of linking each country's cancer registry with census records to garner information on recent occupation. Brain, lymphatic, and hematopoietic cancers have been studied in Irish agricultural workers (Dean, 1994). Kristensen et al. (1997) tested whether cancers or birth defects were increased in the offspring of Norwegian farmers who worked on farms with pesticide usage documented from agricultural censuses. Faustini et al. (1996) evaluated the immune, neurobehavioral, and lung function of residents in an agricultural area of Saskatchewan, Canada, and focused on immunologic changes in 10 farmers who mixed and applied commercial formulations that contained chlorophenoxy herbicides. Mandel et al. (2005) reported results of urinary biomonitoring of farm families in Minnesota and South Carolina as a part of CropLife America's Farm Family Exposure Study. Fritschi et al. (2005) used a computer-assisted telephone interview and occupational histories reviewed by an industrial hygienist to estimate exposures to phenoxy herbicides in an Australian study. Curwin et al. (2005) measured 2,4-D concentrations in urine and hand-wipe samples to characterize exposures of farmers and nonfarmers in Iowa.

Other studies of the agricultural use of pesticides have not provided specific information on exposure to 2,4-D, TCDD, or other compounds relevant to Vietnam veterans' exposure (Bell et al., 2001a,b; Chiu et al., 2004; Duell et al., 2001; Garry et al., 2003; Gorell et al., 2004; Hanke et al., 2003; Van Wijngaarden et al., 2003).

A series of papers from a workshop focused on methods of assessing pesticide exposure in farmworker populations (Arcury et al., 2006; Barr et al., 2006a,b; Hoppin et al., 2006; Quandt et al., 2006). They provide a helpful review of current methodologic issues in exposure science for those populations but do not address the chemicals of interest directly.

Since *Update 2006*, Hansen et al. (2007) have evaluated cancer incidence from May 1975 through 2001 in an occupational cohort of Danish Union of General Workers identified among men working in 1973; their cancer incidence from 1975 to 1984 was reported by Hansen et al. (1992). The cohort of 3,156 male gardeners, whose pesticide exposure was primarily to herbicides, including phenoxy acetic acids, was matched to the Danish Cancer Registry to determine cancer incidence. The expected number of cancers was calculated by using national cancer rates. Standardized incidence ratios were used to control for age and calendar time. The cohort was subdivided by year of birth, a proxy for exposure inasmuch as pesticide use decreased over time. Three subcohorts were evaluated: high exposure, early birth, born before 1915; low exposure, late birth, born after 1934; and medium exposure, born in 1915–1934.

Forestry Workers

Studies have been conducted in forestry workers potentially exposed to the types of herbicides used in Vietnam. A cohort mortality study examined men employed at a Canadian public utility (Green, 1987, 1991), a Dutch study of forestry workers exposed to 2,4,5-T investigated the prevalence of acne and hepatic dysfunction (van Houdt et al., 1983), a study evaluated cancer incidence in a group of New Zealand forestry workers (Reif et al., 1989), and a study examined mortality and cancer incidence in a cohort of Swedish lumberjacks (Thörn et al., 2000).

Other Studies of Herbicide and Pesticide Applicators

Studies of commercial herbicide applicators are relevant because they can be presumed to have had sustained exposure to herbicides. However, because they also are likely to be exposed to a variety of other compounds, assessment of individual or group exposure to specific phenoxy herbicides or TCDD is complicated. Some studies have attempted to measure applicators' exposure on the basis of information from work records on acreage sprayed or on the number of days of spraying. Employment records also can be used to extract information on which compounds are sprayed.

One surrogate indicator of herbicide exposure is the receipt of a license to spray. Several studies have specifically identified licensed or registered pesticide and herbicide applicators (Blair et al., 1983; Smith AH et al., 1981, 1982; Swaen et al., 1992; Wiklund et al., 1988b, 1989). Individual estimates of the intensity and frequency of exposure were rarely reported in the studies that the committee examined, however, and many applicators were known to have applied many kinds of herbicides, pesticides, and other substances. In addition, herbicide spraying is generally a seasonal occupation, and information is not always available on possible exposure-related activities during the rest of the year.

Several studies have evaluated various characteristics of herbicide exposures: type of exposure, routes of entry, and routes of excretion (Ferry et al., 1982; Frank et al., 1985; Kolmodin-Hedman and Erne, 1980; Kolmodin-Hedman et al., 1983; Lavy et al., 1980a,b; Libich et al., 1984). Those studies appear to have shown that the major route of exposure is dermal absorption, with 2–4% of the chemical that contacts the skin being absorbed into the body during a normal workday. Air concentrations of the herbicides were usually less than 0.2 mg/m^3. Absorbed phenoxy acid herbicides are virtually cleared within 1 day, primarily through urinary excretion. Typical measured excretion was 0.1–5 mg/day in ground crews and lower in air crews.

A study of 98 professional turf sprayers in Canada developed new models to predict 2,4-D dose (Harris et al., 2001). Exposure information was gathered from self-administered questionnaires. Urine samples were collected throughout the spraying season (24-hour samples on 2 consecutive days). Estimated 2,4-D doses were developed from the data and used to evaluate the effect of protective clothing and other exposure variables.

Only one study has provided information on serum TCDD concentrations in herbicide applicators. Smith AH et al. (1992) analyzed blood from nine professional spray applicators in New Zealand who first sprayed before 1960 and were spraying in 1984. The duration of spraying varied from 80 to 370 months. Serum TCDD was 3–131 ppt on a lipid basis (mean 53 ppt). The corresponding value for age-matched controls was 2–11 ppt (mean 6 ppt). Serum TCDD was positively correlated with the number of months of professional spraying.

Several additional cohorts of herbicide and pesticide applicators have been assessed for health outcomes: cancer mortality in Swedish railroad workers (Axelson and Sundell, 1974; Axelson et al., 1980), mortality in pesticide applicators in Florida (Blair et al., 1983), prospective general and cancer mortality and morbidity in Finnish men who applied 2,4-D and 2,4,5-T (Asp et al., 1994;

Riihimaki et al., 1982, 1983), cancer in pesticide and herbicide applicators in Sweden (Dich and Wiklund, 1998; Wiklund et al., 1987, 1988b, 1989a,b), mortality from cancer and other causes in Dutch male herbicide applicators (Swaen et al., 1992, 2004), cancer mortality in Minnesota highway-maintenance workers (Bender et al., 1989), birth defects in the offspring of Minnesota pesticide applicators (Garry et al., 1994, 1996a,b), lung-cancer morbidity in male agricultural plant-protection workers in the former German Democratic Republic who spent a portion of their work year in applying pesticides (Barthel, 1981), mortality and reproductive effects in British Columbia sawmill workers potentially exposed to chlorophenate wood preservatives used as fungicides (Dimich-Ward et al., 1996; Heacock et al., 1998; Hertzman et al., 1997), and cancer risk in pesticide users in Iceland (Zhong and Rafnsson, 1996). 't Mannetje et al. (2005) evaluated a study population that included herbicide production workers and is a subcohort of the IARC cohort, which was discussed earlier in the section on production workers. Details of the studies' designs and results are included in *VAO*, *Update 1996*, *Update 1998*, *Update 2000*, *Update 2002*, *Update 2004*, and *Update 2006*.

No new studies relevant to the chemicals of interest have been published on herbicide or pesticide applicators since *Update 2006*.

Paper and Pulp Workers

Workers in the paper and pulp industry can be exposed to TCDD and other dioxins that can be generated by the bleaching process during the production and treatment of paper and paper products. *VAO* described studies of pulp and paper workers potentially exposed to TCDD and various health outcomes, including general mortality in workers at five mills in Washington, Oregon, and California (Robinson et al., 1986), cancer incidence in male paper-mill workers in Finland (Jappinen and Pukkala, 1991), respiratory health in a New Hampshire mill (Henneberger et al., 1989), and cause-specific mortality in white men employed in plants identified by the United Paperworkers International Union (Solet et al., 1989). *Update 2000* described studies of cancer risk in workers in the Danish paper industry (Rix et al., 1998) and oral-cancer risk in occupationally exposed workers in Sweden (Schildt et al., 1999). *Update 2006* included a mortality study by McLean et al. (2006) that used a JEM to estimate individual cumulative exposure to 27 agents, including TCDD.

In the past, workers in sawmills might have been exposed to pentachlorophenates, which are contaminated with higher-chlorinated PCDDs (Cl_6–Cl_8), or to tetrachlorophenates, which are less contaminated with higher-chlorinated PCDDs. Wood is dipped into those chemical preservatives and then cut and planed in the mills. Most exposure is dermal, but some exposure can occur by inhalation (Hertzmann et al., 1997; Teschke et al., 1994). No new studies of those populations have been reported since *Update 2000*.

Case–Control Studies

Numerous case–control studies have been reviewed in previous updates. In 1977, case-series reports in Sweden (Hardell, 1977, 1979) of a potential connection between exposure to phenoxyacetic acids and STS prompted several case–control investigations (Eriksson et al., 1979, 1981, 1990; Hardell and Eriksson, 1988; Hardell and Sandstrom, 1979; Wingren et al., 1990). After the initial STS reports (Hardell, 1977, 1979), case–control studies of other cancer outcomes were conducted in Sweden: of HD and NHL (Hardell and Bengtsson, 1983; Hardell et al., 1980, 1981; Persson et al., 1989, 1993), of NHL (Hardell and Eriksson, 1999; Olsson and Brandt, 1988), of nasal and nasopharyngeal carcinomas (Hardell et al., 1982), of gastric cancer (Ekström et al., 1999), and of primary or unspecified liver cancer (Hardell et al., 1984). To address criticism regarding potential observer bias in some of the case–control series, Hardell (1981) conducted another case–control study of colon cancer. Hardell et al. (1994) also examined the relationship between occupational exposure to phenoxyacetic acids and chlorophenols and various characteristics related to NHL—including histopathologic measures, stage, and anatomic location—on the basis of the NHL cases in a previous study (Hardell et al., 1981).

Prompted by the Swedish studies (Hardell, 1977, 1979), Smith AH and Pearce (1986) and Smith AH et al. (1983, 1984) conducted a set of case–control studies to evaluate the association between phenoxy herbicide and chlorophenol exposure and STS incidence and mortality in New Zealand. An expanded case series was collected, and additional case–control studies of exposure to phenoxy herbicides or chlorophenols and the risks of malignant lymphoma, NHL, and multiple myeloma were conducted (Pearce et al., 1985, 1986a,b, 1987).

Geographic patterns of increased leukemia mortality in white men in the central part of the United States prompted a study of leukemia mortality in Nebraska farmers (Blair and Thomas, 1979). Additional case–control studies of leukemia were later conducted in Nebraska (Blair and White, 1985), in Iowa (Burmeister et al., 1982) on the basis of the cohort study of Burmeister (1981), and in Iowa and Minnesota (Brown et al., 1990). Another study investigated leukemia in association with NHL and 2,4-D in eastern Nebraska (Zahm et al., 1990).

Case–control studies have been conducted in various US populations for associations of herbicides with other cancers, including NHL (Cantor, 1982; Cantor et al., 1992; Hartge et al., 2005; Tatham et al., 1997; Zahm et al., 1993); multiple myeloma (Boffetta et al., 1989; Brown et al., 1993; Morris et al., 1986); gastric cancer, prostate cancer, NHL, and multiple myeloma (Burmeister et al., 1983); STS, HD, and NHL (Hoar et al., 1986); NHL and HD (Dubrow et al., 1988); and STS and NHL (Woods and Polissar, 1989; Woods et al., 1987). In a subset of subjects from the Hartge et al. (2005) study, De Roos et al. (2005a) studied associations between overall TEQs of polychlorinated biphenyls, furans, and dioxins but not dioxin alone.

Other studies outside the United States have examined STS and other cancers in the 15 regional cancer registries that constitute the National Cancer Register in England in connection with the chemicals of interest (Balarajan and Acheson, 1984); ovarian cancer in the Piedmont region of Italy (Donna et al., 1984); STS in rice weeders in northern Italy (Vineis et al., 1986); esophageal cancer, pancreatic cancer, cutaneous melanoma, renal cancer, and brain-cancer mortality in three English counties (Magnani et al., 1987); brain gliomas in two hospitals in Milan, Italy (Musicco et al., 1988); lymphoid cancer in Milan, Italy (LaVecchia et al., 1989); primary lung cancer in pesticide users in Saskatchewan (McDuffie et al., 1990); STS and malignant lymphomas in the Victorian Cancer Registry of Australia (Smith JG and Christophers, 1992); and renal-cell carcinoma in the Denmark Cancer Registry (Mellemgaard et al., 1994). Nanni et al. (1996) conducted a population-based case–control study, based on the work of Amadori et al. (1995), of occupational and chemical risk factors for lymphocytic leukemia and NHL in northeastern Italy.

Noncancer health outcomes also have been investigated in case–control studies: spontaneous abortion (Carmelli et al., 1981); congenital malformations (García et al., 1998); immunosuppression and later decreased host resistance to infection in AIDS patients who had Kaposi's sarcoma (Hardell et al., 1987); mortality in US Department of Agriculture extension agents (Alavanja et al., 1988, 1989); PD associated with occupational risk factors (Semchuk et al., 1993); birth defects in offspring of agriculture workers (Nurminen et al., 1994); mortality from neurodegenerative diseases associated with occupational risk factors (Schulte et al., 1996); PD associated with various rural factors, including exposure to herbicides and wood preservatives (Seidler et al., 1996); spina bifida in offspring associated with paternal occupation (Blatter et al., 1997); PD associated with occupational and environmental risk factors (Liou et al., 1997); and mortality from neurodegenerative diseases, including Alzheimer's disease and presenile dementia, PD, and motor neuron disease associated with occupational factors (Park et al., 2005). Those studies are discussed in detail in previous updates.

Children's Oncology Group

In two related case–control studies, Chen Z et al. (2005, 2006) reported on exposure to pesticides (including "herbicides") and the risk of childhood germ-cell tumors. One focused on parental occupational exposures (Chen Z et al., 2005) and the other on parental exposures to residential pesticides and chemicals (Chen Z et al., 2006), but they are based on the same overall case–control study.

No new studies from the Children's Oncology Group have been published since *Update 2006.*

Cross-Canada Study of Pesticides and Health

In a nationwide case–control study of men who were 19 years old or older in 1991–1994 and lived in six Canadian provinces, Pahwa et al. (2006) investigated whether exposure to phenoxy herbicides and other pesticides was associated with incidence of HD, multiple myeloma, or STS.

McDuffie et al. (2001, 2005) followed an analogous protocol in conducting a case–control study of male NHL cases and controls. McDuffie et al. (2005) and Pahwa et al. (2006) considered the possible interaction of exposure to insect repellents, particularly *N*,*N*-dietheyl-*m*-toluamide (DEET) and phenoxy herbicides in the genesis of the malignancies in question.

No new studies from the Cross-Canada Study of Pesticides and Health that are relevant to the chemicals of interest have been published since the *Update 2006*.

ENVIRONMENTAL STUDIES

The occurrence of industrial accidents has led to the evaluation of the long-term health effects of exposure to the chemicals of interest.

Chapaevsk, Russia

Researchers in the Samara region of Russia have identified a chemical plant in Chapaevsk as a major source of TCDD pollution (Revazova et al., 2001; Revich et al., 2001). From 1967 to 1987, the plant produced γ-hexachlorocyclohexane (lindane) and its derivatives. Since then, the plant has produced various crop-protection products. Dioxins have been detected in air, soil, drinking water, and cows' milk in the region. However, the researchers do not describe air-, soil-, or water-sampling methods. The number of samples analyzed was small for some media (two drinking-water samples, seven breast-milk samples pooled from 40 women, and 14 blood samples) and unreported for others (air, soil, and vegetables). Results of analysis of the samples suggested higher concentrations of dioxin around the center of Chapaevsk than in outlying areas. That conclusion was based primarily on concentrations measured in soil: 141 ng TEQ/kg soil less than 2 km from the plant compared with 37 ng TEQ/kg soil 2–7 km from the plant and 4 ng TEQ/kg soil 7–10 km from the plant. Concentrations outside the city (10–15 km from the plant) were about 1 ng TEQ/kg. The authors also compared measurements from Chapaevsk with those from other Russian cities that had industrial facilities. The data presented do not allow direct comparison of dioxin concentrations in soil as a function of distance from the industrial facilities. However, the highest TCDD concentrations in the Chapaevsk study (those nearest the plant) were higher than the maximum concentrations reported by four other studies referred to in the article. Residence in the city of Chapaevsk was used as a surrogate for exposure in the epidemiologic analyses presented in the report. No attempt was made to create exposure categories based on residential location in the city or on occupational or lifestyle factors that might have influenced TCDD exposure.

Akhmedkhanov et al. (2002) sampled 24 volunteers in the same population for lipid-adjusted serum-dioxin concentrations. Residents living within 5 km of the plant had higher concentrations than those who lived farther from the plant. It was not clear whether the analysis included adjustments for age, BMI, or education, all of which are significant predictors of dioxin concentration. No new studies have been published since *Update 2004*.

Seveso, Italy

Among the largest industrial accidents that have resulted in environmental exposure to TCDD was one in Seveso, Italy, in July 1976 that was caused by an uncontrolled reaction during trichlorophenol production. The degree of TCDD contamination in the soil has been used extensively as a means of imputing exposures of members of the population. Three areas were defined on the basis of soil sampling: Zone A, the most heavily contaminated, from which all residents were evacuated within 20 days; Zone B, an area of lower contamination that all children and women in the first trimester of pregnancy were urged to avoid during daytime; and Zone R, a region with some contamination in which consumption of local crops was prohibited (Bertazzi et al., 1989a,b).

Data on serum TCDD concentrations in Zone A residents have been presented by Mocarelli et al. (1990, 1991) and by CDC (1988a). In those who had severe chloracne (n = 10), TCDD was 828–56,000 ppt of lipid weight. Those without chloracne (n = 10) had TCDD at 1,770–10,400 ppt. TCDD was undetectable in all control subjects but one. The highest of those concentrations exceeded any that had been estimated at the time for TCDD-exposed workers on the basis of backward extrapolation and a half-life of 7 years. Data on nearby soil concentrations, number of days that a person stayed in Zone A, and whether local food was consumed were considered in evaluating TCDD. That none of those data correlated with serum TCDD suggested strongly that the important exposure was from fallout on the day of the accident. The presence and degree of chloracne did correlate with TCDD. Adults seemed much less likely than children to develop chloracne after acute exposure, but surveillance bias could have affected that finding. Recent updates (Bertazzi et al., 1998, 2001) have not changed the exposure-assessment approach.

A number of studies of the Seveso population have used lipid-adjusted serum TCDD concentrations as the primary exposure metric (Baccarelli et al., 2002; Eskenazi et al., 2002a,b, 2003, 2004; Landi et al., 2003). Fattore et al. (2003) measured current air concentrations of PCDDs in Zones A and B and compared them with measurements in a control area near Milan. The authors concluded that release from PCDD-contaminated soil did not add appreciably to air concentrations in the Seveso study area. Finally, Weiss et al. (2003) collected breast milk from 12 mothers in Seveso to compare TCDD concentrations with those in a control population near Milan. The investigators reported that the TCDD concentrations in human milk from mothers in Seveso were twice as high as those in controls. The authors concluded that breastfed children in the Seveso area were likely to have higher body burdens of TCDD than children from other areas.

Several cohort studies have been conducted on the basis of the exposure categories. Seveso residents have had long-term follow-up of their health outcomes, especially cancer. Bertazzi and colleagues conducted 10-year mortality follow-up studies of adults and children who were 1–19 years old at the time of the accident (Bertazzi et al., 1989a,b, 1992), 15-year follow-up studies (Bertazzi et al., 1997, 1998), and a 20-year follow-up study (Bertazzi et al., 2001). Pesatori et al. (1998) also conducted a 15-year follow-up study to update noncancer mortality. The studies were reviewed extensively in *VAO*, *Update 1996*, *Update 1998*, *Update 2000*, *Update 2002*, and *Update 2004* and are summarized here.

In addition to a 2-year prospective controlled study of workers potentially exposed to TCDD during cleanup of the most highly contaminated areas after the accident (Assennato et al., 1989b), studies have examined specific health effects associated with TCDD exposure in Seveso residents: chloracne, birth defects, spontaneous abortion, and crude birth and death rates (Bisanti et al., 1980); chloracne and peripheral nervous system conditions (Barbieri et al., 1988); chloracne among cases and noncases recruited previously by Landi et al., 1997, 1998 (Baccarelli et al., 2005a); hepatic-enzyme–associated conditions (Ideo et al., 1982, 1985); abnormal pregnancy outcomes (Mastroiacovo et al., 1988); cytogenetic abnormalities in maternal and fetal tissues (Tenchini et al., 1983); neurologic disorders (Boeri et al., 1978; Filippini et al., 1981); cancer (Bertazzi et al., 1993; Pesatori et al., 1992, 1993); sex ratio of offspring who were born in Zone A (Mocarelli et al., 1996); breast cancer (Warner et al., 2002); immunologic effects (Baccarelli et al., 2002); aryl hydrocarbon receptor–dependent (AHR-dependent) pathway and toxic effects of TCDD in humans (Baccarelli et al., 2004); effects of TCDD-mediated alterations in the AHR-dependent pathway in people who lived in Zones A and B (Landi et al., 2003); and NHL-related t(14;18) translocations prevalence and frequency in dioxin-exposed healthy people from Seveso (Baccarelli et al., 2006). Baccarelli et al. (2005b) reviewed statistical strategies for handling nondetectable or near the detection limit readings in dioxin measurement datasets. They recommended that a distribution-based multiple-imputation method be used to analyze environmental data when substantial proportions of observations have nondetectable readings.

Caramaschi et al. (1981) presented the distribution of chloracne in Seveso children, and Mocarelli et al. (1986) measured several compounds in the blood and urine of children who had chloracne. In a follow-up study, dermatologic and laboratory tests were conducted in a group of the children with chloracne and compared with results in a group of controls (Assennato et al., 1989a).

Since *Update 2006*, Consonni et al. (2008) have published a 25-year follow-up study of residents ("present") in the Seveso area and reference territory at the time of the Seveso industrial accident and of immigrants and newborns ("nonpresent") in the 10 years thereafter. Mortality in exposed residents—804 in

Zone A (723 present and 81 nonpresent), 5,941 in Zone B (4,821 present and 1,120 nonpresent), and 38,623 in Zone R (31,643 present and 6,980 nonpresent)— was compared with mortality in 232,740 residents of surrounding communities (181,574 present and 51,166 nonpresent). Mortality data were obtained from vital-statistics offices in the study municipalities. For residents who emigrated outside the study area and remained in the Lombardy region, record linkage with population databases traced about 40,000 subjects who either lived in the area or died elsewhere in the region. For residents who were not linked or who did not emigrate outside the region (about 20,000 people), an individual postal follow-up was performed through the vital-statistics offices of municipalities throughout Italy. Cause of death (coded according to ICD-9) was ascertained through record linkage with databases of the National Central Statistics Institute and Lombardy region local health units or through postal contact with other vital-statistics offices and local health units. Cause-specific mortality was determined for each zone and compared with that in the comparison cohort and adjusted for presence at the accident, sex, period (1976–1981, 1982–1986, 1987–1991, 1992–1996, and 1997–2001), age (under 1 years old, 1–4 years old, 5-year categories up to the age of 84 years, and at least 85 years old), and time since the Seveso accident ("latency"; 0–4, 5–9, 10–14, 15–19, and at least 20 years).

Since *Update 2006*, two new studies examining reproductive effects in the Seveso cohort have been published. Baccarelli et al. (2008) reported on crude sex ratios, birth weight, and neonatal thyroid function for all births in 1994–2005 to women who were less than 18 years old at the time of the Seveso accident. Mocarelli et al. (2008) investigated TCDD's effects on reproductive hormones and sperm quality in a comparison of 135 men exposed to TCDD by the 1976 Seveso accident with 184 healthy men not exposed to TCDD or living in the Seveso contamination zones. Both groups were divided into three categories reflecting their age at the time of the Seveso accident: infancy to prepuberty (1–9 years), puberty (10–17 years), and adulthood (18–26 years).

Several studies have used data from the Seveso Women's Health Study (SWHS) to evaluate the association between individual serum TCDD and reproductive effects in women who resided in Seveso at the time of the accident in 1976. The study group consisted of 981 volunteers who were between infancy and 40 years old at the time of the accident, who had resided in Zone A or B, and for whom adequate serum remained from samples collected for TCDD measurements shortly after the explosion.

As part of the SWHS, Eskenazi et al. (2001) tested the validity of exposure classification by zone. Investigators measured serum TCDD in samples collected in 1976–1980 from 601 residents (97 from Zone A and 504 from Zone B). A questionnaire that the women completed in 1996–1998 included age, chloracne history, animal mortality, consumption of homegrown food, and location at the time of the explosion. Participants did not know their TCDD concentrations at the time of the interview, but most knew their zone of residence. Interviewers and TCDD analysts were blinded to participants' zone of residence. Zone of residence explained 24% of the variability in serum TCDD. Addition of the questionnaire data improved the regression model, explaining 42% of the variability. Those findings demonstrate a significant association between zone of residence and serum TCDD, but much of the variability in TCDD concentration is still unexplained by the models.

Previously reviewed studies have examined associations between serum TCDD and menstrual cycle (Eskenazi et al., 2002a), endometriosis (Eskenazi et al., 2002b), pregnancy outcome (Eskenazi et al., 2003), age at exposure of female Seveso residents (Eskenazi et al., 2004), age at menarche and age at menopause (Eskenazi et al., 2005), and age at menarche in women who were premenarcheal at the time of the explosion (Warner et al., 2004). Warner et al. (2005) compared a chemical-activated luciferase-gene expression bioassay with an isotope-dilution high-resolution gas-chromatography–high-resolution mass-spectrometry assay to measure PCDDs, PCDFs, and PCBs in serum of 78 women residing near Seveso to determine average total dioxin-like toxic equivalents; similar results were obtained with the two methods.

Since *Update 2006*, Eskenazi et al. (2007) and Warner et al. (2007) have published new studies of women in the SWHS that examined the incidence of fibroids and ovarian function, respectively. For both studies, women were identified who were 40 years old or younger at the time of the dioxin explosion in 1976; women who lived in the most contaminated zones (A and B) and had adequate stored serum were enrolled in 1996–1998. Eskanazi et al. (2007) excluded women who had received a diagnosis of fibroids before 1976, leaving a total of 956 women for analyses. Fibroids were ascertained in 634 women by self-report, medical records, and ultrasonography. Analyses were adjusted for confounding by parity, family history of fibroids, age at menarche, current BMI, smoking, alcohol consumption, and education.

In the Warner et al. (2007) study of menstrual function, women who were 20–40 years old and not taking oral contraceptives were evaluated by ultrasonography (96 women), serum hormone concentrations (87 women), and the occurrence of ovulation (203 women).

Times Beach and Quail Run Cohorts

Several reports have provided information on environmental exposure to TCDD in the Times Beach area of Missouri (Andrews et al., 1989; Patterson et al., 1986). In 1971, TCDD-contaminated sludge from a hexachlorophene-production facility was mixed with waste oil and sprayed in various community areas for dust control. Soil contamination in some samples exceeded 100 ppb. Among the Missouri sites with the highest soil TCDD concentrations was the Quail Run mobile-home park. Residents were considered exposed if they had lived in the park for at least 6 months during the time when contamination occurred (Hoffman et al., 1986). Other investigations of Times Beach have estimated exposure risk on the basis of residents' reported occupational and recreational activities in the sprayed area. Exposure estimates have been based on duration of residence and soil TCDD concentrations.

Andrews et al. (1989) provided the most extensive data on human adipose-tissue TCDD in 128 nonexposed control subjects compared with concentrations in 51 exposed persons who had ridden or cared for horses at arenas sprayed with TCDD-contaminated oil, who lived in areas where the oil had been sprayed, who were involved in TCP production, or who were involved in non-production TCP activities, such as laboratory or maintenance work. Persons were considered exposed if they lived near, worked with, or had other contact for at least 2 years with soil contaminated with TCDD at 20–100 ppb or for 6 months or more with soil contaminated with TCDD above 100 ppb. Of the exposed-population samples, 87% had adipose-tissue TCDD concentrations below 200 ppt; however, TCDD concentrations in seven of the 51 exposed persons were 250–750 ppt. In nonexposed persons, adipose-tissue TCDD ranged from undetectable to 20 ppt (median, 6 ppt). On the basis of a 7-year half-life, it is calculated that two study participants would have had adipose-tissue TCDD near 3,000 ppt at the time of the last exposure.

Several studies evaluated health effects potentially attributable to exposure (Evans et al., 1988; Hoffman et al., 1986; Stehr et al., 1986; Stehr-Green et al., 1987; Stockbauer et al., 1988; Webb et al., 1987). *VAO* discussed those studies; no further work has been published.

Vietnam

Researchers in Vietnam studied the native population exposed to the spraying that occurred during the Vietnam conflict. In a review paper, Constable and Hatch (1985) summarized the unpublished results of the studies. That article also examined nine reports that focused primarily on reproductive outcomes (Can et al., 1983a,b; Huong and Phuong, 1983; Khoa, 1983; Lang et al., 1983a,b; Nguyen, 1983; Phuong and Huong, 1983; Trung and Chien, 1983). Vietnamese researchers later published results of four additional studies: two on reproductive abnormalities (Phuong et al., 1989a,b), one on mortality (Dai et al., 1990), and one on hepatocellular carcinoma (Cordier et al., 1993). Ngo et al. (2006) published a meta-analysis addressing an association between exposure to Agent Orange and birth defects.

National Health and Nutrition Examination Survey

In the early 1960s, the National Center for Health Statistics of the CDC began the National Health and Nutrition Examination Survey (NHANES) program as a means of monitoring and assessing the health and nutritional status of people of all ages living in the United States. Data, including demographic, socioeconomic, dietary information and medical, dental, and physiological assessments, is collected through in-person interviews and health examinations from a representative sample of adults and children from across the country. Information gleaned from NHANES data is used to determine prevalence rates for diseases, assess nutritional status, and establish national standards of height, weight, and blood pressure. Researchers also conduct analyses of the NHANES data for epidemiologic studies and health science research.

Since *Update 2006*, several studies have been published that draw upon NHANES data as the basis for their analyses. NHANES data from 1999–2002 was used to evaluate cardiovascular disease (Ha et al., 2007) and hypertension (Everett et al., 2008a,b). Lee DH et al. (2006, 2007a,b,c) used data from the same years to evaluate several health outcomes including diabetes, metabolic syndrome, insulin resistance, and arthritis. Turyk et al. (2007) analyzed NHANES data from 1999–2002 and 2001–2002 to evaluate thyroid hormone levels.

Other Environmental Studies

VAO, *Update 1996*, and *Update 1998* reported on numerous studies of reproductive outcomes attendant on environmental exposure to the chemicals of interest in Oregon (EPA, 1979); Arkansas (Nelson et al., 1979); Iowa and Michigan (Gordon and Shy, 1981); New Brunswick, Canada (White et al., 1988); Skaraborg, Sweden (Jansson and Voog, 1989); and Northland, New Zealand (Hanify et al., 1981).

Other studies reviewed in previous updates focused on different outcomes of environmental exposure to the chemicals of interest: STS and connective-tissue cancers in Midland County, Michigan (Michigan Department of Public Health, 1983); NHL in Yorkshire, England (Cartwright et al., 1988); adverse health effects after an electric-transformer fire in Binghamton, New York (Fitzgerald et al., 1989); lymphomas and STS in Italy (Vineis et al., 1991); cancer in Finland (Lampi et al., 1992); early-onset PD in Oregon and Washington (Butterfield et al., 1993); neuropsychologic effects in Germany (Peper et al., 1993); mortality and cancer incidence in two cohorts of Swedish fishermen whose primary exposure route was assumed to be diet (Svensson et al., 1995); immunologic effects of prenatal and postnatal exposure to PCB or TCDD in Dutch infants from birth to 18 months of age (Weisglas-Kuperus et al., 1995); effects of inhalation exposure to TCDD and related compounds in wood preservatives on cell-mediated immunity in German day-care center employees (Wolf and Karmaus, 1995); skin cancer in Alberta, Canada (Gallagher et al., 1996); immunologic effects in hobby fishermen in the Frierfjord in southeastern Norway (Lovik et al., 1996); HD, NHL, multiple myeloma, and acute myeloid leukemia in various regions of Italy (Masala et al., 1996); NHL, HD, and chronic lymphocytic leukemia in a rural Michigan community (Waterhouse et al., 1996); cancer mortality in four northern wheat-producing states (Schreinemachers, 2000); mortality and incinerator dioxin emissions in municipalities in Japan (Fukuda et al., 2003); prevalence of hypertension in Taiwanese who lived near municipal-waste incinerators (Chen HL et al., 2006); and adverse pregnancy outcomes in Japan on the basis of maternal residence at the time of birth (Tango et al., 2004).

Several epidemiologic studies have been conducted in association with industrial-facility emissions or in regions with documented variation in dioxin exposures. Viel et al. (2000) reported on an investigation of apparent clusters of cases of STS and NHL in the vicinity of a municipal solid-waste incinerator in Doubs, France. The presumptive source of TCDD in the region is a municipal solid-waste incinerator in the Besançon electoral ward in western Doubs. Dioxin emissions from the incinerator were measured in international TEQ units at 16.3 ng/m^3, far in excess of the European Union (EU) standard of 0.1 ng/m^3. TCDD concentrations in cow's milk measured at three farms near the incinerator were well below the EU guideline of 6 ng/kg of fat, but the concentrations were highest at the farm closest to the incinerator.

Examining the same population as Viel et al. (2000), Floret et al. (2003) investigated the rates of NHL in Besançon, France. Cases were identified from a cancer registry of people who had a diagnosis of NHL in 1980–1995. Almost all the cases were histologically confirmed. Data on each case included date of birth, sex, age at diagnosis, and address at the time of diagnosis. Control subjects were selected from the population census; because of confidentiality laws and requirements, the only data available to investigators were the age categories (0–19, 20–39, 40–59, 60–74, and 75+ years), sex, and residence in specific blocks. Controls were selected randomly from census lists, according to a 10-to-1 matching that was based on sex and age group.

Exposure was based on geocoding of the distance of each study participant's residence from the plant. Dispersion modeling was used to account for meteorologic effects. The exposure assessment took advantage of an earlier study, conducted in 1999, that developed a model to predict dioxin emissions from the solid-waste incinerator. No other industrial sources of dioxin exposure were found in the area. The study region was divided into four areas of increasing dioxin concentration, from less than 0.0001 pg/m^3 in the low-exposure or reference group to 0.0004–0.0016 pg/m^3 in the highest-exposure category. Although the exposure assessment relied on sophisticated methods for modeling emissions, there was insufficient information on residential history and time–activity patterns, so the duration of exposure could not be included in the analysis.

In a case–control study conducted in France, 434 women who had breast cancer were compared with 2,170 community controls according to the proximity of their residence to emissions from a waste incinerator that generated PCDDs and PCDFs (Viel et al., 2008). Four exposure categories were created on the basis of emission data and a wind dispersion model. Separate analyses were carried out for women 20–59 years old and 60 years old or older. Among older women, the odds ratio was 0.31 (95% confidence interval, 0.08–0.89); however, this was based on only four cases, and there was no evidence of a dose–response trend. Furthermore, the study did not adjust for potential confounders.

Combustion records for the Zeeburg area of Amsterdam in the Netherlands were used as a surrogate for exposure to dioxins in a study of orofacial clefts (ten Tusscher et al., 2000). Location downwind or upwind of an incineration source was used to define exposed and reference groups for the study. A study of STS in the general population was conducted in northern Italy around the city of Mantua (Costani et al., 2000). Several industrial facilities are in Mantua, and residential proximity to them was presumed to result in increased TCDD exposure, but TCDD was not measured in the environment or in human tissues.

A study of dioxin exposure pathways in Belgium focused on long-time residents in the vicinity of two municipal-waste incinerators (Fierens et al., 2003a). Residents near a rural incinerator had significantly higher serum dioxin concentrations than a control group (38 vs 24 TEQ pg/g lipid). Concentrations in residents living near the incinerators increased proportionally with intake of local-animal fat. A second study (Fierens et al., 2003b) measured dioxin body burden in 257 people who had been environmentally exposed, with the object of determining whether dioxin and PCB exposures were associated with type 2 diabetes and endometriosis. No difference in body burden was found between women who had endometriosis and women in a control group, but the risk of type 2 diabetes was significantly higher in those with higher body burdens of dioxin-like compounds and PCBs. Another study of the correlation between dioxin-like compounds in Italian and Belgian women and the risk of endometriosis used measurements of TCDD and other dioxins in blood (De Felip et al., 2004). There was no difference in body burden between women who had endometriosis and a control group, but serum-dioxin concentrations were substantially higher in the Belgian controls than in a similar group from Italy (45 vs 18 TEQ pg/g lipid, respectively).

Bloom et al. (2006) measured serum dioxin in New York sport fishermen as part of a study of thyroid function. A methodologic study by Petreas et al. (2004) found generally quite high correlations between concentrations of dioxins and related compounds in breast and abdominal fat in the same woman, this suggested that they could be used interchangeably in epidemiologic studies. The same study, however, also found that adjusting concentrations according to lipid content rather than weight of the fat samples is important because of the presence of nonlipid components in the samples.

Dioxins and furans were among the soil contaminants at a Superfund site in Pensacola, Florida, resulting from operations at a wood treating company in operation from 1942 until 1982. In 2000, Karouna-Renier et al. (2007) gathered health and exposure histories and measured serum concentrations of 17 PCDD and PCDF congeners for 47 potentially exposed individuals. The study sample was selected in a non-systematic fashion from among former workers, their family, and residents. Logistic analysis of the prevalence of several health problems in terms of TEQs with adjustment for age, race, sex, BMI, tobacco and alcohol use, and worker status permitted investigation of dose–response relationships.

From 2002 to 2006, Ueruma et al. (2008a,b) assembled a stratified sample of 1,374 Japanese aged 15–73 years (627 men and 747 women) representing urban, farming, and fishing areas of the entire country. The subjects completed questionnaires with occupational, medical, smoking and residential histories, plus height and weight. They also provided blood samples that were analyzed by isotope dilution high-resolution gas chromatography/mass spectrometry for PCDDs and PCDFs and dioxin-like PCBs. Ueruma et al. (2008a) investigated relationship of these compounds with the prevalence of diabetes, defined as self-reported physician-diagnosed diabetes or using a value of plasma HbA1c greater than 6.1% as a predictor of fasting plasma glucose above 126 mg/dl. Ueruma et al. (2008b) presented summary statistics on the serum levels of the individual compounds in the blood of the study subjects and of their distributions with respect to various demographic characteristics; they also provided the results of log-transformed correlation analyses of all PCDDs and PCDFs combined (PCDD/Fs), of all dioxin-like PCBs, and of total TEQ with total cholesterol, high-density lipoprotein, and triglycerides.

REFERENCES[1]

Abdelouahab N, Mergler D, Takser L, Vanier C, St-Jean M, Baldwin M, Spear PA, Chan HM. 2008. Gender differences in the effects of organochlorines, mercury, and lead on thyroid hormone levels in lakeside communities of Quebec (Canada). *Environmental Research* 107(3):380–392.

ADVA (Australia, Department of Veterans' Affairs). 2005a. *Cancer Incidence in Australian Vietnam Veteran Study 2005.* Canberra: Department of Veterans' Affairs.

ADVA. 2005b. *The Third Australian Vietnam Veterans Mortality Study 2005.* Canberra: Department of Veterans' Affairs.

ADVA. 2005c. *Australian National Service Vietnam Veterans: Mortality and Cancer Incidence 2005.* Canberra: Department of Veterans' Affairs.

AFHS (Air Force Health Study). 1982. *An Epidemiologic Investigation of Health Effects in Air Force Personnel Following Exposure to Herbicides: Study Protocol, Initial Report.* Brooks AFB, TX: USAF School of Aerospace Medicine. SAM-TR-82-44.

AFHS. 1983. *An Epidemiologic Investigation of Health Effects in Air Force Personnel Following Exposure to Herbicides. Baseline Mortality Study Results.* Brooks AFB, TX: USAF School of Aerospace Medicine. NTIS AD-A130 793.

AFHS. 1984a. *An Epidemiologic Investigation of Health Effects in Air Force Personnel Following Exposure to Herbicides. Baseline Morbidity Study Results.* Brooks AFB, TX: USAF School of Aerospace Medicine. NTIS AD-A138 340.

AFHS. 1984b. *An Epidemiologic Investigation of Health Effects in Air Force Personnel Following Exposure to Herbicides. Mortality Update: 1984.* Brooks AFB, TX: USAF School of Aerospace Medicine.

---

[1]Throughout the report the same alphabetic indicator following year of publication is used consistently for the same article when there were multiple citations by the same first author in a given year. The convention of assigning the alphabetic indicator in order of citation in a given chapter is not followed.

AFHS. 1985. *An Epidemiologic Investigation of Health Effects in Air Force Personnel Following Exposure to Herbicides. Mortality Update: 1985.* Brooks AFB, TX: USAF School of Aerospace Medicine.

AFHS. 1986. *An Epidemiologic Investigation of Health Effects in Air Force Personnel Following Exposure to Herbicides. Mortality Update: 1986.* Brooks AFB, TX: USAF School of Aerospace Medicine. USAFSAM-TR-86-43.

AFHS. 1987. *An Epidemiologic Investigation of Health Effects in Air Force Personnel Following Exposure to Herbicides. First Follow-up Examination Results.* Brooks AFB, TX: USAF School of Aerospace Medicine. USAFSAM-TR-87-27.

AFHS. 1989. *An Epidemiologic Investigation of Health Effects in Air Force Personnel Following Exposure to Herbicides. Mortality Update: 1989.* Brooks AFB, TX: USAF School of Aerospace Medicine. USAFSAM-TR-89-9.

AFHS. 1990. *An Epidemiologic Investigation of Health Effects in Air Force Personnel Following Exposure to Herbicides.* Brooks AFB, TX: USAF School of Aerospace Medicine. USAFSAM-TR-90-2.

AFHS. 1991a. *An Epidemiologic Investigation of Health Effects in Air Force Personnel Following Exposure to Herbicides. Mortality Update: 1991.* Brooks AFB, TX: Armstrong Laboratory. AL-TR-1991-0132.

AFHS. 1991b. *An Epidemiologic Investigation of Health Effects in Air Force Personnel Following Exposure to Herbicides. Serum Dioxin Analysis of 1987 Examination Results.* Brooks AFB, TX: USAF School of Aerospace Medicine.

AFHS. 1992. *An Epidemiologic Investigation of Health Effects in Air Force Personnel Following Exposure to Herbicides. Reproductive Outcomes.* Brooks AFB, TX: Armstrong Laboratory. AL-TR-1992-0090.

AFHS. 1995. *An Epidemiologic Investigation of Health Effects in Air Force Personnel Following Exposure to Herbicides. 1992 Follow-up Examination Results.* Brooks AFB, TX: Epidemiologic Research Division; Armstrong Laboratory.

AFHS. 1996. *An Epidemiologic Investigation of Health Effects in Air Force Personnel Following Exposure to Herbicides. Mortality Update 1996.* Brooks AFB, TX: Epidemiologic Research Division; Armstrong Laboratory. AL/AO-TR-1996-0068.

AFHS. 2000. An *Epidemiologic Investigation of Health Effects in Air Force Personnel Following Exposure to Herbicides. 1997 Follow-up Examination and Results.* Reston, VA: Science Application International Corporation. F41624-96-C1012.

AFHS. 2005. *An Epidemiologic Investigation of Health Effects in Air Force Personnel Following Exposure to Herbicides. 1997 Follow-up Examination and Results.* Brooks AFB, TX: Epidemiologic Research Division. Armstrong Laboratory. AFRL-HE-BR-SR-2005-0003.

Agent Orange Review. 2008. IOM announces new Vietnam veterans and Agent Orange committee to prepare 2008 update. *Department of Veterans Affairs* 20(2):1–8.

AIHW (Australian Institute of Health and Welfare). 1999. *Morbidity of Vietnam Veterans: A Study of the Health of Australia's Vietnam Veteran Community: Volume 3: Validation Study.* Canberra: AIHW.

AIHW. 2000. *Morbidity of Vietnam Veterans. Adrenal Gland Cancer, Leukaemia and non-Hodgkin's Lymphoma: Supplementary Report No. 2.* (AIHW cat. No. PHE 28). Canberra: AIHW.

AIHW. 2001. *Morbidity of Vietnam Veterans. Adrenal Gland Cancer, Leukaemia and non-Hodgkin's Lymphoma: Supplementary Report No. 2.* Revised edition (AIHW cat. No. PHE 34). Canberra: AIHW.

Akhmedkhanov A, Revich B, Adibi JJ, Zeilert V, Masten SA, Patterson DG Jr, Needham LL, Toniolo P. 2002. Characterization of dioxin exposure in residents of Chapaevsk, Russia. *Journal of Exposure Analysis and Environmental Epidemiology* 12(6):409–417.

Akhtar FZ, Garabrant DH, Ketchum NS, Michalek JE. 2004. Cancer in US Air Force veterans of the Vietnam war. *Journal of Occupational and Environmental Medicine* 46(2):123–136.

Alavanja MC, Blair A, Merkle S, Teske J, Eaton B. 1988. Mortality among agricultural extension agents. *American Journal of Industrial Medicine* 14:167–176.

Alavanja MC, Merkle S, Teske J, Eaton B, Reed B. 1989. Mortality among forest and soil conservationists. *Archives of Environmental Health* 44:94–101.

Alavanja MC, Sandler DP, Mcdonnell CJ, Lynch CF, Pennybacker M, Zahm SH, Lubin J, Mage D, Steen WC, Wintersteen W, Blair A. 1998. Factors associated with self-reported, pesticide-related visits to health care providers in the Agricultural Health Study. *Environmental Health Perspectives* 106(7):415–420.

Alavanja MCR, Samanic C, Dosemeci M, Lubin J, Tarone R, Lynch CF, Knott C, Thomas K, Hoppin JA, Barker J, Coble J, Sandler DP, Blair A. 2003. Use of agricultural pesticides and prostate cancer risk in the Agricultural Health Study cohort. *American Journal of Epidemiology* 157(9):800–814.

Alavanja MC, Hoppin JA, Kamel F. 2004. Health effects of chronic pesticide exposure: Cancer and neurotoxicity. *Annual Review of Public Health* 25:155–197.

Alavanja MCR, Sandler DP, Lynch CF, Knott C, Lubin JH, Tarone R, Thomas K, Dosemeci M, Barker J, Hoppin JA, Blair A. 2005. Cancer incidence in the Agricultural Health Study. *Scandinavian Journal of Work, Environment and Health* 31(Suppl 1):39–45.

Alderfer R, Sweeney M, Fingerhut M, Hornung R, Wille K, Fidler A. 1992. Measures of depressed mood in workers exposed to 2,3,7,8-tetrachlorodibenzo-*p*-dioxin (TCDD). *Chemosphere* 25:247–250.

Amadori D, Nanni O, Falcini F, Saragoni A, Tison V, Callea A, Scarpi E, Ricci M, Riva N, Buiatti E. 1995. Chronic lymphocytic leukemias and non-Hodgkin's lymphomas by histological type in farming-animal breeding workers: A population case–control study based on job titles. *Occupational and Environmental Medicine* 52(6):374–379.

Anderson HA, Hanrahan LP, Jensen M, Laurin D, Yick WY, Wiegman P. 1986a. *Wisconsin Vietnam Veteran Mortality Study: Proportionate Mortality Ratio Study Results.* Madison: Wisconsin Division of Health.

Anderson HA, Hanrahan LP, Jensen M, Laurin D, Yick WY, Wiegman P. 1986b. *Wisconsin Vietnam Veteran Mortality Study: Final Report.* Madison: Wisconsin Division of Health.

Andrews JS Jr, Garrett WA, Patterson DG Jr, Needham LL, Roberts DW, Bagby JR, Anderson JE, Hoffman RE, Schramm W. 1989. 2,3,7,8-tetrachlorodibenzo-*p*-dioxin levels in adipose tissue of persons with no known exposure and in exposed persons. *Chemosphere* 18(1-6):499–506.

Arbuckle TE, Ritter L. 2005. Phenoxyacetic acid herbicide exposure for women on Ontario farms. *Journal of Toxicology and Environmental Health, Part A* 68(15):1359–1370.

Arbuckle TE, Schrader SM, Cole D, Hall JC, Bancej CM, Turner LA, Claman P. 1999a. 2,4-Dichlorophenoxyacetic acid (2,4-D) residues in semen of Ontario farmers. *Reproductive Toxicology* 13(6):421–429.

Arbuckle TE, Savitz DA, Mery LS, Curtis KM. 1999b. Exposure to phenoxy herbicides and the risk of spontaneous abortion. *Epidemiology* 10:752–760.

Arbuckle TE, Lin Z, Mery LS. 2001. An exploratory analysis of the effect of pesticide exposure on the risk of spontaneous abortion in an Ontario farm population. *Environmental Health Perspectives* 109(8):851–857.

Arbuckle TE, Burnett R, Cole D, Teschke K, Dosemecci M, Bancej C, Zhang J. 2002. Predictors of herbicide exposure in farm applicators. *International Archives of Occupational and Environmental Health* 75:406–414.

Arbuckle TE, Cole DC, Ritter L, Ripley BD. 2005. Biomonitoring of gerbicides in Ontario farm applicators. *Scandinavian Journal of Work, Environment and Health* 31(Supplement 1):90–97.

Arbuckle TE, Bruce D, Ritter L, Hall JC. 2006. Indirect sources of herbicide exposure for families on Ontario farms. *Journal of Exposure Science and Environmental Epidemiology* 16(1):98–104.

Arcury TA, Quandt SA, Barr DB, Hoppin JA, McCauley L, Grzywacz JG, Robson MG. 2006. Farmworker exposure to pesticides: Methodologic issues for the collection of comparable data. *Environmental Health Perspectives* 114(6):923–928.

Aschengrau A, Monson RR. 1989. Paternal military service in Vietnam and risk of spontaneous abortion. *Journal of Occupational Medicine* 31:618–623.

Aschengrau A, Monson RR. 1990. Paternal military service in Vietnam and the risk of late adverse pregnancy outcomes. *American Journal of Public Health* 80:1218–1224.

Asp S, Riihimaki V, Hernberg S, Pukkala E. 1994. Mortality and cancer morbidity of Finnish chlorophenoxy herbicide applicators: An 18-year prospective follow-up. *American Journal of Industrial Medicine* 26:243–253.

Assennato G, Cervino D, Emmett E, Longo G, Merlo F. 1989a. Follow-up of subjects who developed chloracne following TCDD exposure at Seveso. *American Journal of Industrial Medicine* 16:119–125.

Assennato G, Cannatelli P, Emmett E, Ghezzi I, Merlo F. 1989b. Medical monitoring of dioxin cleanup workers. *American Industrial Hygiene Association Journal* 50:586–592.

ATSDR (Agency for Toxic Substances and Disease Registry). 1998. *Toxicological Profile for Chlorinated Dibenzo-p-dioxins (CDDs).* Atlanta, GA: Centers for Disease Control.

Axelson O, Sundell L. 1974. Herbicide exposure, mortality and tumor incidence. An epidemiological investigation on Swedish railroad workers. *Scandinavian Journal of Work, Environment and Health* 11:21–28.

Axelson O, Sundell L, Andersson K, Edling C, Hogstedt C, Kling H. 1980. Herbicide exposure and tumor mortality: An updated epidemiologic investigation on Swedish railroad workers. *Scandinavian Journal of Work, Environment and Health* 6:73–79.

Aylward LL, Brunet RC, Carrier G, Hays SM, Cushing CA, Needham LL, Patterson DG Jr, Gerthoux PM, Brambilla P, Mocarelli P. 2005a. Concentration-dependent TCDD elimination kinetics in humans: Toxicokinetic modeling for moderately to highly exposed adults from Seveso, Italy, and Vienna, Austria, and impact on dose estimates for the NIOSH cohort. *Journal of Exposure Analysis and Environmental Epidemiology* 15(1):51–65.

Aylward LL, Brunet RC, Starr TB, Carrier G, Delzell E, Cheng H, Beall C. 2005b. Exposure reconstruction for the TCDD-exposed NIOSH cohort using a concentration and age-dependent model of elimination. *Risk Analysis* 25(4):945–956.

Baccarelli A, Mocarelli P, Patterson DG Jr, Bonzini M, Pesatori A, Caporaso N, Landi MT. 2002. Immunologic effects of dioxin: New results from Seveso and comparison with other studies. *Environmental Health Perspectives* 110(12):1169–1173.

Baccarelli A, Pesatori AC, Masten SA, Patterson DG Jr, Needham LL, Mocarelli P, Caporaso NE, Consonni D, Grassman JA, Bertazzi PA, Landi MT. 2004. Aryl-hydrocarbon receptor-dependent pathways and toxic effects of TCDD in humans: A population-based study in Seveso, Italy. *Toxicology Letters* 149(1-3):287–293.

Baccarelli A, Pesatori AC, Consonni D, Mocarelli P, Patterson DG Jr, Caporaso NE, Bertazzi PA, Landi MT. 2005a. Health status and plasma dioxin levels in chloracne cases 20 years after the Seveso, Italy accident. *British Journal of Dermatology* 152(3):459–465.

Baccarelli A, Pfeiffer R, Consonni D, Pesatori AC, Bonzini M, Patterson DG Jr, Bertazzi PA, Landi MT. 2005b. Handling of dioxin measurement data in the presence of non-detectable values: Overview of available methods and their application in the Seveso chloracne study. *Chemosphere* 60(7):898–906.

Baccarelli A, Hirt C, Pesatori AC, Consonni D, Patterson DG Jr, Bertazzi PA, Dölken G, Landi MT. 2006. t(14;18) translocations in lymphocytes of healthy dioxin-exposed individuals from Seveso, Italy. *Carcinogenesis* 27(10):2001–2007.

Baccarelli A, Giacomini SM, Corbetta C, Landi MT, Bonzini M, Consonni D, Grillo P, Patterson DG Jr, Pesatori AC, Bertazzi PA. 2008. Neonatal thyroid function in Seveso 25 years after maternal exposure to dioxin. *PLoS Medicine* 5(7):1133–1142.

Balarajan R, Acheson ED. 1984. Soft tissue sarcomas in agriculture and forestry workers. *Journal of Epidemiology and Community Health* 38:113–116.

Barbieri S, Pirovano C, Scarlato G, Tarchini P, Zappa A, Maranzana M. 1988. Long-term effects of 2,3,7,8-tetrachlorodibenzo-*p*-dioxin on the peripheral nervous system. Clinical and neurophysiological controlled study on subjects with chloracne from the Seveso area. *Neuroepidemiology* 7:29–37.

Barr DB, Landsittel D, Nishioka M, Thomas K, Curwin B, Raymer J, Donnelly KC, McCauley L, Ryan PB. 2006a. A survey of laboratory and statistical issues related to farmworker exposure studies. *Environmental Health Perspectives* 114(6):961–968.

Barr DB, Thomas K, Curwin B, Landsittel D, Raymer J, Lu C, Donnelly KC, Acquavella J. 2006b. Biomonitoring of exposure in farmworker studies. *Environmental Health Perspectives* 114(6): 936–942.

Barrett DH, Morris RD, Akhtar FZ, Michalek JE. 2001. Serum dioxin and cognitive functioning among veterans of Operation Ranch Hand. *Neurotoxicology* 22:491–502.

Barrett DH, Morris RD, Jackson WG Jr, Stat M, Michalek JE. 2003. Serum dioxin and psychological functioning in US Air Force veterans of the Vietnam War. *Military Medicine* 168:153–159.

Barthel E. 1981. Increased risk of lung cancer in pesticide-exposed male agricultural workers. *Journal of Toxicology and Environmental Health* 8:1027–1040.

Bashirov AA. 1969. The health of workers involved in the production of amine and butyl 2,4-D herbicides. *Vrachebnoye Delo* 10:92–95.

Becher H, Flesch-Janys D, Kauppinen T, Kogevinas M, Steindorf K, Manz A, Wahrendorf J. 1996. Cancer mortality in German male workers exposed to phenoxy herbicides and dioxins. *Cancer Causes and Control* 7(3):312–321.

Bell EM, Hertz-Picciotto I, Beaumont JJ. 2001a. Case–cohort analysis of agricultural pesticide applications near maternal residence and selected causes of fetal death. *American Journal of Epidemiology* 154(8):702–710.

Bell EM, Hertz-Picciotto I, Beaumont JJ. 2001b. A case–control study of pesticides and fetal death due to congenital anomalies. *Epidemiology* 12(2):148–156.

Bender AP, Parker DL, Johnson RA, Scharber WK, Williams AN, Marbury MC, Mandel JS. 1989. Minnesota highway maintenance worker study: Cancer mortality. *American Journal of Industrial Medicine* 15:545–556.

Bertazzi PA, Zocchetti C, Pesatori AC, Guercilena S, Sanarico M, Radice L. 1989a. Mortality in an area contaminated by TCDD following an industrial incident. *Medicina Del Lavoro* 80:316–329.

Bertazzi PA, Zocchetti C, Pesatori AC, Guercilena S, Sanarico M, Radice L. 1989b. Ten-year mortality study of the population involved in the Seveso incident in 1976. *American Journal of Epidemiology* 129:1187–1200.

Bertazzi PA, Zocchetti C, Pesatori AC, Guercilena S, Consonni D, Tironi A, Landi MT. 1992. Mortality of a young population after accidental exposure to 2,3,7,8-tetrachlorodibenzodioxin. *International Journal of Epidemiology* 21:118–123.

Bertazzi A, Pesatori AC, Consonni D, Tironi A, Landi MT, Zocchetti C. 1993. Cancer incidence in a population accidentally exposed to 2,3,7,8-tetrachlorodibenzo-*para*-dioxin. *Epidemiology* 4:398–406.

Bertazzi PA, Zochetti C, Guercilena S, Consonni D, Tironi A, Landi MT, Pesatori AC. 1997. Dioxin exposure and cancer risk: A 15-year mortality study after the "Seveso accident." *Epidemiology* 8(6):646–652.

Bertazzi PA, Bernucci I, Brambilla G, Consonni D, Pesatori AC. 1998. The Seveso studies on early and long-term effects of dioxin exposure: A review. *Environmental Health Perspectives* 106(Suppl 2):625–633.

Bertazzi PA, Consonni D, Bachetti S, Rubagotti M, Baccarelli A, Zocchetti C, Pesatori AC. 2001. Health effects of dioxin exposure: A 20-year mortality study. *American Journal of Epidemiology* 153(11):1031–1044.

Bisanti L, Bonetti F, Caramaschi F, Del Corno G, Favaretti C, Giambelluca SE, Marni E, Montesarchio E, Puccinelli V, Remotti G, Volpato C, Zambrelli E, Fara GM. 1980. Experiences from the accident of Seveso. *Acta Morphologica Academiae Scientarum Hungaricae* 28:139–157.

Blair A, Thomas TL. 1979. Leukemia among Nebraska farmers: A death certificate study. *American Journal of Epidemiology* 110:264–273.

Blair A, White DW. 1985. Leukemia cell types and agricultural practices in Nebraska. *Archives of Environmental Health* 40:211–214.

Blair A, Grauman DJ, Lubin JH, Fraumeni JF Jr. 1983. Lung cancer and other causes of death among licensed pesticide applicators. *Journal of the National Cancer Institute* 71:31–37.

Blair A, Mustafa D, Heineman EF. 1993. Cancer and other causes of death among male and female farmers from twenty-three states. *American Journal of Industrial Medicine* 23:729–742.

Blair A, Sandler DP, Tarone R, Lubin J, Thomas K, Hoppin JA, Samanic C, Coble J, Kamel F, Knott C, Dosemeci M, Zahm SH, Lynch CF, Rothman N, Alavanja MC. 2005a. Mortality among participants in the Agricultural Health Study. *Annals of Epidemiology* 15(4):279–285.

Blair A, Sandler D, Thomas K, Hoppin JA, Kamel F, Cobel J, Lee WJ, Rusiecki J, Knott C, Dosemeci M, Lynch CF, Lubin J, Alavanja M. 2005b. Disease and injury among participants in the Agricultural Health Study. *Journal of Agricultural Safety and Health* 11(2):141–150.

Blatter BM, Hermens R, Bakker M, Roeleveld N, Verbeek AL, Zielhuis GA. 1997. Paternal occupational exposure around conception and spina bifida in offspring. *American Journal of Industrial Medicine* 32(3):283–291.

Bloemen LJ, Mandel JS, Bond GG, Pollock AF, Vitek RP, Cook RR. 1993. An update of mortality among chemical workers potentially exposed to the herbicide 2,4-dichlorophenoxyacetic acid and its derivatives. *Journal of Occupational Medicine* 35:1208–1212.

Bloom M, Vena J, Olson J, Moysich K. 2006. Chronic exposure to dioxin-like compounds and thyroid function among New York anglers. *Environmental Toxicology and Pharmacology* 21(3): 260–267.

Bodner KM, Collins JJ, Bloemen LJ, Carson ML. 2003. Cancer risk for chemical workers exposed to 2,3,7,8-tetrachlorodibenzo-*p*-dioxin. *Occupational and Environmental Medicine* 60:672–675.

Boehmer TK, Flanders WD, McGeehin MA, Boyle C, Barrett DH. 2004. Postservice mortality in Vietnam veterans: 30-year follow-up. *Archives of Internal Medicine* 164(17):1908–1916.

Boeri R, Bordo B, Crenna P, Filippini G, Massetto M, Zecchini A. 1978. Preliminary results of a neurological investigation of the population exposed to TCDD in the Seveso region. *Rivista di Patologia Nervosa e Mentale* 99:111–128.

Boffetta P, Stellman SD, Garfinkel L. 1989. A case–control study of multiple myeloma nested in the American Cancer Society prospective study. *International Journal of Cancer* 43:554–559.

Bond GG, Ott MG, Brenner FE, Cook RR. 1983. Medical and morbidity surveillance findings among employees potentially exposed to TCDD. *British Journal of Industrial Medicine* 40:318–324.

Bond GG, Cook RR, Brenner FE, McLaren EA. 1987. Evaluation of mortality patterns among chemical workers with chloracne. *Chemosphere* 16:2117–2121.

Bond GG, Wetterstroem NH, Roush GJ, McLaren EA, Lipps TE, Cook RR. 1988. Cause specific mortality among employees engaged in the manufacture, formulation, or packaging of 2,4-dichlorophenoxyacetic acid and related salts. *British Journal of Industrial Medicine* 45:98–105.

Bond GG, McLaren EA, Lipps TE, Cook RR. 1989a. Update of mortality among chemical workers with potential exposure to the higher chlorinated dioxins. *Journal of Occupational Medicine* 31:121–123.

Bond GG, McLaren EA, Brenner FE, Cook RR. 1989b. Incidence of chloracne among chemical workers potentially exposed to chlorinated dioxins. *Journal of Occupational Medicine* 31:771–774.

Boyle C, Decoufle P, Delaney RJ, DeStefano F, Flock ML, Hunter MI, Joesoef MR, Karon JM, Kirk ML, Layde PM, McGee DL, Moyer LA, Pollock DA, Rhodes P, Scally MJ, Worth RM. 1987. *Postservice Mortality Among Vietnam Veterans*. Atlanta, GA: Centers for Disease Control. CEH 86-0076.

Breslin P, Kang H, Lee Y, Burt V, Shepard BM. 1988. Proportionate mortality study of US Army and US Marine Corps veterans of the Vietnam War. *Journal of Occupational Medicine* 30: 412–419.

Brighina L, Frigerio R, Schneider NK, Lesnick TG, de Andrade M, Cunningham JM, Farrer MJ, Lincoln SJ, Checkoway H, Rocca WA, Maraganore DM. 2008. Alpha-synuclein, pesticides, and Parkinson disease: A case–control study. *Neurology* 70(16 Pt 2):1461–1469.

Brown LM, Blair A, Gibson R, Everett GD, Cantor KP, Schuman LM, Burmeister LF, Van Lier SF, Dick F. 1990. Pesticide exposures and other agricultural risk factors for leukemia among men in Iowa and Minnesota. *Cancer Research* 50:6585–6591.

Brown LM, Burmeister LF, Everett GD, Blair A. 1993. Pesticide exposures and multiple myeloma in Iowa men. *Cancer Causes and Control* 4:153–156.

Bueno de Mesquita HB, Doornbos G, van der Kuip DA, Kogevinas M, Winkelmann R. 1993. Occupational exposure to phenoxy herbicides and chlorophenols and cancer mortality in the Netherlands. *American Journal of Industrial Medicine* 23:289–300.

Bullman TA, Kang HK. 1996. The risk of suicide among wounded Vietnam veterans. *American Journal of Public Health* 86(5):662–667.

Bullman TA, Kang HK, Watanabe KK. 1990. Proportionate mortality among US Army Vietnam veterans who served in Military Region I. *American Journal of Epidemiology* 132:670–674.

Bullman TA, Kang H, Thomas TL. 1991. Posttraumatic stress disorder among Vietnam veterans on the Agent Orange Registry: A case–control analysis. *Annals of Epidemiology* 1:505–512.

Bullman TA, Watanabe KK, Kang HK. 1994. Risk of testicular cancer associated with surrogate measures of Agent Orange exposure among Vietnam veterans on the Agent Orange Registry. *Annals of Epidemiology* 4:11–16.

Burmeister LF. 1981. Cancer mortality in Iowa farmers: 1971–1978. *Journal of the National Cancer Institute* 66:461–464.

Burmeister LF, Van Lier SF, Isacson P. 1982. Leukemia and farm practices in Iowa. *American Journal of Epidemiology* 115:720–728.

Burmeister LF, Everett GD, Van Lier SF, Isacson P. 1983. Selected cancer mortality and farm practices in Iowa. *American Journal of Epidemiology* 118:72–77.

Burns CJ, Beard KK, Cartmill JB. 2001. Mortality in chemical workers potentially exposed to 2,4-dichlorophenoxyacetic acid (2,4-D) 1945–1994: An update. *Occupational and Environmental Medicine* 58:24–30.

Burt VL, Breslin PP, Kang HK, Lee Y. 1987. *Non-Hodgkin's lymphoma in Vietnam veterans*. Washington, DC: Department of Medicine and Surgery, Veterans Administration.

Burton JE, Michalek JE, Rahe AJ. 1998. Serum dioxin, chloracne, and acne in veterans of Operation Ranch Hand. *Archives of Environmental Health* 53(3):199–204.

Butterfield PG, Valanis BG, Spencer PS, Lindeman CA, Nutt JG. 1993. Environmental antecedents of young-onset Parkinson's disease. *Neurology* 43:1150–1158.

Calvert GM, Sweeney MH, Morris JA, Fingerhut MA, Hornung RW, Halperin WE. 1991. Evaluation of chronic bronchitis, chronic obstructive pulmonary disease, and ventilatory function among workers exposed to 2,3,7,8-tetrachlorodibenzo-*p*-dioxin. *American Review of Respiratory Disease* 144:1302–1306.

Calvert GM, Hornung RW, Sweeney MH, Fingerhut MA, Halperin WE. 1992. Hepatic and gastrointestinal effects in an occupational cohort exposed to 2,3,7,8-tetrachlorodibenzo-*para*-dioxin. *Journal of the American Medical Association* 267:2209–2214.

Calvert GM, Sweeney MH, Fingerhut MA, Hornung RW, Halperin WE. 1994. Evaluation of porphyria cutanea tarda in US workers exposed to 2,3,7,8-tetrachlorodibenzo-*p*-dioxin. *American Journal of Industrial Medicine* 25:559–571.

Calvert GM, Wall DK, Sweeney MH, Fingerhut MA. 1998. Evaluation of cardiovascular outcomes among US workers exposed to 2,3,7,8-tetrachlorodibenzo-*p*-dioxin. *Environmental Health Perspectives* 106(Suppl 2):635–643.

Calvert GM, Sweeney MH, Deddens J, Wall DK. 1999. Evaluation of diabetes mellitus, serum glucose, and thyroid function among United States workers exposed to 2,3,7,8-tetrachlorodibenzo-*p*-dioxin. *Occupational and Environmental Medicine* 56(4):270–276.

Can N, Xiem NT, Tong NK, Duong DB. 1983a. A case–control survey of congenital defects in My Van District, Hai Hung Province. Summarized in: Constable JD, Hatch MC. *Reproductive effects of herbicide exposure in Vietnam: Recent studies by the Vietnamese and others.* As cited in Constable and Hatch, 1985.

Can N, Xiem NT, Tong NK, Duong DB. 1983b. An epidemiologic survey of pregnancies in Viet Nam. Summarized in: Constable JD, Hatch MC. *Reproductive effects of herbicide exposure in Vietnam: Recent studies by the Vietnamese and others.* As cited in Constable and Hatch, 1985.

Cantor KP. 1982. Farming and mortality from non-Hodgkin's lymphoma: A case–control study. *International Journal of Cancer* 29:239–247.

Cantor KP, Blair A, Everett G, Gibson R, Burmeister LF, Brown LM, Schuman L, Dick FR. 1992. Pesticides and other agricultural risk factors for non-Hodgkin's lymphoma among men in Iowa and Minnesota. *Cancer Research* 52:2447–2455.

Caramaschi F, Del Corno G, Favaretti C, Giambelluca SE, Montesarchio E, Fara GM. 1981. Chloracne following environmental contamination by TCDD in Seveso, Italy. *International Journal of Epidemiology* 10:135–143.

Carmelli D, Hofherr L, Tomsic J, Morgan RW. 1981. *A Case–control Study of the Relationship Between Exposure to 2,4-D and Spontaneous Abortions in Humans.* SRI International. Prepared for the National Forest Products Association and the US Department of Agriculture, Forest Service.

Carreon T, Butler MA, Ruder AM, Waters MA, Davis-King KE, Calvert GM, Schulte PA, Connally B, Ward EM, Sanderson WT, Heineman EF, Mandel JS, Morton RF, Reding DJ, Rosenman KD, Talaska G, Cancer B. 2005. Gliomas and farm pesticide exposure in women: The Upper Midwest Health Study. *Environmental Health Perspectives* 113(5):546–551.

Cartwright RA, McKinney PA, O'Brien C, Richards IDG, Roberts B, Lauder I, Darwin CM, Bernard SM, Bird CC. 1988. Non-Hodgkin's lymphoma: Case–control epidemiological study in Yorkshire. *Leukemia Research* 12:81–88.

CDC (Centers for Disease Control and Prevention). 1985. *Exposure Assessment for the Agent Orange Study. Interim Report Number 2.* Atlanta, GA: Center for Environmental Health.

CDC. 1987. Postservice mortality among Vietnam veterans. *Journal of the American Medical Association* 257:790–795.

CDC. 1988a. Health status of Vietnam veterans. I. Psychosocial characteristics. *Journal of the American Medical Association* 259:2701–2707.

CDC. 1988b. Health status of Vietnam veterans. II. Physical health. *Journal of the American Medical Association* 259:2708–2714.

CDC. 1988c. Health status of Vietnam veterans. III. Reproductive outcomes and child health. *Journal of the American Medical Association* 259:2715–2717.

CDC. 1989a. *Comparison of Serum Levels of 2,3,7,8-Tetrachlorodibenzo-p-dioxin with Indirect Estimates of Agent Orange Exposure Among Vietnam Veterans: Final Report.* Atlanta, GA: US Department of Health and Human Services.

CDC. 1989b. *Health Status of Vietnam Veterans: Vietnam Experience Study. Vols. I–V, Supplements A–C.* Atlanta, GA: US Department of Health and Human Services.

CDC. 1990a. *The Association of Selected Cancers with Service in the US Military in Vietnam: Final Report.* Atlanta, GA: US Department of Health and Human Services.

CDC. 1990b. The association of selected cancers with service in the US military in Vietnam. I. Non-Hodgkin's lymphoma. *Archives of Internal Medicine* 150:2473–2483.

CDC. 1990c. The association of selected cancers with service in the US military in Vietnam. II. Soft-tissue and other sarcomas. *Archives of Internal Medicine* 150:2485–2492.

CDC. 1990d. The association of selected cancers with service in the US military in Vietnam. III. Hodgkin's disease, nasal cancer, nasopharyngeal cancer, and primary liver cancer. *Archives of Internal Medicine* 150:2495–2505.

CDVA (Commonwealth Department of Veterans' Affairs). 1998a. *Morbidity of Vietnam Veterans: A Study of the Health of Australia's Vietnam Veteran Community. Volume 1: Male Vietnam Veterans Survey and Community Comparison Outcomes.* Canberra, Australia: Department of Veterans' Affairs.

CDVA. 1998b. *Morbidity of Vietnam Veterans: A Study of the Health of Australia's Vietnam Veteran Community. Volume 2: Female Vietnam Veterans Survey and Community Comparison Outcomes.* Canberra, Australia: Department of Veterans' Affairs.

Chamie K, deVere White R, Volpp B, Lee D, Ok J, Ellison L. 2008. Agent Orange exposure, Vietnam War veterans, and the risk of prostate cancer. *Cancer* 113(9):2464–2470.

Chao HR, Wang SL, Lin LY, Lee WJ, Papke O. 2007. Placental transfer of polychlorinated dibenzo-*p*-dioxins, dibenzofurans, and biphenyls in Taiwanese mothers in relation to menstrual cycle characteristics. *Food and Chemical Toxicology* 45(2):259–265.

Chen HL, Su HJ, Guo YL, Liao PC, Hung CF, Lee CC. 2006. Biochemistry examinations and health disorder evaluation of Tiawanese living near incinerators and with low serum PCDD/Fs levels. *Science of the Total Environment* 366:538–548.

Chen Z, Stewart PA, Davies S, Giller R, Krailo M, Davis M, Robison L, Shu XO. 2005. Parental occupational exposure to pesticides and childhood germ-cell tumors. *American Journal of Epidemiology* 162(9):858–867.

Chen Z, Robison L, Giller R, Krailo M, Davis M, Davies S, Shu XO. 2006. Environmental exposure to residential pesticides, chemicals, dusts, fumes, and metals, and risk of childhood germ cell tumors. *International Journal of Hygiene and Environmental Health* 209(1):31–40.

Chevrier J, Eskenazi B, Holland N, Bradman A, Barr DB. 2008. Effects of exposure to polychlorinated biphenyls and organochlorine pesticides on thyroid function during pregnancy. *American Journal of Epidemiology* 168(3):298–310.

Chinh TT, Phi PT, Thuy NT. 1996. Sperm auto-antibodies and anti-nuclear antigen antibodies in chronic dioxin-exposed veterans. *Chemosphere* 32(3):525–530.

Chiu BC, Weisenburger DD, Zahm SH, Cantor KP, Gapstur SM, Holmes F, Burmeister LF, Blair A. 2004. Agricultural pesticide use, familial cancer, and risk of non-Hodgkin lymphoma. *Cancer Epidemiology, Biomarkers and Prevention* 13(4):525–531.

Chiu BC, Dave BJ, Blair A, Gapstur SM, Zahm SH, Weisenburger DD. 2006. Agricultural pesticide use and risk of t(14;18)-defined subtypes of non-Hodgkin lymphoma. *Blood* 108(4):1363–1369.

CIH (Commonwealth Institute of Health). 1984a. Australian Veterans Health Studies. *Mortality Report. Part I. A Retrospective Cohort Study of Mortality Among Australian National Servicemen of the Vietnam Conflict Era, and An Executive Summary of the Mortality Report.* Canberra, Australia: Australian Government Publishing Service.

CIH. 1984b. *Australian Veterans Health Studies. The Mortality Report. Part II. Factors Influencing Mortality Rates of Australian National Servicemen of the Vietnam Conflict Era.* Canberra, Australia: Australian Government Publishing Service.

CIH. 1984c. *Australian Veterans Health Studies. The Mortality Report. Part III. The Relationship Between Aspects of Vietnam Service and Subsequent Mortality Among Australian National Servicemen of the Vietnam Conflict Era.* Canberra, Australia: Australian Government Publishing Service.

Clapp RW. 1997. Update of cancer surveillance of veterans in Massachusetts, USA. *International Journal of Epidemiology* 26(3):679–681.

Clapp RW, Cupples LA, Colton T, Ozonoff DM. 1991. Cancer surveillance of veterans in Massachusetts, 1982–1988. *International Journal of Epidemiology* 20:7–12.

Coggon D, Pannett B, Winter PD, Acheson ED, Bonsall J. 1986. Mortality of workers exposed to 2-methyl-4-chlorophenoxyacetic acid. *Scandinavian Journal of Work, Environment and Health* 12:448–454.

Coggon D, Pannett B, Winter P. 1991. Mortality and incidence of cancer at four factories making phenoxy herbicides. *British Journal of Industrial Medicine* 48:173–178.

Collins JJ, Strauss ME, Levinskas GJ, Conner PR. 1993. The mortality experience of workers exposed to 2,3,7,8-tetrachlorodibenzo-*p*-dioxin in a trichlorophenol process accident. *Epidemiology* 4:7–13.

Collins JJ, Budinsky RA, Burns CJ, Lamparski LL, Carson ML, Martin GD, Wilken M. 2006. Serum dioxin levels in former chlorophenol workers. *Journal of Exposure Science and Environmental Epidemiology* 16(1):76–84.

Consonni D, Pesatori AC, Zocchetti C, Sindaco R, D'Oro LC, Rubagotti M, Bertazzi PA. 2008. Mortality in a population exposed to dioxin after the Seveso, Italy, accident in 1976: 25 years of follow-up. *American Journal of Epidemiology* 167(7):847–858.

Constable JD, Hatch MC. 1985. Reproductive effects of herbicide exposure in Vietnam: Recent studies by the Vietnamese and others. *Teratogenesis, Carcinogenesis, and Mutagenesis* 5:231–250.

Cook RR, Townsend JC, Ott MG, Silverstein LG. 1980. Mortality experience of employees exposed to 2,3,7,8-tetrachlorodibenzo-*p*-dioxin (TCDD). *Journal of Occupational Medicine* 22:530–532.

Cook RR, Bond GG, Olson RA. 1986. Evaluation of the mortality experience of workers exposed to the chlorinated dioxins. *Chemosphere* 15:1769–1776.

Cook RR, Bond GG, Olson RA, Ott MG. 1987. Update of the mortality experience of workers exposed to chlorinated dioxins. *Chemosphere* 16:2111–2116.

Cooney MA, Daniels JL, Ross JA, Breslow NE, Pollock BH, Olshan AF. 2007. Household pesticides and the risk of Wilms tumor. *Environmental Health Perspectives* 115(1):134–137.

Cordier S, Le TB, Verger P, Bard D, Le CD, Larouze B, Dazza MC, Hoang TQ, Abenhaim L. 1993. Viral infections and chemical exposures as risk factors for hepatocellular carcinoma in Vietnam. *International Journal of Cancer* 55:196–201.

Corrao G, Caller M, Carle F, Russo R, Bosia S, Piccioni P. 1989. Cancer risk in a cohort of licensed pesticide users. *Scandinavian Journal of Work, Environment and Health* 15:203–209.

Costani G, Rabitti P, Mambrini A, Bai E, Berrino F. 2000. Soft tissue sarcomas in the general population living near a chemical plant in northern Italy. *Tumori* 86:381–383.

Crane PJ, Barnard DL, Horsley KW, Adena MA. 1997a. *Mortality of Vietnam Veterans: The Veteran Cohort Study. A Report of the 1996 Retrospective Cohort Study of Australian Vietnam Veterans.* Canberra, Australia: Department of Veterans' Affairs.

Crane PJ, Barnard DL, Horsley KW, Adena MA. 1997b. *Mortality of National Service Vietnam Veterans: A Report of the 1996 Retrospective Cohort Study of Australian Vietnam Veterans.* Canberra, Australia: Department of Veterans' Affairs.

Crump KS, Canady R, Kogevinas M. 2003. Meta-analysis of dioxin cancer dose response for three occupational cohorts. *Environmental Health Perspectives* 111(5):681–687.

Curtis K, Savitz D, Weinberg C, Arbuckle T. 1999. The effect of pesticide exposure on time to pregnancy. *Epidemiology* 10(2):112–117. [Comment in *Epidemiology* 1999. 10(3):470.]

Curwin BD, Hein MJ, Sanderson WT, Barr DB, Heederik D, Reynolds SJ, Ward EM, Alavanja MC. 2005. Urinary and hand wipe pesticide levels among farmers and nonfarmers in Iowa. *Journal of Exposure Analysis and Environmental Epidemiology.* 15(6):500–508.

Cypel Y, Kang H. 2008. Mortality patterns among women Vietnam-era veterans: Results of a retrospective cohort study. *Annals of Epidemiology* 18(3):244–252.

Dai LC, Phuong NTN, Thom LH, Thuy TT, Van NTT, Cam LH, Chi HTK, Thuy LB. 1990. A comparison of infant mortality rates between two Vietnamese villages sprayed by defoliants in wartime and one unsprayed village. *Chemosphere* 20:1005–1012.

Dalager NA, Kang HK. 1997. Mortality among Army Chemical Corps Vietnam veterans. *American Journal of Industrial Medicine* 31(6):719–726.

Dalager NA, Kang HK, Burt VL, Weatherbee L. 1991. Non-Hodgkin's lymphoma among Vietnam veterans. *Journal of Occupational Medicine* 33:774–779.

Dalager NA, Kang HK, Thomas TL. 1995a. Cancer mortality patterns among women who served in the military: The Vietnam experience. *Journal of Occupational and Environmental Medicine* 37:298–305.

Dalager NA, Kang HK, Burt VL, Weatherbee L. 1995b. Hodgkin's disease and Vietnam service. *Annals of Epidemiology* 5(5):400–406.

Dankovic DA, Andersen ME, Salvan A, Stayner LT. 1995. A simplified PBPK model describing the kinetics of TCDD in humans (abstract). *Toxicologist* 15:272.

De Felip E, Porpora MG, di Domenico A, Ingelido AM, Cardelli M, Cosmi EV, Donnez J. 2004. Dioxin-like compounds and endometriosis: A study on Italian and Belgian women of reproductive age. *Toxicology Letters* 150(2):203–209.

De Roos AJ, Hartge P, Lubin JH, Colt JS, Davis S, Cerhan JR, Severson RK, Cozen W, Patterson DG Jr, Needham LL, Rothman N. 2005a. Persistent organochlorine chemicals in plasma and risk of non-Hodgkin's lymphoma. *Cancer Research* 65(23):11214–11226.

De Roos AJ, Cooper GS, Alavanja MC, Sandler DP. 2005b. Rheumatoid arthritis among women in the Agricultural Health Study: Risk associated with farming activities and exposures. *Annals of Epidemiology* 15(10):762–770.

Dean G. 1994. Deaths from primary brain cancers, lymphatic and haematopoietic cancers in agricultural workers in the Republic of Ireland. *Journal of Epidemiology and Community Health* 48:364–368.

Decoufle P, Holmgreen P, Boyle CA, Stroup NE. 1992. Self-reported health status of Vietnam veterans in relation to perceived exposure to herbicides and combat. *American Journal of Epidemiology* 135:312–323.

Deprez RD, Carvette ME, Agger MS. 1991. *The Health and Medical Status of Maine Veterans: A Report to the Bureau of Veterans Services, Commission of Vietnam and Atomic Veterans.* Portland, ME: Public Health Resource Group.

Dhooge W, van Larebeke N, Koppen G, Nelen V, Schoeters G, Vlietinck R, Kaufman JM, Comhaire F, Flemish E, Health Study G. 2006. Serum dioxin-like activity is associated with reproductive parameters in young men from the general Flemish population. *Environmental Health Perspectives* 114(11):1670–1676.

Dich J, Wiklund K. 1998. Prostate cancer in pesticide applicators in Swedish agriculture. *Prostate* 34(2):100–112.

Dimich-Ward H, Hertzman C, Teschke K, Hershler R, Marion SA, Ostry A, Kelly S. 1996. Reproductive effects of paternal exposure to chlorophenate wood preservatives in the sawmill industry. *Scandinavian Journal of Work, Environment and Health* 22(4):267–273.

Donna A, Betta PG, Robutti F, Crosignani P, Berrino F, Bellingeri D. 1984. Ovarian mesothelial tumors and herbicides: A case–control study. *Carcinogenesis* 5:941–942.

Donovan JW, Adena MA, Rose G, Battistutta D. 1983. *Case–Control Study of Congenital Anomalies and Vietnam Service: Birth Defects Study. Report to the Minister for Veterans' Affairs.* Canberra, Australia: Australian Government Publishing Service.

Donovan JW, MacLennan R, Adena M. 1984. Vietnam service and the risk of congenital anomalies: A case–control study. *Medical Journal of Australia* 140:394–397.

Dosemeci M, Alavanja MC, Rowland AS, Mage D, Zahm SH, Rothman N, Lubin JH, Hoppin JA, Sandler DP, Blair A. 2002. A quantitative approach for estimating exposure to pesticides in the Agricultural Health Study. *Annals of Occupational Hygiene* 46(2):245–260.

Dubrow R, Paulson JO, Indian RW. 1988. Farming and malignant lymphoma in Hancock County, Ohio. *British Journal of Industrial Medicine* 45:25–28.

Duell EJ, Millikan RC, Savitz DA, Schell MJ, Newman B, Tse CKJ, Sandler DP. 2001. Reproducibility of reported farming activities and pesticide use among breast cancer cases and controls: A comparison of two modes of data collection. *Association of Emergency Physicians* 11(3):178–185.

Egeland GM, Sweeney MH, Fingerhut MA, Wille KK, Schnorr TM, Halperin WE. 1994. Total serum testosterone and gonadotropins in workers exposed to dioxin. *American Journal of Epidemiology* 139:272–281.

Eisen S, Goldberg J, True WR, Henderson WG. 1991. A co-twin control study of the effects of the Vietnam War on the self-reported physical health of veterans. *American Journal of Epidemiology* 134:49–58.

Ekström AM, Eriksson M, Hansson LE, Lindgren A, Signorello LB, Nyren O, Hardell L. 1999. Occupational exposures and risk of gastric cancer in a population-based case–control study. *Cancer Research* 59(23):5932–5937.

Engel LS, Hill DA, Hoppin JA, Lubin JH, Lynch CF, Pierce J, Samanic C, Sandler DP, Blair A, Alavanja MC. 2005. Pesticide use and breast cancer risk among farmers' wives in the Agricultural Health Study. *American Journal of Epidemiology* 161(2):121–135.

EPA (United States Environmental Protection Agency). 1979. *Report of Assessment of a Field Investigation of Six-Year Spontaneous Abortion Rates in Three Oregon Areas in Relation to Forest 2,4,5-T Spray Practices.* Washington, DC: Epidemiologic Studies Program, Human Effects Monitoring Branch.

Erickson JD, Mulinare J, McClain PW, Fitch TG, James LM, McClearn AB, Adams MJ Jr. 1984a. *Vietnam Veterans' Risks for Fathering Babies with Birth Defects.* Atlanta, GA: US Department of Health and Human Services, Centers for Disease Control.

Erickson JD, Mulinare J, McClain PW, Fitch TG, James LM, McClearn AB, Adams MJ Jr. 1984b. Vietnam veterans' risks for fathering babies with birth defects. *Journal of the American Medical Association* 252:903–912.

Eriksson M, Hardell L, Berg NO, Moller T, Axelson O. 1979. Case–control study on malignant mesenchymal tumor of the soft tissue and exposure to chemical substances. *Lakartidningen* 76:3872–3875 [in Swedish].

Eriksson M, Hardell L, Berg NO, Moller T, Axelson O. 1981. Soft-tissue sarcomas and exposure to chemical substances: A case–referent study. *British Journal of Industrial Medicine* 38:27–33.

Eriksson M, Hardell L, Adami HO. 1990. Exposure to dioxins as a risk factor for soft tissue sarcoma: A population-based case–control study. *Journal of the National Cancer Institute* 82:486–490.

Eriksson M, Hardell L, Malker H, Weiner J. 1992. Malignant lymphoproliferative diseases in occupations with potential exposure to phenoxyacetic acids or dioxins: A register-based study. *American Journal of Industrial Medicine* 22:305–312.

Eriksson M, Hardell L, Carlberg M, Akerman M. 2008. Pesticide exposure as risk factor for non-Hodgkin lymphoma including histopathological subgroup analysis. *International Journal of Cancer* 123(7):1657–1663.

Eskenazi B, Mocarelli P, Warner M, Samuels S, Needham L, Patterson D, Brambilla P, Gerthoux PM, Turner W, Casalini S, Cazzaniga M, Chee WY. 2001. Seveso Women's Health Study: Does zone of residence predict individual TCDD exposure? *Chemosphere* 43(4-7):937–942.

Eskenazi B, Warner M, Mocarelli P, Samuels S, Needham LL, Patterson DG Jr, Lippman S, Vercellini P, Gerthoux PM, Brambilla P, Olive D. 2002a. Serum dioxin concentrations and menstrual cycle characteristics. *American Journal of Epidemiology* 156(4):383–392.

Eskenazi B, Mocarelli P, Warner M, Samuels S, Vercellini P, Olive D, Needham LL, Patterson DG Jr, Brambilla P, Gavoni N, Casalini S, Panazza S, Turner W, Gerthoux PM. 2002b. Serum dioxin concentrations and endometriosis: A cohort study. *Environmental Health Perspectives* 110(7):629–634.

Eskenazi B, Mocarelli P, Warner M, Chee W-Y, Gerthoux PM, Samuels S, Needham LL, Patterson DG Jr. 2003. Maternal serum dioxin levels and birth outcomes in women of Seveso, Italy. *Environmental Health Perspectives* 111(7):947–953.

Eskenazi B, Mocarelli P, Warner M, Needham LL, Patterson DG Jr, Samuels S, Turner W, Gerthoux PM, Brambilla P. 2004. Relationship of serum TCDD concentrations and age at exposure of female residents of Seveso, Italy. *Environmental Health Perspectives* 112(1):22–27.

Eskenazi B, Warner M, Marks AR, Samuels S, Gerthoux PM, Vercellini P, Olive DL, Needham L, Patterson D Jr, Mocarelli P. 2005. Serum dioxin concentrations and age at menopause. *Environmental Health Perspectives* 113(7):858–862.

Eskenazi B, Warner M, Samuels S, Young J, Gerthoux PM, Needham L, Patterson D, Olive D, Gavoni N, Vercellini P, Mocarelli P. 2007. Serum dioxin concentrations and risk of uterine leiomyoma in the Seveso Women's Health Study. *American Journal of Epidemiology* 166(1):79–87.

Evans RG, Webb KB, Knutsen AP, Roodman ST, Roberts DW, Bagby JR, Garrett WA Jr, Andrews JS Jr. 1988. A medical follow-up of the health effects of long-term exposure to 2,3,7,8-tetrachlorodibenzo-*p*-dioxin. *Archives of Environmental Health* 43:273–278.

Evatt P. 1985. *Royal Commission on the Use and Effect of Chemical Agents on Australian Personnel in Vietnam, Final Report.* Canberra, Australia: Australian Government Publishing Service.

Everett CJ, Frithsen IL, Diaz VA, Koopman RJ, Simpson WM Jr, Mainous AG 3rd. 2007. Association of a polychlorinated dibenzo-*p*-dioxin, a polychlorinated biphenyl, and DDT with diabetes in the 1999–2002 National Health and Nutrition Examination Survey. *Environmental Research* 103(3):413–418.

Everett CJ, Mainous AG 3rd, Frithsen IL, Player MS, Matheson EM. 2008a. Association of polychlorinated biphenyls with hypertension in the 1999–2002 National Health and Nutrition Examination Survey. *Environmental Research* 108(1):94–97.

Everett CJ, Mainous AG 3rd, Frithsen IL, Player MS, Matheson EM. 2008b. Commentary on association of polychlorinated biphenyls with hypertension. *Environmental Research* 108(3): 428–429.

Farberow NL, Kang H, Bullman T. 1990. Combat experience and postservice psychosocial status as predictors of suicide in Vietnam veterans. *Journal of Nervous and Mental Disease* 178:32–37.

Farr SL, Cooper GS, Cai J, Savitz DA, Sandler DP. 2004. Pesticide use and menstrual cycle characteristics among premenopausal women in the Agricultural Health Study. *American Journal of Epidemiology* 160(12):1194–1204.

Farr SL, Cai J, Savitz DA, Sandler DP, Hoppin JA, Cooper GS. 2006. Pesticide exposure and timing of menopause: The Agricultural Health Study. *American Journal of Epidemiology* 163(8): 731–742.

Fattore E, Di Guardo A, Mariani G, Guzzi A, Benfenati E, Fanelli R. 2003. Polychlorinated dibenzo-*p*-dioxins and dibenzofurans in the air of Seveso, Italy, 26 years after the explosion. *Environmental Science and Technology* 37(8):1503–1508.

Faustini A, Settimi L, Pacifici R, Fano V, Zuccaro P, Forastiere F. 1996. Immunological changes among farmers exposed to phenoxy herbicides: Preliminary observations. *Occupational and Environmental Medicine* 53(9):583–585.

Ferry DG, Gazeley LR, Edwards IR. 1982. 2,4,5-T absorption in chemical applicators. *Proceedings of the University Otago Medical School* 60:31–34.

Fett MJ, Adena MA, Cobbin DM, Dunn M. 1987a. Mortality among Australian conscripts of the Vietnam conflict era. I. Death from all causes. *American Journal of Epidemiology* 126:869–877.

Fett MJ, Nairn JR, Cobbin DM, Adena MA. 1987b. Mortality among Australian conscripts of the Vietnam conflict era. II. Causes of death. *American Journal of Epidemiology* 125:878–884.

Fiedler N, Gochfeld M. 1992. *Neurobehavioral Correlates of Herbicide Exposure in Vietnam Veterans.* New Jersey Agent Orange Commission.

Field B, Kerr C. 1988. Reproductive behaviour and consistent patterns of abnormality in offspring of Vietnam veterans. *Journal of Medical Genetics* 25:819–826.

Fierens S, Mairesse H, Heilier J-F, De Burbure C, Focant J-F, Eppe G, De Pauw E, Bernard A. 2003a. Dioxin/polychlorinated biphenyl body burden, diabetes and endometriosis: Findings in a population-based study in Belgium. *Biomarkers* 8(6):529–534.

Fierens S, Mairesse H, Hermans C, Bernard A, Eppe G, Focant JF, De Pauw E. 2003b. Dioxin accumulation in residents around incinerators. *Journal of Toxicology and Environmental Health Part A* 66(14):1287–1293.

Filippini G, Bordo B, Crenna P, Massetto N, Musicco M, Boeri R. 1981. Relationship between clinical and electrophysiological findings and indicators of heavy exposure to 2,3,7,8-tetrachlorodibenzodioxin. *Scandinavian Journal of Work, Environment and Health* 7:257–262.

Fingerhut MA, Halperin WE, Marlow DA, Piacitelli LA, Honchar PA, Sweeney MH, Greife AL, Dill PA, Steenland K, Suruda AJ. 1991. Cancer mortality in workers exposed to 2,3,7,8-tetrachlorodibenzo-*p*-dioxin. *New England Journal of Medicine* 324:212–218.

Fitzgerald EF, Weinstein AL, Youngblood LG, Standfast SJ, Melius JM. 1989. Health effects three years after potential exposure to the toxic contaminants of an electrical transformer fire. *Archives of Environmental Health* 44:214–221.

Flesch-Janys D. 1997. Analyses of exposure to polychlorinated dibenzo-*p*-dioxins, furans, and hexachlorocyclohexane and different health outcomes in a cohort of former herbicide-producing workers in Hamburg, Germany. *Teratogenesis, Carcinogenesis and Mutagenesis* 17(4-5):257–264.

Flesch-Janys D, Berger J, Gurn P, Manz A, Nagel S, Waltsgott H, Dwyer JH. 1995. Exposure to polychlorinated dioxins and furans (PCDD/F) and mortality in a cohort of workers from a herbicide-producing plant in Hamburg, Federal Republic of Germany. *American Journal of Epidemiology* 142(11):1165–1175.

Flesch-Janys D, Steindorf K, Gurn P, Becher H. 1998. Estimation of the cumulated exposure to polychlorinated dibenzo-*p*-dioxins/furans and standardized mortality ratio analysis of cancer mortality by dose in an occupationally exposed cohort. *Environmental Health Perspectives* 106 (Supplement 2):655–662.

Floret N, Mauny F, Challier B, Arveux P, Cahn J-Y, Viel J-F. 2003. Dioxin emissions from a solid waste incinerator and risk of non-Hodgkin lymphoma. *Epidemiology* 14(4):392–398.

Flower KB, Hoppin JA, Lynch CF, Blair A, Knott C, Shore DL, Sandler DP. 2004. Cancer risk and parental pesticide application in children of Agricultural Health Study participants. *Environmental Health Perspectives* 112(5):631–635.

Forcier L, Hudson HM, Cobbin DM, Jones MP, Adena MA, Fett MJ. 1987. Mortality of Australian veterans of the Vietnam conflict and the period and location of their Vietnam service. *Military Medicine* 152:9–15.

Frank R, Campbell RA, Sirons GJ. 1985. Forestry workers involved in aerial application of 2,4-dichlorophenoxyacetic acid (2,4-D): Exposure and urinary excretion. *Archives of Environment and Contaminant Toxicology* 14:427–435.

Fritschi L, Benke G, Hughes AM, Kricker A, Turner J, Vajdic CM, Grulich A, Milliken S, Kaldor J, Armstrong BK. 2005. Occupational exposure to pesticides and risk of non-Hodgkin's lymphoma. *American Journal of Epidemiology* 162(9):849–857.

Fukuda Y, Nakamura K, Takano T. 2003. Dioxins released from incineration plants and mortality from major diseases: An analysis of statistical data by municipalities. *Journal of Medical and Dental Sciences* 50:249–255.

Gallagher RP, Bajdik CD, Fincham S, Hill GB, Keefe AR, Coldman A, McLean DI. 1996. Chemical exposures, medical history, and risk of squamous and basal cell carcinoma of the skin. *Cancer Epidemiology, Biomarkers and Prevention* 5(6):419–424.

Gambini GF, Mantovani C, Pira E, Piolatto PG, Negri E. 1997. Cancer mortality among rice growers in Novara Province, northern Italy. *American Journal of Industrial Medicine* 31(4):435–441.

Garaj-Vrhovac V, Zeljezic D. 2002. Assessment of genome damage in a population of Croatian workers employed in pesticide production by chromosomal aberration analyis, micronucleus assay and Comet assay. *Journal of Applied Toxicology* 22(4):249–255.

Garcia AM, Benavides FG, Fletcher T, Orts E. 1998. Paternal exposure to pesticides and congenital malformations. *Scandinavian Journal of Work, Environment and Health* 24(6):473–480.

Garry VF, Kelly JT, Sprafka JM, Edwards S, Griffith J. 1994. Survey of health and use characterization of pesticide appliers in Minnesota. *Archives of Environmental Health* 49:337–343.

Garry VF, Tarone RE, Long L, Griffith J, Kelly JT, Burroughs B. 1996a. Pesticide appliers with mixed pesticide exposure: G-banded analysis and possible relationship to non-Hodgkin's lymphoma. *Cancer Epidemiology, Biomarkers and Prevention* 5(1):11–16.

Garry VF, Schreinemachers D, Harkins ME, Griffith J. 1996b. Pesticide appliers, biocides, and birth defects in rural Minnesota. *Environmental Health Perspectives* 104(4):394–399.

Garry VF, Holland SE, Erickson LL, Burroughs BL. 2003. Male reproductive hormones and thyroid function in pesticide applicators in the Red River Valley of Minnesota. *Journal of Toxicology and Environmental Health* 66:965–986.

Goldberg J, True WR, Eisen SA, Henderson WG. 1990. A twin study of the effects of the Vietnam War on posttraumatic stress disorder. *Journal of the American Medical Association* 263:1227–1232.

Gordon JE, Shy CM. 1981. Agricultural chemical use and congenital cleft lip and/or palate. *Archives of Environmental Health* 36:213–221.

Gorell JM, Peterson EL, Rybicki BA, Johnson CC. 2004. Multiple risk factors for Parkinson's disease. *Journal of the Neurological Sciences* 217:169–174.

Goun BD, Kuller LH. 1986. *Final Report: A Case–Control Mortality Study on the Association of Soft Tissue Sarcomas, Non-Hodgkin's Lymphomas, and Other Selected Cancers and Vietnam Military Service in Pennsylvania Males.* Pittsburgh, PA: University of Pittsburgh.

Green LM. 1987. Suicide and exposure to phenoxy acid herbicides. *Scandinavian Journal of Work, Environment and Health* 13(5):460.

Green LM. 1991. A cohort mortality study of forestry workers exposed to phenoxy acid herbicides. *British Journal of Industrial Medicine* 48:234–238.

Greenwald P, Kovasznay B, Collins DN, Therriault G. 1984. Sarcomas of soft tissues after Vietnam service. *Journal of the National Cancer Institute* 73:1107–1109.

Gupta A, Ketchum N, Roehrborn CG, Schecter A, Aragaki CC, Michalek JE. 2006. Serum dioxin, testosterone, and subsequent risk of benign prostatic hyperplasia: A prospective cohort study of Air Force veterans. *Environmental Health Perspectives* 114(11):1649–1654.

Ha MH, Lee DH, Jacobs Jr DR. 2007. Association between serum concentrations of persistent organic pollutants and self-reported cardiovascular disease prevalence: Results from the National Health and Nutrition Examination Survey, 1999–2002. *Environmental Health Perspectives* 115(8):1204–1209.

Halperin W, Kalow W, Sweeney MH, Tang BK, Fingerhut M, Timpkins B, Wille K. 1995. Induction of P-450 in workers exposed to dioxin. *Occupational and Environmental Medicine* 52(2):86–91.

Halperin W, Vogt R, Sweeney MH, Shopp G, Fingerhut M, Petersen M. 1998. Immunological markers among workers exposed to 2,3,7,8-tetrachlorodibenzo-*p*-dioxin. *Occupational and Environmental Medicine* 55(11):742–749.

Hancock DB, Martin ER, Mayhew GM, Stajich JM, Jewett R, Stacy MA, Scott BL, Vance JM, Scott WK. 2008. Pesticide exposure and risk of Parkinson's disease: A family-based case–control study. *BMC Neurology* 8:6.

Hanify JA, Metcalf P, Nobbs CL, Worsley KJ. 1981. Aerial spraying of 2,4,5-T and human birth malformations: An epidemiological investigation. *Science* 212:349–351.

Hanke W, Romitti P, Fuortes L, Sobala W, Mikulski M. 2003. The use of pesticides in a Polish rural population and its effect on birth weight. *International Archives of Occupational and Environmental Health* 76:614–620.

Hansen ES, Hasle H, Lander F. 1992. A cohort study on cancer incidence among Danish gardeners. *American Journal of Industrial Medicine* 21:651–660.

Hansen ES, Lander F, Lauritsen JM. 2007. Time trends in cancer risk and pesticide exposure, a long-term follow-up of Danish gardeners. *Scandinavian Journal of Work, Environment and Health* 33(6):465–469.

Hardell L. 1977. Malignant mesenchymal tumors and exposure to phenoxy acids: A clinical observation. *Lakartidningen* 74:2753–2754 [in Swedish].

Hardell L. 1979. Malignant lymphoma of histiocytic type and exposure to phenoxyacetic acids or chlorophenols. *Lancet* 1(8106):55–56.

Hardell L. 1981. Relation of soft-tissue sarcoma, malignant lymphoma and colon cancer to phenoxy acids, chlorophenols and other agents. *Scandinavian Journal of Work, Environment and Health* 7:119–130.

Hardell L, Bengtsson NO. 1983. Epidemiological study of socioeconomic factors and clinical findings in Hodgkin's disease, and reanalysis of previous data regarding chemical exposure. *British Journal of Cancer* 48:217–225.

Hardell L, Eriksson M. 1988. The association between soft tissue sarcomas and exposure to phenoxyacetic acids: A new case-referent study. *Cancer* 62:652–656.

Hardell L, Eriksson M. 1999. A case–control study of non-Hodgkin lymphoma and exposure to pesticides. *Cancer* 85(6):1353–1360.

Hardell L, Sandstrom A. 1979. Case–control study: Soft-tissue sarcomas and exposure to phenoxyacetic acids or chlorophenols. *British Journal of Cancer* 39:711–717.

Hardell L, Eriksson M, Lenner P. 1980. Malignant lymphoma and exposure to chemical substances, especially organic solvents, chlorophenols and phenoxy acids. *Lakartidningen* 77:208–210.

Hardell L, Eriksson M, Lenner P, Lundgren E. 1981. Malignant lymphoma and exposure to chemicals, especially organic solvents, chlorophenols and phenoxy acids: A case–control study. *British Journal of Cancer* 43:169–176.

Hardell L, Johansson B, Axelson O. 1982. Epidemiological study of nasal and nasopharyngeal cancer and their relation to phenoxy acid or chlorophenol exposure. *American Journal of Industrial Medicine* 3:247–257.

Hardell L, Bengtsson NO, Jonsson U, Eriksson S, Larsson LG. 1984. Aetiological aspects on primary liver cancer with special regard to alcohol, organic solvents and acute intermittent porphyria: An epidemiological investigation. *British Journal of Cancer* 50:389–397.

Hardell L, Moss A, Osmond D, Volberding P. 1987. Exposure to hair dyes and polychlorinated dibenzo-*p*-dioxins in AIDS patients with Kaposi sarcoma: An epidemiological investigation. *Cancer Detection and Prevention Supplement* 1:567–570.

Hardell L, Eriksson M, Degerman A. 1994. Exposure to phenoxyacetic acids, chlorophenols, or organic solvents in relation to histopathology, stage, and anatomical localization of non-Hodgkin's lymphoma. *Cancer Research* 54:2386–2389.

Harris SA, Corey PN, Sass-Kortsak AM, Purdham JT. 2001. The development of a new method to estimate total daily dose of pesticides in professional turf applicators following multiple and varied exposures in occupational settings. *International Archives of Occupational Environmental Health* 74(5):345–358.

Hartge P, Colt JS, Severson RK, Cerhan JR, Cozen W, Camann D, Zahm SH, Davis S. 2005. Residential herbicide use and risk of non-Hodgkin lymphoma. *Cancer Epidemiology, Biomarkers and Prevention* 14(4):934–937.

Hayes HM, Tarone RE, Casey HW, Huxsoll DL. 1990. Excess of seminomas observed in Vietnam service US military working dogs. *Journal of the National Cancer Institute* 82:1042–1046.

Heacock H, Hogg R, Marion SA, Hershler R, Teschke K, Dimich-Ward H, Demers P, Kelly S, Ostry A, Hertzman C. 1998. Fertility among a cohort of male sawmill workers exposed to chlorophenate fungicides. *Epidemiology* 9(1):56–60.

Heilier JF, Donnez J, Defrere S, Van Kerckhove V, Donnez O, Lison D. 2006. Serum dioxin-like compounds and aromatase (CYP19) expression in endometriotic tissues. *Toxicology Letters* 167(3):238–244.

Heilier JF, Donnez J, Nackers F, Rousseau R, Verougstraete V, Rosenkranz K, Donnez O, Grandjean F, Lison D, Tonglet R. 2007. Environmental and host-associated risk factors in endometriosis and deep endometriotic nodules: A matched case–control study. *Environmental Research* 103(1):121–129.

Henneberger PK, Ferris BG Jr, Monson RR. 1989. Mortality among pulp and paper workers in Berlin, New Hampshire. *British Journal of Industrial Medicine* 46:658–664.

Henriksen GL, Michalek JE, Swaby JA, Rahe AJ. 1996. Serum dioxin, testosterone, and gonadotropins in veterans of Operation Ranch Hand. *Epidemiology* 7(4):352–357.

Henriksen GL, Ketchum NS, Michalek JE, Swaby JA. 1997. Serum dioxin and diabetes mellitus in veterans of Operation Ranch Hand. *Epidemiology* 8(3):252–258.

Hertzman C, Teschke K, Ostry A, Hershler R, Dimich-Ward H, Kelly S, Spinelli JJ, Gallagher RP, McBride M, Marion SA. 1997. Mortality and cancer incidence among sawmill workers exposed to chlorophenate wood preservatives. *American Journal of Public Health* 87(1):71–79.

Hertz-Picciotto I, Jusko TA, Willman EJ, Baker RJ, Keller JA, Teplin SW, Charles MJ. 2008. A cohort study of in utero polychlorinated biphenyl (PCB) exposures in relation to secondary sex ratio. *Environmental Health: A Global Access Science Source* 7:37.

Hoar SK, Blair A, Holmes FF, Boysen CD, Robel RJ, Hoover R, Fraumeni JF. 1986. Agricultural herbicide use and risk of lymphoma and soft-tissue sarcoma. *Journal of the American Medical Association* 256:1141–1147.

Hoffman RE, Stehr-Green PA, Webb KB, Evans RG, Knutsen AP, Schramm WF, Staake JL, Gibson BB, Steinberg KK. 1986. Health effects of long-term exposure to 2,3,7,8-tetrachlorodibenzo-*p*-dioxin. *Journal of the American Medical Association* 255:2031–2038.

Holmes AP, Bailey C, Baron RC, Bosanac E, Brough J, Conroy C, Haddy L. 1986. *West Virginia Department of Health Vietnam-Era Veterans Mortality Study, Preliminary Report.* Charleston: West Virginia Health Department.

Hooiveld M, Heederik DJ, Kogevinas M, Boffetta P, Needham LL, Patterson DG Jr, Bueno de Mesquita HB. 1998. Second follow-up of a Dutch cohort occupationally exposed to phenoxy herbicides, chlorophenols, and contaminants. *American Journal of Epidemiology* 147(9):891–901.

Hoppin JA. 2005. Integrating exposure measurements into epidemiologic studies in agriculture. *Scandinavian Journal of Work, Environment and Health* 31(Supplement 1):115–117.

Hoppin JA, Umbach DM, London SJ, Alavanja CR, Sandler DP. 2002. Chemical predictors of wheeze among farmer pesticide applicators in the Agricultural Health Study. *American Journal of Critical Care Medicine* 165:683–689.

Hoppin JA, Umbach DM, London SJ, Lynch CF, Alavanja MC, Sandler DP. 2006a. Pesticides associated with wheeze among commercial pesticide applicators in the Agricultural Health Study. *American Journal of Epidemiology* 163(12):1129–1137.

Hoppin JA, Adgate JL, Eberhart M, Nishioka M, Ryan PB. 2006b. Environmental exposure assessment of pesticides in farmworker homes. *Environmental Health Perspectives* 114(6):929–935.

Hoppin JA, Umbach DM, London SJ, Lynch CF, Alavanja MC, Sandler DP. 2006c. Pesticides and adult respiratory outcomes in the Agricultural Health Study. *Annals of the New York Academy of Sciences* 1076:343–354.

Hoppin JA, Umbach DM, Kullman GJ, Henneberger PK, London SJ, Alavanja MC, Sandler DP. 2007a. Pesticides and other agricultural factors associated with self-reported farmer's lung among farm residents in the Agricultural Health Study. *Occupational and Environmental Medicine* 64(5):334–341.

Hoppin JA, Valcin M, Henneberger PK, Kullman GJ, Limbach DM, London SJ, Alavanja MCR, Sandler DP. 2007b. Pesticide use and chronic bronchitis among farmers in the Agricultural Health Study. *American Journal of Industrial Medicine* 50(12):969–979.

Hoppin JA, Umbach DM, London SJ, Henneberger PK, Kullman GJ, Alavanja MC, Sandler DP. 2008. Pesticides and atopic and nonatopic asthma among farm women in the Agricultural Health Study. *American Journal of Respiratory and Critical Care Medicine* 177(1):11–18.

Hryhorczuk DO, Wallace WH, Persky V, Furner S, Webster JR Jr, Oleske D, Haselhorst B, Ellefson R, Zugerman C. 1998. A morbidity study of former pentachlorophenol-production workers. *Environmental Health Perspectives* 106(7):401–408.

Huong LD, Phuong NTN. 1983. The state of abnormal pregnancies and congenital malformations at the Gyneco-Obstetrical Hospital of Ho Chi Minh City (formerly Tu Du Hospital). Summarized in: Constable JD, Hatch MC. *Reproductive effects of herbicide exposure in Vietnam: Recent studies by the Vietnamese and others.* As cited in Constable and Hatch, 1985.

Huston BL. 1972. Identification of three neutral contaminants in production grade 2,4-D. *Journal of Agricultural and Food Chemistry* 20(3):724–727.

Ideo G, Bellati G, Bellobuono A, Mocarelli P, Marocchi A, Brambilla P. 1982. Increased urinary *d*-glucaric acid excretion by children living in an area polluted with tetrachlorodibenzo-*para*-dioxin (TCDD). *Clinica Chimica Acta* 120:273–283.

Ideo G, Bellati G, Bellobuono A, Bissanti L. 1985. Urinary *d*-glucaric acid excretion in the Seveso area, polluted by tetrachlorodibenzo-*p*-dioxin (TCDD): Five years of experience. *Environmental Health Perspectives* 60:151–157.

IOM (Institute of Medicine). 1994. *Veterans and Agent Orange: Health Effects of Herbicides Used in Vietnam.* Washington, DC: National Academy Press.

IOM. 1996. *Veterans and Agent Orange: Update 1996.* Washington, DC: National Academy Press.

IOM. 1999. *Veterans and Agent Orange: Update 1998.* Washington, DC: National Academy Press.

IOM. 2000. *Veterans and Agent Orange: Herbicide/Dioxin Exposure and Type 2 Diabetes.* Washington, DC: National Academy Press.

IOM. 2001. *Veterans and Agent Orange: Update 2000.* Washington, DC: National Academy Press.

IOM. 2003a. *Veterans and Agent Orange: Update 2002.* Washington, DC: The National Academies Press.

IOM. 2003b. *Characterizing Exposure of Veterans to Agent Orange and Other Herbicides Used in Vietnam: Interim Findings and Recommendations.* Washington, DC: The National Academies Press.

IOM. 2003c. *Characterizing Exposure of Veterans to Agent Orange and Other Herbicides Used in Vietnam: Final Report.* Washington, DC: The National Academies Press.

IOM. 2004. *Veterans and Agent Orange: Length of Presumptive Period for Association Between Exposure and Respiratory Cancer.* Washington, DC: The National Academies Press.

IOM. 2005. *Veterans and Agent Orange: Update 2004.* Washington, DC: The National Academies Press.

IOM. 2006. *Disposition of the Air Force Health Study.* Washington, DC: National Academies Press.

IOM. 2007. *Veterans and Agent Orange: Update 2006.* Washington, DC: The National Academies Press.

Jäger R, Neuberger M, Rappe C, Kundi M, Pigler B, Smith AG. 1998. Chloracne and other symptoms 23 years after dioxin-exposure. *Atemwegs-Und Lungenkrankheiten* 24(Suppl 1):S101–S104.

Jansson B, Voog L. 1989. Dioxin from Swedish municipal incinerators and the occurrence of cleft lip and palate malformations. *International Journal of Environmental Studies* 34:99–104.

Jappinen P, Pukkala E. 1991. Cancer incidence among pulp and paper workers exposed to organic chlorinated compounds formed during chlorine pulp bleaching. *Scandinavian Journal of Work, Environment and Health* 17:356–359.

Jennings AM, Wild G, Ward JD, Ward AM. 1988. Immunological abnormalities 17 years after accidental exposure to 2,3,7,8-tetrachlorodibenzo-*p*-dioxin. *British Journal of Industrial Medicine* 45:701–704.

Jung D, Berg PA, Edler L, Ehrenthal W, Fenner D, Flesch-Janys D, Huber C, Klein R, Koitka C, Lucier G, Manz A, Muttray A, Needham L, Päpke O, Pietsch M, Portier C, Patterson D, Prellwitz W, Rose DM, Thews A, Konietzko J. 1998. Immunological findings in formerly exposed workers to 2,3,7,8-tetrachlorodibenzo-*p*-dioxin (TCDD) and related compounds in pesticide production. *Arbeitsmedizin Sozialmedizin Umweltmedizin, Supplement* 24:38–43.

Kahn PC, Gochfeld M, Nygren M, Hansson M, Rappe C, Velez H, Ghent-Guenther T, Wilson WP. 1988. Dioxins and dibenzofurans in blood and adipose tissue of Agent Orange-exposed Vietnam veterans and matched controls. *Journal of the American Medical Association* 259:1661–1667.

Kahn PC, Gochfeld M, Lewis WW. 1992a. *Dibenzodioxin and Dibenzofuran Congener Levels in Four Groups of Vietnam Veterans Who Did Not Handle Agent Orange.* New Jersey Agent Orange Commission.

Kahn PC, Gochfeld M, Lewis WW. 1992b. *Immune Status and Herbicide Exposure in the New Jersey Pointman I Project.* New Jersey Agent Orange Commission.

Kahn PC, Gochfeld M, Lewis WW. 1992c. *Semen Analysis in Vietnam Veterans with Respect to Presumed Herbicide Exposure.* New Jersey Agent Orange Commission.

Kamel F, Engel LS, Gladen BC, Hoppin JA, Alavanja MC, Sandler DP. 2005. Neurologic symptoms in licensed private pesticide applicators in the Agricultural Health Study. *Environmental Health Perspectives* 113(7):877–882.

Kamel F, Engel LS, Gladen BC, Hoppin JA, Alavanja MC, Sandler DP. 2007a. Neurologic symptoms in licensed pesticide applicators in the Agricultural Health Study. *Human and Experimental Toxicology* 26(3):243–250.

Kamel F, Tanner C, Umbach D, Hoppin J, Alavanja M, Blair A, Comyns K, Goldman S, Korell M, Langston J, Ross G, Sandler D. 2007b. Pesticide exposure and self-reported Parkinson's disease in the Agricultural Health Study. *American Journal of Epidemiology* 165(4):364–374.

Kang HK, Weatherbee L, Breslin PP, Lee Y, Shepard BM. 1986. Soft tissue sarcomas and military service in Vietnam: A case comparison group analysis of hospital patients. *Journal of Occupational Medicine* 28:1215–1218.

Kang HK, Enzinger FM, Breslin P, Feil M, Lee Y, Shepard B. 1987. Soft tissue sarcoma and military service in Vietnam: A case–control study. *Journal of the National Cancer Institute* 79:693–699 [published erratum appears in *Journal of the National Cancer Institute* 79:1173].

Kang HK, Watanabe KK, Breen J, Remmers J, Conomos MG, Stanley J, Flicker M. 1991. Dioxins and dibenzofurans in adipose tissue of US Vietnam veterans and controls. *American Journal of Public Health* 81(3):344–348.

Kang HK, Mahan CM, Lee KY, Magee CA, Mather SH, Matanoski G. 2000a. Pregnancy outcomes among US women Vietnam veterans. *American Journal Industrial Medicine* 38(4):447–454.

Kang HK, Mahan CM, Lee KY, Magee CA, Selvin S. 2000b. Prevalence of gynecologic cancers among female Vietnam veterans. *Journal of Occupational and Environmental Medicine* 42:1121–1127.

Kang HK, Dalager NA, Needham LL, Patterson DG, Matanoski GM, Kanchanaraksa S, Lees PSJ. 2001. US Army chemical corps Vietnam veterans health study: Preliminary results. *Chemosphere* 43:943–949.

Kang HK, Dalager NA, Needham LL, Patterson DG, Lees PSJ, Yates K, Matanoski GM. 2006. Health status of Army Chemical Corps Vietnam veterans who sprayed defoliant in Vietnam. *American Journal of Industrial Medicine* 49(11):875–884.

Kang MJ, Lee DY, Joo WA, Kim CW. 2005. Plasma protein level changes in waste incineration workers exposed to 2,3,7,8-tetrachlorodibenzo-*p*-dioxin. *Journal of Proteome Research* 4(4):1248–1255.

Karouna-Renier NK, Rao KR, Lanza JJ, Davis DA, Wilson PA. 2007. Serum profiles of PCDDs and PCDFs, in individuals near the Escambia Wood Treatment Company Superfund Site in Pensacola, FL. *Chemosphere* 69:1312–1319.

Kayajanian GM. 2002. The J-shaped dioxin dose response curve. *Ecotoxicology and Environmental Safety* 51:1–4.

Kern PA, Said S, Jackson WG Jr, Michalek JE. 2004. Insulin sensitivity following agent orange exposure in Vietnam veterans with high blood levels of 2,3,7,8-tetrachlorodibenzo-*p*-dioxin. *Journal of Clinical Endocrinology and Metabolism* 89(9):4665–4672.

Ketchum NS, Michalek JE. 2005. Postservice mortality of Air Force veterans occupationally exposed to herbicides during the Vietnam War: 20-year follow-up results. *Military Medicine* 170(5):406–413.

Ketchum NS, Michalek JE, Burton JE. 1999. Serum dioxin and cancer in veterans of Operation Ranch Hand. *American Journal of Epidemiology* 149(7):630–639.

Khoa ND. 1983. Some biologic parameters collected on the groups of people in an area affected by chemicals. Summarized in: Constable JD, Hatch MC. *Reproductive effects of herbicide exposure in Vietnam: Recent studies by the Vietnamese and others.* As cited in Constable and Hatch, 1985.

Kim H-A, Kim E-M, Park Y-C, Yu J-Y, Hong S-K, Jeon S-H, Park K-L, Hur S-J, Heo Y. 2003. Immunotoxicological effects of Agent Orange exposure to the Vietnam War Korean veterans. *Industrial Health* 41:158–166.

Kim J-S, Kang H-K, Lim H-S, Cheong H-K, Lim M-K. 2001. A study on the correlation between categorizations of the individual exposure levels to Agent Orange and serum dioxin levels among the Korean Vietnam veterans. *Korean Journal of Preventative Medicine* 34(1):80–88.

Kim J-S, Lim H-S, Cho S-I, Cheong H-K, Lim M-K. 2003. Impact of Agent Orange Exposure among Korean Vietnam Veterans. *Industrial Health* 41:149–157.

Kirrane EF, Hoppin JA, Umbach DM, Samanic C, Sandler DP. 2004. Patterns of pesticide use and their determinants among wives of farmer pesticide applicators in the Agricultural Health Study. *Journal of Occupational and Environmental Medicine* 46(8):856–865.

Kogan MD, Clapp RW. 1985. *Mortality Among Vietnam Veterans in Massachusetts, 1972–1983.* Boston, MA: Massachusetts Office of the Commissioner of Veterans Services, Agent Orange Program.

Kogan MD, Clapp RW. 1988. Soft tissue sarcoma mortality among Vietnam veterans in Massachusetts, 1972–1983. *International Journal of Epidemiology* 17:39–43.

Kogevinas M, Saracci R, Bertazzi PA, Bueno de Mesquita BH, Coggon D, Green LM, Kauppinen T, Littorin M, Lynge E, Mathews JD, Neuberger M, Osman J, Pearce N, Winkelmann R. 1992. Cancer mortality from soft-tissue sarcoma and malignant lymphomas in an international cohort of workers exposed to chlorophenoxy herbicides and chlorophenols. *Chemosphere* 25: 1071–1076.

Kogevinas M, Saracci R, Winkelmann R, Johnson ES, Bertazzi PA, Bueno de Mesquita BH, Kauppinen T, Littorin M, Lynge E, Neuberger M. 1993. Cancer incidence and mortality in women occupationally exposed to chlorophenoxy herbicides, chlorophenols, and dioxins. *Cancer Causes and Control* 4:547–553.

Kogevinas M, Kauppinen T, Winkelmann R, Becher H, Bertazzi PA, Bas B, Coggon D, Green L, Johnson E, Littorin M, Lynge E, Marlow DA, Mathews JD, Neuberger M, Benn T, Pannett B, Pearce N, Saracci R. 1995. Soft tissue sarcoma and non-Hodgkin's lymphoma in workers exposed to phenoxy herbicides, chlorophenols and dioxins: Two nested case–control studies. *Epidemiology* 6:396–402.

Kogevinas M, Becher H, Benn T, Bertazzi PA, Boffetta P, Bueno de Mesquita HB, Coggon D, Colin D, Flesch-Janys D, Fingerhut M, Green L, Kauppinen T, Littorin M, Lynge E, Mathews JD, Neuberger M, Pearce N, Saracci R. 1997. Cancer mortality in workers exposed to phenoxy herbicides, chlorophenols, and dioxins. An expanded and updated international cohort study. *American Journal of Epidemiology* 145(12):1061–1075.

Kolmodin-Hedman B, Erne K. 1980. Estimation of occupational exposure to phenoxy acids (2,4-D and 2,4,5-T). *Archives of Toxicology Supplement* (Suppl 4):318–321.

Kolmodin-Hedman B, Hoglund S, Akerblom M. 1983. Studies on phenoxy acid herbicides. I. Field study: Occupational exposure to phenoxy acid herbicides (MCPA, dichlorprop, mecoprop and 2,4-D) in agriculture. *Archives of Toxicology* 54:257–265.

Kristensen P, Irgens LM, Andersen A, Bye AS, Sundheim L. 1997. Birth defects among offspring of Norwegian farmers, 1967–1991. *Epidemiology* 8(5):537–544.

Kumagai S, Koda S. 2005. Polychlorinated dibenzo-*p*-dioxin and dibenzofuran concentrations in serum samples of workers at an infectious waste incineration plant in Japan. *Journal of Occupational and Environmental Hygiene* 2(2):120–125.

Lampi P, Hakulinen T, Luostarinen T, Pukkala E, Teppo L. 1992. Cancer incidence following chlorophenol exposure in a community in southern Finland. *Archives of Environmental Health* 47:167–175.

Landi MT, Needham LL, Lucier G, Mocarelli P, Bertazzi PA, Caporaso N. 1997. Concentrations of dioxin 20 years after Seveso. *Lancet* 349(9068):1811.

Landi MT, Consonni D, Patterson DG Jr, Needham LL, Lucier G, Brambilla P, Cazzaniga MA, Mocarelli P, Pesatori AC, Bertazzi PA, Caporaso NE. 1998. 2,3,7,8-Tetrachlorodibenzo-*p*-dioxin plasma levels in Seveso 20 years after the accident. *Environmental Health Perspectives* 106(5):273–277.

Landi MT, Bertazzi PA, Baccarelli A, Consonni D, Masten S, Lucier G, Mocarelli P, Needham L, Caporaso N, Grassman J. 2003. TCDD-mediated alterations in the AhR-dependent pathway in Seveso, Italy, 20 years after the accident. *Carcinogenesis* 24(4):673–680.

Lang TD, Tung TT, Van DD. 1983a. Mutagenic effects on the first generation after exposure to "Orange Agent." Summarized in: Constable JD, Hatch MC. *Reproductive effects of herbicide exposure in Vietnam: Recent studies by the Vietnamese and others.* As cited in Constable and Hatch, 1985.

Lang TD, Van DD, Dwyer JH, Flamenbuam C, Dwyer KM, Fantini D. 1983b. Self-reports of exposure to herbicides and health problems: A preliminary analysis of survey data from the families of 432 veterans in northern Vietnam. Summarized in: Constable JD, Hatch MC. *Reproductive effects of herbicide exposure in Vietnam: Recent studies by the Vietnamese and others.* As cited in Constable and Hatch, 1985.

LaVecchia C, Negri E, D'Avanzo B, Franceschi S. 1989. Occupation and lymphoid neoplasms. *British Journal of Cancer* 60:385–388.

Lavy TL, Shepard JS, Bouchard DC. 1980a. Field worker exposure and helicopter spray pattern of 2,4,5-T. *Bulletin of Environmental Contamination and Toxicology* 24:90–96.

Lavy TL, Shepard S, Mattice JD. 1980b. Exposure measurements of applicators spraying (2,4,5-trichlorophenoxy)acetic acid in the forest. *Journal of Agricultural and Food Chemistry* 28:626–630.

Lawrence CE, Reilly AA, Quickenton P, Greenwald P, Page WF, Kuntz AJ. 1985. Mortality patterns of New York State Vietnam veterans. *American Journal of Public Health* 75:277–279.

Lawson CC, Schnorr TM, Whelan EA, Deddens JA, Dankovic DA, Piacitelli LA, Sweeney MH, Connally LB. 2004. Paternal occupational exposure to 2,3,7,8-tetrachlorodibenzo-*p*-dioxin and birth outcomes of offspring: Birth weight, preterm delivery, and birth defects. *Environmental Health Perspectives* 112(14):1403–1408.

Leavy J, Ambrosini G, Fritschi L. 2006. Vietnam military service history and prostate cancer. *BMC Public Health* 6:75.

Lee DH, Lee IK, Song K, Steffes M, Toscano W, Baker BA, Jacobs DR Jr. 2006. A strong dose–response relation between serum concentrations of persistent organic pollutants and diabetes: Results from the National Health and Examination Survey 1999–2002. *Diabetes Care* 29(7):1638–1644.

Lee DH, Steffes M, Jacobs Jr DR. 2007a. Positive associations of serum concentration of polychlorinated biphenyls or organochlorine pesticides with self-reported arthritis, especially rheumatoid type, in women. *Environmental Health Perspectives* 115(6):883–888.

Lee DH, Lee IK, Jin SH, Steffes M, Jacobs Jr DR. 2007b. Association between serum concentrations of persistent organic pollutants and insulin resistance among nondiabetic adults: Results from the National Health and Nutrition Examination Survey 1999–2002. *Diabetes Care* 30(3):622–628.

Lee DH, Lee IK, Porta M, Steffes M, Jacobs Jr DR. 2007c. Relationship between serum concentrations of persistent organic pollutants and the prevalence of metabolic syndrome among nondiabetic adults: Results from the National Health and Nutrition Examination Survey 1999–2002. *Diabetologia* 50(9):1841–1851.

Lee WJ, Lijinsky W, Heineman EF, Markin RS, Weisenburger DD, Ward MH. 2004a. Agricultural pesticide use and adenocarcinomas of the stomach and oesophagus. *Occupational and Environmental Medicine* 61(9):743–749.

Lee WJ, Cantor KP, Berzofsky JA, Zahm SH, Blair A. 2004b. Non-Hodgkin's lymphoma among asthmatics exposed to pesticides. *International Journal of Cancer* 111(2):298–302.

Lee WJ, Colt JS, Heineman EF, McComb R, Weisenburger DD, Lijinsky W, Ward MH. 2005. Agricultural pesticide use and risk of glioma in Nebraska, United States. *Occupational and Environmental Medicine* 62(11):786–792.

Lee WJ, Purdue MP, Stewart P, Schenk M, De Roos AJ, Cerhan JR, Severson RK, Cozen W, Hartge P, Blair A. 2006. Asthma history, occupational exposure to pesticides and the risk of non-Hodgkin's lymphoma. *International Journal of Cancer* 118(12):3174–3176.

Lee WJ, Sandler DP, Blair A, Samanic C, Cross AJ, Alavanja MC. 2007. Pesticide use and colorectal cancer risk in the Agricultural Health Study. *International Journal of Cancer* 121(2):339–346.

Lerda D, Rizzi R. 1991. Study of reproductive function in persons occupationally exposed to 2,4-dichlorophenoxyacetic acid (2,4-D). *Mutation Research* 262:47–50.

Levy CJ. 1988. Agent Orange exposure and posttraumatic stress disorder. *Journal of Nervous and Mental Disorders* 176:242–245.

Libich S, To JC, Frank R, Sirons GJ. 1984. Occupational exposure of herbicide applicators to herbicides used along electric power transmission line right-of-way. *American Industrial Hygiene Association Journal* 45:56–62.

Liou HH, Tsai MC, Chen CJ, Jeng JS, Chang YC, Chen SY, Chen RC. 1997. Environmental risk factors and Parkinson's disease: A case–control study in Taiwan. *Neurology* 48(6):1583–1588.

Longnecker MP, Michalek JE. 2000. Serum dioxin level in relation to diabetes mellitus among Air Force veterans with background levels of exposure. *Epidemiology* 11(1):44–48.

Lovik M, Johansen HR, Gaarder PI, Becher G, Aaberge IS, Gdynia W, Alexander J. 1996. Halogenated organic compounds and the human immune system: Preliminary report on a study in hobby fishermen. *Archives of Toxicology Supplement* 18:15–20.

Lynge E. 1985. A follow-up study of cancer incidence among workers in manufacture of phenoxy herbicides in Denmark. *British Journal of Cancer* 52:259–270.

Lynge E. 1993. Cancer in phenoxy herbicide manufacturing workers in Denmark, 1947–87—an update. *Cancer Causes and Control* 4:261–272.

Magnani C, Coggon D, Osmond C, Acheson ED. 1987. Occupation and five cancers: A case–control study using death certificates. *British Journal of Industrial Medicine* 44(11):769–776.

Mahan CM, Bullman TA, Kang HK, Selvin S. 1997. A case–control study of lung cancer among Vietnam veterans. *Journal of Occupational and Environmental Medicine* 39(8):740–747.

Mandel JS, Alexander BH, Baker BA, Acquavella JF, Chapman P, Honeycutt R. 2005. Biomonitoring for farm families in the Farm Family Exposure Study. *Scandinavian Journal of Work, Environment and Health* 31(Supplement 1):98–104.

Manz A, Berger J, Dwyer JH, Flesch-Janys D, Nagel S, Waltsgott H. 1991. Cancer mortality among workers in chemical plant contaminated with dioxin. *Lancet* 338:959–964.

Masala G, Di Lollo S, Picoco C, Crosignani P, Demicheli V, Fontana A, Funto I, Miligi L, Nanni O, Papucci A, Ramazzotti V, Rodella S, Stagnaro E, Tumino R, Vigano C, Vindigni C, Seniori Costantini A, Vineis P. 1996. Incidence rates of leukemias, lymphomas and myelomas in Italy: Geographic distribution and NHL histotypes. *International Journal of Cancer* 68(2):156–159.

Mastroiacovo P, Spagnolo A, Marni E, Meazza L, Bertollini R, Segni G, Borgna-Pignatti C. 1988. Birth defects in the Seveso area after TCDD contamination. *Journal of the American Medical Association* 259:1668–1672 [published erratum appears in the *Journal of the American Medical Association* 1988, 260:792].

May G. 1982. Tetrachlorodibenzodioxin: A survey of subjects ten years after exposure. *British Journal of Industrial Medicine* 39:128–135.

May G. 1983. TCDD: A study of subjects 10 and 14 years after exposure. *Chemosphere* 12: 771–778.

McDuffie HH, Klaassen DJ, Dosman JA. 1990. Is pesticide use related to the risk of primary lung cancer in Saskatchewan? *Journal of Occupational Medicine* 32(10):996–1002.

McDuffie HH, Pahwa P, McLaughlin JR, Spinelli JJ, Fincham S, Dosman JA, Robson D, Skinnider LF, Choi NW. 2001. Non-Hodgkin's lymphoma and specific pesticide exposures in men: Cross–Canada study of pesticides and health. *Cancer Epidemiology, Biomarkers and Prevention* 10(11):1155–1163.

McDuffie HH, Pahwa P, Robson D, Dosman JA, Fincham S, Spinelli JJ, McLaughlin JR. 2005. Insect repellents, phenoxyherbicide exposure, and non-Hodgkin's lymphoma. *Journal of Occupational and Environmental Medicine* 47(8):806–816.

McKinney WP, McIntire DD, Carmody TJ, Joseph A. 1997. Comparing the smoking behavior of veterans and nonveterans. *Public Health Reports* 112(3):212–217.

McLean D, Pearce N, Langseth H, Jäppinen P, Szadkowska-Stanczyk I, Person B, Wild P, Kishi R, Lynge E, Henneberger P, Sala M, Teschke K, Kauppinen T, Colin D, Kogevinas M, Boffetta P. 2006. Cancer mortality in workers exposed to organochlorine compounds in the pulp and paper industry: An international collaborative study. *Environmental Health Perspectives* 114(7):1007–1012.

Mellemgaard A, Engholm G, McLaughlin JK, Olsen JH. 1994. Occupational risk factors for renal-cell carcinoma in Denmark. *Scandinavian Journal of Work, Environment and Health* 20:160–165.

Meyer KJ, Reif JS, Veeramachaneni DN, Luben TJ, Mosley BS, Nuckols JR. 2006. Agricultural pesticide use and hypospadias in eastern Arkansas. *Environmental Health Perspectives* 114(10): 1589–1595.

Michalek JE, Pavuk M. 2008. Diabetes and cancer in veterans of Operation Ranch Hand after adjustment for calendar period, days of sprayings, and time spent in Southeast Asia. *Journal of Occupational and Environmental Medicine* 50(3):330–340.

Michalek JE, Wolfe WH, Miner JC. 1990. Health status of Air Force veterans occupationally exposed to herbicides in Vietnam. II. Mortality. *Journal of the American Medical Association* 264:1832–1836.

Michalek JE, Wolfe WH, Miner JC, Papa TM, Pirkle JL. 1995. Indices of TCDD exposure and TCDD body burden in veterans of Operation Ranch Hand. *Journal of Exposure Analysis and Environmental Epidemiology* 5(2):209–223.

Michalek JE, Rahe AJ, Boyle CA. 1998a. Paternal dioxin, preterm birth, intrauterine growth retardation, and infant death. *Epidemiology* 9(2):161–167.

Michalek JE, Ketchum NS, Akhtar FZ. 1998b. Postservice mortality of US Air Force veterans occupationally exposed to herbicides in Vietnam: 15-year follow-up. *American Journal of Epidemiology* 148(8):786–792.

Michalek JE, Rahe AJ, Boyle CA. 1998c. Paternal dioxin and the sex of children fathered by veterans of Operation Ranch Hand. *Epidemiology* 9(4):474–475.

Michalek JE, Akhtar FZ, Kiel JL. 1999a. Serum dioxin, insulin, fasting glucose, and sex hormone-binding globulin in veterans of Operation Ranch Hand. *Journal of Clinical Endocrinology and Metabolism* 84(5):1540–1543.

Michalek JE, Ketchum NS, Check IJ. 1999b. Serum dioxin and immunologic response in veterans of Operation Ranch Hand. *American Journal of Epidemiology* 149(11):1038–1046.

Michalek JE, Ketchum N, Longnecker MP. 2001a. Serum dioxin and hepatic abnormalities in veterans of Operation Ranch Hand. *Annals of Epidemiology* 11(5):304–311.

Michalek JE, Akhtar FZ, Arezzo JC, Garabrant DH, Albers JW. 2001b. Serum dioxin and peripheral neuropathy in veterans of Operation Ranch Hand. *Neurotoxicology* 22:479–490.

Michalek JE, Akhtar FZ, Longnecker MP, Burton JE. 2001c. Relation of serum 2,3,7,8-tetrachloro-dibenzo-*p*-dioxin (TCDD) level to hematological examination results in veterans of Operation Ranch Hand. *Archives of Environmental Health* 56(5):396–405.

Michalek JE, Ketchum NS, Tripathi RC. 2003. Diabetes mellitus and 2,3,7,8-tetrachlorodibenzo-*p*-dioxin elimination in veterans of Operation Ranch Hand. *Journal of Toxicology and Environmental Health, Part A*, 66:211–221.

Michigan Department of Public Health. 1983. *Evaluation of Soft and Connective Tissue Cancer Mortality Rates for Midland and Other Selected Michigan Counties*. Michigan Department of Public Health.

Miligi L, Costantini AS, Veraldi A, Benvenuti A, WILL, Vineis P. 2006. Cancer and pesticides: An overview and some results of the Italian multicenter case–control study on hematolymphopoietic malignancies. *Annals of the New York Academy of Sciences* 1076:366–377.

Mills PK, Yang R. 2005b. Breast cancer risk in Hispanic agricultural workers in California. *International Journal of Occupational and Environmental Health* 11(2):123–131.

Mills PK, Yang RC. 2007. Agricultural exposures and gastric cancer risk in Hispanic farm workers in California. *Environmental Research* 104(2):282–289.

Mills PK, Yang R, Riordan D. 2005a. Lymphohematopoietic cancers in the United Farm Workers of America (UFW), 1988–2001. *Cancer Causes and Control* 16(7):823–830.

Mo HJ, Park HJ, Kim JH, Lee JY, Cho BK. 2002. A study about the skin and general disease patterns of the Vietnam veterans exposed to dioxin. *Korean Journal of Dermatology* 40(6):634–638.

Mocarelli P, Marocchi A, Brambilla P, Gerthoux P, Young DS, Mantel N. 1986. Clinical laboratory manifestations of exposure to dioxin in children. A six-year study of the effects of an environmental disaster near Seveso, Italy. *Journal of the American Medical Association* 256:2687–2695.

Mocarelli P, Patterson DG Jr, Marocchi A, Needham LL. 1990. Pilot study (phase II) for determining polychlorinated dibenzo-*p*-dioxin (PCDD) and polychlorinated dibenzofuran (PCDF) levels in serum of Seveso, Italy residents collected at the time of exposure: Future plans. *Chemosphere* 20:967–974.

Mocarelli P, Needham LL, Marocchi A, Patterson DG Jr, Brambilla P, Gerthoux PM, Meazza L, Carreri V. 1991. Serum concentrations of 2,3,7,8-tetrachlorobdibenzo-*p*-dioxin and test results from selected residents of Seveso, Italy. *Journal of Toxicology and Environmental Health* 32:357–366.

Mocarelli P, Brambilla P, Gerthoux PM, Patterson DG Jr, Needham LL. 1996. Change in sex ratio with exposure to dioxin. *Lancet* 348(9024):409.

Mocarelli P, Gerthoux PM, Patterson DG Jr, Milani S, Limonta G, Bertona M, Signorini S, Tramacere P, Colombo L, Crespi C, Brambilla P, Sarto C, Carreri V, Sampson EJ, Turner WE, Needham LL. 2008. Dioxin exposure, from infancy through puberty, produces endocrine disruption and affects human semen quality. *Environmental Health Perspectives* 116(1):70–77.

Monge P, Wesseling C, Guardado J, Lundberg I, Ahlbom A, Cantor KP, Weiderpass E, Partanen T. 2007. Parental occupational exposure to pesticides and the risk of childhood leukemia in Costa Rica. *Scandinavian Journal of Work, Environment and Health* 33(4):293–303.

Montgomery MP, Kamel F, Saldana TM, Alavanja MC, Sandler DP. 2008. Incident diabetes and pesticide exposure among licensed pesticide applicators: Agricultural Health Study, 1993–2003. *American Journal of Epidemiology* 167(10):1235–1246.

Morris PD, Koepsell TD, Daling JR, Taylor JW, Lyon JL, Swanson GM, Child M, Weiss NS. 1986. Toxic substance exposure and multiple myeloma: A case–control study. *Journal of the National Cancer Institute* 76:987–994.

Morrison H, Semenciw RM, Morison D, Magwood S, Mao Y. 1992. Brain cancer and farming in western Canada. *Neuroepidemiology* 11:267–276.

Morrison H, Savitz D, Semenciw RM, Hulka B, Mao Y, Morison D, Wigle D. 1993. Farming and prostate cancer mortality. *American Journal of Epidemiology* 137:270–280.

Morrison HI, Semenciw RM, Wilkins K, Mao Y, Wigle DT. 1994. Non-Hodgkin's lymphoma and agricultural practices in the prairie provinces of Canada. *Scandinavian Journal of Work, Environment and Health* 20:42–47.

Moses M, Lilis R, Crow KD, Thornton J, Fischbein A, Anderson HA, Selikoff IJ. 1984. Health status of workers with past exposure to 2,3,7,8-tetrachlorodibenzo-*p*-dioxin in the manufacture of 2,4,5-trichlorophenoxyacetic acid: Comparison of findings with and without chloracne. *American Journal of Industrial Medicine* 5:161–182.

Musicco M, Sant M, Molinari S, Filippini G, Gatta G, Berrino F. 1988. A case–control study of brain gliomas and occupational exposure to chemical carcinogens: The risks to farmers. *American Journal of Epidemiology* 128:778–785.

Nanni O, Amadori D, Lugaresi C, Falcini F, Scarpi E, Saragoni A, Buiatti E. 1996. Chronic lymphocytic leukæmias and non-Hodgkin's lymphomas by histological type in farming-animal breeding workers: A population case–control study based on a priori exposure matrices. *Occupational and Environmental Medicine* 53(10):652–657.

Nelson CJ, Holson JF, Green HG, Gaylor DW. 1979. Retrospective study of the relationship between agricultural use of 2,4,5-T and cleft palate occurrence in Arkansas. *Teratology* 19:377–383.

Neuberger M, Kundi M, Jäger R. 1998. Chloracne and morbidity after dioxin exposure (preliminary results). *Toxicology Letters* 96/97:347–350.

Neuberger M, Rappe C, Bergek S, Cai H, Hansson M, Jager R, Kundi M, Lim CK, Wingfors H, Smith AG. 1999. Persistent health effects of dioxin contamination in herbicide production. *Environmental Research* 81(3):206–214.

Newell GR. 1984. *Development and Preliminary Results of Pilot Clinical Studies. Report of the Agent Orange Advisory Committee to the Texas Department of Health.* University of Texas System Cancer Center.

Ngo AD, Taylor R, Roberts CL, Nguyen TV. 2006. Association between Agent Orange and birth defects: Systematic review and meta-analysis. *International Journal of Epidemiology* 35:1220–1230.

Nguyen HD. 1983. Pregnancies at the Polyclinic of Tay Ninh Province. Summarized in: Constable JD, Hatch MC. *Reproductive effects of herbicide exposure in Vietnam: Recent studies by the Vietnamese and others.* As cited in Constable and Hatch, 1985.

Nishijo M, Tawara K, Nakagawa H, Honda R, Kido T, Nishijo H, Saito S. 2008. 2,3,7,8-tetrachlorodibenzo-*p*-dioxin in maternal breast milk and newborn head circumference. *Journal of Exposure Science and Environmental Epidemiology* 18(3):246–251.

Norström A, Rappe C, Lindahl R, Buser HR. 1979. Analysis of some older Scandinavioan formulations of 2,4-dichlorophenoxy acetic acid for contents of chlorinated dibenzo-*p*-dioxins and dibenzofurans. *Scandanavian Journal of Work, Environment and Health* 5:375–378.

Nurminen T, Rantala K, Kurppa K, Holmberg PC. 1994. Agricultural work during pregnancy and selected structural malformations in Finland. *Epidemiology* 1:23–30.

O'Brien TR, Decoufle P, Boyle CA. 1991. Non-Hodgkin's lymphoma in a cohort of Vietnam veterans. *American Journal of Public Health* 81:758–760.

Oh E, Lee E, Im H, Kang HS, Jung WW, Won NH, Kim EM, Sul D. 2005. Evaluation of immuno-
and reproductive toxicities and association between immunotoxicological and genotoxicological
parameters in waste incineration workers. *Toxicology* 2(1):65–80.

Olsson H, Brandt L. 1988. Risk of non-Hodgkin's lymphoma among men occupationally exposed to
organic solvents. *Scandinavian Journal of Work, Environment and Health* 14:246–251.

O'Toole BI, Marshall RP, Grayson DA, Schureck RJ, Dobson M, Ffrench M, Pulvertaft B, Meldrum
L, Bolton J, Vennard J. 1996a. The Australian Vietnam Veterans Health Study: I. Study design
and response bias. *International Journal of Epidemiology* 25(2):307–318.

O'Toole BI, Marshall RP, Grayson DA, Schureck RJ, Dobson M, Ffrench M, Pulvertaft B, Meldrum
L, Bolton J, Vennard J. 1996b. The Australian Vietnam Veterans Health Study: II. Self-reported
health of veterans compared with the Australian population. *International Journal of Epidemiology* 25(2):319–330.

O'Toole BI, Marshall RP, Grayson DA, Schureck RJ, Dobson M, Ffrench M, Pulvertaft B, Meldrum
L, Bolton J, Vennard J. 1996c. The Australian Vietnam Veterans Health Study: III. Psychological
health of Australian Vietnam veterans and its relationship to combat. *International Journal of
Epidemiology* 25(2):331–340.

Ott MG, Zober A. 1996. Cause specific mortality and cancer incidence among employees exposed
to 2,3,7,8-TCDD after a 1953 reactor accident. *Occupational and Environmental Medicine*
53(9):606–612.

Ott MG, Holder BB, Olson RD. 1980. A mortality analysis of employees engaged in the manufacture
of 2,4,5-trichlorophenoxyacetic acid. *Journal of Occupational Medicine* 22:47–50.

Ott MG, Olson RA, Cook RR, Bond GG. 1987. Cohort mortality study of chemical workers with
potential exposure to the higher chlorinated dioxins. *Journal of Occupational Medicine* 29:
422–429.

Pahwa P, McDuffie HH, Dosman JA, McLaughlin JR, Spinelli JJ, Robson D, Fincham S. 2006.
Hodgkin lymphoma, multiple myeloma, soft tissue sarcomas, insect repellents, and phenoxyherbicides. *Journal of Occupational and Environmental Medicine* 48(3):264–274.

Park RM, Schulte PA, Bowman JD, Walker JT, Bondy SC, Yost MG, Touchstone JA, Dosemeci M.
2005. Potential occupational risks for neurodegenerative diseases. *American Journal of Industrial Medicine* 48(1):63–77.

Patterson DG Jr, Hoffman RE, Needham LL, Roberts DW, Bagby JR, Pinkle JL, Falk H, Sampson
EJ, Houk VN. 1986. 2,3,7,8-tetrachlorodibenzo-*p*-dioxin levels in adipose tissue of exposed
and control persons in Missouri. *Journal of the American Medical Association* 256(19):
2683–2686.

Pavuk M, Schecter AJ, Akhtar FZ, Michalek JE. 2003. Serum 2,3,7,8-tetrachlorodibenzo-*p*-dioxin
(TCDD) levels and thyroid function in Air Force veterans of the Vietnam War. *Annals of Epidemiology* 13(5):335–343.

Pavuk M, Michalek JE, Schecter A, Ketchum NS, Akhtar FZ, Fox KA. 2005. Did TCDD exposure or
service in Southeast Asia increase the risk of cancer in Air Force Vietnam veterans who did not
spray Agent Orange? *Journal of Occupational and Environmental Medicine* 47(4):335–342.

Pavuk M, Michalek JE, Ketchum NS. 2006. Prostate cancer in US Air Force veterans of the Vietnam
War. *Journal of Exposure Science and Environmental Epidemiology* 16(2):184–190.

Pazderova-Vejlupková J, Lukás E, Nîmcova M, Pícková J, Jirásek L. 1981. The development and
prognosis of chronic intoxication by tetrachlorodibenzo-*p*-dioxin in men. *Archives of Environmental Health* 36:5–11.

Pearce NE, Smith AH, Fisher DO. 1985. Malignant lymphoma and multiple myeloma linked with
agricultural occupations in a New Zealand cancer registry-based study. *American Journal of
Epidemiology* 121:225–237.

Pearce NE, Smith AH, Howard JK, Sheppard RA, Giles HJ, Teague CA. 1986a. Case–control study
of multiple myeloma and farming. *British Journal of Cancer* 54:493–500.

Pearce NE, Smith AH, Howard JK, Sheppard RA, Giles HJ, Teague CA. 1986b. Non-Hodgkin's lymphoma and exposure to phenoxyherbicides, chlorophenols, fencing work, and meat works employment: A case–control study. *British Journal of Industrial Medicine* 43:75–83.

Pearce NE, Sheppard RA, Smith AH, Teague CA. 1987. Non-Hodgkin's lymphoma and farming: An expanded case–control study. *International Journal of Cancer* 39:155–161.

Pelclová D, Fenclová Z, Dlasková Z, Urban P, Lukáš E, Procházka B, Rappe C. 2001. Biochemical, neuropsychological, and neurological abnormalities following 2,3,7,8-tetrachlorodibenzo-*p*-dioxin (TCDD) exposure. *Archives of Environmental Health* 56:493–500.

Pelclová D, Fenclová Z, Preiss J, Procházka B, Spácil J, Dubská Z, Okrouhlík B, Lukáš E, Urban P. 2002. Lipid metabolism and neuropsychological follow-up study of workers exposed to 2,3,7,8-tetrachlordibenzo-*p*-dioxin. *International Archives of Occupational and Environmental Health* 75(Supp l):S60–S66.

Pelclová D, Prazny M, Skrha J, Fenclova Z, Kalousova M, Urban P, Navratil T, Senholdova Z, Smerhovsky Z. 2007. 2,3,7,8-TCDD exposure, endothelial dysfunction and impaired microvascular reactivity. *Human and Experimental Toxicology* 26(9):705–713.

Peper M, Klett M, Frentzel-Beyme R, Heller WD. 1993. Neuropsychological effects of chronic exposure to environmental dioxins and furans. *Environmental Research* 60:124–135.

Persson B, Dahlander A-M, Fredriksson M, Brage HN, Ohlson C-G, Axelson O. 1989. Malignant lymphomas and occupational exposures. *British Journal of Industrial Medicine* 46:516–520.

Persson B, Fredriksson M, Olsen K, Boeryd B, Axelson O. 1993. Some occupational exposures as risk factors for malignant lymphomas. *Cancer* 72:1773–1778.

Pesatori AC, Consonni D, Tironi A, Landi MT, Zocchetti C, Bertazzi PA. 1992. Cancer morbidity in the Seveso area, 1976–1986. *Chemosphere* 25:209–212.

Pesatori AC, Consonni D, Tironi A, Zocchetti C, Fini A, Bertazzi PA. 1993. Cancer in a young population in a dioxin-contaminated area. *International Journal of Epidemiology* 22:1010–1013.

Pesatori AC, Zocchetti C, Guercilena S, Consonni D, Turrini D, Bertazzi PA. 1998. Dioxin exposure and nonmalignant health effects: A mortality study. *Occupational and Environmental Medicine* 55(2):126–131.

Petreas M, Smith D, Hurley S, Jeffrey SS, Gilliss D, Reynolds P. 2004. Distribution of persistent, lipid-soluble chemicals in breast and abdominal adipose tissues: Lessons learned from a breast cancer study. *Cancer Epidemiology, Biomarkers and Prevention* 13(3):416–424.

Phuong NTN, Huong LTD. 1983. The effects of toxic chemicals on the pregnancy of the women living at two localities in the South of Vietnam. Summarized in: Constable JD, Hatch MC. *Reproductive effects of herbicide exposure in Vietnam: Recent studies by the Vietnamese and others.* As cited in Constable and Hatch, 1985.

Phuong NTN, Thuy TT, Phuong PK. 1989a. An estimate of differences among women giving birth to deformed babies and among those with hydatidiform mole seen at the Ob-Gyn hospital of Ho Chi Minh City in the south of Vietnam. *Chemosphere* 18:801–803.

Phuong NTN, Thuy TT, Phuong PK. 1989b. An estimate of reproductive abnormalities in women inhabiting herbicide sprayed and non-herbicide sprayed areas in the south of Vietnam, 1952–1981. *Chemosphere* 18:843–846.

Piacitelli LA, Marlow DA. 1997. NIOSH 2,3,7,8-tetrachlorodibenzo-*p*-dioxin exposure matrix. *Organohalogen Compounds* 33:510–514.

Poland AP, Smith D, Metter G, Possick P. 1971. A health survey of workers in a 2,4-D and 2,4,5-T plant with special attention to chloracne, porphyria cutanea tarda, and psychologic parameters. *Archives of Environmental Health* 22:316–327.

Pollei S, Mettler FA Jr, Kelsey CA, Walters MR, White RE. 1986. Follow-up chest radiographs in Vietnam veterans: Are they useful? *Radiology* 161:101–102.

Polsky JY, Aronson KJ, Heaton JP, Adams MA. 2007. Pesticides and polychlorinated biphenyls as potential risk factors for erectile dysfunction. *Journal of Andrology* 28(1):28–37.

Quandt SA, Hernandez-Valero MA, Grzywacz JG, Hovey JD, Gonzales M, Arcury TA. 2006. Workplace, household, and personal predictors of pesticide exposure for farmworkers. *Environmental Health Perspectives* 114(6):943–952.

Ramlow JM, Spadacene NW, Hoag SR, Stafford BA, Cartmill JB, Lerner PJ. 1996. Mortality in a cohort of pentachlorophenol manufacturing workers, 1940–1989. *American Journal of Industrial Medicine* 30(2):180–194.

Read D, Wright C, Weinstein P, Borman B. 2007. Cancer incidence and mortality in a New Zealand community potentially exposed to 2,3,7,8-tetrachlorodibenzo-*p*-dioxin from 2,4,5-trichlorophenoxyacetic acid manufacture. *Australian and New Zealand Journal of Public Health* 31(1):13–18.

Reif JS, Pearce N, Fraser J. 1989. Occupational risks of brain cancer: A New Zealand cancer registry-based study. *Journal of Occupational Medicine* 31(10):863–867.

Rellahan WL. 1985. *Aspects of the Health of Hawaii's Vietnam-Era Veterans.* Honolulu: Hawaii State Department of Health, Research, and Statistics Office.

Revazova J, Yurchenko V, Katosova L, Platonova V, Sycheva L, Khripach L, Ingel F, Tsutsman T, Zhurkov V. 2001. Cytogenetic investigation of women exposed to different levels of dioxins in Chapaevsk town. *Chemosphere* 43:999–1004.

Revich B, Aksel E, Ushakova T, Ivanova I, Zhuchenko N, Klyuev N, Brodsky B, Sotskov Y. 2001. Dioxin exposure and public health in Chapaevsk, Russia. *Chemosphere* 43:951–966.

Richardson DB, Terschuren C, Hoffmann W. 2008. Occupational risk factors for non-Hodgkin's lymphoma: A population-based case–control study in Northern Germany. *American Journal of Industrial Medicine* 51(4):258–268.

Riihimaki V, Asp S, Hernberg S. 1982. Mortality of 2,4-dichlorophenoxyacetic acid and 2,4,5-trichlorophenoxyacetic acid herbicide applicators in Finland: First report of an ongoing prospective cohort study. *Scandinavian Journal of Work, Environment and Health* 8:37–42.

Riihimaki V, Asp S, Pukkala E, Hernberg S. 1983. Mortality and cancer morbidity among chlorinated phenoxyacid applicators in Finland. *Chemosphere* 12:779–784.

Rix BA, Villadsen E, Engholm G, Lynge E. 1998. Hodgkin's disease, pharyngeal cancer, and soft tissue sarcomas in Danish paper mill workers. *Journal of Occupational and Environmental Medicine* 40(1):55–62.

Robinson CF, Waxweiler RJ, Fowler DP. 1986. Mortality among production workers in pulp and paper mills. *Scandinavian Journal of Work, Environment and Health* 12:552–560.

Ronco G, Costa G, Lynge E. 1992. Cancer risk among Danish and Italian farmers. *British Journal of Industrial Medicine* 49:220–225.

Rubin CS, Holmes AK, Belson MG, Jones RL, Flanders WD, Kieszak SM, Osterloh J, Luber GE, Blount BC, Barr DB, Steinberg KK, Satten GA, McGeehin MA, Todd RL. 2007. Investigating childhood leukemia in Churchill County, Nevada. *Environmental Health Perspectives* 115(1): 151–157.

Rudant J, Menegaux F, Leverger G, Baruchel A, Nelken B, Bertrand Y, Patte C, Pacquement H, Verite C, Robert A, Michel G, Margueritte G, Gandemer V, Hemon D, Clavel J. 2007. Household exposure to pesticides and risk of childhood hematopoietic malignancies: The ESCALE study (SFCE). *Environmental Health Perspectives* 115(12):1787–1793.

Ruder AM, Waters MA, Butler MA, Carreon T, Calvert GM, Davis-King KE, Schulte PA, Sanderson WT, Ward EM, Connally LB, Heineman EF, Mandel JS, Morton RF, Reding DJ, Rosenman KD, Talaska G. 2004. Gliomas and farm pesticide exposure in men: The Upper Midwest Health Study. *Archives of Environmental Health* 59(12):650–657.

Ruder AM, Waters MA, Carreon T, Butler MA, Davis-King KE, Calvert GM, Schulte PA, Ward EM, Connally LB, Lu J, Wall D, Zivkovich Z, Heineman EF, Mandel JS, Morton RF, Reding DJ, Rosenman KD, The Brain Cancer Collaborative Study G. 2006. The Upper Midwest Health Study: A case–control study of primary intracranial gliomas in farm and rural residents. *Journal of Agricultural Safety and Health* 12(4):255–274.

Sagiv SK, Tolbert PE, Altshul LM, Korrick SA. 2007. Organochlorine exposures during pregnancy and infant size at birth. *Epidemiology* 18(1):120–129.

Saldana TM, Basso O, Hoppin JA, Baird DD, Knott C, Blair A, Alavanja MC, Sandler DP. 2007. Pesticide exposure and self-reported gestational diabetes mellitus in the Agricultural Health Study. *Diabetes Care* 30(3):529–534.

Samanic C, Hoppin JA, Lubin JH, Blair A, Alavanja MC. 2005. Factor analysis of pesticide use patterns among pesticide applicators in the Agricultural Health Study. *Journal of Exposure Analysis and Environmental Epidemiology* 15(3):225–233.

Samanic C, Rusiecki J, Dosemeci M, Hou L, Hoppin JA, Sandler DP, Lubin J, Blair A, Alavanja MC. 2006. Cancer incidence among pesticide applicators exposed to dicamba in the Agricultural Health Study. *Environmental Health Perspectives* 114(10):1521–1526.

Samanic CM, De Roos AJ, Stewart PA, Rajaraman P, Waters MA, Inskip PD. 2008. Occupational exposure to pesticides and risk of adult brain tumors. *American Journal of Epidemiology* 167(8):976–985.

Saracci R, Kogevinas M, Bertazzi PA, Bueno de Mesquita BH, Coggon D, Green LM, Kauppinen T, L'Abbe KA, Littorin M, Lynge E, Mathews JD, Neuberger M, Osman J, Pearce N, Winkelmann R. 1991. Cancer mortality in workers exposed to chlorophenoxy herbicides and chlorophenols. *Lancet* 338:1027–1032.

Savitz DA, Arbuckle T, Kaczor D, Curtis K. 1997. Male pesticide exposure and pregnancy outcome. *American Journal of Epidemiology* 146(12):1025–1036.

Schildt EB, Eriksson M, Hardell L, Magnuson A. 1999. Occupational exposures as risk factors for oral cancer evaluated in a Swedish case–control study. *Oncology Reports* 6(2):317–320.

Schreinemachers DM. 2000. Cancer mortality in four northern wheat-producing states. *Environmental Health Perspectives* 108(9):873–881.

Schulte PA, Burnett CA, Boeniger MF, Johnson J. 1996. Neurodegenerative diseases: Occupational occurrence and potential risk factors, 1982 through 1991. *American Journal of Public Health* 86(9):1281–1288.

Seidler A, Hellenbrand W, Robra BP, Vieregge P, Nischan P, Joerg J, Oertel WH, Ulm G, Schneider E. 1996. Possible environmental, occupational, and other etiologic factors for Parkinson's disease: A case–control study in Germany. *Neurology* 46(5):1275–1284.

Semchuk KM, Love EJ, Lee RG. 1993. Parkinson's disease: A test of the multifactorial etiologic hypothesis. *Neurology* 43:1173–1180.

Semenciw RM, Morrison HI, Riedel D, Wilkins K, Ritter L, Mao Y. 1993. Multiple myeloma mortality and agricultural practices in the prairie provinces of Canada. *Journal of Occupational Medicine* 35:557–561.

Semenciw RM, Morrison HI, Morison D, Mao Y. 1994. Leukemia mortality and farming in the prairie provinces of Canada. *Canadian Journal of Public Health* 85:208–211.

Senthilselvan A, McDuffie HH, Dosman JA. 1992. Association of asthma with use of pesticides: Results of a cross-sectional survey of farmers. *American Review of Respiratory Disease* 146: 884–887.

Smith AH, Pearce NE. 1986. Update on soft tissue sarcoma and phenoxyherbicides in New Zealand. *Chemosphere* 15:1795–1798.

Smith AH, Matheson DP, Fisher DO, Chapman CJ. 1981. Preliminary report of reproductive outcomes among pesticide applicators using 2,4,5-T. *New Zealand Medical Journal* 93:177–179.

Smith AH, Fisher DO, Pearce N, Chapman CJ. 1982. Congenital defects and miscarriages among New Zealand 2,4,5-T sprayers. *Archives of Environmental Health* 37:197–200.

Smith AH, Fisher DO, Giles HJ, Pearce N. 1983. The New Zealand soft tissue sarcoma case–control study: Interview findings concerning phenoxyacetic acid exposure. *Chemosphere* 12:565–571.

Smith AH, Pearce NE, Fisher DO, Giles HJ, Teague CA, Howard JK. 1984. Soft tissue sarcoma and exposure to phenoxyherbicides and chlorophenols in New Zealand. *Journal of the National Cancer Institute* 73:1111–1117.

Smith AH, Patterson DG Jr, Warner ML, MacKenzie R, Needham LL. 1992. Serum 2,3,7,8-tetrachlorodibenzo-*p*-dioxin levels of New Zealand pesticide applicators and their implication for cancer hypotheses. *Journal of the National Cancer Institute* 84(2):104–108.

Smith JG, Christophers AJ. 1992. Phenoxy herbicides and chlorophenols: A case–control study on soft tissue sarcoma and malignant lymphoma. *British Journal of Cancer* 65:442–448.

Snow BR, Stellman JM, Stellman SD, Sommer JF. 1988. Post-traumatic stress disorder among American Legionnaires in relation to combat experience in Vietnam: Associated and contributing factors. *Environmental Research* 47:175–192.

Sobel W, Bond GG, Skowronski BJ, Brownson PJ, Cook RR. 1987. A soft tissue sarcoma case–control study in a large multi-chemical manufacturing facility. *Chemosphere* 16:2095–2099.

Solet D, Zoloth SR, Sullivan C, Jewett J, Michaels DM. 1989. Patterns of mortality in pulp and paper workers. *Journal of Occupational Medicine* 31:627–630.

Solomon C, Poole J, Palmer KT, Peveler R, Coggon D. 2007. Neuropsychiatric symptoms in past users of sheep dip and other pesticides. *Occupational and Environmental Medicine* 64(4):259–266.

Spinelli JJ, Ng CH, Weber JP, Connors JM, Gascoyne RD, Lai AS, Brooks-Wilson AR, Le ND, Berry BR, Gallagher RP. 2007. Organochlorines and risk of non-Hodgkin lymphoma. *International Journal of Cancer* 121(12):2767–2775.

Spoonster-Schwartz L. 1987. Women and the Vietnam experience. *Journal of Nursing Scholarship* 19(4):168–173.

Steenland K, Piacitelli L, Deddens J, Fingerhut M, Chang LI. 1999. Cancer, heart disease, and diabetes in workers exposed to 2,3,7,8-tetrachlorodibenzo-*p*-dioxin. *Journal of the National Cancer Institute* 91(9):779–786.

Steenland K, Calvert G, Ketchum N, Michalek J. 2001a. Dioxin and diabetes mellitus: An analysis of the combined NIOSH and Ranch Hand data. *Occupational and Environmental Medicine* 58:641–648.

Steenland K, Deddens J, Piacitelli L. 2001b. Risk assessment for 2,3,7,8-tetrachlorodibenzo-*p*-dioxin (TCDD) based on an epidemiologic study. *American Journal of Epidemiology* 154(5):451–458.

Stehr PA, Stein G, Webb K, Schramm W, Gedney WB, Donnell HD, Ayres S, Falk H, Sampson E, Smith SJ. 1986. A pilot epidemiologic study of possible health effects associated with 2,3,7,8-tetrachlorodibenzo-*p*-dioxin contaminations in Missouri. *Archives of Environmental Health* 41:16–22.

Stehr-Green P, Hoffman R, Webb K, Evans RG, Knusten A, Schramm W, Staake J, Gibson B, Steinberg K. 1987. Health effects of long-term exposure to 2,3,7,8-tetrachlorodibenzo-*p*-dioxin. *Chemosphere* 16:2089–2094.

Stellman JM, Stellman SD. 2003. *Contractor's Final Report: Characterizing Exposure of Veterans to Agent Orange and Other Herbicides in Vietnam.* Submitted to the National Academy of Sciences, Institute of Medicine in fulfillment of Subcontract VA-5124-98-0019, June 30, 2003.

Stellman JM, Stellman SD, Sommer JF. 1988. Social and behavioral consequences of the Vietnam experience among American Legionnaires. *Environmental Research* 47:129–149.

Stellman JM, Stellman SD, Christian R, Weber T, Tomasallo C. 2003a. The extent and patterns of usage of Agent Orange and other herbicides in Vietnam. *Nature* 422:681–687.

Stellman JM, Stellman SD, Weber T, Tomasallo C, Stellman AB, Christian R Jr. 2003b. A geographic information system for characterizing exposure to Agent Orange and other herbicides in Vietnam. *Environmental Health Perspectives* 111(3):321–328.

Stellman SD, Stellman JM. 1986. Estimation of exposure to Agent Orange and other defoliants among American troops in Vietnam: A methodological approach. *American Journal of Industrial Medicine* 9:305–321.

Stellman SD, Stellman JM. 2004. Exposure opportunity models for Agent Orange, dioxin, and other military herbicides used in Vietnam, 1961–1971. *Journal of Exposure Analysis and Environmental Epidemiology* 14(4):354–362.

Stellman SD, Stellman JM, Sommer JF Jr. 1988. Health and reproductive outcomes among American Legionnaires in relation to combat and herbicide exposure in Vietnam. *Environmental Research* 47:150–174.

Stockbauer JW, Hoffman RE, Schramm WF, Edmonds LD. 1988. Reproductive outcomes of mothers with potential exposure to 2,3,7,8-tetrachlorodibenzo-*p*-dioxin. *American Journal of Epidemiology* 128:410–419.

Suskind RR, Hertzberg VS. 1984. Human health effects of 2,4,5-T and its toxic contaminants. *Journal of the American Medical Association* 251:2372–2380.

Svensson BG, Mikoczy Z, Stromberg U, Hagmar L. 1995. Mortality and cancer incidence among Swedish fishermen with a high dietary intake of persistent organochlorine compounds. *Scandinavian Journal of Work, Environment and Health* 21(2):106–115.

Swaen GMH, van Vliet C, Slangen JJM, Sturmans F. 1992. Cancer mortality among licensed herbicide applicators. *Scandinavian Journal of Work, Environment and Health* 18:201–204.

Swaen GMH, van Amelsvoort LGPM, Slangen JJM, Mohren DCL. 2004. Cancer mortality in a cohort of licensed herbicide applicators. *International Archives of Occupational and Environmental Health* 77:293–295.

Sweeney MH, Fingerhut MA, Connally LB, Halperin WE, Moody PL, Marlow DA. 1989. Progress of the NIOSH cross-sectional study of workers occupationally exposed to chemicals contaminated with 2,3,7,8-TCDD. *Chemosphere* 19:973–977.

Sweeney MH, Fingerhut MA, Arezzo JC, Hornung RW, Connally LB. 1993. Peripheral neuropathy after occupational exposure to 2,3,7,8-tetrachlorodibenzo-*p*-dioxin (TCDD). *American Journal of Industrial Medicine* 23:845–858.

Sweeney MH, Calvert G, Egeland GA, Fingerhut MA, Halperin WE, Piacitelli LA. 1996. *Review and update of the results of the NIOSH medical study of workers exposed to chemicals contaminated with 2,3,7,8-tetrachlorodibenzodioxin.* Presented at the symposium Dioxin Exposure and Human Health—An Update, Berlin, June 17.

Sweeney MH, Calvert GM, Egeland GA, Fingerhut MA, Halperin WE, Piacitelli LA. 1997/98. Review and update of the results of the NIOSH medical study of workers exposed to chemicals contaminated with 2,3,7,8-tetrachlorodibenzodioxin. *Teratogenesis, Carcinogenesis, and Mutagenesis* 17(4-5):241–247.

't Mannetje A, McLean D, Cheng S, Boffetta P, Colin D, Pearce N. 2005. Mortality in New Zealand workers exposed to phenoxy herbicides and dioxins. *Occupational and Environmental Medicine* 62(1):34–40.

Tango T, Fujita T, Tanihata T, Minowa M, Doi Y, Kato N, Kunikane S, Uchiyama I, Tanaka M, Uehata T. 2004. Risk of adverse reproductive outcomes associated with proximity to municipal solid waste incinerators with high dioxin emission levels in Japan. *Journal of Epidemiology* 14(3):83–93.

Tarone RE, Hayes HM, Hoover RN, Rosenthal JF, Brown LM, Pottern LM, Javadpour N, O'Connell KJ, Stutzman RE. 1991. Service in Vietnam and risk of testicular cancer. *Journal of the National Cancer Institute* 83:1497–1499.

Tatham L, Tolbert P, Kjeldsberg C. 1997. Occupational risk factors for subgroups of non-Hodgkin's lymphoma. *Epidemiology* 8(5):551–558.

Teitelbaum SL, Gammon MD, Britton JA, Neugut AI, Levin B, Stellman SD. 2007. Reported residential pesticide use and breast cancer risk on Long Island, New York. *American Journal of Epidemiology* 165(6):643–651.

ten Tusscher GW, Stam GA, Koppe JG. 2000. Open chemical combustions resulting in a local increased incidence of orofacial clefts. *Chemosphere* 40:1263–1270.

Tenchini ML, Crimaudo C, Pacchetti G, Mottura A, Agosti S, De Carli L. 1983. A comparative cytogenetic study on cases of induced abortions in TCDD-exposed and nonexposed women. *Environmental Mutagenesis* 5:73–85.

Teschke K, Hertzman C, Fenske RA, Jin A, Ostry A, van NC, Leiss W. 1994. A history of process and chemical changes for fungicide application in the western Canadian lumber industry: What can we learn? *Applied Occupational and Environmental Hygiene* 9:984–993.

Thiess AM, Frentzel-Beyme R, Link R. 1982. Mortality study of persons exposed to dioxin in a tri-chlorophenol-process accident that occurred in the BASF AG on November 17, 1953. *American Journal of Industrial Medicine* 3:179–189.

Thomas TL. 1987. Mortality among flavour and fragrance chemical plant workers in the United States. *British Journal of Industrial Medicine* 44:733–737.

Thomas TL, Kang HK. 1990. Mortality and morbidity among Army Chemical Corps Vietnam veterans: A preliminary report. *American Journal of Industrial Medicine* 18:665–673.

Thomas TL, Kang H, Dalager N. 1991. Mortality among women Vietnam veterans, 1973–1987. *American Journal of Epidemiology* 134:973–980.

Thomaseth K, Salvan A. 1998. Estimation of occupational exposure to 2,3,7,8-tetrachlorodibenzo-*p*-dioxin using a minimal physiologic toxicokinetic model. *Environmental Health Perspectives* 106(Suppl 2):743–753.

Thörn A, Gustavsson P, Sadigh J, Westerlund-Hannestrand B, Hogstedt C. 2000. Mortality and cancer incidence among Swedish lumberjacks exposed to phenoxy herbicides. *Occupational and Environmental Medicine* 57(10):718–720.

Toft G, Long M, Kruger T, Hjelmborg PS, Bonde JP, Rignell-Hydbom A, Tyrkiel E, Hagmar L, Giwercman A, Spano M, Bizzaro D, Pedersen HS, Lesovoy V, Ludwicki JK, Bonefeld-Jorgensen EC. 2007. Semen quality in relation to xenohormone and dioxin-like serum activity among Inuits and three European populations. *Environmental Health Perspectives* 115(Supplement 1):15–20.

Tonn T, Esser C, Schneider EM, Steinmann-Steiner-Haldenstatt W, Gleichmann E. 1996. Persistence of decreased T-helper cell function in industrial workers 20 years after exposure to 2,3,7,8-tetrachlorodibenzo-*p*-dioxin. *Environmental Health Perspectives* 104(4):422–426.

Torchio P, Lepore AR, Corrao G, Comba P, Settimi L, Belli S, Magnani C, di Orio F. 1994. Mortality study on a cohort of Italian licensed pesticide users. *The Science of the Total Environment* 149(3):183–191.

Townsend JC, Bodner KM, Van Peenen PFD, Olson RD, Cook RR. 1982. Survey of reproductive events of wives of employees exposed to chlorinated dioxins. *American Journal of Epidemiology* 115:695–713.

True WR, Goldberg J, Eisen SA. 1988. Stress symptomatology among Vietnam veterans. Analysis of the Veterans Administration Survey of Veterans II. *American Journal of Epidemiology* 128:85–92.

Trung CB, Chien NT. 1983. Spontaneous abortions and birth defects in area exposed to toxic chemical sprays in Giong Trom District. Summarized in: Constable JD, Hatch MC. *Reproductive effects of herbicide exposure in Vietnam: Recent studies by the Vietnamese and others.* As cited in Constable and Hatch, 1985.

Tsuchiya M, Tsukino H, Iwasaki M, Sasaki H, Tanaka T, Katoh T, Patterson DG Jr, Turner W, Needham L, Tsugane S. 2007. Interaction between cytochrome P450 gene polymorphisms and serum organochlorine TEQ levels in the risk of endometriosis. *Molecular Human Reproduction* 13(6):399–404.

Tsukimori K, Tokunaga S, Shibata S, Uchi H, Nakayama D, Ishimaru T, Nakano H, Wake N, Yoshimura T, Furue M. 2008. Long-term effects of polychlorinated biphenyls and dioxins on pregnancy outcomes in women affected by the Yusho incident. *Environmental Health Perspectives* 116(5):626–630.

Turyk ME, Anderson HA, Persky VW. 2007. Relationships of thyroid hormones with polychlorinated biphenyls, dioxins, furans, and DDE in adults. *Environmental Health Perspectives* 115(8):1197–1203.

Uemura H, Arisawa K, Hiyoshi M, Satoh H, Sumiyoshi Y, Morinaga K, Kodama K, Suzuki T, Nagai M, Suzuki T. 2008a. Associations of environmental exposure to dioxins with prevalent diabetes among general inhabitants in Japan. *Environmental Research* 108(1):63–68.

Uemura H, Arisawa K, Hiyoshi M, Satoh H, Sumiyoshi Y, Morinaga K, Kodama K, Suzuki T, Nagai M, Suzuki T. 2008b. PCDDs/PCDFs and dioxin-like PCBs: Recent body burden levels and their determinants among general inhabitants in Japan. *Chemosphere* 73(1):30–37.

Urban P, Pelclová D, Lukas E, Kupka K, Preiss J, Fenclova Z, Smerhovsky Z. 2007. Neurological and neurophysiological examinations on workers with chronic poisoning by 2,3,7,8-TCDD: Follow-up 35 years after exposure. *European Journal of Neurology* 14(2):213–218.

Valcin M, Henneberger PK, Kullman GJ, Umbach DM, London SJ, Alavanja MC, Sandler DP, Hoppin JA. 2007. Chronic bronchitis among nonsmoking farm women in the Agricultural Health Study. *Journal of Occupational and Environmental Medicine* 49(5):574–583.

van Houdt JJ, Fransman LG, Strik JJ. 1983. Epidemiological case–control study in personnel exposed to 2,4,5-T. *Chemosphere* 12(4):575.

van Wijngaarden E, Stewart PA, Olshan AF, Savitz DA, Bunin GR. 2003. Parental occupational exposure to pesticides and childhood brain cancer. *American Journal of Epidemiology* 157(11): 989–997.

Vena J, Boffetta P, Becher H, Benn T, Bueno de Mesquita HB, Coggon D, Colin D, Flesch-Janys D, Green L, Kauppinen T, Littorin M, Lynge E, Mathews JD, Neuberger M, Pearce N, Pesatori AC, Saracci R, Steenland K, Kogevinas M. 1998. Exposure to dioxin and nonneoplastic mortality in the expanded IARC international cohort study of phenoxy herbicide and chlorophenol production workers and sprayers. *Environmental Health Perspectives* 106(Supplement 2):645–653.

Viel JF, Clement MC, Hagi M, Grandjean S, Challier B, Danzon A. 2008. Dioxin emissions from a municipal solid waste incinerator and risk of invasive breast cancer: A population-based case–control study with GIS-derived exposure. *International Journal of Health Geographics [Electronic Resource]* 7:4.

Vineis P, Terracini B, Ciccone G, Cignetti A, Colombo E, Donna A, Maffi L, Pisa R, Ricci P, Zanini E, Comba P. 1986. Phenoxy herbicides and soft-tissue sarcomas in female rice weeders. A population-based case-referent study. *Scandinavian Journal of Work, Environment and Health* 13:9–17.

Vineis P, Faggiano F, Tedeschi M, Ciccone G. 1991. Incidence rates of lymphomas and soft-tissue sarcomas and environmental measurements of phenoxy herbicides. *Journal of the National Cancer Institute* 83:362–363.

Visintainer PF, Barone M, McGee H, Peterson EL. 1995. Proportionate mortality study of Vietnam-era veterans of Michigan. *Journal of Occupational and Environmental Medicine* 37(4):423–428.

Warner M, Eskenazi B, Mocarelli P, Gerthoux PM, Samuels S, Needham L, Patterson D, Brambilla P. 2002. Serum dioxin concentrations and breast cancer risk in the Seveso Women's Health Study. *Environmental Health Perspectives* 110(7):625–628.

Warner M, Samuels S, Mocarelli P, Gerthoux PM, Needham L, Patterson DG Jr, Eskenazi B. 2004. Serum dioxin concentrations and age at menarche. *Environmental Health Perspectives* 112(13):1289–1292.

Warner M, Eskenazi B, Olive DL, Samuels S, Quick-Miles S, Vercellini P, Gerthoux PM, Needham L, Patterson DG, Mocarelli P. 2007. Serum dioxin concentrations and quality of ovarian function in women of Seveso. *Environmental Health Perspectives* 115(3):336–340.

Watanabe KK, Kang HK. 1995. Military service in Vietnam and the risk of death from trauma and selected cancers. *Annals of Epidemiology* 5(5):407–412.

Watanabe KK, Kang HK. 1996. Mortality patterns among Vietnam veterans: A 24-year retrospective analysis. *Journal of Occupational and Environmental Medicine* 38(3):272–278.

Watanabe KK, Kang HK, Thomas TL. 1991. Mortality among Vietnam veterans: With methodological considerations. *Journal of Occupational Medicine* 33:780–785.

Waterhouse D, Carman WJ, Schottenfeld D, Gridley G, McLean S. 1996. Cancer incidence in the rural community of Tecumseh, Michigan: A pattern of increased lymphopoietic neoplasms. *Cancer* 77(4):763–770.

Webb K, Evans RG, Stehr P, Ayres SM. 1987. Pilot study on health effects of environmental 2,3,7,8-TCDD in Missouri. *American Journal of Industrial Medicine* 11:685–691.

Weisglas-Kuperus N, Sas TC, Koopman-Esseboom C, van der Zwan CW, De Ridder MA, Beishuizen A, Hooijkaas H, Sauer PJ. 1995. Immunologic effects of background prenatal and postnatal exposure to dioxins and polychlorinated biphenyls in Dutch infants. *Pediatric Research* 38(3):404–410.

Weiss J, Papke O, Bignert A, Jensen S, Greyerz E, Agostoni C, Besana R, Riva E, Giovannini M, Zetterstrom R. 2003. Concentrations of dioxins and other organochlorines (PCBs, DDTs, HCHs) in human milk from Seveso, Milan and a Lombardian rural area in Italy: A study performed 25 years after the heavy dioxin exposure in Seveso. *Acta Paediatrica* 92(4):467–472.

Wendt AS. 1985. *Iowa Agent Orange Survey of Vietnam Veterans.* Iowa State Department of Health.

Weselak M, Arbuckle TE, Wigle DT, Krewski D. 2007. In utero pesticide exposure and childhood morbidity. *Environmental Research* 103(1):79–86.

White FMM, Cohen FG, Sherman G, McCurdy R. 1988. Chemicals, birth defects and stillbirths in New Brunswick: Associations with agricultural activity. *Canadian Medical Association Journal* 138:117–124.

Wigle DT, Semenciw RB, Wilkins K, Riedel D, Ritter L, Morrison HI, Mao Y. 1990. Mortality study of Canadian male farm operators: Non-Hodgkin's lymphoma mortality and agricultural practices in Saskatchewan. *Journal of the National Cancer Institute* 82:575–582.

Wiklund K. 1983. Swedish agricultural workers: A group with a decreased risk of cancer. *Cancer* 51:566–568.

Wiklund K, Holm LE. 1986. Soft tissue sarcoma risk in Swedish agricultural and forestry workers. *Journal of the National Cancer Institute* 76:229–234.

Wiklund K, Dich J, Holm LE. 1987. Risk of malignant lymphoma in Swedish pesticide appliers. *British Journal of Cancer* 56:505–508.

Wiklund K, Lindefors BM, Holm LE. 1988a. Risk of malignant lymphoma in Swedish agricultural and forestry workers. *British Journal of Industrial Medicine* 45:19–24.

Wiklund K, Dich J, Holm LE. 1988b. Soft tissue sarcoma risk in Swedish licensed pesticide applicators. *Journal of Occupational Medicine* 30:801–804.

Wiklund K, Dich J, Holm LE, Eklund G. 1989a. Risk of cancer in pesticide applicators in Swedish agriculture. *British Journal of Industrial Medicine* 46:809–814.

Wiklund K, Dich J, Holm LE. 1989b. Risk of soft tissue sarcoma, Hodgkin's disease and non-Hodgkin lymphoma among Swedish licensed pesticide applicators. *Chemosphere* 18:395–400.

Wingren G, Fredrikson M, Brage HN, Nordenskjold B, Axelson O. 1990. Soft tissue sarcoma and occupational exposures. *Cancer* 66:806–811.

Wolf N, Karmaus W. 1995. Effects of inhalative exposure to dioxins in wood preservatives on cell-mediated immunity in day-care center teachers. *Environmental Research* 68(2):96–105.

Wolfe WH, Michalek JE, Miner JC, Rahe A, Silva J, Thomas WF, Grubbs WD, Lustik MB, Karrison TG, Roegner RH, Williams DE. 1990. Health status of Air Force veterans occupationally exposed to herbicides in Vietnam. I. Physical health. *Journal of the American Medical Association* 264:1824–1831.

Wolfe WH, Michalek JE, Miner JC, Rahe AJ, Moore CA, Needham LL, Patterson DG. 1995. Paternal serum dioxin and reproductive outcomes among veterans of Operation Ranch Hand. *Epidemiology* 6(1):17–22.

Woods JS, Polissar L. 1989. Non-Hodgkin's lymphoma among phenoxy herbicide-exposed farm workers in western Washington State. *Chemosphere* 18:401–406.

Woods JS, Polissar L, Severson RK, Heuser LS, Kulander BG. 1987. Soft tissue sarcoma and non-Hodgkin's lymphoma in relation to phenoxy herbicide and chlorinated phenol exposure in western Washington. *Journal of the National Cancer Institute* 78:899–910.

Xu JX, Hoshida Y, Yang WI, Inohara H, Kubo T, Kim GE, Yoon JH, Kojya S, Bandoh N, Harabuchi Y, Tsutsumi K, Koizuka I, Jia XS, Kirihata M, Tsukuma H, Aozasa K. 2007. Life-style and environmental factors in the development of nasal NK/T-cell lymphoma: A case–control study in East Asia. *International Journal of Cancer* 120(2):406–410.

Yeboah J, Crouse JR, Hsu FC, Burke GL, Herrington DM. 2007. Brachial flow-mediated dilation predicts incident cardiovascular events in older adults: The Cardiovascular Health Study. *Circulation* 115(18):2390–2397.

Yoshida J, Kumagai S, Tabuchi T, Kosaka H, Akasaka S, Kasai H, Oda H. 2006. Negative association between serum dioxin level and oxidative DNA damage markers in municipal waste incinerator workers. *International Archives of Occupational and Environmental Health* 79(2):115–122.

Young AL. 2004. TCDD biomonitoring and exposure to Agent Orange: Still the gold standard. *Environmental Science and Pollution Research* 11(3):143–146.

Young AL, Newton M. 2004. Long overlooked historical information on Agent Orange and TCDD following massive applications of 2,4,5-T–containing herbicides, Eglin Air Force Base, Florida. *Environmental Science and Pollution Research* 11(4):209–221.

Young AL, Cecil PF Sr, Guilmartin JF Jr. 2004a. Assessing possible exposures of ground troops to Agent Orange during the Vietnam War: The use of contemporary military records. *Environmental Science and Pollution Research* 11(6):349–358.

Young AL, Giesy JP, Jones P, Newton M, Guilmartin JF Jr, Cecil PF Sr. 2004b. Assessment of potential exposure to Agent Orange and its associated TCDD. *Environmental Science and Pollution Research* 11(6):347–348.

Zack JA, Gaffey WR. 1983. A mortality study of workers employed at the Monsanto company plant in Nitro, West Virginia. *Environmental Science Research* 26:575–591.

Zack JA, Suskind RR. 1980. The mortality experience of workers exposed to tetrachlorodibenzo-dioxin in a trichlorophenol process accident. *Journal of Occupational Medicine* 22:11–14.

Zahm SH, Weisenburger DD, Babbitt PA, Saal RC, Vaught JB, Cantor KP, Blair A. 1990. A case–control study of non-Hodgkin's lymphoma and the herbicide 2,4-dichlorophenoxyacetic acid (2,4-D) in eastern Nebraska. *Epidemiology* 1:349–356.

Zahm SH, Weisenburger DD, Saal RC, Vaught JB, Babbitt PA, Blair A. 1993. The role of agricultural pesticide use in the development of non-Hodgkin's lymphoma in women. *Archives of Environmental Health* 48:353–358.

Zambon P, Ricci P, Bovo E, Casula A, Gattolin M, Fiore AR, Chiosi F, Guzzinati S. 2007. Sarcoma risk and dioxin emissions from incinerators and industrial plants: A population-based case–control study (Italy). *Environmental Health: A Global Access Science Source* 6(19).

Zhong Y, Rafnsson V. 1996. Cancer incidence among Icelandic pesticide users. *International Journal of Epidemiology* 25(6):1117–1124.

Zober A, Messerer P, Huber P. 1990. Thirty-four-year mortality follow-up of BASF employees exposed to 2,3,7,8-TCDD after the 1953 accident. *International Archives of Occupational and Environmental Health* 62:139–157.

Zober A, Ott MG, Messerer P. 1994. Morbidity follow-up study of BASF employees exposed to 2,3,7,8-tetrachlorodibenzo-*p*-dioxin (TCDD) after a 1953 chemical reactor incident. *Occupational and Environmental Medicine* 51:479–486.

Zober A, Messerer P, Ott MG. 1997. BASF studies: Epidemiological and clinical investigations on dioxin-exposed chemical workers. *Teratogenesis, Carcinogenesis, and Mutagenesis* 17(4-5): 249–256.

6

Cancer

Cancer is the second-leading cause of death in the United States. Among men 50–64 years old, the group that includes most Vietnam veterans (see Table 6-1), however, the risk of dying from cancer exceeds the risk of dying from heart disease, the main cause of death in the United States, and does not fall to second place until after the age of 75 years (Heron et al., 2009). About 565,650 Americans of all ages were expected to die from cancer in 2008—more than 1,500 per day. In the United States, one-fourth of all deaths are from cancer (Jemal et al., 2008a).

This chapter summarizes and presents conclusions about the strength of the evidence from epidemiologic studies regarding associations be-

TABLE 6-1 Age Distribution of Vietnam-Era and Vietnam-Theater Male Veterans, 2004–2005 (numbers in thousands)

Age Group (Years)	Vietnam Era		Vietnam Theater	
	n	(%)	n	(%)
All ages	7,938		3,852	
≤ 49	133	(1.7)	32	(0.8)
50–54	1,109	(14.0)	369	(9.6)
55–59	3,031	(38.2)	1,676	(43.5)
60–64	2,301	(29.0)	1,090	(28.3)
65–69	675	(8.5)	280	(7.3)
70–79	511	(6.4)	322	(8.4)
≥ 80	178	(2.2)	83	(2.2)

SOURCE: IOM, 1994, Table 3-3, updated by 15 years.

tween exposure to the chemicals of interest—2,4-dichlorophenoxyacetic acid (2,4-D), 2,4,5-trichlorophenoxyacetic acid (2,4,5-T) and its contaminant 2,3,7,8-tetrachlorodibenzo-*p*-dioxin (TCDD), picloram, and cacodylic acid—and various types of cancer. If a new study reported on only a single type of cancer and did not revisit a previously studied population, its design information is summarized here with its results; design information on all other new studies can be found in Chapter 4.

In an evaluation of a possible connection between herbicide exposure and risk of cancer, the approach used to assess study subjects is of critical importance in determining the overall relevance and usefulness of findings. As noted in Chapter 5, there is great variety in detail and accuracy of exposure assessment among studies. A few studies used biologic markers of exposure, such as the presence of a compound in serum or tissues; some developed an index of exposure from employment or activity records; and some used other surrogate measures of exposure, such as presence in a locale when herbicides were used. As noted in Chapter 2, inaccurate assessment of exposure can obscure the relationship between exposure and disease.

Each section on a type of cancer opens with background information, including data on its incidence in the general US population and known or suspected risk factors. Cancer-incidence data on the general US population are included in the background material to provide a context for consideration of cancer risk in Vietnam veterans; the figures presented are estimates of incidence in the entire US population, however, not predictions for the Vietnam-veteran cohort. The data reported are for 2000–2005 and are from the most recent dataset available (NCI, 2008). Incidence data are given for all races combined and separately for blacks and whites. The age range of 50–64 years now includes about 80% of Vietnam-era veterans, so incidences are presented for three 5-year age groups: 50–54 years, 55–59 years, and 60–64 years. The data were collected for the Surveillance, Epidemiology, and End Results (SEER) program of the National Cancer Institute and are categorized by sex, age, and race, all of which can have profound effects on risk. For example, the incidence of prostate cancer is about 4.1 times as high as men who are 60–64 years old than in men 50–54 years old and about twice as high in blacks 50–64 years old as in whites in the same age group (NCI, 2008). Many other factors can influence cancer incidence, including screening methods, tobacco and alcohol use, diet, genetic predisposition, and medical history. Those factors can make someone more or less likely than the average to contract a given kind of cancer; they also need to be taken into account in epidemiologic studies of the possible contributions of the chemicals of interest.

Each section of this chapter pertaining to a specific type of cancer includes a summary of the findings described in the previous Agent Orange reports: *Veterans and Agent Orange: Health Effects of Herbicides Used in Vietnam*, hereafter referred to as *VAO* (IOM, 1994); *Veterans and Agent Orange: Update 1996*, referred to as *Update 1996* (IOM, 1996); *Update 1998* (IOM, 1999); *Update*

2000 (IOM, 2001); *Update 2002* (IOM, 2003); *Update 2004* (IOM, 2005); and *Update 2006* (IOM, 2007). That is followed by a discussion of the most recent scientific literature, a discussion of biologic plausibility, and a synthesis of the material reviewed. When it is appropriate, the literature is discussed by exposure type (service in Vietnam, occupational exposure, or environmental exposure). Each section ends with the committee's conclusion regarding the strength of the evidence from epidemiologic studies. The categories of association and the committee's approach to categorizing the health outcomes are discussed in Chapters 1 and 2.

Biologic plausibility corresponds to the third element of the committee's congressionally mandated statement of task. In fact, the degree of biologic plausibility itself influences whether the committee perceives positive findings to be indicative of an association or the product of statistical fluctuations (chance) or bias.

Information on biologic mechanisms by which exposure to TCDD could contribute to the generic (rather than tissue-specific or organ-specific) carcinogenic potential of the chemicals of interest is summarized in Chapter 4. It distills toxicologic information concerning the mechanisms by which TCDD affects the basic process of carcinogenesis; such information, of course, applies to all the cancer sites discussed individually in this chapter. When biologic plausibility is discussed in this chapter's sections on particular cancer types, the generic information is implicit, and only experimental data peculiar to carcinogenesis at the site in question is presented.

Considerable uncertainty remains about the magnitude of potential risk posed by exposure to the chemicals of interest. Many of the veteran, occupational, and environmental studies reviewed by the committee did not control fully for important confounders. There is not enough information about the exposure experience of individual Vietnam veterans to permit combining exposure estimates for them with any potency estimates that might be derived from scientific research studies in order to quantify risk. The committee therefore cannot accurately estimate the risk to Vietnam veterans that is attributable to exposure to the chemicals of interest. The (at least currently) insurmountable problems of deriving useful quantitative estimates of the risks of various health outcomes to Vietnam veterans are explained in Chapter 1 and the summary of this report, but the point is not reiterated for every health outcome addressed.

ORGANIZATION OF CANCER GROUPINGS

For *Update 2006*, a system for addressing cancer types was described to clarify how specific cancer diagnoses were grouped for evaluation by the committee and to ensure that the full array of cancer types would be considered.

As described in *Update 2006*, the organization of cancer groups follows major and minor categories of cause of death related to cancer sites established by the National Institute for Occupational Safety and Health (NIOSH). The NIOSH groups map the full range of *International Classification of Diseases, Revision 9* (ICD-9) codes for malignant neoplasms (140–208). The ICD system is used by physicians and researchers to group related diseases and procedures in a standard form for statistical evaluation. Revision 10 (ICD-10) came into use in 1999 and constitutes a marked change from the previous four revisions that evolved into the ninth ICD-9. ICD-9 was in effect from 1979 to 1998; because ICD-9 is the version most prominent in the research reviewed in this series, it has been used when codes are given for a specific health outcome. Appendix B describes the correspondence between the NIOSH cause-of-death groupings and ICD-9 codes (Table B-1); the groupings for mortality are largely congruent with those of the SEER program for cancer incidence (see Table B-2, which presents equivalences between the ICD-9 and ICD-10 systems).

The system of organization used by the committee simplifies the process for locating a particular cancer for readers and facilitated the committee's identification of ICD codes for malignancies that had not been explicitly addressed in previous updates. *VAO* reports' default category for any health outcome for which no epidemiologic research findings have been recovered has always been "inadequate evidence" of association, which in principle is applicable to specific cancers. Failure to review a specific cancer or other condition separately reflects the paucity of information, so there is indeed inadequate or insufficient information to categorize such a disease outcome.

BIOLOGIC PLAUSIBILITY

The studies considered with respect to the biologic plausibility of an association between exposure to the chemicals of interest and human cancers have been performed primarily in either laboratory animals (rats, mice, hamsters, and monkeys) or cultured cells. Collectively, the evidence obtained from studies of TCDD indicates that a connection between human exposure to this compound and cancers is biologically plausible, as will be discussed more fully in a generic sense below and more specifically in the biologic-plausibility sections on individual cancers.

With respect to 2,4-D, 2,4,5-T, and picloram, several studies have been performed in laboratory animals. In general, the results were negative although some would not meet current standards for cancer bioassays; for instance, there is some question whether the highest doses (generally 30–50 mg/kg) in some of these studies achieved a maximum tolerated dose (MTD). It is not possible to have absolute confidence that these compounds have no carcinogenic potential. Further evidence of a lack of carcinogenic potential is provided, however, by negative findings for genotoxic effects in assays conducted primarily in vitro. The evidence indicates that 2,4-D is genotoxic only at very high concentrations. Although 2,4,5-T was shown to increase the formation of DNA adducts by cytochrome P450–derived metabolites of benzo[*a*]pyrene, most available evidence indicates that 2,4,5-T is genotoxic only at high concentrations.

There is some evidence that cacodylic acid is carcinogenic. Studies performed in laboratory animals have shown that it can induce neoplasms of the kidney (Yamamoto et al., 1995) and bladder (Arnold et al., 2006; Wei et al., 2002). In the lung, treatment with cacodylic acid induced formation of neoplasms when administered to mouse strains that are genetically susceptible to them (Hayashi et al., 1998). Other studies have used the two-stage model of carcinogenesis in which animals are exposed first to a known genotoxic agent and then to a suspected tumor-promoting agent. With that model, cacodylic acid has been shown to act as a tumor-promoter with respect to lung cancer (Yamanaka et al., 1996).

Studies in laboratory animals in which only TCDD has been administered have reported that it can increase the incidence of a number of neoplasms, most notably of the liver, lung, thyroid, and oral mucosa (Kociba et al., 1978; NTP, 2006). Some studies have used the two-stage model of carcinogenesis and shown that TCDD can act as a tumor-promoter and increase the incidence of ovarian (Davis et al., 2000), liver (Beebe et al., 1995), and skin cancers (Wyde et al., 2004). As to the mechanisms by which TCDD exerts its carcinogenic effects, it is thought to act primarily as a tumor-promoter. In many of the animal studies reviewed, treatment with TCDD has resulted in hyperplasia or metaplasia of epithelial tissues. In addition, in both laboratory animals and cultured cells, TCDD has been shown to exhibit a wide array of effects on growth regulation, hormone systems, and other factors associated with the regulation of cellular processes that involve growth, maturation, and differentiation. Thus, it may be that TCDD increases the incidence or progression of human cancers through an interplay between multiple cellular factors. Tissue-specific protective cellular mechanisms may also affect the response to TCDD and complicate our understanding of its site-specific carcinogenic effects.

As shown with long-term bioassays in both sexes of several strains of rats, mice, hamsters, and fish, there is adequate evidence that TCDD is a carcinogen in laboratory animals, increasing the incidence of tumors at sites distant from the site of treatment at doses well below the maximum tolerated. On the basis of animal studies, TCDD has been characterized as a nongenotoxic carcinogen because it does not have obvious DNA-damaging potential, but it is a potent "promoter" and a weak initiator in two-stage initiation–promotion models for liver, skin, and lung. Early studies demonstrated that TCDD is 2 orders of magnitude more potent than the "classic" promoter tetradecanoyl phorbol acetate and that TCDD skin-tumor promotion depends on the aryl hydrocarbon receptor (AHR). For many years, it has been known that TCDD is a potent tumor-promoter. Recent evidence has shown that AHR activation by TCDD in human breast and endocervical cell lines induces sustained high concentrations of the interleukin–6 (IL–6) cytokine, which has tumor-promoting effects in numerous tissues—including breast, prostate, ovarian, and malignant cholangiocytes—and opens up the possibility that TCDD would promote carcinogenesis in these and possibly other tissues (Hollingshead et al., 2008).

In vitro work with mouse hepatoma cells has shown that activation of the AHR results in increased concentrations of 8-hydroxydeoxyguanosine—a product of DNA-base oxidation and later excision repair and a marker of DNA damage. Induction of cytochrome P4501A1 (CYP1A1) by TCDD or indolo(3,2-b)carbazole is associated with oxidative DNA damage (Park et al., 1996). In vivo experiments in mice corroborated those findings by showing that TCDD caused a sustained oxidative stress, as determined by measurements of urinary 8-hydroxydeoxyguanosine (Shertzer et al., 2002), involving AHR-dependent uncoupling of mitochondrial respiration (Senft et al., 2002). Mitochondrial reactive oxygen production depends on the AHR. Recent work designed to measure DNA damage in humans has also found high urinary 8-hydroxydeoxyguanosine in workers dismantling electronic equipment who were exposed to high concentrations of dioxins and dioxin-like compounds (Wen et al., 2008).

In a recent study of New Zealand Vietnam War veterans (Rowland et al., 2007), clastogenic genetic disturbances arising as a consequence of confirmed exposure to Agent Orange were determined by analyzing sister-chromatid exchanges (SCEs) in lymphocytes from a group of 24 New Zealand Vietnam War veterans and 23 control volunteers. The results showed a highly significant difference ($p < 0.001$) between the mean of the experimental group and the mean of the control group. The Vietnam War veterans also had a much higher proportion of cells with SCE frequencies above the 95th percentile than the controls (11.0 and 0.07%, respectively).

The weight of evidence that TCDD and dioxin-like polychlorinated biphenyls make up a group of compounds with carcinogenic potential includes unequivocal animal carcinogenesis and biologic plausibility based on mode-of-action data. Although the specific mechanisms by which dioxin causes cancer remain to be established, the intracellular factors and mechanistic pathways involved in dioxin's cancer-promotion mode of action all have parallels between animals and humans. No qualitative differences have been reported to indicate that humans should be considered as fundamentally different from the multiple animal species in which bioassays have demonstrated dioxin-induced neoplasia.

In conclusion, the toxicologic evidence indicates that a connection of TCDD and perhaps cacodylic acid with cancer in humans is, in general, biologically plausible, but (as discussed below) it must be determined case-by-case whether such potential is realized in a given tissue. Experiments with 2,4-D, 2,4,5-T, and picloram in animals and cells have not provided a strong biologic basis of the presence or absence of carcinogenic effects.

The Committee's View of "General" Human Carcinogens

In order to address its charge, the committee weighed the scientific evidence linking the chemicals of interest to specific individual cancer sites. That was appropriate given the different susceptibilities of various tissues and organs to cancer development and the various genetic and environmental factors that can influence the occurrence of a particular type of cancer. Before considering each site in turn, however, it is important to address the concept that cancers share certain features among organ sites and to clarify the committee's view regarding the implications of a compound's being a "general" human carcinogen. All cancers share phenotypic features: uncontrolled cell proliferation, increased cell survival, invasion outside normal tissue boundaries, and eventually metastasis. The current model for understanding cancer development holds that a cell or group of cells must acquire a series of sufficient genetic mutations to progress and that particular epigenetic events (events that affect gene function but do not involve a change in gene coding sequence) must occur to accelerate the mutational process and provide growth advantages for the more aggressive clones of cells. That means that a carcinogen can stimulate the process of cancer development by either genetic (mutational) or epigenetic (nonmutational) activities.

In classic experiments based on the induction of cancer in mouse skin that were conducted over 40 years ago, carcinogens were categorized as initiators, those capable of causing an initial genetic insult to the target tissue, and promoters, those capable of promoting the growth of initiated tumor cells, generally through nonmutational events. Some carcinogens, such as those found in tobacco smoke, were considered "whole carcinogens"; that is, they were capable of both initiation and promotion. Today, cancer researchers recognize that the acquisition of important mutations is a continuing process in tumors, and that promoters, or epigenetic processes that favor cancer growth, influence the accumulation of genotoxic damage and vice versa.

As discussed above and in Chapter 4, 2,4-D, 2,4,5-T, and picloram have shown little evidence of genotoxicity in laboratory studies, except at very high doses, and little ability to facilitate cancer growth in laboratory animals. However, cacodylic acid and TCDD have shown the capacity to increase cancer development in animal experiments, particularly as promoters rather than as pure genotoxic agents. Extrapolating organ-specific results from animal experiments to humans is problematic because of important differences between species in overall susceptibility of various organs to cancer development and in organ-specific responses to particular putative carcinogens. Therefore, judgments about the general carcinogenicity of a compound are based heavily on the results of epidemiologic studies, particularly on the question of whether there is evidence of excess cancer risk at multiple organ sites. As the cancer-type evaluations indicate in the remainder of this chapter, the committee finds that TCDD in particular appears to be a multisite carcinogen. That finding is in agreement with the International Agency for Research on Cancer (IARC), which has determined that TCDD is a category 1 "known human carcinogen," and with the US Environmental Protection Agency (EPA), which has concluded that TCDD is "likely to be carcinogenic to humans." It is important to emphasize that the goals and methodology of the IARC and EPA in making their determinations were different from those of this committee; the mission of those organizations focuses on evaluating risk to minimize future exposure, whereas this committee focuses on risk after exposure.

Furthermore, recognition that TCDD and cacodylic acid are multisite carcinogens does not imply that they cause human cancer at every organ site.

The distinction between *general carcinogen* and *site-specific carcinogen* is more difficult to grasp in light of the common practice of beginning analyses of epidemiologic cohorts with a category of "all malignant neoplasms," which is a routine first screen for any unusual cancer activity in the study population rather than a test of a biologically-based hypothesis. When the distribution of cancers among anatomic sites is lacking in the report of a cohort study, a statistical test for an increase in all cancers is not meaningless, but it is usually less scientifically supportable than analyses based on specific sites, for which more substantial biologically based hypotheses can be developed. The size of a cohort and the length of the observation period often constrain the number of cases of individual cancer types observed and the extent to which specific cancer types can be analyzed. For instance, this present update includes an analysis of cumulative results on diabetes and cancer from a report of the prospective Air Force Health Study (Michalek and Pavuk, 2008). For the fairly common condition of diabetes, that publication represents important information summarizing previous findings, but the cancer analysis does not go beyond "all cancers." The committee does not accept those findings as an indication that exposure to Agent Orange increases the risk of every variety of cancer. The committee acknowledges that the highly stratified analyses conducted suggest that some increase in the incidence of some cancers did occur in some of the Ranch Hand subjects, but it views the "all cancers" results as a conglomeration containing information on specific cancers—most important, melanoma and prostate cancer—for which provocative results have been published (Akhtar et al., 2004; Pavuk et al., 2006) and which merit individual longitudinal analysis to resolve outstanding questions.

The remainder of this chapter deals with the committee's review of the evidence on each individual cancer site in accordance with its charge to evaluate the statistical association between exposure and cancer occurrence, the biologic plausibility and potential causal nature of that association, and the relevance to US veterans of the Vietnam War.

ORAL, NASAL, AND PHARYNGEAL CANCER

Oral, nasal, and pharyngeal cancers are found in many anatomic subsites, including the structures of the mouth (inside lining of the lips, cheeks, gums, tongue, and hard and soft palate) (ICD-9 140–145), oropharynx (ICD-9 146), nasopharynx (ICD-9 147), hypopharynx (ICD-9 148), other buccal cavity and pharynx (ICD-9 149), and nasal cavity and paranasal sinuses (ICD-9 160). Although those sites are anatomically diverse, cancers that occur in the nasal cavity, oral cavity, and pharynx are for the most part similar in descriptive epidemiology and risk factors. The exception is cancer of the nasopharynx, which has a different epidemiologic profile.

The American Cancer Society (ACS) estimated that about 35,310 men and women would receive diagnoses of oral, nasal, or pharyngeal cancer in the United States in 2006 and 7,590 men and women would die from these diseases (Jemal et al., 2008a). Almost 91% of those cancers originate in the oral cavity or oropharynx. Most oral, nasal, and pharyngeal cancers are squamous-cell carcinomas. Nasopharyngeal carcinoma (NPC) is the most common malignant epithelial tumor of the nasopharynx although it is relatively rare in the United States. There are three types of NPC: keratinizing squamous-cell carcinoma, nonkeratinizing carcinoma, and undifferentiated carcinoma.

The average annual incidences reported in Table 6-2 show that men are at greater risk than women for those cancers and that the incidences increase with age although there are few cases, and care should be exercised in interpreting the numbers. Tobacco and alcohol use are established risk factors for oral and pharyngeal cancers. Reported risk factors for nasal cancer include occupational exposure to nickel and chromium compounds (Hayes, 1997), wood dust (Demers et al., 1995), and formaldehyde (Blair and Kazerouni, 1997).

Conclusions from *VAO* and Previous Updates

The committee responsible for *VAO* concluded that there was inadequate or insufficient information to determine whether there is an association between exposure to the chemicals of interest and oral, nasal, and pharyngeal cancers. Additional information available to the committees responsible for *Update 1996*,

TABLE 6-2 Average Annual Incidence (per 100,000) of Nasal, Nasopharyngeal, Oral-Cavity and Pharyngeal, and Oropharyngeal Cancers in United States[a]

	50–54 Years Old			55–59 Years Old			60–64 Years Old		
	All Races	White	Black	All Races	White	Black	All Races	White	Black
Nose, Nasal Cavity, and Middle Ear:									
Men	1.3	1.2	1.5	1.5	1.4	1.5	2.2	2.3	2.7
Women	0.5	0.5	0.5	1.0	1.1	0.0	1.1	1.1	1.3
Nasopharynx:									
Men	1.8	1.0	1.3	2.6	1.4	2.4	2.8	1.6	3.1
Women	0.7	0.3	0.8	0.7	0.3	0.4	1.1	0.5	0.6
Oral Cavity and Pharynx:									
Men	29.4	29.2	38.3	39.0	38.3	50.4	48.9	49.5	56.1
Women	9.0	8.7	11.7	12.6	12.6	13.9	16.0	16.3	17.5
Oropharynx:									
Men	1.9	1.0	2.3	1.6	1.4	3.2	2.0	1.9	4.7
Women	0.2	0.1	0.6	0.5	0.4	1.1	0.2	0.2	0.6

[a] Surveillance, Epidemiology, and End Results program, nine standard registries, crude age-specific rates, 2000–2005.

Update 1998, *Update 2000*, *Update 2002*, *Update 2004*, and *Update 2006* did not change that conclusion.

For *Update 2006*, the Department of Veterans Affairs (VA) made the specific request that the committee screened studies that had reported the number of tonsil-cancer cases observed. Given the small number of cases diagnosed in the general population, it is often not possible to evaluate tonsil-cancer cases separately in epidemiologic studies; therefore, they are grouped in the more general category of oral, nasal, and pharyngeal cancers. The committee was able to identify only three cohort studies that provided the number of tonsil-cancer cases in their study populations and concluded that these studies did not provide sufficient evidence to determine whether an association existed between exposure to the chemicals of interest and tonsil cancer. The committee responsible for *Update 2006* recommended that VA evaluate the possibility of studying health outcomes, including tonsil cancer, in Vietnam-era veterans by using existing administrative and health-services databases. Anecdotal evidence provided to the present committee by the veterans suggests a potential association between the exposures in Vietnam and tonsil cancer, so this committee strongly reiterates the 2006 recommendation that VA develop a strategy for evaluating tonsil cancer in Vietnam-era veterans with existing databases.

Studies evaluated previously and in this report are summarized in Table 6-3.

Update of the Epidemiologic Literature

No studies of Vietnam veterans or of populations exposed to the chemicals of interest environmentally and oral, nasal, or pharyngeal cancers have been published since *Update 2006*.

Occupational Studies

Hansen et al. (2007) evaluated cancer incidence from May 1975 through 2001 in an occupational cohort of the Danish Union of General Workers identified from men working in 1973; their cancer incidence from 1975 to 1984 was reported in Hansen et al. (1992). The cohort of 3,156 male gardeners—whose pesticide exposure was primarily to herbicides, including phenoxyacetic acids—was matched to the Danish Cancer Registry to determine the observed cancer incidence; cancer cases were coded with ICD-7. The expected number of cancers was calculated by using national cancer incidences. The standardized incidence ratios (SIRs) were controlled for age and calendar time. The cohort was divided by year of birth, a proxy for exposure because pesticide use decreased over time. Three subcohorts were evaluated: high, early-birth cohort (born before 1915); low, late-birth cohort (born after 1934); and medium (born in 1915–1934). A total of 521 cancer cases were identified; nine were classified as originating in the buccal cavity or pharynx (ICD-7 140–148). The observed incidence of pharyngeal cancers was

TABLE 6-3 Selected Epidemiologic Studies—Oral, Nasal, and Pharyngeal
Cancer

Reference	Study Population[a]	Exposed Cases[b]	Estimated Relative Risk (95% CI)[b]
VIETNAM VETERANS			
Studies Reviewed in *Update 2006*			
ADVA, 2005a	Australian Vietnam veterans vs Australian population—incidence		
	Head and neck	247	1.5 (1.3–1.6)
	Navy	56	1.6 (1.1–2.0)
	Army	174	1.6 (1.3–1.8)
	Air Force	17	0.9 (0.5–1.5)
ADVA, 2005b	Australian Vietnam veterans vs Australian population—mortality		
	Head and neck	101	1.4 (1.2–1.7)
	Navy	22	1.5 (0.9–2.1)
	Army	69	1.5 (1.1–1.8)
	Air Force	9	1.1 (0.5–2.0)
	Nasal	3	0.8 (0.2–2.2)
ADVA, 2005c	Australian conscripted Army National Service Vietnam-era veterans: deployed vs nondeployed		
	Head and neck		
	Incidence	44	2.0 (1.2–3.4)
	Mortality	16	1.8 (0.8–4.3)
	Nasal		
	Mortality	0	0.0 (0.0–48.2)
Boehmer et al., 2004	Follow-up of CDC Vietnam Experience Cohort (ICD-9 140–149)	6	nr
Studies Reviewed in *Update 2004*			
Akhtar et al., 2004	White AFHS subjects vs national rates (buccal cavity)		
	Ranch Hand veterans		
	Incidence	6	0.9 (0.4–1.9)
	With tours in 1966–1970	6	1.1 (0.5–2.3)
	Mortality	0	0.0 (nr)
	Comparison veterans		
	Incidence	5	0.6 (0.2–1.2)
	With tours in 1966–1970	4	0.6 (0.2–1.4)
	Mortality	1	0.5 (nr)
Studies Reviewed in *Update 2000*			
AFHS, 2000	Air Force veterans participating in 1997 examination cycle, Ranch Hands vs comparisons (oral cavity, pharynx, and larynx)	4	0.6 (0.2–2.4)
Studies Reviewed in *Update 1998*			
CDVA, 1997a	Australian Vietnam veterans vs Australian population—incidence		
	Lip (ICD-9 140)	0	nr
	Nasopharyngeal cancer (ICD-9 147)	2	0.5 (0.1–1.7)
	Nasal cavities (ICD-9 160)	2	1.2 (0.1–4.1)

TABLE 6-3 Continued

Reference	Study Population[a]	Exposed Cases[b]	Estimated Relative Risk (95% CI)[b]
CDVA, 1997b	Australian conscripted Army National Service Vietnam-era veterans—deployed vs nondeployed		
	Nasopharyngeal cancer	1	1.3 (0.0– > 10)
	Nasal cavities	0	0.0 (0.0– > 10)
Visintainer et al., 1995	PM study of deaths (1974–1989) of Michigan Vietnam-era veterans—deployed vs nondeployed		
	Lip, oral cavity, and pharynx	12	1.0 (0.5–1.8)
Studies Reviewed in *VAO*			
CDC, 1990a	Case–control study of US males born 1929–1953		
	89 nasopharyngeal carcinomas		
	Vietnam service	3	0.5 (0.2–1.8)
	62 nasal carcinomas		
	Vietnam service	2	0.7 (0.2–2.9)
OCCUPATIONAL			
New Studies			
Hansen et al., 2007	Danish gardeners—incidence (buccal cavity and pharynx, ICD-7 140–148)		
	10-year follow-up (1975–1984) reported in Hansen et al. (1992)	6	1.1 (0.4–2.5)
	25-year follow-up (1975–2001)		
	Born before 1915 (high exposure)	3	0.7 (0.2–2.3)
	Born 1915–1934 (medium exposure)	6	0.7 (0.3–1.4)
	Born after 1934 (low exposure)	0	0.0 (0.0–1.0)
Studies Reviewed in *Update 2006*			
Alavanja et al., 2005	US AHS—incidence (buccal cavity)		
	Private applicators (men and women)	66	0.7 (0.5–0.8)
	Lip	25	1.4 (0.9–2.1)
	Spouses of private applicators (> 99% women)	14	0.7 (0.4–1.2)
	Lip	2	1.4 (0.2–5.1)
	Commercial applicators (men and women)	5	0.9 (0.3–2.2)
	Lip	3	2.7 (0.6–8.0)
Blair et al., 2005a	US AHS (buccal cavity, and pharynx)		
	Private applicators (men and women)	5	0.3 (0.1–0.7)
	Spouses of private applicators (> 99% women)	0	0.0 (0.0–25.4)
McLean et al., 2006	IARC cohort of pulp and paper workers		
	Exposure to nonvolatile organochlorine compounds (oral cavity, and pharynx)		
	Never	33	0.9 (0.6–1.3)
	Ever	15	0.5 (0.3–0.9)
't Mannetje et al., 2005	Phenoxy herbicide producers (men and women) (ICD-9 140–149)	2	2.8 (0.3–9.9)
	Lip (ICD-9 140)	0	nr
	Mouth (ICD-9 141–145)	2	5.4 (0.7–20)
	Oropharynx (ICD-9 146)	0	nr
	Nasopharynx (ICD-9 147)	0	0.0 (0.0–42)

continued

TABLE 6-3 Continued

Reference	Study Population[a]	Exposed Cases[b]	Estimated Relative Risk (95% CI)[b]
	Hypopharynx, other (ICD-9 148–149)	0	nr
	Phenoxy herbicide sprayers (> 99% men) (ICD-9 140–149)	1	1.0 (0.0–5.7)
	Lip (ICD-9 140)	0	nr
	Mouth (ICD-9 141–145)	0	0.0 (0.0–7.5)
	Oropharynx (ICD-9 146)	0	nr
	Nasopharynx (ICD-9 147)	1	8.3 (0.2–46)
	Hypopharynx, other (ICD-9 148–149)	0	nr
Torchio et al., 1994	Italian licensed pesticide users		
	Buccal cavity, pharynx	18	0.3 (0.2–0.5)
Reif et al., 1989	New Zealand forestry workers—incidence		
	Buccal cavity	3	0.7 (0.2–2.2)
	Nasopharynx	2	5.6 (1.6–19.5)
Studies Reviewed in *Update 2004*			
Nordby et al., 2004	Norwegian farmers born 1925–1971—incidence, lip		
	Reported pesticide use	nr	0.7 (0.4–1.0)
Swaen et al., 2004	Dutch licensed herbicide applicators		
	Nose	0	nr
	Mouth, pharynx	0	nr
Studies Reviewed in *Update 2000*			
Caplan et al., 2000	Case–control study of US males born 1929–1953, all 70 nasal cancers (carcinomas, 11 lymphomas, 5 sarcomas) in CDC (1990a) study population		
	Selected landscaping, forestry occupations	26	1.8 (1.1–3.1)
	Living, working on farm	23	0.5 (0.3–0.8)
	Herbicides, pesticides	19	0.7 (0.4–1.3)
	Phenoxy herbicides	5	1.2 (0.4–3.3)
Studies Reviewed in *Update 1998*			
Hooiveld et al., 1998	Dutch chemical production workers included in IARC cohort (lip, oral cavity, pharynx)		
	All working any time in 1955–1985	1	2.3 (0.1–12.4)
	Cleaned up 1963 explosion	1	7.1 (0.2–39.6)
Rix et al., 1998	Danish male, female paper-mill workers		
	Buccal cavity (ICD-7 140–144)		
	Men	24	1.0 (0.7–1.5)
	Women	4	1.5 (0.4–3.8)
	Pharynx (ICD-7 145–149)		
	Men	15	2.0 (1.1–3.3)
	Women	2	2.1 (0.2–7.6)
	Tonsil cancers among pharyngeal cancers	11	nr
Kogevinas et al., 1997	IARC cohort, male and female workers exposed to any phenoxy herbicide or chlorophenol		
	Oral cavity, pharynx cancer (ICD-9 140–149)	26	1.1 (0.7–1.6)
	Exposed to highly chlorinated PCDDs	22	1.3 (0.8–2.0)
	Not exposed to highly chlorinated PCDDs	3	0.5 (0.1–1.3)

TABLE 6-3 Continued

Reference	Study Population[a]	Exposed Cases[b]	Estimated Relative Risk (95% CI)[b]
	Nose, nasal sinus cancer (ICD-9 160)	3	1.6 (0.3–4.7)
	Exposed to highly chlorinated PCDDs	0	0.0 (0.0–3.5)
	Not exposed to highly chlorinated PCDDs	3	3.8 (0.8–11.1)
Studies Reviewed in *Update 1996*			
Becher et al., 1996	German phenoxy herbicide production workers (included in IARC cohort)		
	Buccal cavity, pharynx (ICD-9 140–149)	9	3.0 (1.4–5.6)
	Tongue	3	nr
	Floor of mouth	2	nr
	Tonsil	2	nr
	Pharynx	2	nr
Asp et al., 1994	Finnish herbicide applicators		
	Buccal, pharynx (ICD-8 140–149)		
	Incidence	5	1.0 (0.3–2.3)
	Mortality	0	0.0 (0.0–3.0)
	"Other respiratory" (ICD-8 160, 161, 163)— nose, larynx, pleura		
	Incidence	4	1.1 (0.3–2.7)
	Mortality	1	0.5 (0.0–2.9)
Studies Reviewed in *VAO*			
Blair et al., 1993	White male farmers in 23 states—deaths 1984–1988		
	Lip	21	2.3 (1.4–3.5)
Ronco et al., 1992	Italian farmers (lip, tongue, salivary glands, mouth, pharynx)—mortality		
	Self-employed	13	0.9 (nr)
	Employees	4	0.5 (nr)
	Danish self-employed farmers—incidence		
	Lip	182	1.8 (p < 0.05)
	Tongue	9	0.6 (nr)
	Salivary glands	13	0.9 (nr)
	Mouth	14	0.5 (p < 0.05)
	Pharynx	13	0.3 (p < 0.05)
	Nasal cavities, sinuses	11	0.6 (nr)
	Danish farming employees—incidence		
	Lip	43	2.1 (p < 0.05)
	Tongue	2	0.6 (nr)
	Salivary glands	0	0.0 (nr)
	Mouth	0	0.0 (p < 0.05)
	Pharynx	9	1.1 (nr)
	Nasal cavities and sinuses	5	1.3 (nr)
Saracci et al., 1991	IARC cohort—exposed subcohort (males, females)		
	Buccal cavity, pharynx (ICD-8 140–149)	11	1.2 (0.6–2.1)
	Nose, nasal cavities (ICD-8 160)	3	2.9 (0.6–8.5)
Zober et al., 1990	BASF Aktiengesellschaft accident cohort—33 cancers in 247 workers at 34-year follow-up		
	Squamous-cell carcinoma of tonsil	1	nr

continued

TABLE 6-3 Continued

Reference	Study Population[a]	Exposed Cases[b]	Estimated Relative Risk (95% CI)[b]
Wiklund et al., 1989a	Licensed Swedish pesticide applicators—incidence		
	Lip	14	1.8 (1.0–2.9)
Coggon et al., 1986	British MCPA production workers (included in IARC cohort)		
	Lip (ICD-9 140)	0	nr
	Tongue (ICD-9 141)	1	1.1 (0.0–6.2)
	Pharynx (ICD-9 146–149)	1	0.5 (0.0–3.0)
	Nose (ICD-9 160)	3	4.9 (1.0–14.4)
Robinson et al., 1986	Northwestern US paper and pulp workers		90% CI
	Buccal cavity, pharynx (ICD-7 140–148)	1	0.1 (0.0–0.7)
	Nasal (ICD-7 160)	0	nr
Wiklund, 1983	Swedish male and female agricultural workers—incidence		99% CI
	Lip	508	1.8 (1.6–2.1)
	Tongue	32	0.4 (0.2–0.6)
	Salivary glands	68	1.0 (0.7–1.4)
	Mouth	70	0.6 (0.5–0.8)
	Throat	84	0.5 (0.4–0.7)
	Nose, nasal sinuses	64	0.8 (0.6–1.2)
Hardell et al., 1982	Residents of northern Sweden (44 nasal, 27 nasopharyngeal cancers)		
	Phenoxy acid exposure	8	2.1 (0.9–4.7)
	Chlorophenol exposure	9	6.7 (2.8–16.2)
Burmeister et al., 1981	Iowa farmers—deaths in 1971–1978		
	Lip	20	2.1 (p < 0.01)
ENVIRONMENTAL			
Studies Reviewed in *VAO*			
Bertazzi et al., 1993	Seveso residents—10-year follow-up—incidence		
	Buccal cavity (ICD-9 140–149)		
	Zone B—Men	6	1.7 (0.8–3.9)
	Women	0	nr
	Zone R—Men	28	1.2 (0.8–1.7)
	Women	0	nr
	Nose, nasal cavities (ICD-9 160)		
	Zone R—Men	0	nr
	Women	2	2.6 (0.5–13.3)

ABBREVIATIONS: AFHS, Air Force Health Study; AHS, Agricultural Health Study; CDC, Centers for Disease Control and Prevention; CI, confidence interval; IARC, International Agency for Research on Cancer; ICD, International Classification of Diseases; MCPA, 2 methyl-4-chlorophenoxyacetic acid; nr, not reported; PCDDs, chlorinated dibenzo-*p*-dioxins (highly chlorinated, if four or more chlorines); PM, proportionate mortality; TCDD, 2,3,7,8-tetrachlorodibenzo-*p*-dioxin.

[a] Subjects are male and outcome is mortality unless otherwise noted.

[b] Given when available; results other than estimated risk explained individually.

Studies in italics have been superseded by newer studies of same cohort.

lower than the expected incidence for all birth cohorts examined. For men born before 1915, the SIR was 0.74 (95% confidence interval [CI] 0.24–2.29). A reduced incidence was also observed in men born in 1915–1934 (SIR = 0.65, 95% CI 0.29–1.44). No cases were observed in men born after 1934. Nasal cancers were grouped in the respiratory-cancer category (ICD-7 160–165). The SIRs for respiratory cancers were also lower than expected, with SIRs of 0.90 (95% CI 0.64–1.26), 0.98 (95% CI 0.78–1.23), and 0.84 (95% CI 0.42–1.69) in the early-, intermediate-, and late-birth cohorts, respectively. The study was limited by the inability to examine incidence by pesticide class (for example, herbicides) and the lack of confounder data.

Biologic Plausibility

Long-term animal studies have examined the effect of exposure to the chemicals of interest on tumor incidences (Charles et al., 1996; Stott et al., 1990; Walker et al., 2006; Wanibuchi et al., 2004). A recent National Toxicology Program study (Yoshizawa et al., 2005a) reported an increase in the incidence of gingival squamous-cell carcinoma in female rats treated orally (by gavage) with TCDD at 100 ng/kg 5 days/week for 104 weeks. Incidences of gingival squamous-cell hyperplasia were significantly increased in all groups treated at 3–46 ng/kg. In addition, squamous-cell carcinoma in the oral mucosa of the palate was increased. Increased neoplasms of the oral mucosa were previously observed and described as carcinomas of the hard palate and nasal turbinates (Kociba et al., 1978). Kociba et al. (1978) also reported a small increase in the incidence of tongue squamous-cell carcinoma. A similar 2-year study performed in female rats failed to reveal a pathologic effect of TCDD on nasal tissues (Nyska et al., 2005).

The biologic plausibility of the carcinogenicity of the chemicals of interest is discussed in general at the beginning of this chapter.

Synthesis

The single study reporting on oral, nasal, and pharyngeal cancers found nothing suggestive of an association with the herbicides sprayed in Vietnam.

Conclusion

On the basis of the evidence reviewed here and in previous VAO reports, the committee concludes that there is inadequate or insufficient evidence to determine whether there is an association between exposure to the chemicals of interest and oral, nasal, or pharyngeal cancers.

CANCERS OF THE DIGESTIVE ORGANS

Until *Update 2006*, VAO committees had reviewed "gastrointestinal tract tumors" as a group consisting of stomach, colorectal, and pancreatic cancers, with esophageal cancer being formally factored in only since *Update 2002*. With more evidence from occupational studies available, VAO updates now address cancers of the digestive organs individually. Findings on cancers of the digestive organs as a group (ICD-9 150–159) are too broad for useful etiologic analysis and will no longer be considered.

Esophageal cancer (ICD-9 150), stomach cancer (ICD-9 151), colon cancer (ICD-9 153), rectal cancer (ICD-9 154), and pancreatic cancer (ICD-9 157) are among the most common cancers. ACS estimated that about 224,460 people would receive diagnoses of those cancers in the United States in 2008 and 109,410 people would die from them (Jemal et al., 2008a). When other digestive cancers (for example, small intestine, anal, and hepatobiliary) were included, the 2008 estimates for the United States were about 271,290 new diagnoses and 135,130 deaths (Jemal et al., 2008a). Collectively, tumors of the digestive organs were expected to account for 19% of new diagnoses and 24% of cancer deaths in 2008. The average annual incidences of gastrointestinal cancers are presented in Table 6-4.

TABLE 6-4 Average Annual Incidence (per 100,000) of Selected Gastrointestinal Cancers in United States[a]

	50–54 Years Old			55–59 Years Old			60–64 Years Old		
	All Races	White	Black	All Races	White	Black	All Races	White	Black
Stomach:									
Men	9.2	8.0	16.8	15. 8	14.0	22.3	24.1	21.0	44.1
Women	4.7	3.8	7.9	7.0	5.7	11.7	9.5	7.6	17.5
Esophagus:									
Men	9.4	9.5	12.8	16.8	16.9	25.2	23.9	24.2	33.7
Women	1.7	1.5	4.6	3.2	2.8	8.0	4.9	5.0	9.4
Colon (excluding rectum):									
Men	35.8	34.2	50.0	57.1	54.9	85.6	94.9	91.1	144.4
Women	28.5	26.3	44.1	43.9	39.8	77.3	69.9	66.5	112.4
Rectum and rectosigmoid junction:									
Men	25.0	23.9	27.3	33.6	32.6	31.3	49.5	49.3	47.2
Women	15.1	14.6	19.5	21.0	20.4	27.0	26.5	25.8	34.6
Liver and intrahepatic bile duct:									
Men	19.0	15.3	34.3	21.2	15.7	49.6	24.9	18.0	44.1
Women	3.4	2.5	6.6	5.1	4.1	9.1	8.1	5.8	11.2
Pancreas:									
Men	13.1	12.6	20.7	21.4	20.7	32.1	34.6	33.5	48.0
Women	8.1	7.7	12.5	14.2	13.5	18.6	24.2	23.3	39.0

TABLE 6-4 Continued

	50–54 Years Old			55–59 Years Old			60–64 Years Old		
	All Races	White	Black	All Races	White	Black	All Races	White	Black
Small Intestine:									
Men	3.3	3.1	5.5	5.1	4.8	10.3	5.9	5.6	8.5
Women	2.0	1.9	4.0	3.2	3.2	4.6	4.4	4.2	8.1
Anus, anal canal, and anorectum:									
Men	2.4	2.3	4.3	2.7	2.9	2.6	3.5	3.8	2.3
Women	3.2	3.6	3.5	3.7	3.8	5.5	4.3	4.7	3.2
Other digestive organs:									
Men	0.7	0.6	0.9	1.1	1.0	2.1	1.3	1.4	1.2
Women	0.6	0.6	0.8	0.8	0.8	0.9	1.2	1.2	1.3
Gallbladder:									
Men	0.4	0.4	0.2	1.0	0.8	1.3	1.6	1.6	1.6
Women	1.1	1.0	1.6	2.1	1.9	2.2	2.9	2.8	2.8
Other Biliary:									
Men	1.4	1.2	2.1	2.6	2.4	3.7	4.7	4.6	4.3
Women	1.1	1.1	1.3	1.6	1.5	1.3	3.1	3.1	2.8

[a] Surveillance, Epidemiology, and End Results program, nine standard registries, crude age-specific rates, 2000–2005.

The incidences of stomach, colon, rectal, and pancreatic cancers increase with age. In general, incidence is higher in men than in women and higher in blacks than in whites. Other risk factors for the cancers vary but always include family history of the same form of cancer, some diseases of the affected organ, and diet. Tobacco use is a risk factor for pancreatic cancer and possibly stomach cancer (Miller et al., 1996). Infection with the bacterium *Helicobacter pylori* increases the risk of stomach cancer. Type 2 diabetes is associated with an increased risk of cancers of the colon and pancreas (ACS, 2006).

Esophageal Cancer

Epithelial tumors of the esophagus (squamous-cell carcinomas and adenocarcinomas) are responsible for more than 95% of all esophageal cancers (ICD-9 150); 16,470 newly diagnosed cases and 14,280 deaths were estimated for 2008 (Jemal et al., 2008a). The considerable geographic variation in the incidence of esophageal tumors suggests a multifactorial etiology. Rates of esophageal cancer have been increasing in the last 2 decades. Adenocarcinoma of the esophagus has slowly replaced squamous-cell carcinoma as the most common type of esophageal malignancy in the United States and western Europe (Blot and McLaughlin, 1999). Squamous-cell esophageal carcinoma rates are higher in blacks than in whites and in men than in women. Smoking and alcohol ingestion are associated with the development of squamous-cell carcinoma; these risk factors have been less thoroughly studied for esophageal adenocarcinoma, but they appear to be associated. The rapid increase in obesity in the United States has been linked to increasing rates of gastroesophageal reflux disease (GERD), and the resulting rise in chronic inflammation has been hypothesized to explain the link between GERD and esophageal adenocarcinoma.

Conclusions from *VAO* and Previous Updates

The committee responsible for *VAO* explicitly excluded esophageal cancer from the group of gastrointestinal tract tumors, for which it was concluded that there was limited or suggestive evidence of *no* association with exposure to the herbicides used by the US military in Vietnam. Esophageal cancers were not separately evaluated and were not categorized with this group until *Update 2004*. For *Update 2006*, the committee concluded that there was not enough evidence on each of the chemicals of interest to sustain this negative conclusion for any of the cancers in the gastrointestinal group and that, because these various types of cancer are generally regarded as separate disease entities, the evidence on each should be evaluated separately. Esophageal cancer was thus reclassified to the default category of inadequate or insufficient evidence to determine whether there is an association. Table 6-5 summarizes the results of the relevant studies concerning esophageal cancer.

Update of the Epidemiologic Literature

No studies concerning exposure to the chemicals of interest and esophageal cancer have been published since *Update 2006*.

Biologic Plausibility

Long-term animal studies have examined the effect of exposure to the chemicals of interest on tumor incidence (Charles et al., 1996; Stott et al., 1990; Walker et al., 2006; Wanibuchi et al., 2004). No increase in the incidence of esophageal cancer has been reported in laboratory animals after exposure to them.

The biologic plausibility of the carcinogenicity of the chemicals of interest is discussed in general at the beginning of this chapter.

TABLE 6-5 Selected Epidemiologic Studies—Esophageal Cancer

Reference	Study Population[a]	Exposed Cases[b]	Estimated Relative Risk (95% CI)[b]
VIETNAM VETERANS			
Studies Reviewed in *Update 2006*			
ADVA, 2005a	Australian male Vietnam veterans vs Australian population—incidence	70	1.2 (0.9–1.5)
	Navy	19	1.6 (0.9–2.4)
	Army	40	1.1 (0.7–1.4)
	Air Force	11	1.5 (0.8–2.8)
ADVA, 2005b	Australian male Vietnam veterans vs Australian population—mortality	67	1.1 (0.8–1.3)
	Navy	13	1.0 (0.5–1.7)
	Army	42	1.0 (0.7–1.3)
	Air Force	12	1.5 (0.8–2.6)
ADVA, 2005c	Australian male conscripted Army National Service Vietnam-era veterans: deployed vs nondeployed		
	Incidence	9	1.9 (0.6–6.6)
	Mortality	10	1.3 (0.5–3.6)
Boehmer et al., 2004	Follow-up of CDC Vietnam Experience Cohort	6	1.2 (0.4–4.0)
Studies Reviewed in *Update 1998*			
CDVA, 1997a	Australian military Vietnam veterans	23	1.2 (0.7–1.7)
CDVA, 1997b	Australian National Service Vietnam veterans	1	1.3 (0.0– > 10)
Visintainer et al., 1995	PM study of deaths (1974–1989) of Michigan Vietnam-era veterans—deployed vs nondeployed	9	0.9 (0.4–1.6)
OCCUPATIONAL			
Studies Reviewed in *Update 2006*			
McLean et al., 2006	IARC cohort of pulp and paper workers		
	Exposure to nonvolatile organochlorine compounds		
	Never	27	0.7 (0.4–1.0)
	Ever	26	0.8 (0.5–1.2)
't Mannetje et al., 2005	Phenoxy herbicide producers (men and women)	2	2.0 (0.2–7.0)
	Phenoxy herbicide sprayers (> 99% men)	1	0.7 (0.0–4.0)
Blair et al., 2005a	US AHS		
	Private applicators (men and women)	16	0.5 (0.3–0.9)
	Spouses of private applicators (> 99% women)	1	0.3 (0.1–1.9)
Lee et al., 2004a	Population-based case–control—agricultural pesticide use and adenocarcinoma of the esophagus	137	
	Insecticides		0.7 (0.4–1.1)
	Herbicides		0.7 (0.4–1.2)
Reif et al., 1989	New Zealand forestry workers—nested case–control (incidence) correspondence	4	1.8 (0.7–4.8)
Magnani et al., 1987	UK case–control		
	Herbicides	nr	1.6 (0.7–3.6)
	Chlorophenols	nr	1.2 (0.7–2.2)

continued

TABLE 6-5 Continued

Reference	Study Population[a]	Exposed Cases[b]	Estimated Relative Risk (95% CI)[b]
Studies Reviewed in *Update 1998*			
Kogevinas et al., 1997	IARC cohort, male and female workers exposed to any phenoxy herbicide or chlorophenol	28	1.0 (0.7–1.4)
	Exposed to highly chlorinated PCDDs	20	1.3 (0.8–1.9)
	Not exposed to highly chlorinated PCDDs	6	0.5 (0.2–1.1)
Studies Reviewed in *Update 1996*			
Asp et al., 1994	Finnish herbicide applicators—incidence	3	1.6 (0.3–4.6)
	Finnish herbicide applicators—mortality	2	1.3 (0.2–4.7)
Studies Reviewed in *VAO*			
Ronco et al., 1992	Danish farm workers—incidence		
	Male—Self-employed	32	0.4 (p < 0.05)
	Employee	13	0.9 (nr)
	Female—Self-employed	1	1.4 (nr)
	Family worker	2	0.4 (nr)
Saracci et al., 1991	IARC cohort—exposed subcohort (men and women)	8	0.6 (0.3–1.2)
Coggon et al., 1986	British MCPA production workers (included in IARC cohort)	8	0.9 (0.4–1.9)
Wiklund, 1983	Swedish male and female agricultural workers—incidence	169	99% CI 0.6 (0.5–0.7)

ENVIRONMENTAL

None

ABBREVIATIONS: AHS, Agricultural Health Study; CDC, Centers for Disease Control and Prevention; CI, confidence interval; IARC, International Agency for Research on Cancer; MCPA, methyl-4-chlorophenoxyacetic acid; nr, not reported; PCDD, polychlorinated dibenzo-*p*-dioxin (highly chlorinated, if four or more chlorines).

[a] Subjects are male and outcome is mortality unless otherwise noted.

[b] Given when available; results other than estimated risk explained individually.

Studies in italics have been superseded by newer studies of same cohort.

Synthesis

No epidemiologic evidence concerning the chemicals of interest and esophageal cancer has been published since *Update 2006*. No toxicologic studies provide evidence of the biologic plausibility of an association between the chemicals of interest and tumors of the esophagus.

Conclusion

On the basis of the evidence reviewed here and in previous VAO reports, the committee concludes that there is inadequate or insufficient evidence to determine whether there is an association between exposure to the chemicals of interest and esophageal cancer.

Stomach Cancer

The incidence of stomach cancer (ICD-9 151) increases in people 50–64 years old. ACS estimated that 13,190 men and 8,310 women would develop new cases of stomach cancer in the United States in 2008 and 6,450 men and 4,430 women would die from it (Jemal et al., 2008a). In general, the incidence is higher in men than in women and higher in blacks than in whites. Other risk factors include family history of this cancer, some diseases of the stomach, and diet. Infection with the bacterium *Helicobacter pylori* increases the risk of stomach cancer. Tobacco use and consumption of nitrite- and salt-preserved food may also increase the risk of stomach cancer (Brenner et al., 2009; Key et al., 2004; Miller et al., 1996).

Conclusions from *VAO* and Previous Updates

Update 2006 considered stomach cancer independently for the first time. Prior updates developed a table of results for stomach cancer, but conclusions about the adequacy of the evidence of its association with herbicide exposure had been reached in the context of gastrointestinal tract cancers. The committee responsible for *VAO* concluded that there was limited or suggestive evidence of *no* association between exposure to the herbicides used by the US military in Vietnam and gastrointestinal tract tumors, including stomach cancer. The committee responsible for *Update 2006* concluded that there was not enough evidence on each of the chemicals of interest to sustain this negative conclusion for any of the cancers in the gastrointestinal group and that, because these various types of cancer are generally regarded as separate disease entities, the evidence on each should be evaluated separately. Stomach cancer was thus reclassified to the default category of inadequate or insufficient evidence to determine whether there was an association. Table 6-6 summarizes the results of the relevant studies concerning stomach cancer.

Update of the Epidemiologic Literature

Vietnam-Veteran Studies   No studies of exposure to the chemicals of interest and stomach cancer in Vietnam veterans have been published since *Update 2006*.

Occupational Studies   Mills and Yang (2007) conducted a nested case–control study of gastric cancer in the United Farm Workers of America (UFW) cohort and identified 100 cases of gastic cancer newly diagnosed during 1988–2003.

TABLE 6-6 Selected Epidemiologic Studies—Stomach Cancer

Reference	Study Population[a]	Exposed Cases[b]	Estimated Relative Risk (95% CI)[b]
VIETNAM VETERANS			
Studies reviewed in *Update 2006*			
ADVA, 2005a	Australian male Vietnam veterans vs Australian population—incidence	104	0.9 (0.7–1.1)
	Navy	28	1.1 (0.7–1.6)
	Army	66	0.9 (0.7–1.1)
	Air Force	10	0.7 (0.3–1.3)
ADVA, 2005b	Australian male Vietnam veterans vs Australian population—mortality	76	0.9 (0.7–1.2)
	Navy	22	1.3 (0.8–1.8)
	Army	50	0.9 (0.7–1.2)
	Air Force	4	0.4 (0.1–1.0)
ADVA, 2005c	Australian male conscripted Army National Service Vietnam-era veterans: deployed vs nondeployed		
	Incidence	11	0.6 (0.2–1.2)
	Mortality	7	0.7 (0.2–2.0)
Pavuk et al., 2005	Comparison subjects only from AFHS (digestive system)—incidence		
	Serum TCDD (pg/g) based on model with exposure variable $\log_e$(TCDD)		
	Per unit increase of $-\log_e$(TCDD) (pg/g)	24	1.8 (0.8–3.9)
	Quartiles (pg/g)		
	0.4–2.6	4	nr
	2.6–3.8	3	1.0 (0.2–4.8)
	3.8–5.2	7	2.0 (0.5–8.2)
	> 5.2	10	3.3 (0.9–12.5)
	Number of years served in SEA		
	Per year of service	24	1.2 (1.0–1.4)
	Quartiles (years in SEA)		
	0.8–1.3	4	nr
	1.3–2.1	4	1.0 (0.2–3.8)
	2.1–3.7	5	1.1 (0.3–4.2)
	3.7–16.4	11	2.1 (0.6–7.3)
Boehmer et al., 2004	Follow-up of CDC Vietnam Experience Cohort (stomach)	5	nr
Studies Reviewed in *Update 2004*			
Akhtar et al., 2004	White AFHS subjects vs national rates (digestive system)		
	Ranch Hand veterans		
	Incidence	16	0.6 (0.4–1.0)
	Tours 1966–1970	14	0.6 (0.4–1.1)
	Mortality	6	0.4 (0.2–0.9)
	Comparison veterans		
	Incidence	31	0.9 (0.6–1.2)
	Tours 1966–1970	24	0.9 (0.6–1.3)
	Mortality	14	0.7 (0.4–1.1)

TABLE 6-6 Continued

Reference	Study Population[a]	Exposed Cases[b]	Estimated Relative Risk (95% CI)[b]
Studies Reviewed in *Update 1998*			
CDVA, 1997a	Australian military Vietnam veterans	32	1.1 (0.7–1.4)
CDVA, 1997b	Australian National Service Vietnam veterans	4	1.7 (0.3– > 10)
Studies Reviewed in *VAO*			
Breslin et al., 1988	Army Vietnam veterans	88	1.1 (0.9–1.5)
	Marine Vietnam veterans	17	0.8 (0.4–1.6)
Anderson et al., 1986	Wisconsin Vietnam veterans	1	nr
OCCUPATIONAL			
New Studies			
Mills and Yang, 2007	Nested case–control study of agricultural exposure and gastric cancer in UFW cohort		
	Ever worked in area where 2,4-D used	42	1.9 (1.1–3.3)
	Quartile of lifetime exposure to 2,4-D (lb)		
	0	58	1.0
	1–14	17	2.2 (1.0–4.6)
	15–85	14	1.6 (0.7–3.5)
	86–1,950	11	2.1 (0.9–5.1)
Ekström et al., 1999	Case–control study of Swedish residents with gastric adenocarcinoma		
	All occupational herbicide exposure	75	1.6 (1.1–2.2)
	Phenoxyacetic acid exposure	62	1.8 (1.3–2.6)
	Hormoslyr (2,4-D and 2,4,5-T)	48	1.7 (1.2–2.6)
	2,4-D only	3	nr (vs 0 controls)
	MCPA	11	1.8 (0.8–4.1)
	Duration of exposure		
	Nonexposed to all herbicides	490	1.0
	< 1 month	11	1.6 (0.7–3.5)
	1–6 months	30	1.9 (1.1–3.2)
	7–12 months	7	1.7 (0.6–4.7)
	> 1 year	13	1.4 (0.6–3.0)
	Other herbicide exposure	13	1.0 (0.5–1.9)
Studies Reviewed in *Update 2006*			
McLean et al., 2006	IARC cohort of pulp and paper workers		
	Exposure to nonvolatile organochlorine compounds		
	Never	146	0.9 (0.8–1.1)
	Ever	98	0.9 (0.7–1.1)
't Mannetje et al., 2005	Phenoxy herbicide producers (men and women)	2	1.1 (0.1–4.0)
	Phenoxy herbicide sprayers (> 99% men)	3	1.4 (0.3–4.0)

continued

TABLE 6-6 Continued

Reference	Study Population[a]	Exposed Cases[b]	Estimated Relative Risk (95% CI)[b]
Alavanja et al., 2005	AHS—incidence (all digestive cancers)		
	Private applicators (men and women)	462	0.8 (0.8–0.9)
	Spouses of private applicators (> 99% women)	161	0.9 (0.7–1.0)
	Commercial applicators (men and women)	24	1.0 (0.6–1.4)
Blair et al., 2005a	AHS (stomach cancers)		
	Private applicators (men and women)	10	0.5 (0.2–1.0)
	Spouses of private applicators (> 99% women)	4	1.1 (0.3–2.8)
Lee et al., 2004a	Population-based case–control—agricultural pesticide use and adenocarcinoma of stomach	170	
	Insecticides		0.9 (0.6–1.4)
	Herbicides		0.9 (0.5–1.4)
Torchio et al., 1994	Italian licensed pesticide users	126	0.7 (0.6–0.9)
Reif et al., 1989	New Zealand forestry workers—nested case–control (incidence)	13	2.2 (1.3–3.9)
Studies Reviewed in *Update 2004*			
Bodner et al., 2003	Dow production workers (included in the IARC cohort, NIOSH Dioxin Registry)	nr	1.5 (0.7–2.7)
Swaen et al., 2004	Dutch licensed herbicide applicators (stomach and small intestine)	3	0.4 (0.1–1.3)
Studies Reviewed in *Update 2002*			
Burns et al., 2001	Dow 2,4-D production workers (included in the IARC cohort, NIOSH Dioxin Registry)		
	Digestive organs, peritoneum	16	0.7 (0.4–1.2)
Studies Reviewed in *Update 2000*			
Steenland et al., 1999	US chemical production workers (included in IARC cohort, NIOSH Dioxin Registry)	13	1.0 (0.6–1.8)
Hooiveld et al., 1998	Dutch chemical production workers (included in IARC cohort)	3	1.0 (0.2–2.9)
Rix et al., 1998	Danish paper-mill workers—incidence		
	Men	48	1.1 (0.8–1.4)
	Women	7	1.0 (0.4–2.1)
Studies Reviewed in *Update 1998*			
Gambini et al., 1997	Italian rice growers	39	1.0 (0.7–1.3)
Kogevinas et al., 1997	IARC cohort, male and female workers exposed to any phenoxy herbicide or chlorophenol	72	0.9 (0.7–1.1)
	Exposed to highly chlorinated PCDDs	42	0.9 (0.7–1.2)
	Not exposed to highly chlorinated PCDDs	30	0.9 (0.6–1.3)
Becher et al., 1996	German production workers (included in IARC cohort)		
	Plant I	12	1.3 (0.7–2.2)
	Plant II	0	nr
	Plant III	0	nr
	Plant IV	2	0.6 (0.1–2.3)

TABLE 6-6 Continued

Reference	Study Population[a]	Exposed Cases[b]	Estimated Relative Risk (95% CI)[b]
Ott and	BASF employees—incidence	3	1.0 (0.2–2.9)
Zober, 1996	TCDD < 0.1 µg/kg of body weight	0	0.0 (0.0–3.4)
	TCDD 0.1–0.99 µg/kg of body weight	1	1.3 (0.0–7.0)
	TCDD ≥ 1 µg/kg of body weight	2	1.7 (0.2–6.2)
Ramlow	Dow pentachlorophenol production workers		
et al., 1996	(included in IARC cohort, NIOSH Dioxin Registry)		
	0-year latency	4	1.7 (0.5–4.3)
	15-year latency	3	1.8 (0.4–5.2)
Studies Reviewed in *Update 1996*			
Blair et al.,	US farmers in 23 states		
1993	White men	657	1.0 (1.0–1.1)
	White women	12	1.2 (0.6–2.0)
Bueno de	Dutch phenoxy herbicide workers (included in		
Mesquita	IARC cohort)	2	0.7 (0.1–2.7)
et al., 1993			
Collins	Monsanto Company workers (included in NIOSH		
et al., 1993	cohort)	0	0.0 (0.0–1.1)
Kogevinas	IARC cohort—women		
et al., 1993		1	1.4 (nr)
Studies Reviewed in *VAO*			
Ronco et al.,	Danish farm workers—incidence		
1992	Men	286	0.9 (nr)
	Women	5	1.0 (nr)
Swaen	Dutch licensed herbicide applicators (stomach and		
et al., 1992	small intestine)	1	0.5 (0.0–2.7)
Fingerhut	NIOSH—entire cohort	10	1.0 (0.5–1.9)
et al., 1991	≥ 1-year exposure, ≥ 20-year latency	4	1.4 (0.4–3.5)
Manz et al.,	German production workers—men, women		
1991	(included in IARC cohort)		
	Men	12	1.2 (0.6–2.1)
Saracci	IARC cohort—exposed subcohort (men and women)	40	0.9 (0.6–1.2)
et al., 1991			
Wigle et al.,	Canadian farmers	246	0.9 (0.8–1.0)
1990			
Zober et al.,			90% CI
1990	BASF employees—basic cohort	3	3.0 (0.8–7.7)
Alavanja	USDA forest, soil conservationists	9	0.7 (0.3–1.3)
et al., 1989			
Henneberger	New Hampshire pulp and paper workers	5	1.2 (0.4–2.8)
et al., 1989			
Solet et al.,	US paper and pulp workers	1	0.5 (0.1–3.0)
1989			
Alavanja	USDA agricultural extension agents	10	0.7 (0.4–1.4)
et al., 1988			

continued

TABLE 6-6 Continued

Reference	Study Population[a]	Exposed Cases[b]	Estimated Relative Risk (95% CI)[b]
Bond et al., 1988	Dow 2,4-D production workers (included in IARC cohort, NIOSH Dioxin Registry)	0	nr (0.0–3.7)
Thomas, 1987	US flavor and fragrance chemical plant workers	6	Expected exposed cases 4.2
Coggon et al., 1986	British MCPA production workers (included in IARC cohort)	26	0.9 (0.6–1.3)
Robinson et al., 1986	Northwestern US paper and pulp workers	17	90% CI 1.2 (0.8–1.9)
Lynge, 1985	Danish production workers—incidence (included in IARC cohort)		
	Men	12	1.3 (nr)
	Women	1	0.7 (nr)
Blair et al., 1983			Expected exposed cases
	Florida pesticide applicators	4	3.3
Burmeister et al., 1983	Iowa residents—farming exposures	1,812	1.3 (p < 0.05)
Wiklund, 1983	Swedish male and female agricultural workers—incidence	2,599	99% CI 1.1 (1.0–1.2)
Burmeister, 1981	Iowa farmers	338	1.1 (p < 0.01)
Axelson et al., 1980	Swedish railroad workers—total exposure	3	2.2 (nr)
ENVIRONMENTAL			
New Studies			
Consonni et al., 2008	Seveso residents—25-year follow-up—men, women		
	Zone A	3	0.7 (0.2–2.0)
	Zone B	24	0.8 (0.5–1.2)
	Zone R	212	1.0 (0.8–1.1)
Studies Reviewed in *Update 2004*			
Fukuda et al., 2003	Residents of Japanese municipalities with and without waste-incineration plants		Age-adjusted mortality (per 100,000)
	Men		
	With		38.2 ± 7.8 vs 39.0
	Without		± 8.8 (p = 0.29)
	Women		
	With		20.7 ± 5.0 vs 20.7
	Without		± 5.8 (p = 0.92)
Studies Reviewed in *Update 2002*			
Revich et al., 2001	Residents of Chapaevsk, Russia		
	Men	59	1.7 (1.3–2.2)
	Women	45	0.7 (0.5–0.9)
Studies Reviewed in *Update 2000*			

TABLE 6-6 Continued

Reference	Study Population[a]	Exposed Cases[b]	Estimated Relative Risk (95% CI)[b]
Bertazzi	Seveso residents—20-year follow-up		
et al., 2001	Zones A, B—men	16	0.9 (0.5–1.5)
	women	11	1.0 (0.6–1.9)
Studies Reviewed in *Update 1998*			
Bertazzi	Seveso residents—15-year follow-up		
et al., 1997	Zone A—women	1	0.9 (0.0–5.3)
	Zone B—men	10	0.8 (0.4–1.5)
	women	7	1.0 (0.4–2.1)
	Zone R—men	76	0.9 (0.7–1.1)
	women	58	1.0 (0.8–1.3)
Svensson	Swedish fishermen—mortality (men and women)		
et al., 1995	East coast	17	1.4 (0.8–2.2)
	West coast	63	0.9 (0.7–1.2)
	Swedish fishermen—incidence (men and women)		
	East coast	24	1.6 (1.0–2.4)
	West coast	71	0.9 (0.7–1.2)
Studies Reviewed in *Update 1996*			
Bertazzi	Seveso residents—10-year follow-up—incidence		
et al., 1993	Zone B—men	7	1.0 (0.5–2.1)
	women	2	0.6 (0.2–2.5)
	Zone R—men	45	0.9 (0.7–1.2)
	women	25	1.0 (0.6–1.5)
Studies Reviewed in *VAO*			
Pesatori	Seveso residents—incidence		
et al., 1992	Zones A, B—men	7	0.9 (0.4–1.8)
	women	3	0.8 (0.3–2.5)
Bertazzi	Seveso residents—10-year follow-up		
et al., 1989a	Zones A, B, R—men	40	0.8 (0.6–1.2)
	women	22	1.0 (0.6–1.5)
Bertazzi	Seveso residents—10-year follow-up		
et al., 1989b	Zone B—men	7	1.2 (0.6–2.6)

ABBREVIATIONS: 2,4-D, 2,4-dichlorophenoxyacetic acid; 2,4,5-T, 2,4,5-trichlorophenoxyacetic acid; AFHS, Air Force Health Study; AHS, Agricultural Health Study; CDC, Centers for Disease Control and Prevention; CI, confidence interval; IARC, International Agency for Research on Cancer; MCPA, 2-methyl-4-chlorophenoxyacetic acid; NIOSH, National Institute for Occupational Safety and Health; nr, not reported; PCDDs, chlorinated dibenzo-*p*-dioxins (highly chlorinated, if four or more chlorines); SEA, Southeast Asia; TCDD, 2,3,7,8-tetrachlorodibenzo-*p*-dioxin; UFW, United Farm Workers of America; USDA, US Department of Agriculture.

[a] Subjects are male and outcome is mortality unless otherwise noted.

[b] Given when available; results other than estimated risk explained individually.

Studies in italics have been superseded by newer studies of same cohort.

California has maintained a pesticide-reporting program since the early 1970s for many restricted-use chemicals and implemented full-use reporting in 1990. Union records indicate when and where the workers were employed, and grower contracts indicate in what crop or commodity the workers were involved. Linkages with the Department of Pesticide Regulation were used to determine what pesticides were applied to the crops in a given county or month and year. Controls (n = 210) were matched on age, sex, ethnicity (predominantly Hispanic), and being alive and a California resident up to the date of the cases' diagnoses. Ever working in areas with high use of 2,4-D was associated with gastric cancer (odds ratio [OR], 1.85, 95% CI 1.05–3.25). The ORs for 2,4-D exposure and gastric cancer were about twice as high in the second and fourth quartiles of use as in the nonexposed (first quartile), but a pattern of increased risk was not seen when the low-exposure group (second quartile) was used as the referent. Gastric cancer was also associated with use of the insecticide chlordane (OR = 2.96, 95% CI 1.48–5.94), use of the acaricide propargite (OR = 2.86, 95% CI 1.56–5.23), use of the herbicide triflurin (OR = 1.69, 95% CI 0.99–2.89), and citrus-crop employment (OR = 2.88, 95% CI 1.02–8.12). The authors were not able to adjust their data for socioeconomic status (SES), alcohol intake, or smoking. The association with 2,4-D did not differ between cardia and noncardia gastric cancers or between diffuse and intestinal cancers.

Mills and Yang (2007) compared their results with those of Ekström et al. (1999). The publication by Ekström et al. was reviewed with the epidemiologic studies in *Update 2000*, but specific results for gastric cancer were not included in the cancer chapter of that review. The Ekström et al. study included all Swedish-born people who were 40–79 years old and living in either of two areas with different rates of gastric cancer (total population, 1.3 million) during 1989–1995. In-person interviews were conducted with 567 people who had histologically confirmed gastric adnenocarcinoma newly diagnosed in the study period and 1,165 population-based controls who were frequency-matched for age and sex. All employment of at least 1 year's duration was coded with a five-digit classification of occupational titles. Work in each industry was analyzed as ever vs never and stratified by duration (1–10 years vs more than 10 years). Interviewers asked open-ended questions about exposures to occupational chemicals, including pesticides. Occupational epidemiologists who were blinded to case–control status assigned exposure status to subjects and estimated cumulative duration of exposure to each agent. Pesticides were divided into herbicides (phenoxyacetic acids and others), insecticides (DDT and others) and fungicides, and the year of withdrawal or banning was considered when applicable.

The risk of gastric cancer was increased after exposure to herbicides (OR = 1.56, 95% CI 1.13–2.15). Further stratification by herbicide type revealed that those ever exposed to phenoxyacetic acids had an 80% excess risk (OR = 1.80, 95% CI 1.26–2.57) after adjustment for age and sex. With additional adjustment for SES, place of residence, number of siblings, and diet, the results of exposure to phenoxyacetic acid herbicides were similar among tumor subtypes and were not affected by smoking, alcohol consumption, body-mass index, or *Helicobacter pylori* status. The maximum risk was observed in cases exposed to both *H. pylori* and phenoxyacetic acids (OR = 3.42, 95% CI 1.41–8.26). The cases that had been exposed to Hormoslyr, a combination of 2,4-D and 2,4,5-T, had a risk (OR = 1.73, 95% CI 1.16–2.58) similar to that of the smaller number who had been exposed to 2-methyl-4-chlorophenoxyacetic acid (OR = 1.84, 95% CI 0.82–4.10). Although there was a marginally significant trend (p = 0.03) with duration of exposure to phenoxyacetic acid herbicides, there was no marked indication of a dose–response relationship. There was no association between exposure to other herbicides or insecticides and gastric cancer.

An earlier study by Cocco et al. (1999) was reviewed by the current committee. This case–control study focused on gastric-cancer mortality in 24 US states in 1984–1996. "Herbicide" was one of 12 workplace exposures encoded from occupation and industry information on death certificates. Type and intensity of exposure was determined by applying job exposure matrices to the occupation and industry combinations. Intensity of exposure was estimated on the basis of industrial-hygiene and occupational-health references and NIOSH and Occupational Safety and Health Administration databases. The ORs for men (white or black) and for black women fluctuated around 1.0, but findings were significant for white women with high *probability* of exposure to herbicides (OR = 1.71, 95% CI 1.18–2.46) or medium (OR = 3.26, 95% CI 1.07–9.99) or high (OR = 1.60, 95% CI 1.11–2.31) *intensity* of exposure to herbicides. No specific information was obtained regarding the specificity of the herbicides and whether the cases were exposed to any of the chemicals of interest for this review.

Environmental Studies   Consonni et al. (2008) reported on a mortality follow-up of the Seveso cohort of 273,108 subjects resident at the time of the accident or immigrating or born in the 10 years thereafter. Analyses were performed according to three zones with increasing TCDD contamination in the soil. In the overall sample, no statistically significant increases in deaths related to stomach cancer were observed. In the zone with greatest TCDD contamination, three stomach-cancer deaths were observed (relative risk [RR] = 0.65, 95% CI 0.21–2.03). The middle-contamination zone had 24 stomach-cancer deaths (RR = 0.78, 95% CI 0.52–1.17), and the lowest-contamination zone had 212 stomach-cancer deaths (RR = 0.95, 95% CI 0.82–1.09).

Biologic Plausibility

Long-term animal studies have examined the effect of exposure to the chemicals of interest (2-4-D and TCDD) on tumor incidences (Charles et al., 1996; Stott et al., 1990; Walker et al., 2006; Wanibuchi et al., 2004). No increase in the incidence of gastrointestinal cancer has been reported in laboratory animals.

However, studies performed in laboratory animals have observed dose-dependent increases in the incidence of squamous-cell hyperplasia of the forestomach or fundus of the stomach after administration of TCDD (Hebert et al., 1990; Walker et al., 2006). Similarly, in a long-term TCDD-treatment study performed in monkeys, hypertrophy, hyperplasia, and metaplasia were observed in the gastric epithelium (Allen et al., 1977). In addition, a transgenic mouse bearing a constitutively active form of the AHR has been shown to develop stomach tumors (Andersson et al., 2002a). The tumors are neither dysplastic nor metaplastic but are indicative of both squamous and intestinal metaplasia (Andersson et al., 2005). The validity of the transgenic-animal model is indicated by the similarities in the phenotype of the transgenic animal (increased relative weight of the liver and heart, decreased weight of the thymus, and increased expression of the AHR target gene CYP1A1) and animals treated with TCDD (Brunnberg et al., 2006).

The biologic plausibility of the carcinogenicity of the chemicals of interest is discussed in general at the beginning of this chapter.

Synthesis

The two occupational studies reporting significant findings regarding a relationship between stomach cancer and exposure to phenoxyacetic acid herbicides considered in this review have several strengths. The Swedish study by Ekström et al. (1999) is based on a large number of cases on which data were available for dietary factors, lifetime SES, smoking, alcohol intake, and infection by *H. pylori*. Data were available for specific pesticide groups, and the increased risk was observed for the phenoxyacetic acids and not other herbicides. The Mills and Yang (2007) case–control study also included employment history on dates, location, and primary crop. Pesticide reporting in California was used to determine what pesticides a worker was most likely to be exposed to and thereby avoided potential errors in self-reporting but resulted in a somewhat ecologic exposure assessment. The exposures occurred in the 2 decades before the diagnosis of cancer and are used extensively in California agriculture. The significant findings were dampened somewhat by the reported findings of a significant relationship of gastric cancer with agents not included in the chemicals of interest for this review, including the insecticide chlordane, the acaricide propargite and the herbicide triflurin. The study by Cocco et al. (1999) was not specific as to type of herbicide, and *Update 2006* reviewed a study by Reif et al. (1989) that reported a significant relationship between stomach cancer and the nonspecific exposure of being a forestry worker.

The Mills and Yang (2007) and Ekström et al. (1999) occupational studies are well done and indicative of an association between the chemicals of interest and stomach cancer, but there has been no suggestion of an association between the chemicals of interest and stomach cancer in the studies of Vietnam-veteran cohorts, the IARC cohort studies, or the US Agricultural Health Study (AHS).

There is some evidence of biologic plausibility in animal models, but overall the epidemiologic studies do not support an association between exposure to the chemicals of interest and stomach cancer.

Conclusion

On the basis of the evidence reviewed here and in previous VAO reports, the committee concludes that there is inadequate or insufficient evidence to determine whether there is an association between exposure to the chemicals of interest and stomach cancer.

Colorectal Cancer

Colorectal cancers include malignancies of the colon (ICD-9 153) and of the rectum and anus (ICD-9 154); less prevalent tumors of the small intestine (ICD-9 152) are often included. Findings on cancers of the retroperitoneum and other unspecified digestive organs (ICD-9 159) are considered in this category. Colorectal cancers account for about 55% of digestive tumors; ACS estimated that 159,990 people would develop new cases in the United States in 2008 and 51,750 would die from the cancers (Jemal et al., 2008a). Excluding basal-cell and squamous-cell skin cancers, colorectal cancer is the third-most common form of cancer both in men and in women.

The incidence of colorectal cancer increases with age; it is higher in men than in women and higher in blacks than in whites. Because it is recommended that all persons over 50 years old receive colon-cancer screening, screening can affect the incidence. Other risk factors include family history of this form of cancer, some diseases of the intestines, and diet. Type 2 diabetes is associated with an increased risk of cancer of the colon (ACS, 2007a).

Conclusions from *VAO* and Previous Updates

Update 2006 considered colorectal cancer independently for the first time. Prior updates developed tables of results on colon and rectal cancer, but conclusions about the adequacy of the evidence of their association with herbicide exposure had been reached only in the context of gastrointestinal tract cancers. The committee responsible for *VAO* concluded that there was limited or suggestive evidence of *no* association between exposure to the herbicides used by the US military in Vietnam and gastrointestinal tract tumors, including colorectal cancer. The committee responsible for *Update 2006* concluded that there was not enough evidence on each of the chemicals of interest to sustain this negative conclusion for any of the cancers in the gastrointestinal group and that, because these various types of cancer are generally regarded as separate disease entities, the evidence on each should be evaluated separately. Colorectal cancer was thus reclassified to the default category of inadequate or insufficient evidence to determine whether there is an association. Table 6-7 summarizes the results of the relevant studies concerning colon and rectal cancers.

Update of the Epidemiologic Literature

Vietnam-Veteran Studies   Cypel and Kang (2008) compiled and analyzed data on two cohorts of female veterans who served in Vietnam (the Vietnam-veteran cohort, n = 4,586) or served elsewhere during the Vietnam War (the era-veteran cohort, n = 5,325). All-causes mortality and cause-specific mortality in the Vietnam-veteran and era-veteran cohorts, the US population, and earlier research were compared. Similar analyses were performed for nurses only. Eleven cases of large intestine–cancer deaths were observed in the Vietnam veterans (crude rate, 0.75/10,000) compared with 29 in the era veterans, for an adjusted standardized mortality ratio (SMR) of 0.50 (95% CI 0.24–1.04). No excess risk was observed in the nurses-only analysis (SMR = 0.59, 95% CI 0.26–1.37).

Occupational Studies   Lee WJ et al. (2007) analyzed 305 incident cases of colorectal cancer (212 colon and 93 rectal) diagnosed in 1993–2005 in the AHS. The association with self-reported exposures to 50 pesticides (including 2,4-D, 2,4,5-T, and 2,4,5-trichlorophenoxypropionic acid) was studied. Some, including chlorpyrifos and aldicarb, were associated with an increased risk for rectal cancer and colon cancer, respectively. 2,4-D had a significant inverse association with colon cancer. The lack of a monotonic exposure–response pattern with lifetime exposure weakens somewhat the argument for a true protective relationship, but further evaluation of this inverse association in the AHS cohort is planned.

Samanic et al. (2006) reported on the incidence of all cancers, including those of the colon, in male pesticide applicators in the AHS with respect to re-ported exposures to dicamba (3,6-dichloro-2-methoxybenzoic acid), a benzoic acid herbicide with a chemical structure similar to that of phenoxy herbicides. Dicamba is used in combination with other herbicides, such as 2,4-D. The au-thors reported significant trends of increasing risk of colon cancer with lifetime exposure days and with intensity-weighted lifetime days when the referent group comprised low-exposed applicators. Only the RRs for the highest-exposure cat-egory were significant (lifetime days RR = 3.29, 95% CI 1.40–7.73; p trend, 0.02; intensity-weighted lifetimes days RR = 2.57, 95% CI 1.28–5.17; p trend, 0.002). That trend was not observed when the referent group comprised applicators who never used dicamba. There were no differences when analysis was restricted to only applicators who first applied dicamba before 1990.

Hansen et al. (2007) included colorectal-cancer deaths in their historical co-hort study of 3,156 male gardeners followed from 1975 until 2002. Although their study did not include specific types of pesticide exposure, the Danish National Environmental Board reports that 2,4-D and other chlorophenoxy acids were

TABLE 6-7 Selected Epidemiologic Studies—Colon and Rectal Cancer

Reference	Study Population[a]	Exposed Cases[b]	Estimated Relative Risk (95% CI)[b]
VIETNAM VETERANS			
New Studies			
Cypel and	US Vietnam veterans—women	29	0.5 (0.2–1.0)
Kang, 2008	Vietnam-veteran nurses	11	0.6 (0.2–1.4)
Studies Reviewed in *Update 2006*			
ADVA, 2005a	Australian male Vietnam veterans vs Australian population		
	Colon—incidence	376	1.1 (1.0–1.2)
	Navy	91	1.3 (1.0–1.5)
	Army	239	1.1 (0.9–1.2)
	Air Force	47	1.1 (0.8–1.5)
	Rectum—incidence		
	Navy	54	1.1 (0.8–1.4)
	Army	152	1.0 (0.8–1.1)
	Air Force	28	1.0 (0.6–1.4)
ADVA, 2005b	Australian male Vietnam veterans vs Australian population		
	Colon—mortality	176	1.0 (0.8–1.1)
	Navy	49	1.3 (0.9–1.6)
	Army	107	0.9 (0.7–1.0)
	Air Force	21	0.9 (0.5–1.3)
	Rectum—mortality		
	Navy	13	0.8 (0.4–1.4)
	Army	44	0.9 (0.6–1.1)
	Air Force	12	1.3 (0.6–2.2)
ADVA, 2005c	Australian male conscripted Army National Service Vietnam-era veterans: deployed vs nondeployed		
	Colon		
	Incidence	54	0.9 (0.7–1.4)
	Mortality	29	0.8 (0.5–1.3)
	Rectum		
	Incidence	46	1.4 (0.9–2.2)
	Mortality	10	1.8 (0.6–5.6)
Boehmer et al., 2004	Follow-up of CDC Vietnam Experience Cohort—mortality		
	Colon, rectum, and anus	9	1.0 (0.4–2.6)
Studies Reviewed in *Update 2000*			
AFHS, 2000	Ranch Hand veterans from AFHS—mortality		
	Colon, rectum combined	7	1.5 (0.4–5.5)
AIHW, 1999	Australian Vietnam veterans (men)—incidence (validation study)		Expected number of exposed cases (95% CI)
	Colorectal cancer	188	221 (191–251)
CDVA, 1998a	Australian Vietnam veterans (men)—incidence		
	Self-reported colon cancer	405	117 (96–138)

continued

TABLE 6-7 Continued

Reference	Study Population[a]	Exposed Cases[b]	Estimated Relative Risk (95% CI)[b]
CDVA, 1998b	Australian Vietnam veterans (women)—incidence		
	Self-reported colon cancer	1	1.0 (0–5)
Studies Reviewed in Update 1998			
CDVA, 1997a	Australian military Vietnam veterans—mortality		
	Colon	78	1.2 (0.9–1.5)
	Rectum	16	0.6 (0.4–1.0)
CDVA, 1997b	Australian National Service Vietnam veterans—mortality		
	Colon	6	0.6 (0.2–1.5)
	Rectum	3	0.7 (0.2–9.5)
Studies Reviewed in Update 1996			
Dalager et al., 1995	US Vietnam veterans (women)—mortality		
	Colon	4	0.4 (0.1–1.2)
	Vietnam-veteran nurses—mortality		
	Colon	4	0.5 (0.2–1.7)
Studies Reviewed in VAO			
Breslin et al., 1988	Army and Marine Vietnam veterans—mortality		
	Army Vietnam veterans		
	Colon, other gastrointestinal (ICD-8 152–154, 158, 159)	209	1.0 (0.7–1.3)
	Marine Vietnam veterans		
	Colon, other gastrointestinal (ICD-8 152–154, 158, 159)	33	1.3 (0.7–2.2)
Anderson et al., 1986	Wisconsin Vietnam veterans—mortality		
	Colon	6	1.0 (0.4–2.2)
	Rectum	1	nr
OCCUPATIONAL			
New Studies			
Lee WJ et al., 2007	Pesticide applicators (men and women) in AHS—colorectal-cancer incidence (enrollment–2002) and any use before enrollment of:		
	2,4-D	204	0.7 (0.2–0.9)
	2,4,5-T	65	0.9 (0.5–1.5)
	2,4,5-TP	24	0.8 (0.4–1.5)
	Dicamba	110	0.9 (0.7–1.2)
Samanic et al., 2006	Pesticide applicators in AHS—colon-cancer incidence (enrollment–2002)		
	Dicamba—days of use		
	None	76	1.0
	1– < 20	9	0.4 (0.2–0.9)
	20– < 56	20	0.9 (0.5–1.5)
	56– < 116	13	0.8 (0.4–1.5)
	≥ 116	17	1.4 (0.8–2.9)
			p-trend = 0.10

TABLE 6-7 Continued

Reference	Study Population[a]	Exposed Cases[b]	Estimated Relative Risk (95% CI)[b]
	Dicamba—intensity-weighted quartiles		
	None	76	1.0
	Lowest	16	0.6 (0.4–1.1)
	Second	17	0.7 (0.4–1.2)
	Third	6	0.5 (0.2–1.2)
	Highest	20	1.8 (1.0–3.1)
			p-trend = 0.02
Studies Reviewed in *Update 2006*			
McLean et al., 2006	IARC cohort of pulp and paper workers—mortality		
	Ever exposed to nonvolatile organochlorine compounds		
	Colon	62	0.7 (0.6–1.0)
	Rectum	60	0.9 (0.7–1.1)
't Mannetje et al., 2005	Phenoxy herbicide producers, sprayers—mortality		
	Phenoxy herbicide producers (men and women)		
	Colon	2	0.6 (0.0–2.3)
	Rectum, rectosigmoid junction, anus	5	2.5 (0.8–5.7)
	Phenoxy herbicide sprayers (> 99% men)		
	Colon	8	1.9 (0.8–3.8)
	Rectum, rectosigmoid junction, anus	4	1.5 (0.4–3.8)
Alavanja et al., 2005	US AHS—incidence		
	Colon		
	Private applicators (men and women)	208	0.9 (0.8–1.0)
	Spouses of private applicators (> 99% women)	87	0.9 (0.7–1.1)
	Commercial applicators (men and women)	12	1.2 (0.6–2.1)
	Rectum		
	Private applicators (men and women)	94	0.8 (0.7–1.0)
	Spouses of private applicators (> 99% women)	23	0.6 (0.4–0.9)
	Commercial applicators (men and women)	7	1.3 (0.5–2.6)
Blair et al., 2005a	US AHS—mortality		
	Colon		
	Private applicators (men and women)	56	0.7 (0.6–1.0)
	Spouses of private applicators (> 99% women)	31	1.2 (0.8–1.6)
	Rectum		
	Private applicators (men and women)	nr	nr
	Spouses of private applicators (> 99% women)	nr	nr
Torchio et al., 1994	Italian licensed pesticide users—mortality		
	Colon	84	0.6 (0.5–0.7)
	Rectum	nr	nr
Reif et al., 1989	New Zealand forestry workers—nested case–control (incidence)		
	Colon	7	0.5 (0.2–1.1)
	Small intestine	2	5.2 (1.4–18.9)
	Rectum	10	1.2 (0.6–2.3)

continued

TABLE 6-7 Continued

Reference	Study Population[a]	Exposed Cases[b]	Estimated Relative Risk (95% CI)[b]
Studies Reviewed in *Update 2004*			
Swaen	Dutch licensed herbicide applicators—mortality		
et al., 2004	Colon	7	1.0 (0.4–2.1)
	Rectum	5	2.1 (0.7–4.8)
Studies Reviewed in *Update 2000*			
Steenland	US chemical production workers (included in IARC		
et al., 1999	cohort, NIOSH Dioxin Registry)		
	Small intestine and colon	34	1.2 (0.8–1.6)
	Rectum	6	0.9 (0.3–1.9)
Hooiveld	Dutch chemical production workers (included in		
et al., 1998	IARC cohort)		
	Intestine (except rectum)	3	1.4 (0.3–4.0)
	Rectum	1	1.0 (0.0–5.6)
Rix et al.,	Danish paper-mill workers—incidence		
1998	Men		
	Colon	58	1.0 (0.7–1.2)
	Rectum	43	0.9 (0.6–1.2)
	Women		
	Colon	23	1.1 (0.7–1.7)
	Rectum	15	1.5 (0.8–2.4)
Studies Reviewed in *Update 1998*			
Gambini	Italian rice growers—mortality		
et al., 1997	Intestines	27	1.1 (0.7–1.6)
Kogevinas	IARC cohort, male and female workers exposed to		
et al., 1997	any phenoxy herbicide or chlorophenol		
	Colon	86	1.1 (0.9–1.3)
	Rectum	44	1.1 (0.8–1.4)
	Exposed to highly chlorinated PCDDs		
	Colon	52	1.0 (0.8–1.3)
	Rectum	29	1.3 (0.9–1.9)
	Not exposed to highly chlorinated PCDDs		
	Colon	33	1.2 (0.8–1.6)
	Rectum	14	0.7 (0.4–1.2)

TABLE 6-7 Continued

Reference	Study Population[a]	Exposed Cases[b]	Estimated Relative Risk (95% CI)[b]
Becher et al., 1996	German production workers (included in IARC cohort)—mortality		
	Plant I		
	Colon	2	0.4 (0.1–1.4)
	Rectum	6	1.9 (0.7–4.0)
	Plant II		
	Colon	0	nr
	Rectum	0	nr
	Plant III		
	Colon	1	2.2 (0.1–12.2)
	Rectum	0	nr
	Plant IV		
	Colon	0	nr
	Rectum	1	0.9 (0.0–4.9)
Ott and Zober, 1996	BASF employees—colorectal—incidence	5	1.0 (0.3–2.3)
	TCDD < 0.1 µg/kg of body weight	2	1.1 (0.1–3.9)
	TCDD 0.1–0.99 µg/kg of body weight	2	1.4 (0.2–5.1)
	TCDD ≥ 1 µg/kg of body weight	1	0.5 (0.0–3.0)
Ramlow et al., 1996	Dow pentachlorophenol production workers (included in IARC cohort, NIOSH Dioxin Registry) —mortality		
	0-year latency		
	Colon	4	0.8 (0.2–2.1)
	Rectum	0	nr
	15-year latency		
	Colon	4	1.0 (0.3–2.6)
	Rectum	0	nr
Studies Reviewed in *Update 1996*			
Blair et al., 1993	US farmers in 23 states—mortality		
	White men		
	Colon	2,291	1.0 (0.9–1.0)
	Rectum	367	1.0 (0.9–1.1)
	White women		
	Colon	59	1.0 (0.8–1.3)
	Rectum	4	0.5 (0.1–1.3)
Bueno de Mesquita et al., 1993	Dutch phenoxy herbicide workers (included in IARC cohort)—mortality		
	Colon	3	1.8 (0.4–5.4)
	Rectum	0	nr
Collins et al., 1993	Monsanto Company workers (included in NIOSH cohort)—mortality		
	Colon	3	0.5 (0.1–1.3)
Studies Reviewed in *VAO*			
Swaen et al., 1992	Dutch licensed herbicide applicators—mortality		
	Colon	4	2.6 (0.7–6.5)

continued

TABLE 6-7 Continued

Reference	Study Population[a]	Exposed Cases[b]	Estimated Relative Risk (95% CI)[b]
Ronco et al., 1992	Danish workers—incidence		
	Men—self-employed		
	Colon	277	0.7 (p < 0.05)
	Rectum	309	0.8 (p < 0.05)
	Men—employees		
	Colon	45	0.6 (p < 0.05)
	Rectum	55	0.8 (nr)
	Women—self-employed		
	Colon	14	0.9 (nr)
	Rectum	5	0.6 (nr)
	Women—employees		
	Colon	112	0.9 (nr)
	Rectum	55	0.8 (nr)
	Women—family worker		
	Colon	2	0.2 (p < 0.05)
	Rectum	2	0.4 (nr)
Fingerhut et al., 1991	NIOSH cohort—mortality		
	Entire NIOSH cohort		
	Small intestine, colon	25	1.2 (0.8–1.8)
	Rectum	5	0.9 (0.3–2.1)
	≥ 1-year exposure, ≥ 20-year latency		
	Small intestine, colon	13	1.8 (1.0–3.0)
	Rectum	2	1.2 (0.1–4.2)
Manz et al., 1991	German production workers (included in IARC cohort)—mortality		
	Colon	8	0.9 (0.4–1.8)
Saracci et al., 1991	IARC cohort—exposed subcohort (men and women)—mortality		
	Colon (except rectum)	41	1.1 (0.8–1.5)
	Rectum	24	1.1 (0.7–1.6)
Zober et al., 1990	BASF employees—basic cohort—mortality		90% CI
	Colon, rectum	2	2.5 (0.4–7.8)
Alavanja et al., 1989	USDA forest or soil conservationists—mortality		
	Colon	44	1.5(1.1–2.0)
	Rectum	9	1.0 (0.5–1.9)
Henneberger et al., 1989	New Hampshire pulp and paper workers—mortality		
	Colon	9	1.0 (0.5–2.0)
	Rectum	1	0.4 (0.0–2.1)
Solet et al., 1989	US pulp and paper workers—mortality		
	Colon	7	1.5 (0.6–3.0)
Alavanja et al., 1988	USDA agricultural extension agents—mortality		
	Colon	41	1.0 (0.7–1.5)
	Rectum	5	nr

TABLE 6-7 Continued

Reference	Study Population[a]	Exposed Cases[b]	Estimated Relative Risk (95% CI)[b]
Bond et al., 1988	Dow 2,4-D production workers (included in IARC cohort, NIOSH Dioxin Registry)—mortality		
	Colon	4	2.1 (0.6–5.4)
	Rectum	1	1.7 (0.0–9.3)
Thomas, 1987	US flavor and fragrance chemical plant workers—mortality		
	Colon	4	0.6 (nr)
	Rectum	6	2.5 (nr)
Coggon et al., 1986	British MCPA production workers (included in the IARC cohort)—mortality		
	Colon	19	1.0 (0.6–1.6)
	Rectum	8	0.6 (0.3–1.2)
Robinson et al., 1986	Northwestern US pulp and paper workers Intestines (ICD-7 152, 153)	7	0.4 (0.2–0.7)
Lynge, 1985	Danish production workers (included in IARC cohort)—incidence		
	Men		
	Colon	10	1.0 (nr)
	Rectum	14	1.4 (nr)
	Women		
	Colon	1	0.3 (nr)
	Rectum	2	1.0 (nr)
Blair et al., 1983	Florida pesticide applicators—mortality		
	Colon	5	0.8 (nr)
	Rectum	2	nr
Wiklund, 1983	Swedish male and female agricultural workers—incidence		99% CI
	Colon	1,332	0.8 (0.7–0.8)
	Rectum	1,083	0.9 (0.9–1.0)
Thiess et al., 1982	BASF production workers—mortality		
	Colon	1	0.4 (nr)
Burmeister, 1981	Iowa farmers—mortality		
	Colon	1,064	1.0 (nr)
Hardell, 1981	Swedish residents—incidence		
	Colon		
	Exposed to phenoxy acids	11	1.3 (0.6–2.8)
	Exposed to chlorophenols	6	1.8 (0.6–5.3)

continued

TABLE 6-7 Continued

Reference	Study Population[a]	Exposed Cases[b]	Estimated Relative Risk (95% CI)[b]
ENVIRONMENTAL			
New Studies			
Consonni	Seveso residents—25-year follow-up—men, women		
et al., 2008	Zone A		
	Colon	3	1.0 (0.3–3.0)
	Rectum	1	0.9 (0.1–6.4)
	Zone B		
	Colon	12	0.6 (0.3–1.1)
	Rectum	11	1.5 (0.8–2.8)
	Zone R		
	Colon	137	0.9 (0.7–1.3)
	Rectum	50	0.9 (0.7–1.3)
Studies Reviewed in *Update 2002*			
Revich	Residents of Chapaevsk, Russia—mortality		
et al., 2001	Men		
	Colon	17	1.3 (0.8–2.2)
	Rectum	21	1.5 (1.0–2.4)
	Women		
	Colon	24	1.0 (0.7–1.5)
	Rectum	24	0.9 (0.6–1.4)
Studies Reviewed in *Update 2000*			
Bertazzi	Seveso residents—20-year follow-up—mortality		
et al., 2001	Zones A, B—men		
	Colon	10	1.0 (0.5–1.9)
	Rectum	9	2.4 (1.2–4.6)
	Zones A, B—men		
	Colon	5	0.6 (0.2–1.4)
	Rectum	3	1.1 (0.4–3.5)
Studies Reviewed in *Update 1998*			
Bertazzi	Seveso residents—15-year follow-up—mortality		
et al., 1997	Zone A—women		
	Colon	2	2.6 (0.3–9.4)
	Zone B—men		
	Colon	5	0.8 (0.3–2.0)
	Rectum	7	2.9 (1.2–5.9)
	Zone B—women		
	Colon	3	0.6 (0.1–1.8)
	Rectum	2	1.3 (0.1–4.5)
	Zone R—men		
	Colon	34	0.8 (0.6–1.1)
	Rectum	19	1.1 (0.7–1.8)
	Zone R—women		
	Colon	33	0.8 (0.6–1.1)
	Rectum	12	0.9 (0.5–1.6)

TABLE 6-7 Continued

Reference	Study Population[a]	Exposed Cases[b]	Estimated Relative Risk (95% CI)[b]
Svensson et al., 1995	Swedish fishermen—mortality (men and women)		
	East coast		
	Colon	1	0.1 (0.0–0.7)
	Rectum	4	0.7 (0.2–1.9)
	West coast		
	Colon	58	1.0 (0.8–1.3)
	Rectum	31	1.0 (0.7–1.5)
	Swedish fishermen—incidence (men and women)		
	East coast		
	Colon	5	0.4 (0.1–0.9)
	Rectum	9	0.9 (0.4–1.6)
	West coast		
	Colon	82	1.0 (0.8–1.2)
	Rectum	59	1.1 (0.8–1.4)
Studies Reviewed in *Update 1996*			
Bertazzi et al., 1993	Seveso residents—10-year follow-up—morbidity		
	Zone B—men		
	Colon	2	0.5 (0.1–2.0)
	Rectum	3	1.4 (.04–4.4)
	Zone B—women		
	Colon	2	0.6 (0.1–2.3)
	Rectum	2	1.3 (0.3–5.4)
	Zone R—men		
	Colon	32	1.1 (0.8–1.6)
	Rectum	17	1.1 (0.7–1.9)
	Zone R—women		
	Colon	23	0.8 (0.5–1.3)
	Rectum	7	0.6 (.03–1.3)
Studies Reviewed in *VAO*			
Lampi et al., 1992	Finnish community exposed to chlorophenol contamination—incidence		
	Colon—men, women	9	1.1 (0.7–1.8)
Pesatori et al., 1992	Seveso residents—incidence		
	Zones A, B—men		
	Colon	3	0.6 (0.2–1.9)
	Rectum	3	1.2 (0.4–3.8)
	Zones A, B—women		
	Colon	3	0.7 (0.2–2.2)
	Rectum	2	1.2 (0.3–4.7)
Bertazzi et al., 1989a	Seveso residents—10-year follow-up—mortality		
	Zones A, B, R—men		
	Colon	20	1.0 (0.6–1.5)
	Rectum	10	1.0 (0.5–2.7)
	Zones A, B, R—women		
	Colon	12	0.7 (0.4–1.2)
	Rectum	7	1.2 (0.5–2.7)

continued

TABLE 6-7 Continued

Reference	Study Population[a]	Exposed Cases[b]	Estimated Relative Risk (95% CI)[b]
Bertazzi et al., 1989b	Seveso residents—10-year follow-up—mortality Zone B—men		
	Rectum	2	1.7 (0.4–7.0)

ABBREVIATIONS: 2,4-D, 2,4-dichlorophenoxyacetic acid; 2,4,5-T, 2,4,5-trichlorophenoxyacetic acid; 2,4,5-TP, 2-(2,4,5-trichlorophenoxy) propionic acid; AFHS, Air Force Health Study; AHS, Agricultural Health Study; CDC, Centers for Disease Control and Prevention; CI, confidence interval; IARC, International Agency for Research on Cancer; ICD, International Classification of Diseases; MCPA, methyl-4-chlorophenoxyacetic acid; NIOSH, National Institute for Occupational Safety and Health; nr, not reported; PCDDs, chlorinated dibenzo-*p*-dioxins (highly chlorinated, if four or more chlorines); TCDD, 2,3,7,8-tetrachlorodibenzo-*p*-dioxin; USDA, US Department of Agriculture.
[a]Subjects are male and outcome is mortality unless otherwise noted.
[b]Given when available; results other than estimated risk explained individually.
Studies in italics have been superseded by newer studies of same cohort.

used during the periods when the older members of the cohort were working. No excess deaths from digestive cancers were found in any of the three age cohorts in the study.

Environmental Studies   Consonni et al. (2008) reported on a mortality follow-up of the Seveso, Italy, cohort exposed to large amounts of environmental contamination with TCDD. The study cohort of 273,108 subjects resident at the time of the accident or immigrating or born in the 10 years thereafter were analyzed according to three zones with increasing levels of soil TCDD. In the overall sample, no statistically significant increases in deaths related to colon or rectal cancer were observed. In the zone with intermediate TCDD contamination, there was a 50% nonsignificant increase in rectal-cancer mortality; the excesses were in males (eight deaths; RR = 1.81, 95% CI 0.89–3.67).

Biologic Plausibility

Long-term animal studies have examined the effect of exposure to the chemicals of interest on tumor incidences (Charles et al., 1996; Stott et al., 1990; Walker et al., 2006; Wanibuchi et al., 2004). No increase in the incidence of colorectal cancer in laboratory animals exposed to the chemicals of interest has been reported.

The biologic plausibility of the carcinogenicity of the chemicals of interest is discussed in general at the beginning of this chapter.

Synthesis

The epidemiologic studies reviewed yielded no evidence to suggest an association between the chemicals of interest and colorectal cancer. There is no evidence of biologic plausibility of an association between exposure to any of the chemicals of interest and the development of tumors of the colon or rectum. Overall, the available evidence does not support an association between the chemicals of interest and colorectal cancer.

Conclusion

On the basis of the evidence reviewed here and in previous VAO reports, the committee concludes that there is inadequate or insufficient evidence to determine whether there is an association between exposure to the chemicals of interest and colorectal cancer.

Hepatobiliary Cancers

Hepatobiliary cancers include cancers of the liver (ICD-9 155.0, 155.2) and the intrahepatic bile duct (ICD-9 155.1). ACS estimated that 15,190 men and 6,180 women would receive diagnoses of liver cancer or intrahepatic bile duct cancer in the United States in 2008 and 12,570 men and 5,840 women would die from these cancers (Jemal et al., 2008a). Gallbladder cancer and extrahepatic bile duct cancer (ICD-9 156) are fairly uncommon and are often grouped with liver cancers when they are addressed.

In the United States, liver cancers account for about 1.5% of new cancer cases and 3.3% of cancer deaths. Misclassification of metastatic cancers as primary liver cancer can lead to overestimation of the number of deaths attributable to liver cancer (Percy et al., 1990). In developing countries, especially those in sub-Saharan Africa and Southeast Asia, liver cancers are common and are among the leading causes of death. The known risk factors for liver cancer include chronic infection with hepatitis B or C virus and exposure to the carcinogens aflatoxin and vinyl chloride. Alcohol cirrhosis and obesity-associated metabolic syndrome may also contribute to the risk of liver cancer. In the general population, the incidence of liver and intrahepatic bile duct cancer increases slightly with age; at the ages of 50–64 years, it is greater in men than in women and greater in blacks than in whites. The average annual incidence of hepatobiliary cancers is shown in Table 6-4.

Conclusions from *VAO* and Previous Updates

The committee responsible for *VAO* concluded that there was inadequate or insufficient information to determine whether there is an association between exposure to the chemicals of interest and hepatobiliary cancers. Additional information available to the committees responsible for *Update 1996*, *Update 1998*, *Update 2000*, *Update 2002*, *Update 2004*, and *Update 2006* did not change that conclusion. Table 6-8 summarizes the results of the relevant studies.

Update of the Epidemiologic Literature

No Vietnam-veteran or occupational studies addressing exposure to the chemicals of interest and hepatobiliary cancer have been published since *Update 2006*.

Environmental Studies   Consonni et al. (2008) reported on a mortality follow-up of the Seveso, Italy, cohort exposed to large amounts of environmental contamination with TCDD. The study cohort of 273,108 subjects resident at the time of the accident or immigrating or born in the 10 years thereafter were analyzed according to three zones with increasing levels of soil TCDD. In the overall sample, no statistically significant increases in deaths related to biliary tract cancer or liver cancer were observed. In Zone A (very high TCDD contamination), no biliary tract cancer deaths were observed; there were three liver-cancer deaths (RR = 1.03, 95% CI 0.33–3.20). The middle-contamination zone (Zone B, high TCDD contamination) had two biliary cancer deaths (RR = 0.56, 95% CI 0.14–2.26) and 16 liver-cancer deaths (RR = 0.86, 95% CI 0.52–1.40). The lowest-contamination zone (Zone R) had 31 biliary cancer deaths (RR = 1.16, 95% CI 0.79–1.70) and 107 liver-cancer deaths (RR = 0.80, 95% CI 0.65–0.98).

Biologic Plausibility

Long-term animal studies have examined the effect of exposure to the chemicals of interest on tumor incidences (Charles et al., 1996; Stott et al., 1990; Walker et al., 2006; Wanibuchi et al., 2004). Studies performed in laboratory animals have consistently demonstrated that long-term exposure to TCDD results in the formation of liver adenomas and carcinomas (Knerr and Schrenk, 2006; Walker et al., 2006). Furthermore, TCDD increases the growth of hepatic tumors that are initiated by the treatment with a complete carcinogen. In addition, changes in liver pathology have been observed after exposure to TCDD and include nodular hyperplasia and massive inflammatory cell infiltration (Walker et al., 2006; Yoshizawa et al., 2007). Inflammation and cancer are strongly intertwined in the development and progression of many cancers, including liver cancers (Mantovani et al., 2008). Similarly, in monkeys treated with TCDD, hyperplasia and an increase in cells that stain positive for alpha-smooth muscle actin have been observed (Korenaga et al., 2007). Postive staining for alpha-smooth muscle actin is thought to be indicative of a process (epithelial–mesenchymal transition) that is associated with the progression of malignant tumors (Weinberg, 2008).

TABLE 6-8 Selected Epidemiologic Studies—Hepatobiliary Cancer

Reference	Study Population[a]	Exposed Cases[b]	Estimated Relative Risk (95% CI)[b]
VIETNAM VETERANS			
Studies Reviewed in *Update 2006*			
ADVA, 2005a	Australian male Vietnam veterans vs Australian population—incidence	27	0.7 (0.4–1.0)
	Navy	8	1.0 (0.4–1.9)
	Army	18	0.7 (0.4–1.1)
	Air Force	1	0.2 (0.0–1.2)
ADVA, 2005b	Australian male Vietnam veterans vs Australian population—mortality (liver, gallbladder)	48	0.9 (0.6–1.1)
	Navy	11	1.0 (0.5–1.7)
	Army	33	0.9 (0.6–1.2)
	Air Force	4	0.6 (0.2–1.5)
ADVA, 2005c	Australian male conscripted Army National Service Vietnam-era veterans: deployed vs nondeployed		
	Incidence	2	2.5 (0.1–147.2)
	Mortality (liver, gallbladder)	4	2.5 (0.4–27.1)
Boehmer et al., 2004	Follow-up of CDC Vietnam Experience Cohort (liver, intrahepatic bile ducts [ICD-9 155])	5	nr
Studies Reviewed in *Update 2000*			
AFHS, 2000	Air Force Ranch Hand veterans—incidence	2	1.6 (0.2–11.4)
Studies Reviewed in *Update 1998*			
CDVA, 1997a	Australian military Vietnam veterans		
	Liver (ICD-9 155)	8	0.6 (0.2–1.1)
	Gallbladder (ICD-9 156)	5	1.3 (0.4–2.8)
CDVA, 1997b	Australian National Service Vietnam veterans	1	nr
Studies Reviewed in *VAO*			
CDC, 1990a	US men born 1921–1953—incidence	8	1.2 (0.5–2.7)
Breslin et al., 1988	Army Vietnam veterans (liver, bile duct)	34	1.0 (0.8–1.4)
	Marine Vietnam veterans (liver, bile duct)	6	1.2 (0.5–2.8)
Anderson et al., 1986	Wisconsin Vietnam veterans	0	nr
OCCUPATIONAL			
Studies Reviewed in *Update 2006*			
McLean et al., 2006	IARC cohort of pulp and paper workers Exposure to nonvolatile organochlorine compounds		
	Never	27	0.9 (0.6–1.3)
	Ever	16	0.7 (0.4–1.1)
't Mannetje et al., 2005	New Zealand phenoxy herbicide workers (ICD-9 155)		
	Producers (men and women)	1	1.6 (0.0–8.8)
	Sprayers (> 99% men)	0	0.0 (0.0–4.2)

continued

TABLE 6-8 Continued

Reference	Study Population[a]	Exposed Cases[b]	Estimated Relative Risk (95% CI)[b]
Alavanja et al., 2005	US AHS—incidence		
	Liver		
	Private applicators (men and women)	35	1.0 (0.7–1.4)
	Spouses of private applicators (> 99% women)	3	0.9 (0.2–2.5)
	Commercial applicators (men and women)	nr	0.0 (0.0–4.2)
	Gallbladder		
	Private applicators (men and women)	8	2.3 (1.0–4.5)
	Spouses of private applicators (> 99% women)	3	0.9 (0.2–2.5)
	Commercial applicators (men and women)	nr	0.0 (0.0–35.8)
Blair et al., 2005a	US AHS		
	Liver		
	Private applicators (men and women)	8	0.6 (0.2–1.1)
	Spouses of private applicators (> 99% women)	4	1.7 (0.4–4.3)
	Gallbladder		
	Private applicators (men and women)	3	2.0 (0.4–5.7)
	Spouses of private applicators (> 99% women)	2	1.3 (0.1–4.6)
Torchio et al., 1994	Italian licensed pesticide users		
	Liver	15	0.6 (0.3–0.9)
Reif et al., 1989	New Zealand forestry workers—nested case–control —incidence		
	Liver	1	0.8 (0.1–5.8)
	Gallbladder	3	4.1 (1.4–12.0)
Studies Reviewed in *Update 2004*			
Swaen et al., 2004	Dutch licensed herbicide applicators	0	nr
Studies Reviewed in *Update 2000*			
Steenland et al., 1999	US chemical production workers (included in IARC cohort, NIOSH Dioxin Registry)		
	Liver, biliary tract (ICD-9 155–156)	7	0.9 (0.4–1.6)
Rix et al., 1998	Danish paper mill workers—incidence		
	Liver—men	10	1.1 (0.5–2.0)
	women	1	0.6 (0.0–3.2)
	Gallbladder—men	9	1.6 (0.7–3.0)
	women	4	1.4 (0.4–3.7)
Studies Reviewed in *Update 1998*			
Gambini et al., 1997	Italian rice growers	7	1.3 (0.5–2.6)
Kogevinas et al., 1997	IARC cohort, male and female workers exposed to any phenoxy herbicide or chlorophenol	15	0.7 (0.4–1.2)
	Exposed to highly chlorinated PCDDs	12	0.9 (0.5–1.5)
	Not exposed to highly chlorinated PCDDs	3	0.4 (0.1–1.2)
Becher et al., 1996	German production workers (included in IARC cohort)		
	Liver and biliary tract	1	1.2 (0.0–6.9)

TABLE 6-8 Continued

Reference	Study Population[a]	Exposed Cases[b]	Estimated Relative Risk (95% CI)[b]
Ott and	BASF employees—incidence	2	2.1 (0.3–7.5)
Zober, 1996	Liver, gallbladder, and bile duct		
	TCDD < 0.1 μg/kg of body weight	1	2.8 (0.1–15.5)
	TCDD 0.1–0.99 μg/kg of body weight	0	0.0 (0.0–15.4)
	TCDD ≥ 1 μg/kg of body weight	1	2.8 (0.1–15.5)
Ramlow	Dow pentachlorophenol production workers		
et al., 1996	(included in IARC cohort, NIOSH Dioxin Registry)		
	Liver, primary (ICDA-8 155–156)		
	0-year latency	0	nr
	15-year latency	0	nr
Studies Reviewed in *Update 1996*			
Asp et al.,	Finnish herbicide applicators—liver, biliary tract		
1994	Incidence	3	0.9 (0.2–2.6)
	Mortality	2	0.6 (0.1–2.2)
Blair et al.,	US farmers in 23 states		
1993	White men	326	1.0 (0.9–1.1)
	White women	6	0.7 (0.3–1.6)
Collins	Monsanto Company 2,4-D production workers		
et al., 1993	(included in NIOSH cohort)		
	Liver, biliary tract	2	1.4 (0.2–5.2)
Studies Reviewed in *VAO*			
Ronco et al.,	Danish farm workers—incidence		
1992	Liver		
	Men—self-employed	23	0.4 (p < 0.05)
	employees	9	0.8 (nr)
	Women—family workers	5	0.5 (nr)
	Gallbladder		
	Men—self-employed	35	0.8 (nr)
	employees	7	0.8 (nr)
	Women—self-employed	7	2.7 (p < 0.05)
	employees	1	0.7 (nr)
	family workers	17	1.0 (nr)
Fingerhut	NIOSH—entire cohort (liver, biliary tract)—	6	1.2 (0.4–2.5)
et al., 1991	≥ 1-year exposure, ≥ 20-year latency	1	0.6 (0.0–3.3)
Saracci	IARC cohort—exposed subcohort (men and women)		
et al., 1991	Liver, gallbladder, bile duct (ICD-8 155–156)	4	0.4 (0.1–1.1)
Solet et al.,	US pulp and paper workers (ICD-8 155–156)	2	2.0 (0.2–7.3)
1989			
Bond et al.,	Dow 2,4-D production workers (included in IARC		
1988	cohort, NIOSH Dioxin Registry)		
	Liver, biliary tract (ICDA-8 155–156)	0	1.2 (nr)
Lynge, 1985	Danish production workers (included in IARC		
	cohort)—incidence		
	Men	3	1.0 (nr)
	Women	0	nr

continued

TABLE 6-8 Continued

Reference	Study Population[a]	Exposed Cases[b]	Estimated Relative Risk (95% CI)[b]
Hardell et al., 1984	Swedish residents—incidence, mortality combined	102	1.8 (0.9–4.0)
Wiklund, 1983	Swedish male and female agricultural workers—incidence		99% CI
	Liver (primary)	103	0.3 (0.3–0.4)
	Biliary tract	169	0.6 (0.5–0.7)
	Liver (unspecified)	67	0.9 (0.7–1.3)
Zack and Suskind, 1980	Monsanto Company production workers (included in NIOSH cohort)	0	nr
ENVIRONMENTAL			
New Studies			
Consonni et al., 2008	Seveso residents—25-year follow-up—men, women		
	Liver (ICD-9 155)		
	Zone A	3	1.0 (0.3–3.2)
	Zone B	16	0.9 (0.5–1.4)
	Zone R	107	0.8 (0.7–1.0)
	Biliary tract (ICD-9 156)		
	Zone A	0	0.0 (nr)
	Zone B	2	0.6 (0.1–2.3)
	Zone R	31	1.2 (0.8–1.7)
Studies Reviewed in *Update 2000*			
Bertazzi et al., 2001	Seveso residents—20-year follow-up		
	Zone A, B—men (liver, gallbladder)	6	0.5 (0.2–1.0)
	(liver)	6	0.5 (0.2–1.1)
	women (liver, gallbladder)	7	1.0 (0.5–2.2)
	(liver)	6	1.3 (0.6–2.9)
Studies Reviewed in *Update 1998*			
Bertazzi et al., 1997	Seveso residents—15-year follow-up		
	Zone B—men (liver, gallbladder)	4	0.6 (0.2–1.4)
	(liver)	4	0.6 (0.2–1.6)
	women (liver, gallbladder)	4	1.1 (0.3–2.9)
	(liver)	3	1.3 (0.3–3.8)
	Zone R—men (liver, gallbladder)	35	0.7 (0.5–1.0)
	(liver)	31	0.7 (0.5–1.0)
	women (liver, gallbladder)	25	0.8 (0.5–1.3)
	(liver)	12	0.6 (0.3–1.1)
Svensson et al., 1995	Swedish fishermen (men and women)—mortality		
	East coast	1	0.5 (0.0–2.7)
	West coast (liver, bile ducts)	9	0.9 (0.4–1.7)
	Swedish fishermen (men and women)—incidence		
	East coast	6	1.3 (0.5–2.9)
	West coast (liver, bile ducts)	24	1.0 (0.6–1.5)

TABLE 6-8 Continued

Reference	Study Population[a]	Exposed Cases[b]	Estimated Relative Risk (95% CI)[b]
Studies Reviewed in *Update 1996*			
Bertazzi	Seveso residents—10-year follow-up—incidence		
et al., 1993	Zone B—men (liver)	4	2.1 (0.8–5.8)
	(gallbladder—ICD-9 156)	1	2.3 (0.3–17.6)
	women (gallbladder—ICD-9 156)	4	4.9 (1.8–13.6)
	Zone R—men (liver)	3	0.2 (0.1–0.7)
	(gallbladder—ICD-9 156)	3	1.0 (0.3–3.4)
	women (liver)	2	0.5 (0.1–2.1)
	(gallbladder—ICD-9 156)	7	1.0 (0.5–2.3)
Cordier	Military service in South Vietnam for ≥ 10 years		
et al., 1993	after 1960	11	8.8 (1.9–41.0)
Studies Reviewed in *VAO*			
Pesatori	Seveso residents—incidence		
et al., 1992	Zone A, B—men (liver)	4	1.5 (0.5–4.0)
	(gallbladder—ICD-9 156)	1	2.1 (0.3–15.6)
	women (liver)	1	1.2 (0.2–9.1)
	(gallbladder—ICD-9 156)	5	5.2 (2.1–13.2)
	Zone R—men (liver)	8	0.5 (0.2–0.9)
	(gallbladder—ICD-9 156)	3	1.0 (0.3–3.4)
	women (liver)	5	0.8 (0.3–2.1)
	(gallbladder—ICD-9 156)	7	1.0 (0.5–2.3)
Bertazzi	Seveso residents—10-year follow-up		
et al., 1989b	Zone A—women (gallbladder—ICD-9 156)	1	12.1 (1.6–88.7)
	Zone B—men (liver)	3	1.2 (0.4–3.8)
	women (gallbladder—ICD-9 156)	2	3.9 (0.9–16.2)
	Zone R—men (liver)	7	0.4 (0.2–0.8)
	women (liver)	3	0.4 (0.1–1.4)
	(gallbladder—ICD-9 156)	5	1.2 (0.5–3.1)
Hoffman	Residents of Quail Run Mobile Home Park (men		
et al., 1986	and women)	0	nr

ABBREVIATIONS: 2,4-D, 2,4-dichlorophenoxyacetic acid; AHS, Agricultural Health Study; CDC, Centers for Disease Control and Prevention; CI, confidence interval; IARC, International Agency for Research on Cancer; ICD, International Classification of Diseases; ICDA, International Classification of Diseases, Adapted for Use in the United States; NIOSH, National Institute for Occupational Safety and Health; nr, not reported; PCDDs, chlorinated dibenzo-*p*-dioxins (highly chlorinated, if four or more chlorines); TCDD, 2,3,7,8-tetrachlorodibenzo-*p*-dioxin.

[a]Subjects are male and outcome is mortality unless otherwise noted.
[b]Given when available; results other than estimated risk explained individually.
Studies in italics have been superseded by newer studies of the same cohort.

With respect to cancers of the bile duct, bile duct hyperplasia, but not tumors, has been reported (Knerr and Schrenk, 2006; Walker et al., 2006; Yoshizawa et al., 2007). Similarly, monkeys treated with TCDD developed metaplasia, hyperplasia, and hypertrophy of the bile duct (Allen et al., 1977). Hollingshead et al. (2008) recently showed that TCDD-activated AHR in human breast and endocervical cell lines induces sustained high concentrations of the IL–6 cytokine, which has tumor-promoting effects in numerous tissues, including cholangiocytes, so TCDD might promote carcinogenesis in biliary tissue.

The biologic plausibility of the carcinogenicity of the chemicals of interest is discussed in general at the beginning of this chapter.

Synthesis

For this update, no new reports of a definitive link between exposure to the chemicals of interest and hepatobiliary tumors were found. Despite the evidence of TCDD's activity as a hepatocarcinogen in animals, the evidence from epidemiologic studies remains inadequate to link the chemicals of interest with hepatobiliary cancer, which occurs at a relatively low incidence in Western populations.

Conclusion

On the basis of the evidence reviewed here and in previous VAO reports, the committee concludes that there is inadequate or insufficient evidence to determine whether there is an association between exposure to the chemicals of interest and hepatobiliary cancer.

Pancreatic Cancer

The incidence of pancreatic cancer (ICD-9 157) increases with age. ACS estimated that 18,770 men and 18,910 women would develop pancreatic cancer in the United States in 2008 and that 17,500 men and 16,790 women would die from it (Jemal et al., 2008a). The incidence is higher in men than in women and higher in blacks than in whites. Other risk factors include family history, diet, and tobacco use; the incidence is about twice as high in smokers as in nonsmokers (Miller et al., 1996). Chronic pancreatitis, obesity, and type 2 diabetes are also associated with an increased risk of pancreatic cancer (ACS, 2006).

Conclusions from *VAO* and Previous Updates

Update 2006 considered pancreatic cancer independently for the first time. Prior updates developed tables of results for pancreatic cancer but reached conclusions about the adequacy of the evidence of its association with herbicide exposure in the context of gastrointestinal tract cancers. The committee responsible for *VAO* concluded that there was limited or suggestive evidence of *no* association between exposure to the herbicides used by the US military in Vietnam and gastrointestinal tract tumors, including pancreatic cancer. The committee responsible for *Update 2006* concluded that there was not enough evidence on each of the chemicals of interest to sustain that negative conclusion for any of the cancers in the gastrointestinal group and that, because these various types of cancer are generally regarded as separate disease entities, the evidence on each should be evaluated separately. Pancreatic cancer was thus reclassified to the default category inadequate or insufficient evidence of an association. That committee reviewed the increased rates of pancreatic cancer in Australian National Service Vietnam veterans but concluded that the increased rates could be attributed to the rates of smoking in the cohort (ADVA, 2005c). The committee also noted the report of increased rates of pancreatic cancer in US female Vietnam nurse veterans (Dalager et al., 1995). Table 6-9 summarizes the results of the relevant studies concerning pancreatic cancer.

Update of the Epidemiologic Literature

Vietnam-Veteran Studies   Cypel and Kang (2008) compiled and analyzed the data on two cohorts of female veterans who served in Vietnam (the Vietnam-veteran cohort, n = 4,586) or served elsewhere during the Vietnam War (the era-veteran cohort, n = 5,325). All-causes mortality and cause-specific mortality through 2004 in the Vietnam-veteran and era-veteran cohorts and earlier research were compared. Similar analyses were performed for nurses only. Seventeen deaths from pancreatic cancer were observed in the Vietnam-veteran groups and 16 in the era-veteran group, for an adjusted RR of 2.12 (95% CI 0.99–4.51). The nurse-only group had 14 cases compared with 11 in the corresponding era group (adjusted RR = 2.45, 95% CI 1.00–6.00). A limitation of the study was the inability to control for diet and smoking behavior.

Occupational Studies   No occupational studies concerning exposure to the chemicals of interest and pancreatic cancer have been published since *Update 2006*.

Environmental Studies   Consonni et al. (2008) reported on a mortality follow-up of the Seveso, Italy, cohort exposed to large amounts of environmental contamination with TCDD. The study cohort of 273,108 subjects resident at the time of the accident or immigrating or born in the 10 years thereafter were analyzed according to three zones with increasing levels of soil TCDD. In the overall sample, no statistically significant increase in deaths related to pancreatic cancer was observed. In Zone A (very high TCDD contamination), two pancreatic-cancer deaths were observed (RR = 1.17, 95% CI 0.29–4.68). The middle-contamination

TABLE 6-9 Selected Epidemiologic Studies—Pancreatic Cancer

Reference	Study Population[a]	Exposed Cases[b]	Estimated Relative Risk (95% CI)[b]
VIETNAM VETERANS			
New Studies			
Cypel and	US Vietnam veterans—women	17	2.1 (1.0–4.5)
Kang, 2008	Vietnam-veteran nurses	14	2.5 (1.0–6.0)
Studies Reviewed in *Update 2006*			
ADVA,	Australian male Vietnam veterans vs Australian		
2005a	population—incidence	86	1.2 (0.9–1.4)
	Navy	14	0.9 (0.5–1.5)
	Army	60	1.2 (0.9–1.5)
	Air Force	12	1.3 (0.7–2.3)
ADVA,	Australian male Vietnam veterans vs Australian		
2005b	population—mortality	101	1.2 (1.0–1.5)
	Navy	18	1.0 (0.6–1.6)
	Army	71	1.3 (1.0–1.6)
	Air Force	11	1.1 (0.5–1.8)
ADVA,	Australian male conscripted Army National Service		
2005c	Vietnam-era veterans: deployed vs nondeployed		
	Incidence	17	2.5 (1.0–6.3)
	Mortality	19	3.1 (1.3–8.3)
Boehmer	Follow-up of CDC Vietnam Experience Cohort	5	1.0 (0.3–3.5)
et al., 2004			
Studies Reviewed in *Update 1998*			
CDVA,	Australian military Vietnam veterans	38	1.4 (0.9–1.8)
1997a			
CDVA,	Australian National Service Vietnam veterans	6	1.5 (nr)
1997b			
Studies Reviewed in *Update 1996*			
Dalager	US Vietnam veterans—women	7	2.8 (0.8–10.2)
et al., 1995	Vietnam-veteran nurses	7	5.7 (1.2–27.0)
Visintainer	PM study of deaths (1974–1989) of Michigan		
et al., 1995	Vietnam-era veterans—deployed vs nondeployed	14	1.0 (0.6–1.7)
	Non-black	9	0.7 (0.3–1.3)
	Black	5	9.1 (2.9–21.2)
Studies Reviewed in *VAO*			
Thomas	US Vietnam veterans—women	5	2.7 (0.9–6.2)
et al., 1991			
Breslin	Army Vietnam veterans	82	0.9 (0.6–1.2)
et al., 1988	Marine Vietnam veterans	18	1.6 (0.5–5.8)
Anderson	Wisconsin Vietnam veterans		
et al., 1986		4	nr
OCCUPATIONAL			
Studies Reviewed in *Update 2006*			
McLean	IARC cohort of pulp and paper workers		
et al., 2006	Exposure to nonvolatile organochlorine		
	compounds		
	Never	67	0.8 (0.7–1.1)
	Ever	69	1.1 (0.9–1.4)

TABLE 6-9 Continued

Reference	Study Population[a]	Exposed Cases[b]	Estimated Relative Risk (95% CI)[b]
't Mannetje	Phenoxy herbicide producers (men and women)	3	2.1 (0.4–6.1)
et al., 2005	Phenoxy herbicide sprayers (> 99% men)	0	0.0 (0.0–2.1)
Alavanja	US AHS—incidence		
et al., 2005	Private applicators (men and women)	46	0.7 (0.5–1.0)
	Spouses of private applicators (> 99% women)	20	0.9 (0.6–1.4)
	Commercial applicators (men and women)	3	1.1 (0.2–3.2)
Blair et al.,	US AHS		
2005a	Private applicators (men and women)	29	0.6 (0.4–0.9)
	Spouses of private applicators (> 99% women)	10	0.7 (0.3–1.2)
Torchio	Italian licensed pesticide users	32	0.7 (0.5–1.0)
et al., 1994			
Reif et al.,	New Zealand forestry workers—nested case–control		
1989	—incidence	6	1.8 (0.8–4.1)
Magnani	UK case–control		
et al., 1987	Herbicides	nr	0.7 (0.3–1.5)
	Chlorophenols	nr	0.8 (0.5–1.4)
Studies Reviewed in *Update 2004*			
Swaen	Dutch licensed herbicide applicators	5	1.2 (0.4–2.7)
et al., 2004			
Studies Reviewed in *Update 2000*			
Steenland	US chemical production workers (included in IARC		
et al., 1999	cohort, NIOSH Dioxin Registry)	16	1.0 (0.6–1.6)
Hooiveld	Dutch chemical production workers (included in		
et al., 1998	IARC cohort)	4	2.5 (0.7–6.3)
Rix et al.,	Danish paper-mill workers—incidence		
1998	Men	30	1.2 (0.8–1.7)
	Women	2	0.3 (0.0–1.1)
Studies Reviewed in *Update 1998*			
Gambini	Italian rice growers	7	0.9 (0.4–1.9)
et al., 1997			
Kogevinas	IARC cohort, male and female workers exposed to		
et al., 1997	any phenoxy herbicide or chlorophenol	47	0.9 (0.7–1.3)
	Exposed to highly chlorinated PCDDs	30	1.0 (0.7–1.4)
	Not exposed to highly chlorinated PCDDs	16	0.9 (0.5–1.4)
Becher	German production workers (included in IARC		
et al., 1996	cohort)		
	Plant I	2	0.6 (0.1–2.3)
	Plant II	0	nr
	Plant III	0	nr
	Plant IV	2	1.7 (0.2–6.1)
Ramlow	Dow pentachlorophenol production workers		
et al., 1996	(included in IARC cohort, NIOSH Dioxin Registry)		
	0-year latency	2	0.7 (0.1–2.7)
	15-year latency	2	0.9 (0.1–3.3)

continued

TABLE 6-9 Continued

Reference	Study Population[a]	Exposed Cases[b]	Estimated Relative Risk (95% CI)[b]
Studies Reviewed in *Update 1996*			
Blair et al., 1993	US farmers in 23 states		
	White men	1,133	1.1 (1.1–1.2)
	White women	23	1.0 (0.6–1.5)
Bueno de Mesquita et al., 1993	Dutch phenoxy herbicide workers (included in IARC cohort)	3	2.2 (0.5–6.3)
Studies Reviewed in *VAO*			
Ronco et al., 1992	Danish farm workers—incidence		
	Men—self-employed	137	0.6 (p < 0.05)
	employees	23	0.6 (p < 0.05)
	Women—self-employed	7	1.2 (nr)
	employees	4	1.3 (nr)
	family workers	27	0.7 (p < 0.05)
Swaen et al., 1992	Dutch licensed herbicide applicators	3	2.2 (0.4–6.4)
Fingerhut et al., 1991	NIOSH—entire cohort	10	0.8 (0.4–1.6)
	≥ 1-year exposure, ≥ 20-year latency	4	1.0 (0.3–2.5)
Saracci et al., 1991	IARC cohort—exposed subcohort (males, females)	26	1.1 (0.7–1.6)
Alavanja et al., 1989	USDA forest, soil conservationists	22	1.5 (0.9–2.3)
Henneberger et al., 1989	New Hampshire paper and pulp workers	9	1.9 (0.9–3.6)
Solet et al., 1989	US pulp and paper workers	1	0.4 (0.0–2.1)
Alavanja et al., 1988	USDA agricultural extension agents	21	1.3 (0.8–1.9)
Thomas, 1987	US flavor and fragrance chemical plant workers	6	1.4 (nr)
Coggon et al., 1986	British MCPA production workers (included in IARC cohort)	9	0.7 (0.3–1.4) 90% CI
Robinson et al., 1986	Northwestern US paper and pulp workers	4	0.3 (0.1–0.8)
Lynge, 1985	Danish production workers (included in IARC cohort)—incidence		
	Men	3	0.6 (nr)
	Women	0	nr
Blair et al., 1983			Expected exposed cases
	Florida pesticide applicators	4	4.0
Wiklund, 1983	Swedish male and female agricultural workers—incidence	777	99% CI 0.8 (0.8–0.9)
Burmeister, 1981	Iowa farmers	416	1.1 (nr)

TABLE 6-9 Continued

Reference	Study Population[a]	Exposed Cases[b]	Estimated Relative Risk (95% CI)[b]
ENVIRONMENTAL			
New Studies			
Consonni et al., 2008	Seveso residents (men and women)—25-year follow-up		
	Zone A	2	1.2 (0.3–4.7)
	Zone B	5	0.5 (0.2–1.1)
	Zone R	76	1.0 (0.7–1.7)
Studies Reviewed in *Update 2000*			
Bertazzi et al., 2001	Seveso residents—20-year follow-up		
	Zones A, B—men	4	0.7 (0.3–1.9)
	women	1	0.3 (0.0–2.0)
Studies Reviewed in *Update 1998*			
Bertazzi et al., 1997	Seveso residents—15-year follow-up		
	Zone A—men	1	1.9 (0.0–10.5)
	Zone B—men	2	0.6 (0.1–2.0)
	women	1	0.5 (0.0–3.1)
	Zone R—men	20	0.8 (0.5–1.2)
	women	11	0.7 (0.4–1.3)
Svensson et al., 1995	Swedish fishermen (men and women)—mortality		
	East coast	5	0.7 (0.2–1.6)
	West coast	33	0.8 (0.6–1.2)
	Swedish fishermen (men and women)—incidence		
	East coast	4	0.6 (0.2–1.6)
	West coast	37	1.0 (0.7–1.4)
Studies Reviewed in *VAO*			
Pesatori et al., 1992	Seveso residents—incidence		
	Zones A, B—men	2	1.0 (0.3–4.2)
	women	1	1.6 (0.2–12.0)
Bertazzi et al., 1989a	Seveso residents—10-year follow-up		
	Zones A, B, R—men	9	0.6 (0.3–1.2)
	women	4	1.0 (0.3–2.7)
Bertazzi et al., 1989b	Seveso residents—10-year follow-up		
	Zone B—men	2	1.1 (0.3–4.5)

ABBREVIATIONS: AHS, Agricultural Health Study; CDC, Centers for Disease Control and Prevention; CI, confidence interval; IARC, International Agency for Research on Cancer; MCPA, methyl-4-chlorophenoxyacetic acid; NIOSH, National Institute for Occupational Safety and Health; nr, not reported; PCDDs, chlorinated dibenzo-*p*-dioxins (highly chlorinated, if four or more chlorines); PM, proportionate mortality; TCDD, 2,3,7,8-tetrachlorodibenzo-*p*-dioxin; USDA, US Department of Agriculture.

[a]Subjects are male and outcome is mortality unless otherwise noted.
[b]Given when available; results other than estimated risk explained individually.
Studies in italics have been superseded by newer studies of same cohort.

zone (Zone B, high TCDD contamination) had five pancreatic-cancer deaths (RR = 0.45, 95% CI 0.19–1.09), and the lowest-contamination zone (Zone R) had 76 (RR = 0.95, 95% CI 0.74–1.21).

Biologic Plausibility

Long-term animal studies have examined the effect of exposure to the chemicals of interest on tumor incidences (Charles et al., 1996; Stott et al., 1990; Walker et al., 2006; Wanibuchi et al., 2004). No increase in the incidence of pancreatic cancer in laboratory animals after the administration of cadodylic acid, 2-4-D, or picloram has been reported. A 2-year study of female rats has reported increased incidences of pancreatic adenomas and carcinomas after treatment at the highest dose of TCDD (100 ng/kg per day) (Nyska et al., 2004). Other studies have observed chronic active inflammation, acinar-cell vacuolation, and an increase in proliferation of the acinar cells surrounding the vacuolated cells (Yoshizawa et al., 2005b). As previously discussed, both chronic inflammation and hyperproliferation are closely linked to the formation and progression of cancers, including that of the pancreas (Hahn and Weinberg, 2002; Mantovani et al., 2008). Metaplastic changes in the pancreatic ducts were also observed in female monkeys treated with TCDD (Allen et al., 1977).

The biologic plausibility of the carcinogenicity of the chemicals of interest is discussed in general at the beginning of this chapter.

Synthesis

The large excess of pancreatic cancers in female Vietnam veterans vs their nondeployed counterparts observed by Thomas et al. (1991) and Dalager et al. (1995) has prevailed and is now significant for all the female Vietnam veterans, as well as for the nursing subset. The committee responsible for *Update 2006* also reported a higher incidence of and mortality from pancreatic cancer in deployed Australian National Service veterans than in nondeployed veterans (ADVA, 2005c). No increase in risk has been reported to date in US male Vietnam veterans or in agricultural cohorts or IARC follow-up studies. A limitation of all of the veteran studies has been the lack of control for the effect of smoking and a lack of supportive data from occupational or environmental studies. The association that has been observed, particularly in women, is moderately plausible.

Conclusion

On the basis of the evidence reviewed here and in previous VAO reports, the committee concludes that there is inadequate or insufficient evidence to determine whether there is an association between exposure to the chemicals of interest and pancreatic cancer.

LARYNGEAL CANCER

ACS estimated that 9,680 men and 2,570 women would receive diagnoses of cancer of the larynx (ICD-9 161) in the United States in 2008 and that 2,910 men and 760 women would die from it (Jemal et al., 2008a). Those numbers constitute a little more than 0.9% of new cancer diagnoses and 0.7% of cancer deaths. The incidence of cancer of the larynx increases with age, and it is more common in men than in women, with a sex ratio in the United States of about 4:1 in people 50–64 years old. The average annual incidence of laryngeal cancer is shown in Table 6-10.

Established risk factors for laryngeal cancer are tobacco use and alcohol use, which are independent and act synergistically. Occupational exposures—long and intense exposures to wood dust, paint fumes, and some chemicals used in the metalworking, petroleum, plastics, and textile industries—also could increase risk (ACS, 2007b). An Institute of Medicine committee recently concluded that asbestos is a causal factor in laryngeal cancer (IOM, 2006); infection with human papilloma virus might also raise the risk of laryngeal cancer (Hobbs and Birchall, 2004).

Conclusions from *VAO* and Previous Updates

The committee responsible for *VAO* concluded that there was limited or suggestive evidence of an association between exposure to at least one of the chemicals of interest and laryngeal cancer. Additional information available to the committees responsible for *Update 1996*, *Update 1998*, *Update 2000*, *Update 2002*, *Update 2004*, and *Update 2006* did not change that conclusion. Table 6-11 summarizes the results of the relevant studies.

TABLE 6-10 Average Annual Cancer Incidence (per 100,000) of Laryngeal Cancer in United States[a]

	50–54 Years Old			55–59 Years Old			60–64 Years Old		
	All Races	White	Black	All Races	White	Black	All Races	White	Black
Men	9.4	9.0	18.3	14.6	13.7	29.7	21.8	21.3	39.9
Women	2.2	2.1	3.7	3.2	3.1	7.1	4.7	4.8	7.5

[a]Surveillance, Epidemiology, and End Results program, nine standard registries, crude age-specific rates, 2000–2005.

Update of the Epidemiologic Literature

No Vietnam-veteran or occupational studies addressing exposure to the chemicals of interest and laryngeal cancer have been published since *Update 2006*.

Environmental Studies

Investigators in Italy completed a 25-year mortality follow-up of people exposed to the industrial accident in Seveso (Consonni et al., 2008). Mortality from respiratory cancer (ICD 160–165) in residents in three exposure zones—very high (Zone A), high (Zone B), and low (Zone R)—was compared with that in a nonexposed reference population. Laryngeal-cancer mortality was not evaluated independently; however, excluding lung-cancer cases (ICD-162) from all respiratory-cancer cases results in a maximum of no, eight, and 49 deaths in Zones A, B, and R, respectively, that could possibly be attributed to laryngeal cancer. There was no evidence of increased mortality in any of the exposure groups.

Biologic Plausibility

Long-term animal studies have examined the effect of exposure to the chemicals of interest on tumor incidences (Charles et al., 1996; Stott et al., 1990; Walker et al., 2006; Wanibuchi et al., 2004). No increase in the incidence of laryngeal cancer in laboratory animals after the administration of any of the chemicals of interest have been reported.

The biologic plausibility of the carcinogenicity of the chemicals of interest is discussed in general at the beginning of this chapter.

Synthesis

The present committee, as part of its reassessment of all health outcomes, had concerns that the conclusion of limited/suggestive evidence for classifying the associations for laryngeal cancer did not meet the current criterion. The original *VAO* committee had few studies to draw on (see *VAO* Table 8-10, reproduced here). It stated that "positive associations were found consistently only in those studies in which TCDD or herbicide exposures were probably high and prolonged, especially the largest, most heavily exposed cohorts of chemical production workers exposed to TCDD (Zober et al., 1990; Fingerhut et al., 1991; Manz et al., 1991; Saracci et al., 1991) and herbicide applicators (Axelson and Sundell, 1974; Riihimaki et al., 1982; Blair et al., 1983; Green, 1991)." Moreover, the committee conducted a pooled analysis of the data in the table and stated that "although the numbers are too small to draw strong conclusions, the consistency

TABLE 6-11 Selected Epidemiologic Studies—Laryngeal Cancer

Reference	Study Population[a]	Exposed Cases[b]	Estimated Relative Risk (95% CI)[b]
VIETNAM VETERANS			
Studies Reviewed in *Update 2006*			
ADVA, 2005a	Australian Vietnam veterans vs Australian population—incidence	97	1.5 (1.2–1.8)
	Navy	21	1.5 (0.9–2.1)
	Army	69	1.6 (1.2–1.9)
	Air Force	7	0.8 (0.3–1.7)
ADVA, 2005b	Australian Vietnam veterans vs Australian population—mortality	28	1.1 (0.7–1.5)
	Navy	6	1.1 (0.4–2.4)
	Army	19	1.1 (0.7–1.7)
	Air Force	3	0.9 (0.2–2.5)
ADVA, 2005c	Australian men conscripted Army National Service Vietnam-era veterans: deployed vs nondeployed		
	Incidence	8	0.7 (0.2–1.6)
	Mortality	2	0.4 (0.0–2.4)
Boehmer et al., 2004	CDC Vietnam Experience Cohort	0	0.0 (nr)
Studies Reviewed in *Update 2000*			
AFHS, 2000	Air Force Ranch Hand veterans—incidence		
	Oral cavity, pharynx, larynx	4	0.6 (0.2–2.4)
Studies Reviewed in *Update 1998*			
CDVA, 1997a	Australian military Vietnam veterans	12	1.3 (0.7–2.2)
CDVA, 1997b	Australian National Service Vietnam veterans	0	0 (0– > 10)
Watanabe and Kang, 1996	Army Vietnam veterans compared with US men	50	1.3 (nr)
	Marine Vietnam veterans	4	0.7 (nr)
	Army Vietnam veterans	50	1.4 (p < 0.05)
OCCUPATIONAL			
Studies Reviewed in *Update 2006*			
McLean et al., 2006	IARC cohort of pulp and paper workers Exposure to nonvolatile organochlorine chemicals		
	Never	18	0.9 (0.5–1.5)
	Ever	20	1.2 (0.8–1.9)
't Mannetje et al., 2005	Phenoxy herbicide producers (men and women)	0	nr
	Phenoxy herbicide sprayers (> 99% men)	0	nr
Torchio et al., 1994	Italian farmers licensed to use pesticides	25	0.5 (0.3–0.7)
Reif et al., 1989	New Zealand forestry workers—nested case–control —incidence	2	1.1 (0.3–4.7)
Studies Reviewed in *Update 2004*			
Swaen et al., 2004	Dutch licensed herbicide applicators	1	1.0 (0.0–5.1)

continued

TABLE 6-11 Continued

Reference	Study Population[a]	Exposed Cases[b]	Estimated Relative Risk (95% CI)[b]
Studies Reviewed in *Update 2002*			
Thörn et al., 2000	Swedish lumberjacks exposed to phenoxyacetic herbicides		
	Foremen—incidence	0	nr
Studies Reviewed in *Update 1998*			
Gambini et al., 1997	Italian rice growers	7	0.9 (0.4–1.9)
Kogevinas et al., 1997	IARC cohort, male and female workers exposed to any phenoxy herbicide or chlorophenol	21	1.6 (1.0–2.5)
	Exposed to highly chlorinated PCDDs	15	1.7 (1.0–2.8)
	Not exposed to highly chlorinated PCDDs	5	1.2 (0.4–2.9)
Ramlow et al., 1996	Dow pentachlorophenol production workers (included in IARC cohort, NIOSH Dioxin Registry)	2	2.9 (0.3–10.3)
	0-year latency	2	2.9 (0.4–10.3)
	15-year latency	1	nr
Studies Reviewed in *Update 1996*			
Blair et al., 1993	US farmers in 23 states		
	White men	162	0.7 (0.6–0.8)
	White women	0	nr (0.0–3.3)
Studies Reviewed in *VAO*			
Fingerhut et al., 1991	NIOSH—entire cohort	7	2.1 (0.8–4.3)
	≥ 1-year exposure, ≥ 20-year latency	3	2.7 (0.6–7.8)
Manz et al., 1991	German production workers—men, women (included in IARC cohort)	2	2.0 (0.2–7.1)
Saracci et al., 1991	IARC cohort (men and women)—exposed subcohort	8	1.5 (0.6–2.9)
Bond et al., 1988	Dow 2,4-D production workers (included in IARC cohort, NIOSH Dioxin Registry)	1	3.0 (0.0–16.8)
Coggon et al., 1986	British MCPA production workers (included in IARC cohort)	4	1.7 (0.5–4.5)
ENVIRONMENTAL			
New Studies			
Consonni et al., 2008	Seveso residents (men and women)—25-year follow-up—all respiratory cancers (ICD-9 160–165) excluding reported lung cancers (ICD-9 162)		
	Zone A	0	nr
	Zone B	≤ 8	nr
	Zone R	≤ 49	nr
Studies Reviewed in *Update 2002*			
Revich et al., 2001	Residents of Chapaevsk, Russia		
	Men	13	2.3 (1.2–3.8)
	Women	1	0.1 (0.0–0.6)

TABLE 6-11 Continued

Reference	Study Population[a]	Exposed Cases[b]	Estimated Relative Risk (95% CI)[b]
Studies Reviewed in *Update 2000*			
Bertazzi et al., 2001	Seseso residents (men and women)—20-year follow-up—all respiratory cancers (ICD-9 160–165) excluding reported lung cancers (ICD-9 162)		
	Zone A	0	nr
	Zone B	8	nr
Bertazzi et al., 1998	Seveso residents—15-year follow-up—all respiratory cancers (ICD-9 160–165) excluding reported lung cancers (ICD-9 162)		
	Zone B—men	6	nr
	women	0	nr
	Zone R—males	32	nr
	women	6	nr

ABBREVIATIONS: CDC, Centers for Disease Control and Prevention; CI, confidence interval; IARC, International Agency for Research on Cancer; ICD, International Classification of Diseases; MCPA, methyl-4-chlorophenoxyacetic acid; NIOSH, National Institute for Occupational Safety and Health; nr = not reported; PCDDs, chlorinated dibenzo-*p*-dioxins (highly chlorinated, if four or more chlorines); TCDD, 2,3,7,8-tetrachlorodibenzo-*p*-dioxin.

[a]Subjects are male and outcome is mortality unless otherwise noted.
[b]Given when available; results other than estimated risk explained individually.
Studies in italics have been superseded by newer studies of same cohorts.

of a mild elevation in relative risk is suggestive of an association for laryngeal cancer. Pooling all but the Coggon data (Coggon et al., 1986, 1991) yields an OR of 1.8 (95% CI 1.0–3.2)."

Since then, a combined analysis of many of the separate cohorts has been conducted (the IARC study, Kogevinas et al., 1997) and has shown significant effects in workers exposed to any phenoxyacetic acid herbicide or chlorophenol (RR = 1.6, 95% CI 1.0–2.5; 21 deaths), especially workers exposed to TCDD (or higher-chlorinated dioxins) (RR = 1.7, 95% CI 1.0–2.8; 15 deaths). Those RRs are remarkably close to the pooled estimate computed by the committee responsible for *VAO*. The study by Kogevinas et al. was a high-quality study that used an excellent method for assessing exposure, and its results were unlikely to be affected by confounding, because the distribution of smoking in working cohorts is not likely to differ in exposure (Siemiatycki et al., 1988). Another cohort of pulp and paper workers also showed an increase in risk (RR = 1.2, 95% CI 0.8–1.9; 20 deaths; McLean et al., 2006).

With regard to veteran studies, a positive association was found in the study of veterans in Australia that compared mortality with that in the general population (ADVA, 2005a) but not in the study that compared Australian veterans of the Vietnam conflict with nondeployed soldiers (ADVA, 2005c). In contrast, Watanabe and Kang (1996) found a significant 40% excess of mortality in Army personnel deployed to the Vietnam theater. The Ranch Hand study is not large enough to have sufficient power to detect an association if one exists.

An environmental study (Revich et al., 2001) of residents of Chapaevsk, Russia, which was heavily contaminated by many industrial pollutants, including dioxin, showed an association in men (RR = 2.3, 95% CI 1.2–3.8).

Conclusion

On the basis of the evidence reviewed here and in previous VAO reports, the committee concludes that there is limited or suggestive evidence of an association between exposure to at least one chemical of interest and laryngeal cancer.

LUNG CANCER

Lung cancer (carcinoma of the lung or bronchus, ICD-9 162.2–162.9) is the leading cause of cancer death in the United States. ACS estimated that 114,690 men and 100,330 women would receive diagnoses of lung cancer in the United States in 2008 and that about 90,810 men and 71,030 women would die from it (Jemal et al., 2008a). Those numbers represent roughly 15% of new cancer diagnoses and 29% of cancer deaths in 2008. The principal types of lung neoplasms are identified collectively as bronchogenic carcinoma (the bronchi are the two main branches of the trachea) and carcinoma of the lung. Cancer of the trachea (ICD-9 162.0) is often grouped with cancer of the lung and bronchus under ICD-9 162. The lung is also a common site of the development of metastatic tumors.

In men and women, the incidence of lung cancer increases greatly beginning at about the age of 40 years. The incidence in people 50–54 years old is double that in people 45–49 years old, and it doubles again in those 55–59 years old. The incidence is consistently higher in black men than in women or white men. The average annual incidence of lung cancer in the United States is shown in Table 6-12.

ACS estimates that 85–90% of lung-cancer deaths are attributable to cigarette-smoking (Jemal et al., 2008b). Smoking increases the risk of all histologic types of lung cancer, but the associations with squamous-cell and small-cell carcinomas are strongest. Other risk factors include exposure to asbestos, uranium, vinyl chloride, nickel chromates, coal products, mustard gas, chloromethyl ethers, gasoline, diesel exhaust, and inorganic arsenic. The latter statement does not imply that cacodylic acid, which is a metabolite of inorganic arsenic, can be assumed to be a risk factor. Important environmental risk factors include exposure to tobacco smoke and radon (ACS, 2007c).

TABLE 6-12 Average Annual Incidence (per 100,000) of Lung and Bronchial Cancer in United States[a]

	50–54 Years Old			55–59 Years Old			60–64 Years Old		
	All Races	White	Black	All Races	White	Black	All Races	White	Black
Men	56.7	52.8	110.5	115.7	107.0	222.4	213.7	208.5	333.4
Women	45.2	44.6	66.8	89.7	90.8	116.5	154.5	162.5	172.0

[a]Surveillance, Epidemiology, and End Results program, nine standard registries, crude age-specific rates, 2000–2005).

Conclusions from *VAO* and Previous Updates

The committee responsible for *VAO* concluded that there was limited or suggestive evidence of an association between exposure to at least one chemical of interest and lung cancer. Additional information available to the committees responsible for *Update 1996*, *Update 1998*, *Update 2000*, *Update 2002*, *Update 2004*, and *Update 2006* did not change that conclusion.

Table 6-13 summarizes the results of the relevant studies.

Update of the Epidemiologic Literature

Vietnam-Veteran Studies

Cypel and Kang (2008) compiled and analyzed the data on two cohorts of female veterans who served in Vietnam (the Vietnam-veteran cohort, n = 4,586) or served elsewhere during the Vietnam War (the era-veteran cohort, n = 5,325). All-cause mortality and cause-specific mortality in the Vietnam-veteran and era-veteran cohorts, the US population, and earlier research were compared. Similar analyses were performed for nurses only. Fifty lung-cancer deaths were observed in the Vietnam veterans (crude rate per 10,000, 3.4) and 66 in the era veterans, for an adjusted SMR of 0.96 (95% CI 0.65–1.42). No excess risk was observed in the nurses-only analysis (SMR = 0.76, 95% CI 0.48–1.18).

Occupational Studies

Hansen et al. (2007) conducted a historical-cohort study of 3,156 male gardeners who were members of a Danish union (the study was first reported in *VAO* as Hansen et al., 1992). Subjects were then followed up with population and cancer registries, and the incidence of cancer was ascertained from 1975 until the end of 2001. Birth date served as a surrogate for potential exposure to pesticides and herbicides, with earlier cohorts representing higher potential exposures. No

TABLE 6-13 Selected Epidemiologic Studies—Lung and Bronchus Cancer

Reference	Study Population[a]	Exposed Cases[b]	Estimated Relative Risk (95% CI)[b]
VIETNAM VETERANS			
New Studies			
Cypel and	US Vietnam veterans—women (lung)	50	1.0 (0.7–1.4)
Kang, 2008	Vietnam veteran nurses	35	0.8 (0.5–1.2)
Studies Reviewed in *Update 2006*			
ADVA,	Australian male Vietnam veterans vs Australian		
2005a	population—incidence	576	1.2 (1.1–1.3)
	Branch of service		
	Navy	141	1.4 (1.2–1.7)
	Army	372	1.2 (1.1–1.3)
	Air Force	63	1.0 (0.7–1.2)
	Histologic type—all service branches combined		
	Adenocarcinoma	188	1.5 (1.2–1.7)
	Squamous	152	1.2 (1.0–1.4)
	Small-cell	87	1.2 (0.97–1.5)
	Large-cell	79	1.1 (0.8–1.3)
	Other	70	1.1 (0.8–1.3)
ADVA,	Australian male Vietnam veterans vs Australian		
2005b	population—mortality	544	1.2 (1.1–1.3)
	Branch of service		
	Navy	135	1.4 (1.2–1.6)
	Army	339	1.1 (1.0–1.3)
	Air Force	71	1.1 (0.9–1.4)
ADVA,	Australian male conscripted Army National Service		
2005c	Vietnam-era veterans: deployed vs nondeployed		
	Incidence (1982–2000)	78	1.2 (1.0–1.5)
	Histologic type		
	Adenocarcinoma	27	1.4 (0.8–1.9)
	Squamous	19	1.5 (0.9–2.3)
	Small-cell	14	1.4 (0.8–2.4)
	Large-cell	8	0.7 (0.3–1.3)
	Other	10	1.2 (0.6–2.2)
	Mortality (1966–2001)	67	1.8 (1.2–2.7)
Pavuk et al.,	Comparison subjects only from AFHS (respiratory		
2005	system)—incidence		
	Serum TCDD (pg/g) based on model with		
	exposure variable $\log_e$(TCDD)		
	Per unit increase of $-\log_e$(TCDD) (pg/g)	36	1.7 (0.9–3.2)
	Quartiles (pg/g)		
	0.4–2.6	6	1.0 (nr)
	2.6–3.8	8	1.1 (0.3–3.4)
	3.8–5.2	9	1.2 (0.4–3.5)
	> 5.2	13	1.9 (0.7–5.5)

TABLE 6-13 Continued

Reference	Study Population[a]	Exposed Cases[b]	Estimated Relative Risk (95% CI)[b]
	Number of years served in SEA		
	Per year of service	36	1.1 (0.9–1.2)
	Quartiles (years in SEA)		
	0.8–1.3	8	1.0 (nr)
	1.3–2.1	4	0.5 (0.2–1.8)
	2.1–3.7	11	0.7 (0.3–2.0)
	3.7–16.4	13	0.7 (0.3–2.0)
Boehmer et al., 2004	Follow-up of CDC Vietnam Experience Cohort (trachea, bronchus, and lung)	41	1.0 (0.6–1.5)
	Low pay grade at time of discharge	nr	1.6 (0.9–3.0)
Studies Reviewed in *Update 2004*			
Akhtar et al., 2004	White AFHS subjects vs national rates (respiratory system)		
	Ranch Hand veterans		
	Incidence	33	1.1 (0.8–1.6)
	With tours between 1966–1970	26	1.1 (0.7–1.6)
	Mortality	21	0.9 (0.6–1.3)
	Comparison veterans		
	Incidence	48	1.2 (0.9–1.6)
	With tours 1966–1970	37	1.2 (0.9–1.6)
	Mortality	38	1.1 (0.8–1.5)
Studies Reviewed in *Update 2000*			
AFHS, 2000	Ranch Hand veterans from AFHS (lung and bronchus)—incidence	10	3.7(0.8–17.1)
			Expected number of exposed cases (95% CI)
AIHW, 1999	Australian Vietnam veterans—(lung cancer)— incidence (validation study)	46	65 (49–81)
CDVA, 1998a	Australian Vietnam veterans (lung)—incidence	120	65 (49–89)
Studies Reviewed in *Update 1998*			
CDVA, 1997a	Australian Vietnam veterans—mortality		
	Lung (ICD-9 162)	212	1.3 (1.1–1.4)
	Respiratory systems (ICD-9 163–165)	13	1.8 (1.0–3.0)
CDVA, 1997b	Australian National Service Vietnam veterans (lung)—mortality	27	2.2 (1.1–4.3)
Dalager and Kang, 1997	Army Chemical Corps veterans (respiratory system)—mortality	11	1.4 (0.4–5.4)
Mahan et al., 1997	Case–control of Vietnam-era Vietnam veterans (lung)—incidence	134	1.4 (1.0–1.9)
Watanabe and Kang, 1996	US Army and Marine Corps Vietnam veterans (lung)—mortality		
	Army Vietnam service	1,139	1.1 (nr) (p < 0.05)
	Non-Vietnam	1,141	1.1 (nr) (p < 0.05)
	Marine Vietnam service	215	1.2 (1.0–1.3)
	Non-Vietnam	77	0.9 (nr)

continued

TABLE 6-13 Continued

Reference	Study Population[a]	Exposed Cases[b]	Estimated Relative Risk (95% CI)[b]
Watanabe and Kang, 1995	Marine Vietnam service vs non-Vietnam (lung)	42	1.3 (0.8–2.1)
Visintainer et al., 1995	PM study of deaths (1974–1989) of Michigan Vietnam-era veterans—deployed vs nondeployed (lung)	80	0.9 (0.7–1.1)
OCCUPATIONAL			
New Studies			
Hansen et al., 2007	Danish gardeners (nasal, laryngeal, lung, and bronchus, ICD-7 160–165)—incidence		
	10-year follow-up (1975–1984) reported in Hansen et al. (1992)	41	1.0 (0.7–1.3)
	25-year follow-up (1975–2001)		
	Born before 1915 (high exposure)	34	0.9 (0.6–1.3)
	Born 1915–1934 (medium exposure)	72	1.0 (0.8–1.2)
	Born after 1934 (low exposure)	8	0.8 (0.4–1.7)
Samanic et al., 2006	Pesticide applicators in AHS—lung-cancer incidence from enrollment through 2002		
	Dicamba—lifetime days exposure		
	None	95	1.0
	1– < 20	14	0.8 (0.5–1.5)
	20– < 56	11	0.6 (0.3–1.3)
	56– < 116	12	1.0 (0.5–1.9)
	≥ 116	15	1.5 (0.8–2.7)
			p-trend = 0.13
Studies Reviewed in *Update 2006*			
McLean et al., 2006	IARC cohort of pulp and paper workers—exposure to nonvolatile organochlorine compounds		
	Lung (ICD-9 162)		
	Never	356	1.0 (0.9–1.1)
	Ever	314	1.0 (0.9–1.2)
	Pleura (ICD-9 163)		
	Never	17	2.8 (1.6–4.5)
	Ever	4	0.8 (0.2–2.0)
	Other respiratory (ICD-9 164–165)		
	Never	8	2.1 (0.9–4.2)
	Ever	2	0.7 (0.1–2.4)
Alavanja et al., 2005	US AHS—incidence		
	Private applicators (men and women)		
	Lung	266	0.5 (0.4–0.5)
	Respiratory system	294	0.5 (0.4–0.5)
	Spouses of private applicators (> 99% women)		
	Lung	68	0.4 (0.3–0.5)
	Respiratory system	71	0.4 (0.3–0.5)

TABLE 6-13 Continued

Reference	Study Population[a]	Exposed Cases[b]	Estimated Relative Risk (95% CI)[b]
	Commercial applicators (men and women)		
	Lung	12	0.6 (0.3–1.0)
	Respiratory system	14	0.6 (0.3–1.0)
Blair et al., 2005a	US AHS (lung)—mortality		
	Private applicators (men and women)	129	0.4 (0.3–0.4)
	Years handled pesticides		
	≤ 10 years	25	0.4 (nr) (p < 0.05)
	> 10 years	80	0.3 (nr) (p < 0.05)
	Spouses of private applicators (> 99% women)	29	0.3 (0.2–0.5)
't Mannetje et al., 2005	New Zealand phenoxy herbicide workers—mortality		
	Producers (men and women)		
	Trachea, bronchus, lung (ICD-9 162)	12	1.4 (0.7–2.4)
	Other respiratory system sites (ICD-9 163–165)	1	3.9 (0.1–21.5)
	Sprayers (> 99% men)		
	Trachea, bronchus, lung (ICD-9 162)	5	0.5 (0.2–1.1)
	Other respiratory system sites (ICD-9 163–165)	1	2.5 (0.1–13.7)
Torchio et al., 1994	Italian licensed pesticide users—mortality		
	Lung	155	0.5 (0.4–0.5)
Reif et al., 1989	New Zealand forestry workers—incidence (nested case–control)		
	Lung	30	1.3 (0.8–1.9)
Studies Reviewed in *Update 2004*			
Bodner et al., 2003	Dow chemical production workers (included in IARC cohort, NIOSH Dioxin Registry)—mortality		
	Lung	54	0.8 (0.6–1.1)
Swaen et al., 2004	Dutch licensed herbicide applicators (trachea, and lung)—mortality	27	0.7 (0.5–1.0)
Studies Reviewed in *Update 2002*			
Burns et al., 2001	Dow 2,4-D production workers (included in IARC cohort, NIOSH Dioxin Registry)—mortality		
	Respiratory system (ICD-8 160–163)	31	0.9 (0.6–1.3)
Thörn et al., 2000	Swedish lumberjacks exposed to phenoxy herbicides		
	Foremen (bronchus and lung)—incidence	1	4.2 (0.0–23.2)
Studies Reviewed in *Update 2000*			
Steenland et al., 1999	US chemical production workers (included in IARC cohort, NIOSH Dioxin Registry)—mortality		
	Lung	125	1.1 (0.9–1.3)
Studies Reviewed in *Update 1998*			
Gambini et al., 1997	Italian rice growers—mortality		
	Lung	45	0.8 (0.6–1.1)
	Pleura	2	2.2 (0.2–7.9)
Kogevinas et al., 1997	IARC cohort, male and female workers exposed to any phenoxy herbicide or chlorophenol		
	Lung (ICD-9 162)	380	1.1 (1.0–1.2)
	Other respiratory organs (ICD-9 163–165)	12	2.3 (1.2–3.9)

continued

TABLE 6-13 Continued

Reference	Study Population[a]	Exposed Cases[b]	Estimated Relative Risk (95% CI)[b]
	Exposed to highly chlorinated PCDDs		
	Lung (ICD-9 162)	225	1.1 (1.0–1.3)
	Other respiratory organs (ICD-9 163–165)	9	3.2 (1.5–6.1)
	Not exposed to highly chlorinated PCDDs		
	Lung (ICD-9 162)	148	1.0 (0.9–1.2)
	Other respiratory organs (ICD-9 163–165)	3	1.2 (0.3–3.6)
Becher et al., 1996	German production workers (included in IARC cohort) (lung)	47	1.4 (1.1–1.9)
Ott and Zober, 1996	BASF employees—incidence		
	Respiratory system	13	1.2 (0.6–2.0)
	TCDD 0.1–0.99 µg/kg of body weight	2	0.7 (0.1–2.5)
	TCDD ≥ 1 µg/kg of body weight	8	2.0 (0.9–3.9)
	Lung, bronchus	11	1.1 (0.6–2.0)
	TCDD 0.1–0.99 µg/kg of body weight	2	0.8 (0.1–2.8)
	TCDD ≥ 1 µg/kg of body weight	8	2.2 (1.0–4.3)
Ramlow et al., 1996	Dow pentachlorophenol production workers (Included in IARC cohort, NIOSH Dioxin Registry)—mortality		
	0-year latency		
	Respiratory system (ICD-8 160–163)	18	1.0 (0.6–1.5)
	Lung (ICD-8 162)	16	0.9 (0.5–1.5)
	15-year latency		
	Respiratory system (ICD-8 160–163)	17	1.1 (0.6–1.8)
	Lung (ICD-8 162)	16	1.1 (0.6–1.8)
Studies Reviewed in *Update 1996*			
Asp et al., 1994	Finnish herbicide applicators, 1972–1989		
	Incidence		
	Trachea, bronchus, lung (ICD-8 162)	39	0.9 (0.7–1.3)
	Other respiratory (ICD-8 160, 161, 163)	4	1.1 (0.7–1.3)
	Mortality		
	Trachea, bronchus, lung (ICD-8 162)	37	1.0 (0.7–1.4)
	Other respiratory (ICD-8 160, 161, 163)	1	0.5 (0.0–2.9)
Blair et al., 1993	US farmers in 23 states (lung)—mortality		
	White men	6,473	0.9 (0.9–0.9)
	White women	57	0.8 (0.6–1.1)
Bloemen et al., 1993	Dow 2,4-D production workers (included in IARC cohort, NIOSH Dioxin Registry)		
	Respiratory system (ICD-8 162–163)	9	0.8 (0.4–1.5)
Kogevinas et al., 1993	IARC cohort, women (lung)—incidence	2	1.4 (0.2–4.9)
Lynge, 1993	Danish production workers (included in IARC cohort)—incidence		
	Lung	13	1.6 (0.9–2.8)

TABLE 6-13 Continued

Reference	Study Population[a]	Exposed Cases[b]	Estimated Relative Risk (95% CI)[b]
Studies Reviewed in *VAO*			
Bueno de Mesquita et al., 1993	Dutch phenoxy herbicide workers (included in IARC cohort)—mortality		
	Trachea, bronchus, lung (ICD-8 162)	9	0.8 (0.4–1.5)
	Respiratory system (ICD-8 160–163)	9	1.7 (0.5–6.3)
Swaen et al., 1992	Dutch herbicide applicators—mortality		
	Trachea and lung	12	1.1 (0.6–1.9)
Coggon et al., 1991	British phenoxy herbicide workers (included in IARC cohort)—mortality		
	Lung	19	1.3 (0.8–2.1)
	Workers with exposure above background	14	1.2 (0.7–2.1)
Fingerhut et al., 1991	NIOSH workers exposed to TCDD—mortality		
	Entire cohort		
	Trachea, bronchus, lung (ICD-9 162)	89	1.1 (0.9–1.4)
	Respiratory system (ICD-9 160–165)	96	1.1 (0.9–1.4)
	≥ 1-year exposure, ≥ 20-year latency		
	Trachea, bronchus, lung (ICD-9 162)	40	1.4 (1.0–1.9)
	Respiratory system (ICD-9 160–165)	43	1.4 (1.0–1.9)
Green, 1991	Herbicide sprayers in Ontario (lung)—mortality	5	nr
Manz et al., 1991	German production workers (included in IARC cohort)—mortality		
	Lung	26	1.7 (1.1–2.4)
Saracci et al., 1991	IARC cohort, men, women—mortality		
	Trachea, bronchus, lung	173	1.0 (0.9–1.2)
McDuffie et al., 1990	Saskatchewan farmers applying herbicides—incidence		
	Lung	103	0.6 (nr)
Zober et al., 1990	BASF employees—incidence		90% CI
	Trachea, bronchus, lung	4	2.0 (0.7–4.6)
Bender et al., 1989	Herbicide sprayers in Minnesota—mortality		
	Trachea, bronchus, lung (ICD-9 162.0–162.8)	54	0.7 (0.5–0.9)
	All respiratory (ICD-9 160.0–165.9)	57	0.7 (0.5–0.9)
Wiklund et al., 1989a	Swedish pesticide applicators—incidence		
	Trachea, bronchus, lung	38	0.5 (0.4–0.7)
Bond et al., 1988	Dow 2,4-D production workers (included in IARC cohort, NIOSH Dioxin Registry)—mortality		
	Lung (ICD-8 162–163)	8	1.0 (0.5–2.0)
	Respiratory (ICD-8 160–163) (exposure lagged 15 years)		
	Low cumulative exposure	1	0.7 (nr)
	Medium cumulative exposure	2	1.0 (nr)
	High cumulative exposure	5	1.7 (nr)

continued

TABLE 6-13 Continued

Reference	Study Population[a]	Exposed Cases[b]	Estimated Relative Risk (95% CI)[b]
Coggon et al., 1986	British MCPA production workers (included in IARC cohort)—mortality		
	Lung, pleura, mediastinum (ICD-8 162–164)	117	1.2 (1.0–1.4)
	Background exposure	39	1.0 (0.7–1.4)
	Low-grade exposure	35	1.1 (0.8–1.6)
	High-grade exposure	43	1.3 (1.0–1.8)
Lynge, 1985	Danish production workers (included in IARC cohort)—incidence		
	Lung		
	Men	38	1.2 (nr)
	Women	6	2.2 (nr)
Blair et al., 1983	Licensed pesticide applicators in Florida, lawn, ornamental pest category only—mortality		
	Lung (ICD-8 162–163)	7	0.9 (nr)
Axelson et al., 1980	Swedish herbicide sprayers (lung)—mortality	3	1.4 (nr)
ENVIRONMENTAL			
New Studies			
Consonni et al., 2008	Seveso residents—25-year follow-up—men, women (lung ICD-9 162)		
	Zone A	11	1.1 (0.6–2.0)
	Zone B	62	1.1 (0.9–1.4)
	Zone R	383	1.0 (0.8–1.1)
Studies Reviewed in *Update 2004*			
Fukuda et al., 2003	Residents of Japanese municipalities with and without waste-incineration plants		Age-adjusted mortality (per 100,000)
	Men		
	With		39.0 ± 6.7 vs 41.6
	Without		± 9.1 (p = 0.001)
	Women		
	With		13.7 ± 3.8 vs 14.3
	Without		± 4.6 (p = 0.11)
Studies Reviewed in *Update 2002*			
Revich et al., 2001	Residents of Chapaevsk, Russia (lung)		
	Men	168	3.1 (2.6–3.5)
	Women	40	0.4 (0.3–0.6)
Studies Reviewed in *Update 2000*			
Bertazzi et al., 2001	Seveso residents—20-year follow-up (lung)—incidence		
	Zones A, B—men	57	1.3 (1.0–1.7)
	women	4	0.6 (0.2–1.7)
Bertazzi et al., 1998	Seveso residents—15-year follow-up (lung)—incidence		
	Zone A—men	4	1.0 (0.4–2.6)
	women	0	nr

TABLE 6-13 Continued

Reference	Study Population[a]	Exposed Cases[b]	Estimated Relative Risk (95% CI)[b]
	Zone B—men	34	1.2 (0.9–1.7)
	women	2	0.6 (0.1–2.3)
	Zone R—men	176	0.9 (0.8–1.1)
	women	29	1.0 (0.7–1.6)
Studies Reviewed in *Update 1998*			
Bertazzi et al., 1997	Seveso residents—15-year follow-up (lung)—incidence		
	Zone A—men	4	1.0 (0.3–2.5)
	Zone B—men	34	1.2 (0.9–1.7)
	women	2	0.6 (0.1–2.1)
	Zone R—men	176	0.9 (0.8–1.0)
	women	29	1.0 (0.7–1.5)
Svensson et al., 1995	Swedish fishermen		
	East coast (lung, larynx)	16	0.8 (0.5–1.3)
	West coast (lung, larynx)	77	0.9 (0.7–1.1)
Studies Reviewed in *VAO*			
Bertazzi et al., 1993	Seveso residents—10-year follow-up (trachea, bronchus, lung)—incidence		
	Zone A—men	2	0.8 (0.2–3.4)
	Zone B—men	18	1.1 (0.7–1.8)
	Zone R—men	96	0.8 (0.7–1.0)
	women	16	1.5 (0.8–2.5)

ABBREVIATIONS: 2,4-D, 2,4-dichlorophenoxyacetic acid; AFHS, Air Force Health Study; AHS, Agricultural Health Study; CDC, Centers for Disease Control and Prevention; CI, confidence interval; IARC, International Agency for Research on Cancer; ICD, International Classification of Diseases; MCPA, methyl-4-chlorophenoxyacetic acid; NIOSH, National Insitute for Occupational Safety and Health; nr = not reported; PCDD, polychlorinated dibenzo-*p*-dioxin (highly chlorinated, if four or more chlorines); PM, proportionate mortality; SEA, Southeast Asia; TCDD, 2,3,7,8-tetrachlorodibenzo-*p*-dioxin.
[a]Subjects are male and outcome is mortality unless otherwise noted.
[b]Given when available; results other than estimated risk explained individually.

associations between the exposures and all respiratory cancers were found; RRs were roughly unity.

In a report on the US AHS, Samanic et al. (2006) conducted an analysis of the incidence of lung cancer and exposure to dicambin male pesticide applicators. When a metric defined as lifetime exposure–days was used, rate ratios comparing subjects exposed to dicamba were less than unity for all categories of exposure except the highest quintile, at least 166 exposure–days (RR = 1.47, 95% CI 0.79–2.72), and there was no trend with increasing exposure (p for linear trend = 0.13).

When a metric defined as "intensity-weighted lifetime exposure–days" (data not shown) was used, there was no evidence of a monotonic association with mortality from lung cancer (p for linear trend = 0.58), and the largest RR was 1.10 (for the category *of at least* 739.2 weighted exposure–days vs no exposure).

Environmental Studies

Investigators in Italy completed a 25-year mortality follow-up of people exposed to the industrial accident in Seveso (Consonni et al., 2008). Mortality from lung cancer in residents in three exposure zones—very high (Zone A), high (Zone B), and low (Zone R)—was compared with that in a nonexposed reference population. The RRs for lung-cancer mortality in the exposure groups were 1.26 (95% CI 0.7–2.29) in Zone A, 1.11 (95% CI 0.87–1.43) in Zone B, and 0.98 (95% CI 0.88–1.09) in Zone R. There were 11, 62, and 383 lung-cancer deaths during the follow-up period in Zones A, B, and R, respectively.

Biologic Plausibility

Long-term animal studies have examined the effect of exposure to the chemicals of interest on tumor incidences (Charles et al., 1996; Stott et al., 1990; Walker et al., 2006; Wanibuchi et al., 2004). As noted in previous VAO reports, there is evidence of increased incidence of squamous-cell carcinoma of the lung in male and female rats exposed to TCDD at high concentrations (Kociba et al., 1978; Van Miller et al., 1977). A more recent study reported a significant increase in cystic keratinizing epitheliomas in female rats exposed to TCDD for 2 years (NTP, 2006; Walker et al., 2006) and increases in the incidences of bronchiolar metaplasia, acinar vacuolization, and inflammation in the high-dose (100 ng/kg) group.

A recent 2-year study of F344 rats exposed to cacodylic acid at 0–100 ppm and B6C3F1 mice exposed at 0–500 ppm failed to detect neoplasms in the lung at any dose (Arnold et al., 2006); this finding is consistent with those of previous studies. However, exposure to cacodylic acid has previously been shown to increase tumor multiplicity in mouse strains susceptible to developing lung tumors (for example, A/J strain; Hayashi et al., 1998) or mice pretreated with an intitiating agent (4-nitroquinoline 1-oxide; Yamanaka et al., 1996). The data indicate that cacodylic acid may act as a tumor promoter in the lung.

The biologic plausibility of the carcinogenicity of the chemicals of interest is discussed in general at the beginning of this chapter.

Synthesis

The evidence remains limited but suggestive of an association between exposure to at least one chemical of interest and the risk of developing or dying from lung cancer. The most compelling evidence comes from studies of heavily exposed occupational cohorts, including British 2-methyl-4-chlorophenoxyacetic acid production workers (Coggon et al., 1986), German production workers (Becher et al., 1996; Manz et al., 1991), a BASF cohort (Ott and Zober, 1996), a NIOSH cohort (Fingerhut et al., 1991; Steenland et al., 1999), and Danish production workers (Lynge, 1993). The latest findings from the US Air Force Health Study suggest an increase in risk with the concentration of serum TCDD even in subjects who made up the comparison group, whose TCDD exposure was considerably lower (but not zero) than that of the Ranch Hand cohort. The American and Australian cohort studies of Vietnam veterans, which presumably cover a large proportion of exposed soldiers, show higher than expected incidence of and mortality from lung cancer. The main limitations of those studies are that there was no assessment of exposure—as there was in, for example, the Ranch Hand study—and that some potential confounding variables, notably smoking, could not be accounted for. The committee believes that it is unlikely that the distribution of smoking differed greatly between the two cohorts of veterans, so confounding by smoking is probably minimal. The studies therefore lend support to the findings of the Ranch Hand study. The methodologically sound AHS did not show any increased risks of lung cancer, but, although there was substantial 2,4-D exposure in this cohort (Blair et al., 2005b), dioxin exposure of the contemporary farmers was probably negligible. Results of the environmental studies were mostly consistent with no association.

Also supportive of an association are the numerous lines of mechanistic evidence, discussed in the section on biologic plausibility, which provide further support for the conclusion that the evidence of an association is limited or suggestive.

Conclusion

On the basis of the evidence reviewed here and in previous VAO reports, the committee concludes that there is limited or suggestive evidence of an association between exposure to at least one chemical of interest and carcinomas of the lung, bronchus, and trachea.

BONE AND JOINT CANCER

ACS estimated that about 1,270 men and 1,110 women would receive diagnoses of bone or joint cancer (ICD-9 170) in the United States in 2008 and that 820 men and 650 women would die from these cancers (Jemal et al., 2008a). Primary bone cancers are among the least common malignancies, but the bones are frequent sites of tumors secondary to cancers that have metastasized. Only primary bone cancer is considered here. The average annual incidence of bone and joint cancer is shown in Table 6-14.

TABLE 6-14 Average Annual Incidence (per 100,000) of Bone and Joint Cancer in United States[a]

	50–54 Years Old			55–59 Years Old			60–64 Years Old		
	All Races	White	Black	All Races	White	Black	All Races	White	Black
Men	0.9	0.9	0.8	1.2	1.2	0.5	1.2	1.2	1.6
Women	0.9	1.0	0.3	1.0	1.1	0.4	1.2	1.1	1.6

[a]Surveillance, Epidemiology, and End Results program, nine standard registries, crude age-specific rates, 2000–2005.

Bone cancer is more common in teenagers than in adults. It is rare among people in the age groups of most Vietnam veterans (50–64 years). Among the risk factors for adults' contracting of bone or joint cancer are exposure to ionizing radiation in treatment for other cancers and a history of some noncancer bone diseases, including Paget disease.

Conclusions from *VAO* and Previous Updates

The committee responsible for *VAO* concluded that there was inadequate or insufficient information to determine whether there is an association between exposure to the chemicals of interest and bone and joint cancer. Additional information available to the committees responsible for *Update 1996*, *Update 1998*, *Update 2000*, *Update 2002*, *Update 2004*, and *Update 2006* did not change that conclusion. Table 6-15 summarizes the results of the relevant studies.

Update of the Epidemiologic Literature

No studies concerning exposure to the chemicals of interest and bone and joint cancers have been published since *Update 2006*.

Biologic Plausibility

No animal studies have reported an increased incidence of bone and joint cancers after exposure to the chemicals of interest. The biologic plausibility of the carcinogenicity of the chemicals of interest is discussed in general at the beginning of this chapter.

TABLE 6-15 Selected Epidemiologic Studies—Bone and Joint Cancer

Reference	Study Population[a]	Exposed Cases[b]	Estimated Relative Risk (95% CI)[b]
VIETNAM VETERANS			
Studies Reviewed in *Update 1998*			
Clapp, 1997	Massachusetts Vietnam veterans	4	0.9 (0.1–11.3)
AFHS, 1996	Air Force Ranch Hand veterans	0	nr
Studies Reviewed in *VAO*			
Breslin	Army Vietnam veterans	27	0.8 (0.4–1.7)
et al., 1988	Marine Vietnam veterans	11	1.4 (0.1–21.5)
Anderson	Wisconsin Vietnam veterans	1	nr
et al., 1986			
Lawrence	New York Vietnam veterans	8	1.0 (0.3–3.0)
et al., 1985			
OCCUPATIONAL			
Studies Reviewed in *Update 2006*			
Merletti	Association between occupational exposure and risk		
et al., 2006	of bone sarcoma	18	2.6 (1.5–4.6)
't Mannetje	Phenoxy herbicide producers and sprayers (men and		
et al., 2005	women)	0	nr
Torchio	Italian licensed pesticide users	10	0.8 (0.4–1.4)
et al., 1994			
Reif et al.,	New Zealand forestry workers—nested case–control		
1989	—incidence	1	1.7 (0.2–13.3)
Studies Reviewed in *Update 2004*			
Swaen	Dutch licenced herbicide applicators	0	nr
et al., 2004			
Studies Reviewed in *Update 2000*			
Rix et al.,	Danish paper-mill workers—incidence		
1998	Men	1	0.5 (0.0–2.7)
	Women	0	nr
Studies Reviewed in *Update 1998*			
Gambini	Italian rice growers	1	0.5 (0.0–2.6)
et al., 1997			
Hertzman	British Columbia sawmill workers		
et al., 1997	Mortality	5	1.3 (0.5–2.7)
	Incidence	4	1.1 (0.4–2.4)
Kogevinas	IARC cohort, male and female workers exposed to		
et al., 1997	any phenoxy herbicide or chlorophenol	5	1.2 (0.4–2.8)
	Exposed to highly chlorinated PCDDs	3	1.1 (0.2–3.1)
	Not exposed to highly chlorinated PCDDs	2	1.4 (0.2–5.2)
Ramlow	Dow pentachlorophenol production workers		
et al., 1996	(included in IARC cohort, NIOSH Dioxin Registry)	0	nr
	0-year latency	0	nr
	15-year latency	0	nr
Studies Reviewed in *Update 1996*			
Blair et al.,	US farmers in 23 states		
1993	White men	49	1.3 (1.0–1.8)
	White women	1	1.2 (0.0–6.6)

continued

TABLE 6-15 Continued

Reference	Study Population[a]	Exposed Cases[b]	Estimated Relative Risk (95% CI)[b]
Collins et al., 1993	Monsanto Company workers (included in NIOSH cohort)	2	5.0 (0.6–18.1)
Studies Reviewed in VAO			
Ronco et al., 1992	Danish, Italian farm workers		
	Male Danish farmers	9	0.9 (nr)
	Female Danish farmers	0	nr
Fingerhut et al., 1991	NIOSH—entire cohort	2	2.3 (0.3–8.2)
	≥ 1-year exposure, ≥ 20-year latency	1	5.5 (0.1–29.0)
Zober et al., 1990			90% CI
	BASF employees—basic cohort	0	0 (0.0–65.5)
Bond et al., 1988	Dow 2,4-D production workers (included in IARC cohort, NIOSH Dioxin Registry)	0	nr (0.0–31.1)
Coggon et al., 1986	British MCPA production workers (included in IARC cohort)	1	0.9 (0.0–5.0)
Wiklund, 1983	Swedish male and female agricultural workers—incidence	44	99% CI 1.0 (0.6–1.4)
Burmeister, 1981	Iowa farmers	56	1.1 (nr)
ENVIRONMENTAL			
Studies Reviewed in Update 2002			
Revich et al., 2001	Residents of Chapaevsk, Russia Mortality standardized to Samara region (bone, soft-tissue cancer)		
	Men	7	2.1 (0.9–4.4)
	Women	7	1.4 (0.6–3.0)
Studies Reviewed in Update 2000			
Bertazzi et al., 1998	Seveso residents—15-year follow-up		
	Zone B women	1	2.6 (0.3–19.4)
	Zone R men	2	0.5 (0.1–2.0)
	Zone R women	7	2.4 (1.0–5.7)
Studies Reviewed in Update 1998			
Bertazzi et al., 1997	Seveso residents—15-year follow-up		
	Zone B women	1	2.6 (0.0–14.4)
	Zone R men	2	0.5 (0.1–1.7)
	Zone R women	7	2.4 (1.0–4.9)

ABBREVIATIONS: 2,4-D, 2,4-dichlorophenoxyacetic acid; CI, confidence interval; IARC, International Agency for Research on Cancer; MCPA, methyl-4-chlorophenoxyacetic acid; NIOSH, National Institute for Occupational Safety and Health; nr, not reported; PCDDs, chlorinated dibenzo-p-dioxins (highly chlorinated, if four or more chlorines); TCDD, 2,3,7,8-tetrachlorodibenzo-p-dioxin.
[a]Subjects are male and outcome is mortality unless otherwise noted.
[b]Given when available; results other than estimated risk explained individually.
Studies in italics have been superseded by newer studies of the same cohorts.

Synthesis

There are no new data concerning the chemicals of interest and bone cancer, and the previous body of results summarized in Table 6-15 does not indicate an association between exposure to the chemicals of interest and bone cancer.

Conclusion

On the basis of the evidence reviewed here and in previous VAO reports, the committee concludes that there is inadequate or insufficient evidence to determine whether there is an association between exposure to the chemicals of interest and bone and joint cancers.

SOFT-TISSUE SARCOMAS

Soft-tissue sarcoma (STS) (ICD-9 164.1, 171) arises in soft somatic tissues in and between organs. Three of the most common types of STS—liposarcoma, fibrosarcoma, and rhabdomyosarcoma—occur in similar numbers in men and women. Because of the diverse characteristics of STS, accurate diagnosis and classification can be difficult. ACS estimated that about 5,720 men and 4,670 women would receive diagnoses of STS in the United States in 2008 and that about 1,880 men and 1,800 women would die from it (Jemal et al., 2008a). The average annual incidence of STS is shown in Table 6-16.

Among the risk factors for STS are exposure to ionizing radiation during treatment for other cancers and some inherited conditions, including Gardner syndrome, Li-Fraumeni syndrome, and neurofibromatosis. Several chemical exposures have been identified as possible risk factors (Zahm and Fraumeni, 1997).

Conclusions from *VAO* and Previous Updates

The committee responsible for *VAO* judged that the strong findings in the IARC and NIOSH cohorts and the extensive Scandinavian case–control studies, complemented by consistency in preliminary reports on the Seveso population

TABLE 6-16 Average Annual Incidence (per 100,000) of Soft-Tissue Sarcoma (Including Malignant Neoplasms of the Heart) in United States[a]

	50–54 Years Old			55–59 Years Old			60–64 Years Old		
	All Races	White	Black	All Races	White	Black	All Races	White	Black
Men	4.5	4.5	4.0	5.0	4.8	7.4	6.7	7.2	3.5
Women	3.1	3.2	3.9	4.3	4.1	6.4	5.1	4.8	7.2

[a]Surveillance, Epidemiology, and End Results program, nine standard registries, crude age-specific rates, 2000–2005.

and one statistically significant finding in a state study of Vietnam veterans, constituted sufficient information to determine that there is an association between exposure to at least one of the chemicals of interest and STS. Additional information available to the committees responsible for *Update 1996*, *Update 1998*, *Update 2000*, *Update 2002*, *Update 2004*, and *Update 2006* did not change that conclusion. Table 6-17 summarizes the relevant studies.

Update of the Epidemiologic Literature

Vietnam-Veteran Studies

No Vietnam-veteran studies concerning exposure to the chemicals of interest and soft tissue sarcomas have been published since *Update 2006*.

Occupational Studies

Hansen et al. (2007) conducted a historical-cohort study of 3,156 male gardeners who were members of a Danish union. The study by Hansen et al. (1992), which followed the cohort for 10 years through 1984, was reported in *VAO*. Subjects were followed-up by using population and cancer registries, and the incidence of cancer was ascertained from 1975 until the end of 2001. Birth date served as a surrogate for potential exposure to pesticides and herbicides, with earlier cohorts representing higher potential exposures. Although the analysis was based on only three cases, the risk of dying from STS was 6 times higher in men born before 1915 (RR = 5.9, 95% CI 1.9–18.2).

Environmental Studies

Consonni et al. (2008) conducted a follow-up of the population in the area of the accident that occurred in Seveso in 1976. The follow-up was extended until 2001, and no associations with deaths from STS were found in any of the three exposure zones. There were only four deaths from STS, all of which occurred in Zone R (RR = 0.76, 95% CI 0.27–2.14).

Read et al. (2007) conducted a study of residents of the coastal community of Paritutu, New Plymouth, New Zealand, near the Ivon Watkins-Dow Limited plant, which had manufactured the herbicide 2,4,5-T during 1962–1987. It was reported that the body burden of TCDD was comparable with that in residents living in Zone B of the Seveso area. Incidence and mortality were ascertained for the period 1970–2001. No association between exposure to 2,4,5-T or TCDD and the incidence of STS was found, but there was a 20% increase in mortality (95% CI 0.8–1.8).

Zambon et al. (2007) conducted a population-based case–control study in Venice, Italy. Confirmed cases of sarcoma (ICD-9 171, 173, 158) were identified from a population cancer registry. The cases were divided by anatomic site

TABLE 6-17 Selected Epidemiologic Studies—Soft-Tissue Sarcoma

Reference	Study Population[a]	Exposed Cases[b]	Estimated Relative Risk (95% CI)[b]
VIETNAM VETERANS			
Studies Reviewed in *Update 2006*			
ADVA, 2005a	Australian Vietnam veterans vs Australian population—incidence	35	1.0 (0.7–1.3)
	Navy	6	0.8 (0.3–1.7)
	Army	29	1.2 (0.8–1.6)
	Air Force	0	0.0 (0.0–1.1)
ADVA, 2005b	Australian Vietnam veterans vs Australian population—mortality	12	0.8 (0.4–1.3)
	Navy	3	0.9 (0.2–2.4)
	Army	9	0.8 (0.4–1.5)
	Air Force	0	0.0 (0.0–2.3)
ADVA, 2005c	Australian men conscripted Army National Service Vietnam era veterans—deployed vs nondeployed		
	Incidence	10	1.0 (0.4–2.4)
	Mortality	3	0.5 (0.1–2.0)
Studies Reviewed in *Update 2000*			
AFHS, 2000	Air Force Ranch Hand veterans	1	0.8 (0.1–12.8)
AIHW, 1999			Expected number of exposed cases (95% CI)
	Male Australian Vietnam veterans—incidence (validation study)	14	27 (17–37)
CDVA, 1998a	Male Australian Vietnam veterans—self-reported incidence	398	27 (17–37)
CDVA, 1998b	Female Australian Vietnam veterans—self-reported incidence	2	0 (0–4)
Studies Reviewed in *Update 1998*			
Clapp, 1997	Massachusetts Vietnam veterans	18	1.6 (0.5–5.4)
CDVA, 1997a	Australian military Vietnam veterans	9	1.0 (0.4–1.8)
CDVA, 1997b	Australian National Service Vietnam veterans	2	0.7 (0.6–4.5)
AFHS, 1996	Ranch Hand veterans	0	nr
Watanabe and Kang, 1995	US Marines in Vietnam	0	nr
Studies Reviewed in *Update 1996*			
Visintainer et al., 1995	PM study of deaths (1974–1989) of Michigan Vietnam-era veterans—deployed vs nondeployed	8	1.1 (0.5–2.2)
Studies Reviewed in *VAO*			
Watanabe et al., 1991	Army Vietnam veterans	43	1.1
	Marine Vietnam veterans	11	0.7
Bullman et al., 1990	Army I Corps Vietnam veterans	10	0.9 (0.4–1.6)
Michalek et al., 1990	Ranch Hand veterans	1	nr
	Comparisons	1	nr

continued

TABLE 6-17 Continued

Reference	Study Population[a]	Exposed Cases[b]	Estimated Relative Risk (95% CI)[b]
Breslin	Army Vietnam veterans	30	1.0 (0.8–1.2)
et al., 1988	Marine Vietnam veterans	8	0.7 (0.4–1.3)
Kogan and Clapp, 1988	Massachusetts Vietnam veterans	9	5.2 (2.4–11.1)
Fett et al., 1987	Australian Vietnam veterans	1	1.3 (0.1–20.0)
Anderson et al., 1986	Wisconsin Vietnam veterans	4	nr
Breslin	US Vietnam veterans		
et al., 1986	Army	30	1.0 (nr)
	Marines	8	0.7 (nr)
Kang et al., 1986	Vietnam veterans vs Vietnam-era veterans	86	0.8 (0.6–1.1)
Lawrence et al., 1985	New York State Vietnam veterans	2	1.1 (0.2–6.7)
Greenwald et al., 1984	New York State Vietnam veterans	10	0.5 (0.2–1.3)

OCCUPATIONAL
New Studies

Hansen et al., 2007	Danish gardeners (ICD-7 197)—incidence		
	10-year follow-up (1975–1984) reported in		
	Hansen et al. (1992)	3	5.3 (1.1–15.4)
	25-year follow-up (1975–2001)		
	Born before 1915 (high exposure)	3	5.9 (1.9–18.2)
	Born 1915–1934 (medium exposure)	0	0.0 (0.0–3.8)
	Born after 1934 (low exposure)	1	1.8 (0.3–12.9)

Studies Reviewed in *Update 2006*

McLean et al., 2006	IARC cohort of pulp and paper workers		
	Exposure to nonvolatile organochlorine compounds		
	Never	8	1.2 (0.5–2.4)
	Ever	4	0.8 (0.2–2.0)
't Mannetje	Phenoxy herbicide producers (men and women)	0	0.0 (0.0–19.3)
et al., 2005	Phenoxy herbicide sprayers (> 99% men)	1	4.3 (0.1–23.8)
Alavanja	US AHS—incidence		
et al., 2005	Private applicators (men and women)	10	0.7 (0.3–1.2)
	Spouses of private applicators (> 99% women)	3	0.5 (0.1–1.4)
	Commercial applicators (men and women)	nr	0.0 (0.0–3.8)
Blair et al.,	US AHS		
2005a	Private applicators (men and women)	4	0.7 (0.2–1.8)
	Spouses of private applicators (> 99% women)	3	1.4 (0.3–4.1)
Torchio et al., 1994	Italian licensed pesticide users	2	1.0 (0.1–3.5)
Reif et al., 1989	New Zealand forestry workers—nested case–control —incidence	4	3.2 (1.2–9.0)

TABLE 6-17 Continued

Reference	Study Population[a]	Exposed Cases[b]	Estimated Relative Risk (95% CI)[b]
Studies Reviewed in *Update 2004*			
Bodner et al., 2003	Dow chemical production workers (included in IARC cohort, NIOSH Dioxin Registry)	2	2.4 (0.3–8.6)
Studies Reviewed in *Update 2000*			
Steenland et al., 1999	US chemical production workers (included in IARC cohort, NIOSH Dioxin Registry)	0	nr
Hooiveld et al., 1998	Dutch chemical production workers (included in IARC cohort)	0	nr
Rix et al., 1998	Danish paper-mill workers—incidence		
	Women employed in sorting and packing	8	4.0 (1.7–7.8)
	Men employed in sorting and packing	12	1.2 (0.6–2.0)
Studies Reviewed in *Update 1998*			
Hertzman et al., 1997	Canadian sawmill workers	11	1.0 (0.6–1.7)
Kogevinas et al., 1997	IARC cohort, male and female workers exposed to any phenoxy herbicide or chlorophenol	9	2.0 (0.9–3.8)
	Exposed to highly chlorinated PCDDs	6	2.0 (0.8–4.4)
	Not exposed to highly chlorinated PCDDs	2	1.4 (0.2–4.9)
Ott and Zober, 1996			Expected number of exposed cases
	BASF employees—incidence	0	0.2
Ramlow et al., 1996	Dow pentachlorophenol production workers (included in IARC cohort, NIOSH Dioxin Registry)	0	Expected number of exposed cases 0.2
Studies Reviewed in *Update 1996*			
Kogevinas et al., 1995	IARC cohort (men and women)—incidence	11	nr
Mack, 1995	US cancer registry data (SEER program) review		
	Men	3,526	nr
	Women	2,886	nr
Blair et al., 1993	US farmers in 23 states	98	0.9 (0.8–1.1)
Lynge, 1993	Danish production workers (included in the IARC cohort)—updated incidence for men, women	5	2.0 (0.7–4.8)
Kogevinas et al., 1992	IARC cohort (men and women)		
	10–19 years since first exposure	4	6.1 (1.7–15.5)
Studies Reviewed in *VAO*			
Bueno de Mesquita et al., 1993	Dutch phenoxy herbicide workers (included in IARC cohort)	0	0.0 (0.0–23.1)
Hansen et al., 1992	Danish gardeners—incidence	3	5.3 (1.1–15.4)
Smith and Christophers, 1992	Australia residents	30	1.0 (0.3–3.1)

continued

TABLE 6-17 Continued

Reference	Study Population[a]	Exposed Cases[b]	Estimated Relative Risk (95% CI)[b]
Fingerhut	NIOSH cohort—entire cohort	4	3.4 (0.9–8.7)
et al., 1991	≥ 1-year exposure, ≥ 20-year latency	3	9.2 (1.9–27.0)
Manz et al.,	German production workers (included in IARC		
1991	cohort)—men, women	0	nr
Saracci	IARC cohort—exposed subcohort (men and		
et al., 1991	women)	4	2.0 (0.6–5.2)
Zober et al.,	BASF employees—basic cohort	0	nr
1990			
Alavanja	USDA forest and soil conservationists	2	1.0 (0.1–3.6)
et al., 1989			
Bond et al.,	Dow 2,4-D production workers (included in IARC		
1988	cohort, NIOSH Dioxin Registry)	0	nr
Wiklund			
et al., 1988,			99% CI
1989b	Swedish agricultural workers (men and women)	7	0.9 (0.4–1.9)
Woods et al.,	Washington state residents—incidence		
1987	High phenoxy exposure	nr	0.9 (0.4–1.9)
	Self-reported chloracne	nr	3.3 (0.8–14.0)
Coggon	British MCPA chemical workers (included in IARC		
et al., 1986	cohort)	1	1.1 (0.03–5.9)
Hoar et al.,	Kansas residents—incidence		
1986	All farmers	95	1.0 (0.7–1.6)
	Farm use of herbicides	22	0.9 (0.5–1.6)
Smith and			90% CI
Pearce, 1986	Reanalysis of New Zealand workers	133	1.1 (0.7–1.8)
Vineis et al.,	Italian rice growers		
1986	Among all living females	5	2.4 (0.4–16.1)
Smith et al.,			90% CI
1984	Update of New Zealand workers	17	1.6 (0.7–3.8)
Lynge, 1985	Danish production workers (included in IARC		
	cohort)—incidence		
	Men	5	2.7 (0.9–6.3)
	Women	0	nr
Balarajan	Agricultural workers in England		
and	Overall	42	1.7 (1.0–2.9)
Acheson,	Under 75 years old		
1984		33	1.4 (0.8–2.6)
Blair et al.,	Florida pesticide applicators		
1983		0	nr
Smith et al.,			90% CI
1983	New Zealand workers exposed to herbicides	17	1.6 (0.8–3.2)
Hardell,	Swedish residents		
1981	Exposed to phenoxy acids	13	5.5 (2.2–13.8)
	Exposed to chlorophenols	6	5.4 (1.3–22.5)

TABLE 6-17 Continued

Reference	Study Population[a]	Exposed Cases[b]	Estimated Relative Risk (95% CI)[b]
Eriksson et al., 1979, 1981	Swedish workers	25	(2.5–10.4) 5:1 matched
ENVIRONMENTAL			
New Studies			
Consonni et al., 2008	Seveso residents—25-year follow-up—men, women		
	Zone A	0	nr
	Zone B	0	nr
	Zone R	4	0.8 (0.3–2.1)
Read et al., 2007	Residents of New Plymouth Territorial Authority, New Zealand near plant manufacturing 2,4,5-T in 1962–1987		
	Incidence	56	1.0 (0.8–1.4)[c]
	1970–1974	7	1.0 (0.4–2.1)
	1975–1979	3	0.4 (0.1–2.1)
	1980–1984	10	1.3 (0.6–2.4)
	1985–1989	11	1.2 (0.6–2.2)
	1990–1994	9	0.9 (0.4–1.7)
	1995–1999	14	1.3 (0.7–2.2)
	2000–2001	2	0.8 (0.1–3.0)
	Mortality	27	1.2 (0.8–1.8)[c]
	1970–1974	5	1.8 (0.6–4.3)
	1975–1979	1	0.4 (0.0–2.0)
	1980–1984	4	1.1 (0.3–2.9)
	1985–1989	5	1.5 (0.5–3.6)
	1990–1994	5	1.3 (0.4–3.0)
	1995–1999	5	1.3 (0.4–3.0)
	2000–2001	2	0.9 (0.1–3.1)
Zambon et al., 2007	Population-based Veneto Tumour Registry, Italy, average exposure based on duration and distance of residence from 33 industrial sources—incidence		
	Sarcoma (ICD-9 158, 171, 173, visceral sites)		
	Men		
	< 4 TCDD (fg/m^3)	31	1.0
	4–6	39	1.1 (0.6–2.0)
	≥ 6	17	1.9 (0.9–4.0)
			p-trend = 0.15
	Women		
	< 4 TCDD (fg/m^3)	24	1.0
	4–6	44	1.5 (0.8–2.7)
	≥ 6	17	2.4 (1.0–5.6)
			p-trend = 0.04

continued

TABLE 6-17 Continued

Reference	Study Population[a]	Exposed Cases[b]	Estimated Relative Risk (95% CI)[b]
	Men, women combined		
	Connective, other soft tissue (ICD-9 171)		
	< 4 TCDD (fg/m³)	25	1.0
	4–6	39	1.4 (0.7–2.5)
	≥ 6	17	3.3 (1.4–7.9)
			p-trend = 0.01
	Skin (ICD-9 173)		
	< 4 TCDD (fg/m³)	5	1.0
	4–6	10	0.0 (0.3–4.7)[d]
	≥ 6	2	0.3 (0.0–3.4)
			p-trend = 0.48
	Retroperitoneum, peritoneum (ICD-9 158)		
	< 4 TCDD (fg/m³)	6	1.0
	4–6	12	1.1 (0.3–3.4)
	≥ 6	3	0.8 (0.1–4.5)
			p-trend = 0.86
	Visceral sites		
	< 4 TCDD (fg/m³)	19	1.0
	4–6	22	1.2 (0.6–2.6)
	≥ 6	12	2.5 (1.0–6.3)
			p-trend = 0.08
Studies Reviewed in *Update 2006*			
Pahwa et al., 2006	Any phenoxyherbicide	46	1.1 (0.7–1.5)
	2,4-D	41	1.0 (0.6–1.5)
	Mecoprop	12	1.0 (0.5–1.9)
	MCPA	12	1.1 (0.5–2.2)
Studies Reviewed in *Update 2004*			
Comba et al., 2003	Residents near industrial-waste incinerator in Mantua, Italy—incidence		
	Residence within 2 km of incinerator	5	31.4 (5.6–176.1)
Tuomisto et al., 2004	Finnish STS patients vs controls within quintiles based on TEQ in subcutaneous fat—incidence	110	
	Quintile 1 (median, ~12 ng/kg TEQ)	nr	1.0
	Quintile 2 (median, ~20 ng/kg TEQ)	nr	0.4 (0.2–1.1)
	Quintile 3 (median, ~28 ng/kg TEQ)	nr	0.6 (0.2–1.7)
	Quintile 4 (median, ~40 ng/kg TEQ)	nr	0.5 (0.2–1.3)
	Quintile 5 (median, ~62 ng/kg TEQ)	nr	0.7 (0.2–2.0)
Studies Reviewed in *Update 2002*			
Costani et al., 2000	Residents near chemical plant in Mantua, Italy—incidence	20	2.3 (1.3–3.5)
Studies Reviewed in *Update 2000*			
Bertazzi et al., 2001	Seveso—20-year follow-up (men and women)	0	nr

TABLE 6-17 Continued

Reference	Study Population[a]	Exposed Cases[b]	Estimated Relative Risk (95% CI)[b]
Viel et al., 2000	Residents near French solid-waste incinerator—incidence		
	Spatial cluster	45	1.4 (p = 0.004)
	1994–1995	12	3.4 (p = 0.008)
Bertazzi et al., 1998	Seveso—15-year follow-up (men and women)		
	Zone R men	4	2.1 (0.7–6.5)
Studies Reviewed in *Update 1998*			
Bertazzi et al. 1997	Seveso residents—15-year follow-up (men and women)		
	Zone R men	4	2.1 (0.6–5.4)
Gambini et al., 1997	Italian rice growers	1	4.0 (0.1–22.3)
Svensson et al., 1995	Swedish fishermen—incidence (men and women)		
	West coast	3	0.5 (0.1–1.4)
Studies Reviewed in *Update 1996*			
Bertazzi et al., 1993	Seveso residents—10-year follow-up—morbidity		
	Zone R men	6	2.8 (1.0–7.3)
	Zone R women	2	1.6 (0.3–7.4)
Studies Reviewed in *VAO*			
Lampi et al., 1992	Finnish community exposed to chlorophenol contamination (men and women)	6	1.6 (0.7–3.5)
Bertazzi et al., 1989a	Seveso residents—10-year follow-up		
	Zone A, B, R men	2	5.4 (0.8–38.6)
	Zone A, B, R women	1	2.0 (0.2–1.9)
Bertazzi et al., 1989b	Seveso residents—10-year follow-up		
	Zone R men	2	6.3 (0.9–45.0)
	Zone B women	1	17.0 (1.8–163.6)

ABBREVIATIONS: 2,4-D, 2,4-dichlorophenoxyacetic acid; 2,4,5-T, 2,4,5-trichlorophenoxyacetic acid; AHS, Agricultural Health Study; CI, confidence interval; IARC, International Agency for Research on Cancer; ICD, International Classification of Diseases; MCPA, methyl-4-chlorophenoxyacetic acid; NIOSH, National Institute for Occupational Safety and Health; nr, not reported; PCDDs, chlorinated dibenzo-*p*-dioxins (highly chlorinated, if four or more chlorines); PM, proportionate mortality; SEER, Surveillance, Epidemiology, and End Results; STS, soft-tissue sarcoma; TCDD, 2,3,7,8-tetrachlorodibenzo-*p*-dioxin; TEQ, toxicity equivalent; USDA, US Department of Agriculture.

[a]Subjects are male and outcome is mortality unless otherwise noted.

[b]Given when available; results other than estimated risk explained individually.

[c]Committee computed total SMR and SIR by dividing sum of observed values by sum of expected values over all years; 95% CIs on these total ratios were computed with exact methods.

[d]There appears to be an error in this entry because lower 95% CL (0.3) is not smaller than odds ratio (0.0).

Studies in italics have been superseded by newer studies of same cohorts.

(connective and soft tissue, skin, peritoneum, and viscera) and by morphologic type (fibrosarcoma, myxosarcoma, liposarcoma, myosarcoma, mixed mesen-chymal sarcoma, synovial sarcoma, blood vessel sarcoma, lymphatic vessel sar-coma, nerve sheath sarcoma, alveolar sarcoma, and not otherwise specified). Three controls, individually matched on sex and age at the time of diagnosis, were sought from the population for each of the identified 205 cases; 172 cases and 405 controls met all eligibility criteria and were included in the analyses. Residential histories were obtained from a population registry and were linked to assessments of exposure to dioxin that made use of the locations of incinerators. The exposures were attributed by estimating total emissions from the incinerators and the proportion of TCDD emitted. Environmental estimates of exposure were derived by using EPA's Industrial Source Complex Model, which is a dispersion model that provides estimates of deposition at different places. The estimates were linked to subjects' addresses. With a metric defined by average exposure at each subject's address, monotonic increases in risk of all types of sarcoma were found in both men and women and of sarcomas of the connective and other soft tissue and in organs in the cavities of the body (visceral sites) in men and women combined.

Biologic Plausibility

In a 2-year study, dermal application of TCDD to Swiss-Webster mice led to an increase in fibrosarcomas in females but not males (NTP, 1982b). There is some concern that the increase in fibrosarcomas may be associated with the treatment protocol rather than with TCDD. The National Toxicology Progam gavage study (1982a) also found increased incidences of fibrosarcomas in male and female rats and in female mice.

The biologic plausibility of the carcinogenicity of the chemicals of interest is discussed in general at the beginning of this chapter.

Synthesis

Previous committees have concluded that the occupational, environmental, and Vietnam-veteran studies showed sufficient evidence to link herbicide expo-sure to STS. That conclusion is strengthened by one of the new studies (Zambon et al., 2007), which showed an increased risk in persons living in the vicinity of incinerators in Venice, Italy.

Conclusion

On the basis of the evidence reviewed here and in previous VAO reports, the committee concludes that there is sufficient evidence of an association between exposure to at least one of the chemicals of interest and STS.

SKIN CANCER—MELANOMA

Skin cancers are generally divided into two broad categories: neoplasms that develop from melanocytes (malignant melanoma, or simply melanoma) and neoplasms that do not. Nonmelanoma skin cancers (primarily basal-cell and squamous-cell carcinomas) have a far higher incidence than melanoma but are considerably less aggressive and therefore more treatable. The average annual incidence of melanoma is shown in Table 6-18. The committee responsible for *Update 1998* first chose to address melanoma studies separately from those of non-melanoma skin cancer. Some researchers report results by combining all types of skin cancer without specifying type. The present committee believes that such information is not interpretable (although there is a supposition that mortality figures refer predominantly to melanoma and that sizable incidence figures refer to nonmelanoma skin cancer); therefore, the committee is interpreting data only on results that are specified as applying to melanoma or to non-melanoma skin cancer.

ACS estimated that about 34,950 men and 27,530 women would receive diagnoses of cutaneous melanoma (ICD-9 172) in the United States in 2008 and that about 5,400 men and 3,020 women would die from it (Jemal et al., 2008a). More than a million cases of nonmelanoma skin cancer (ICD-9 173), primarily basal-cell and squamous-cell carcinomas, are diagnosed in the United States each year (ACS, 2006); it is not required to report them to registries, so the numbers of cases are not as precise as those of other cancers. ACS reports that although melanoma accounts for only about 4% of skin-cancer cases, it is responsible for about 79% of skin-cancer deaths (2006). It estimates that 1,000–2,000 people die each year from nonmelanoma skin cancer.

Melanoma occurs more frequently in fair-skinned people than in dark-skinned people; the risk in whites is roughly 20 times that in dark-skinned blacks. The incidence increases with age; the increase is more striking in males than in females. Other risk factors include the presence of particular kinds of moles on

TABLE 6-18 Average Annual Cancer Incidence (per 100,000) of Skin Cancers (Excluding Basal-Cell and Squamous-Cell Cancers) in United States[a]

	50–54 Years Old			55–59 Years Old			60–64 Years Old		
	All Races	White	Black	All Races	White	Black	All Races	White	Black
Melanomas of the Skin:									
Men	34.4	41.3	1.1	48.5	57.3	3.2	63.3	74.4	5.0
Women	26.9	33.1	2.1	30.1	36.7	3.3	32.7	39.6	2.2

[a]Surveillance, Epidemiology, and End Results program, nine standard registries, crude age-specific rates, 2000–2005. SEER incidence data not available for nonmelanocytic skin cancer.

the skin, suppression of the immune system, and excessive exposure to ultraviolet (UV) radiation, typically from the sun. A family history of the disease has been identified as a risk factor, but it is unclear whether that is attributable to genetic factors or to similarities in skin type and sun-exposure patterns.

Excessive exposure to UV radiation is the most important risk factor for nonmelanoma skin cancer; some skin diseases and chemical exposures have also been identified as potential risk factors. Exposure to inorganic arsenic is a risk factor for skin cancer; this does not imply that exposure to cacodylic acid, which is a metabolite of inorganic arsenic, can be assumed to be a risk factor.

Conclusions from *VAO* and Previous Updates

The committee responsible for *VAO* concluded that there was inadequate or insufficient information to determine whether there is an association between exposure to the chemicals of interest and skin cancer. Additional information available to the committee responsible for *Update 1996* did not change that conclusion. The committee responsible for *Update 1998* considered the literature on melanoma separately from that of nonmelanoma skin cancer. It found that there was inadequate or insufficient information to determine whether there is an association between the chemicals of interest and melanoma. The committees responsible for *Update 2000*, *Update 2002*, and *Update 2004* concurred with the findings of *Update 1998*. The committee responsible for *Update 2006* was unable to reach a consensus as to whether there was limited or suggestive evidence of an association between exposure to the chemicals of interest and melanoma or inadequate or insufficient evidence to determine whether there is an association, so melanoma was left in the lower category. Table 6-19 summarizes the relevant melanoma studies.

Update of the Epidemiologic Literature

Vietnam-Veteran Studies

No Vietnam-veteran studies concerning exposure to the chemicals of interest and melanoma have been published since *Update 2006*.

Occupational Studies

Samanic et al. (2006) observed no strong association with melanoma and exposure to dicamba in the AHS cohort. When exposure was defined as the number of lifetime days of applications, Poisson regression found the largest association for applications of 20–56 days, with a rate ratio of 1.59 (95% CI 0.84–3.00). The association decreased as the number of exposure days increased, with an estimated risk of 0.83 (95% CI 0.33–2.13) for greater than 116 lifetime days of

TABLE 6-19 Selected Epidemiologic Studies—Melanoma

Reference	Study Population[a]	Exposed Cases[b]	Estimated Relative Risk (95% CI)[b]
VIETNAM VETERANS			
Studies Reviewed in *Update 2006*			
Pavuk et al., 2005	White Air Force comparison subjects only—incidence		
	Serum TCDD (pg/g), based on model with exposure variable $\log_e$(TCDD)		
	Per unit increase of $-\log_e$(TCDD)	25	2.7 (1.1–6.3)
	Quartiles (pg/g)		
	0.4–2.6	3	1.0
	2.6–3.8	5	2.1 (0.4–11.0)
	3.8–5.2	8	3.2 (0.7–15.5)
	> 5.2	9	3.6 (0.7–17.2)
	Number years served SEA		
	Per year of service	25	1.1 (0.9–1.3)
	Quartiles (years in SEA)		
	0.8–1.3	3	1.0
	1.3–2.1	4	1.9 (0.3–10.3)
	2.1–3.7	8	3.2 (0.7–15.3)
	3.7–16.4	10	4.1 (0.9–19.7)
ADVA, 2005a	Australian male Vietnam veterans vs Australian population—incidence	756	1.3 (1.2–1.4)
	Navy	173	1.4 (1.2–1.6)
	Army	510	1.2 (1.2–1.4)
	Air Force	73	1.4 (1.1–1.7)
ADVA, 2005b	Australian male Vietnam veterans vs Australian population—mortality	111	1.1 (0.9–1.3)
	Navy	35	1.6 (1.0–2.1)
	Army	66	1.0 (0.7–1.2)
	Air Force	10	1.0 (0.5–1.8)
ADVA, 2005c	Australian male conscripted Army National Service Vietnam-era veterans—deployed vs nondeployed		
	Incidence	204	1.1 (0.9–1.4)
	Mortality	14	0.6 (0.3–1.1)
Boehmer et al., 2004	Follow-up of CDC Vietnam Experience Cohort	6	1.4 (0.4–4.9)
Studies Reviewed in *Update 2004*			
Akhtar et al., 2004	AFHS subjects vs national rates		
	White AFHS Ranch Hand veterans		
	Incidence	17	2.3 (1.4–3.7)
	With tours between 1966–1970	16	2.6 (1.5–4.1)
	Mortality	nr	
	White AFHS comparison veterans		
	Incidence	15	1.5 (0.9–2.4)
	With tours between 1966–1970	12	1.5 (0.8–2.6)
	Mortality	nr	

continued

TABLE 6-19 Continued

Reference	Study Population[a]	Exposed Cases[b]	Estimated Relative Risk (95% CI)[b]
	White AFHS subjects—incidence		
	Who spent at most 2 years in SEA		
	Per unit increase of $-\log_e$(TCDD) (pg/g)	14	2.2 (1.3–3.9)
	Comparison group	3	1.0
	Ranch Hand— < 10 TCDD pg/g in 1987	4	3.0 (0.5–16.8)
	Ranch Hand— < 118.5 TCDD pg/g at end of service	4	7.4 (1.3–41.0)
	Ranch Hand— > 118.5 TCDD pg/g at end of service	3	7.5 (1.1–50.2)
	Only Ranch Hands with 100% service in Vietnam, comparisons with 0% service in Vietnam		
	Per unit increase of $-\log_e$(TCDD) in pg/g	14	1.7 (1.0–2.8)
	Comparison group	2	1.0
	Ranch Hand— < 10 TCDD pg/g in 1987	5	3.9 (0.4–35.3)
	Ranch Hand— < 118.5 TCDD pg/g at end of service	4	7.2 (0.9–58.8)
	Ranch Hand— > 118.5 TCDD pg/g at end of service	3	5.5 (0.6–46.1)
Studies Reviewed in *Update 2000*			
AFHS, 2000	Air Force Ranch Hand veterans—incidence	16	1.8 (0.8–3.8)
Ketchum et al., 1999	Ranch Hand veterans, comparisons through June 1997—incidence		
	Comparisons	9	1.0
	Ranch Hand background exposure	4	1.1 (0.3–4.5)
	Ranch Hand low exposure	6	2.6 (0.7–9.1)
	Ranch Hand high exposure	2	0.9 (0.2–5.6)
AIHW, 1999			Expected number of exposed cases (95% CI)
	Australian Vietnam veterans—incidence (validation study)	483	380 (342–418)
CDVA, 1998a	Australian Vietnam veterans (men)—self-reported incidence	2,689	380 (342–418)
CDVA, 1998b	Australian Vietnam veterans (women)—self-reported incidence	7	3 (1–8)
Studies Reviewed in *Update 1998*			
CDVA, 1997a	Australian Vietnam veterans (men)	51	1.3 (0.9–1.7)
CDVA, 1997b	Australian national service Vietnam veterans	16	0.5 (0.2–1.3)
Clapp, 1997	Massachusetts Vietnam veterans—incidence	21	1.4 (0.7–2.9)
Studies Reviewed in *VAO*			
Wolfe et al., 1990	Air Force Ranch Hand veterans—incidence	4	1.3 (0.3–5.2)
Breslin et al., 1988	Army Vietnam veterans	145	1.0 (0.9–1.1)
	Marine Vietnam veterans	36	0.9 (0.6–1.5)

TABLE 6-19 Continued

Reference	Study Population[a]	Exposed Cases[b]	Estimated Relative Risk (95% CI)[b]
OCCUPATIONAL			
New Studies			
Hansen et al., 2007	Danish gardeners—incidence (skin, ICD-7 190–191)		
	10-year follow-up (1975–1984) reported in Hansen et al. (1992)	31	1.3 (0.9–1.8)
	25-year follow-up (1975–2001)		
	Born before 1915 (high exposure)	28	0.9 (0.6–1.4)
	Born 1915–1934 (medium exposure)	36	0.6 (0.4–0.9)
	Born after 1934 (low exposure)	5	0.3 (0.1–0.7)
Samanic et al., 2006	Pesticide applicators in AHS—melanoma incidence from enrollment through 2002		
	Dicamba—lifetime days exposure		
	None	32	1.0
	1– < 20	10	1.0 (0.5–2.1)
	20– < 56	18	1.6 (0.8–3.0)
	56– < 116	6	0.7 (0.3–1.8)
	≥ 116	6	0.8 (0.3–2.1)
			p-trend = 0.51
Studies Reviewed in *Update 2006*			
McLean et al., 2006	IARC cohort of pulp and paper workers		
	Exposure to nonvolatile organochlorine compounds		
	Never	20	0.8 (0.5–1.3)
	Ever	21	1.2 (0.7–1.8)
't Mannetje et al., 2005	Phenoxy herbicide producers (men and women)	0	0.0 (0.0–3.0)
	Phenoxy herbicide sprayers (> 99% men)	1	0.6 (0.0–3.4)
Alavanja et al., 2005	US AHS—incidence		
	Private applicators (men and women)	100	1.0 (0.8–1.2)
	Spouses of private applicators (> 99% women)	67	1.6 (1.3–2.1)
	Commercial applicators (men and women)	7	1.1 (0.4–2.2)
Blair et al., 2005a	US AHS		
	Private applicators (men and women)	13	0.7 (0.4–1.3)
	Spouses of private applicators (> 99% women)	2	0.4 (0.1–1.6)
Torchio et al., 1994	Italian licensed pesticide users	9	1.2 (0.6–2.3)
Magnani et al., 1987	UK case–control		
	Herbicides	nr	1.2 (0.4–4.0)
	Chlorophenols	nr	0.9 (0.4–2.3)
Studies Reviewed in *Update 2004*			
Swaen et al., 2004	Dutch licensed herbicide applicators		
	Melanoma, squamous-cell carcinoma, unknown skin cancer (mortality presumably attributable to melanoma)	5	3.6 (1.2–8.3)

continued

TABLE 6-19 Continued

Reference	Study Population[a]	Exposed Cases[b]	Estimated Relative Risk (95% CI)[b]
Studies Reviewed in *Update 2002*			
Thörn et al., 2000	Swedish lumberjack workers exposed to phenoxyacetic herbicides—incidence		
	Women	1	3.5 (0.1–19.2)
	Men	0	nr
Studies Reviewed in *Update 2000*			
Hooiveld et al., 1998	Dutch chemical production workers (included in IARC cohort)	1	2.9 (0.1–15.9)
Studies Reviewed in *Update 1998*			
Hertzman et al., 1997	British Columbia sawmill workers		
	Incidence	38	1.0 (0.7–1.3)
	Mortality	17	1.4 (0.9–2.0)
Kogevinas et al., 1997	IARC cohort, male and female workers exposed to any phenoxy herbicide or chlorophenol	9	0.6 (0.3–1.2)
	Exposed to highly chlorinated PCDDs	5	0.5 (0.2–3.2)
	Not exposed to highly chlorinated PCDDs	4	0.0 (0.3–2.4)
Studies Reviewed in *Update 1996*			
Blair et al., 1993	US farmers in 23 states		
	White men	244	1.0 (0.8–1.1)
	White women	5	1.1 (0.4–2.7)
Lynge, 1993	Danish production workers (included in IARC cohort)—updated incidence	4	4.3 (1.2–10.9)
Studies Reviewed in *VAO*			
Ronco et al., 1992	Danish workers—incidence		
	Men	72	0.7 (p < 0.05)
	Women	5	1.2 (nr)
Wigle et al., 1990	Canadian farmers	24	1.1 (0.7–1.6)
Wiklund, 1983	Swedish male and female agricultural workers—incidence	268	99% CI 0.8 (0.7–1.0)
ENVIRONMENTAL			
New Studies			
Consonni et al., 2008	Seveso residents—25-year follow-up—men, women		
	Zone A	1	3.1 (0.4–22.0)
	Zone B	2	1.0 (0.2–3.9)
	Zone R	12	0.8 (0.4–1.5)
Studies Reviewed in *Update 2000*			
Bertazzi et al., 2001	Seveso residents—20-year follow-up		
	Zones A, B—men	1	1.5 (0.2–12.5)
	women	2	1.8 (0.4–7.3)
Studies Reviewed in *Update 1998*			
Bertazzi et al., 1997	Seveso residents—15-year follow-up		
	Zone A—women	1	9.4 (0.1–52.3)
	Zone R—men	3	1.1 (0.2–3.2)
	women	3	0.6 (0.1–1.8)

TABLE 6-19 Continued

Reference	Study Population[a]	Exposed Cases[b]	Estimated Relative Risk (95% CI)[b]
Svensson et al., 1995	Swedish fishermen (men and women)		
	East coast		
	Incidence	0	0.0 (0.0–0.7)
	Mortality	0	0.0 (0.0–1.7)
	West coast		
	Incidence	20	0.8 (0.5–1.2)
	Mortality	6	0.7 (0.3–1.5)
Studies Reviewed in *VAO*			
Bertazzi	Seveso residents—10-year follow-up		
et al., 1989a	Zones A, B, R—men	3	3.3 (0.8–13.9)
	women	1	0.3 (0.1–2.5)

ABBREVIATIONS: 2,4-D, 2,4-dichlorophenoxyacetic acid; AFHS, Air Force Health Study; AHS, Agricultural Health Study; CDC, Centers for Disease Control and Prevention; CI, confidence interval; IARC, International Agency for Research on Cancer; ICD, International Classification of Diseases; nr, not reported; PCDDs, chlorinated dibenzo-*p*-dioxins (highly chlorinated, if four or more chlorines); SEA, Southeast Asia; TCDD, 2,3,7,8-tetrachlorodibenzo-*p*-dioxin.
[a]Cohorts are male and outcome mortality unless otherwise noted.
[b]Given when available; results other than estimated risk explained individually.
Studies in italics have been superseded by newer studies of same cohorts.

exposure. A similar inverse pattern with increasing exposure was observed when exposure categories were weighted by intensity.

Hansen et al. (2007) evaluated cancer incidence from May 1975 through 2001 in an occupational cohort of Danish union workers identified from men working in 1973; their incidence from 1975 to 1984 was reported earlier by Hansen et al. (1992). The cohort of 3,156 male gardeners was matched to the Danish Cancer Registry to measure cancer incidence in the cohort. All skin cancers (ICD-7 190–191) were examined as one group. SIRs, with control for age and calendar time, were calculated by using the national cancer incidences as the standards. Given the reduction in pesticide use over time, birth cohorts were used as a proxy definition of exposure. Three subcohorts were evaluated: high exposure, early-birth cohort (born before 1915); low exposure, late-birth cohort (born after 1935); and medium exposure (births in 1915–1935). Overall, 521 cancer cases were identified, of which 69 were coded as skin cancer. The SIRs decreased with birth-cohort period (the SIRs were lowest in the late-birth cohort), but the observed incidence for all skin cancers combined was lower than the expected incidence in all birth cohorts examined. In men born before 1915, the cohort assumed to have the greatest exposure potential, the SIR was 0.93 (95% CI 0.64–1.35). A lower incidence than expected was also observed in men born after 1935, when exposures were hypothesized to be lower because there were fewer applications and better safety measures (SIR = 0.28, 95% CI 0.12–0.67).

Environmental Studies

The 25-year follow-up of the Seveso cohort was reported by Consonni et al. (2008). Person-years were calculated for 278,108 cohort members from July 10, 1976 (or entry date), until death or the end of the study (December 31, 2001) for all 278,108 study members. A total of 15 melanoma deaths were identified, of which 12 occurred in residents in the low-exposure zone (Zone R). Compared with the incidence in the reference zone, melanoma incidence was decreased in the high exposure Zone B (RR = 0.97, 95% CI 0.24–3.93) and low-exposure Zone R (RR = 0.83, 95% CI 0.45–1.51). One melanoma death was observed in Zone A, which had the highest TCDD exposure (RR = 3.06, 95% CI 0.43–22.01).

Fortes et al. (2007) examined residential use of pesticides and melanoma in a hospital-based case–control study; however, the lack of exposure specificity in the study precluded inclusion of its results in this review.

Biologic Plausibility

There have been no new studies of animal models of skin cancer. TCDD and related herbicides have not been found to cause melanoma in animal models. In general, rodents, which are used in most toxicology studies, are not a good model for studying melanoma. TCDD does produce nonmelanoma skin cancers in animal models (Wyde et al., 2004). As discussed elsewhere in this chapter, TCDD is a known tumor-promoter and could act as a promoter for skin-cancer initiators, such as UV radiation. However, no experiments have been conducted specifically to examine that potential mechanism.

The biologic plausibility of the carcinogenicity of the chemicals of interest is discussed in general at the beginning of this chapter.

Synthesis

No association between the chemicals of interest and melanoma was observed in either of the two new occupational studies. Of the two new environmental studies, that by Fortes et al. observed a weak association between self-reported residential use of pesticides and melanoma, but the numbers were not sufficient to examine herbicides separately. Finally, although the risk of melanoma was increased in those living in the highest-exposure zone in the Seveso cohort, this finding was based on only one melanoma death. The new studies do not provide evidence to support moving melanoma to the category of limited or suggestive evidence.

The committee responsible for *Update 2006* was unable to reach a consensus as to whether there was limited or suggestive evidence of an association between exposure to the chemicals of interest and melanoma or inadequate or insufficient evidence to determine whether there is an association. That committee recognized that the findings from the Air Force Health Study (AFHS), including the evaluation of TCDD measurements and melanoma (Akhtar et al., 2004; Pavuk et al., 2005), were of prime interest. However, the data from the final AFHS examination cycle indicate that many more melanoma cases were diagnosed in the comparison veterans than in the Ranch Hand subjects, so the committee responsible for *Update 2006* recommended that the Akhtar et al. analyses be rerun on the final AFHS dataset. The final data on the Ranch Hand and comparison subjects still have not been analyzed in a satisfactory and uniform manner, so the present committee also strongly encourages that such an analysis be performed and published to provide documentation of the full melanoma experience revealed by the AFHS and to permit definitive evaluation of the possible association between the chemicals of interest and melanoma.

Conclusion

On the basis of the evidence reviewed here and in previous VAO reports, the committee concludes that there is inadequate or insufficient evidence to determine whether there is an association between exposure to the chemicals of interest and melanoma.

SKIN CANCER—BASAL-CELL CANCER AND SQUAMOUS-CELL CANCER (NONMELANOMA SKIN CANCERS)

The preceding section on melanoma presented background information on nonmelanoma skin cancers (ICD-9 173).

Conclusions from *VAO* and Previous Updates

The committee responsible for *VAO* concluded that there was inadequate or insufficient information to determine whether there is an association between exposure to the chemicals of interest and skin cancer, and additional information available to the committee responsible for *Update 1996* did not change that conclusion. The committee responsible for *Update 1998* considered the literature on nonmelanocytic skin cancer separately from that on melanoma and concluded that there was inadequate or insufficient information to determine whether there is an association between exposure to the chemicals of interest and basal-cell or squamous-cell cancer. The committees responsible for *Update 2000*, *Update 2002*, *Update 2004*, and *Update 2006* did not change that conclusion. Table 6-20 summarizes the relevant studies.

Update of the Epidemiologic Literature

No Vietnam-veteran studies or environmental studies concerning exposure to the chemicals of interest and basal-cell or squamous-cell cancer have been published since *Update 2006*.

TABLE 6-20 Selected Epidemiologic Studies—Other Nonmelanoma (Basal-Cell and Squamous-Cell) Skin Cancer

Reference	Study Population[a]	Exposed Cases[b]	Estimated Relative Risk (95% CI)[b]
VIETNAM VETERANS			
Studies Reviewed in *Update 2006*			
Pavuk et al., 2005	White Air Force comparison subjects only (basal cell and squamous cell)—incidence		
	Serum TCDD (pg/g), based on model with exposure variable $\log_e$(TCDD)		
	Per unit increase of $-\log_e$(TCDD)	253	1.2 (0.9–1.4)
	Quartiles (pg/g)		
	0.4–2.6	50	nr
	2.6–3.8	59	1.2 (0.8–1.8)
	3.8–5.2	71	1.5 (1.1–2.3)
	> 5.2	73	1.4 (0.9–2.0)
	Number of years served in SEA		
	Per year of service	253	1 (0.9–1.1)
	Quartiles (years in SEA)		
	0.8–1.3	55	nr
	1.3–2.1	50	0.9 (0.6–1.4)
	2.1–3.7	73	1.1 (0.8–1.6)
	3.7–16.4	75	1.2 (0.8–1.7)
Studies Reviewed in *Update 2000*			
AFHS, 2000	Air Force Ranch Hand veterans—incidence		
	Basal-cell carcinoma	121	1.2 (0.9–1.6)
	Squamous-cell carcinoma	20	1.5 (0.8–2.8)
CDVA, 1998a	Australian Vietnam veterans (men)—self-reported incidence	6,936	nr
CDVA, 1998b	Australian Vietnam veterans (women)—self-reported incidence	37	nr
Studies Reviewed in *VAO*			
Wolfe et al., 1990	Air Force Ranch Hand veterans—incidence		
	Basal-cell carcinoma	78	1.5 (1.0–2.1)
	Squamous-cell carcinoma	6	1.6 (0.5–5.1)
OCCUPATIONAL			
New Studies			
Hansen et al., 2007	Danish gardeners—incidence (skin, ICD-7 190–191)		
	10-year follow-up (1975–1984) reported in Hansen et al. (1992)	31	1.3 (0.9–1.8)
	25-year follow-up (1975–2001)		
	Born before 1915 (high exposure)	28	0.9 (0.6–1.4)
	Born 1915–1934 (medium exposure)	36	0.6 (0.4–0.9)
	Born after 1934 (low exposure)	5	0.3 (0.1–0.7)
Studies Reviewed in *Update 2006*			
Torchio et al., 1994	Italian licensed pesticide users	3	0.6 (0.1–1.8)

TABLE 6-20 Continued

Reference	Study Population[a]	Exposed Cases[b]	Estimated Relative Risk (95% CI)[b]
Studies Reviewed in *Update 2004*			
Swaen et al., 2004	Dutch licensed herbicide applicators		
	Melanoma, squamous-cell carcinoma, unknown skin cancer (mortality presumably attributable to melanoma)	5	3.6 (1.2–8.3)
Studies Reviewed in *Update 2002*			
Burns et al., 2001	Dow 2,4-D production workers (included in IARC cohort, NIOSH Dioxin Registry)		
	Nonmelanoma skin cancer	0	nr
Thörn et al., 2000	Swedish lumberjacks exposed to phenoxyacetic herbicides—incidence		
	Foremen	1	16.7 (0.2–92.7)
Studies Reviewed in *Update 1998*			
Kogevinas et al., 1997	IARC cohort, male and female workers exposed to any phenoxy herbicide or chlorophenol	4	0.9 (0.3–2.4)
	Exposed to highly chlorinated PCDDs	4	1.3 (0.3–3.2)
	Not exposed to highly chlorinated PCDDs	0	0.0 (0.0–3.4)
Zhong and Rafnsson, 1996	Icelandic pesticide users (men, women—incidence)		
	Men	5	2.8 (0.9–6.6)
Studies Reviewed in *Update 1996*			
Blair et al., 1993	US farmers in 23 states		
	Skin (including melanoma)		
	White men	425	1.1 (1.0–1.2)
	White women	6	1.0 (0.4–2.1)
Studies Reviewed in *VAO*			
Ronco et al., 1992	Danish workers—incidence		
	Men—self-employed	493	0.7 (p < 0.05)
	employee	98	0.7 (p < 0.05)
	Women—self-employed	5	0.3 (p < 0.05)
	employee	10	0.9 (nr)
	family worker	90	0.6 (p < 0.05)
Coggon et al., 1986	British MCPA production workers (included in IARC cohort)	3	3.1 (0.6–9.0)
ENVIRONMENTAL			
Studies Reviewed in *Update 1998*			
Gallagher et al., 1996	Alberta, Canada, residents—squamous-cell carcinoma—incidence		
	All herbicide exposure	79	1.5 (1.0–2.3)
	Low herbicide exposure	33	1.9 (1.0–3.6)
	High herbicide exposure	46	3.9 (2.2–6.9)
	Alberta, Canada, residents—basal-cell carcinoma		
	All herbicide exposure	70	1.1 (0.8–1.7)

continued

TABLE 6-20 Continued

Reference	Study Population[a]	Exposed Cases[b]	Estimated Relative Risk (95% CI)[b]
Svensson et al., 1995	Swedish fishermen		
	East coast		
	Incidence	22	2.3 (1.5–3.5)
	Mortality	0	0.0 (0.0–15.4)
	West coast		
	Incidence	69	1.1 (0.9–1.4)
	Mortality	5	3.1 (1.0–7.1)
Studies Reviewed in ***Update 1996***			
Bertazzi et al., 1993	Seveso residents—10-year follow-up—incidence		
	Zone A—men	1	2.4 (0.3–17.2)
	women	1	3.9 (0.5–28.1)
	Zone B—men	2	0.7 (0.2–2.9)
	women	2	1.3 (0.3–5.1)
	Zone R—men	20	1.0 (0.6–1.6)
	women	13	1.0 (0.6–1.9)
Studies Reviewed in *VAO*			
Pesatori et al., 1992	Seveso residents—incidence		
	Zones A, B—men	3	1.0 (0.3–3.0)
	women	3	1.5 (0.5–4.9)
	Zone R—men	20	1.0 (0.6–1.6)
	women	13	1.0 (0.5–1.7)
Wiklund, 1983	Swedish male and female agricultural workers—incidence	708	99% CI 1.1 (1.0–1.2)

ABBREVIATIONS: CI, confidence interval; IARC, International Agency for Research on Cancer; ICD, International Classification of Diseases; MCPA, 2-methyl-4-chlorophenoxyacetic acid; NIOSH, National Institute for Occupational Safety and Health; nr, not reported; PCDDs, chlorinated dibenzo-*p*-dioxins (highly chlorinated, if four or more chlorines); SEA, Southeast Asia; TCDD, 2,3,7,8-tetrachlorodibenzo-*p*-dioxin.

[a]Subjects are male and outcome is mortality unless otherwise noted.
[b]Given when available; results other than estimated risk explained individually.
Studies in italics have been superseded by newer studies of same cohorts.

Occupational Studies

The study by Hansen et al. (2007), which examined the incidence of all skin cancers combined (see section on melanoma above), is the only new one related to skin cancer published since *Update 2006*. No association was observed in this occupational cohort of Danish gardeners when cancer incidence was compared with national rates by birth cohort (a proxy for pesticide exposure). The study was limited by the inability to examine incidence by pesticide class (such as herbicides) and to evaluate nonmelanoma cancer separately from melanoma.

Biologic Plausibility

There are no new studies on animal models of skin cancer to report. TCDD does produce nonmelanoma skins cancers in animal models (Wyde et al., 2004). As discussed elsewhere in this chapter, TCDD is a known tumor-promoter and could act as a promoter for skin-cancer initiators, such as UV radiation, but no experiments have been conducted specifically to support this potential mechanism.

The biologic plausibility of the carcinogenicity of the chemicals of interest is discussed in general at the beginning of this chapter.

Synthesis

In accord with the results of reports previously assessed, the committee concludes that there is inadequate or insufficient evidence to determine whether there is an association between exposure to the chemicals of interest and basal-cell or squamous-cell cancer.

Conclusion

On the basis of the evidence reviewed here and in previous VAO reports, the committee concludes that there is inadequate or insufficient evidence to determine whether there is an association between exposure to the chemicals of interest and basal-cell or squamous-cell cancer.

BREAST CANCER

Breast cancer (ICD-9 174 for females, ICD-9 175 for males) is the second-most common type of cancer (after nonmelanoma skin cancer) in women in the United States. ACS estimated that 182,460 women would receive diagnoses of breast cancer in the United States in 2008 and that 40,480 would die from it (Jemal et al., 2008a). Overall, those numbers represent about 26% of the new cancers and 15% of cancer deaths in women. Incidence data on breast cancer are presented in Table 6-21.

Breast-cancer incidence generally increases with age. In the age groups of most Vietnam veterans, the incidence is higher in whites than in blacks. Established risk factors other than age include personal or family history of breast cancer and some characteristics of reproductive history—specifically, early menarche, late onset of menopause, and either no pregnancies or first full-term pregnancy after the age of 30 years. A pooled analysis of six large-scale prospective studies of invasive breast cancer showed that alcohol consumption over the range of consumption reported by most women was associated with a small, linear increase in incidence in women (Smith-Warner et al., 1998). It is now generally accepted that breast-cancer risk is increased by prolonged use of hormone-replacement therapy, particularly use of preparations that combine es-

TABLE 6-21 Average Annual Incidence (per 100,000) of Breast Cancer in Females in United States[a]

	50–54 Years Old			55–59 Years Old			60–64 Years Old		
	All Races	White	Black	All Races	White	Black	All Races	White	Black
Men	1.2	1.3	1.7	2.3	2.9	4.5	3.5	3.5	6.6
Women	240.5	248.2	224.6	309.0	321.5	270.7	372.4	391.0	321.8

[a]Surveillance, Epidemiology, and End Results program, nine standard registries, crude age-specific rates, 2000–2005.

trogen and progestins (Chlebowski et al., 2003). The potential of other personal behavioral and environmental factors (including use of exogenous hormones) to affect breast-cancer incidence is being studied extensively.

Most of the roughly 10,000 female Vietnam veterans who were potentially exposed to herbicides in Vietnam are approaching or have recently reached menopause. Given the high incidence of breast cancer in older and postmenopausal women in general, on the basis of demographics alone it is expected that the breast-cancer burden in female Vietnam veterans will increase in the near future.

The vast majority of breast-cancer epidemiologic studies involve women, but the disease also occurs rarely in men, with 1,990 new cases expected in 2008 (Jemal et al., 2008a). Reported instances of male breast cancer are noted, but the committee's conclusions are based on the studies in women.

Conclusions from *VAO* and Previous Updates

The committee responsible for *VAO* concluded that there was inadequate or insufficient information to determine whether there is an association between exposure to the chemicals of interest and breast cancer. Additional information available to the committees responsible for *Update 1996*, *Update 1998*, *Update 2000*, *Update 2002*, and *Update 2004* did not change that conclusion. The committee responsible for *Update 2006* was unable to reach consensus as to whether there was limited or suggestive evidence of an association between the chemicals of interest and breast cancer or inadequate or insufficient evidence to determine whether an association exists, and so breast cancer was left in the lower category. Table 6-22 summarizes the relevant research.

Update of the Epidemiologic Literature

Vietnam-Veteran Studies

Cypel and Kang (2008) compared breast-cancer mortality in female veterans who served in Vietnam with that in veterans, matched on rank and type of du-

TABLE 6-22 Selected Epidemiologic Studies—Breast Cancer

Reference	Study Population[a]	Exposed Cases[b]	Estimated Relative Risk (95% CI)[b]
VIETNAM VETERANS			
New Studies			
Cypel and	US Vietnam veterans—women	57	1.0 (0.7–1.4)
Kang, 2008	Vietnam-veteran nurses	44	0.9 (0.6–1.4)
Studies Reviewed in *Update 2006*			
Boehmer	Follow-up of CDC Vietnam Experience Cohort		
et al., 2004		0	nr
ADVA,	Australian male Vietnam veterans vs Australian		
2005a	population—incidence	7	0.9 (0.4–1.9)
	Navy	1	0.6 (0.0–3.3)
	Army	5	1.0 (0.3–2.2)
	Air Force	1	1.1 (0.0–6.3)
ADVA,	Australian male Vietnam veterans vs Australian		
2005b	population—mortality	4	2.2 (0.6–5.4)
	Navy	1	2.5 (0.0–13.5)
	Army	3	2.5 (0.5–7.2)
	Air Force	0	0.0 (0.0–14.6)
ADVA,	Australian male conscripted Army National Service		
2005c	Vietnam era veterans—deployed vs nondeployed	0	nr
	Incidence	0	0.0 (0.0–2.4)
	Mortality	nr	
Studies Reviewed in *Update 2002*			
Kang et al.,	Female US Vietnam veterans		
2000		170	1.2 (0.9–1.5)
CDVA,			<u>Expected number</u>
1998b			<u>of exposed cases</u>
	Australian Vietnam veterans (women)—self-reported		<u>(95% CI)</u>
	incidence	17	5 (2–11)
Studies Reviewed in *Update 1998*			
CDVA,	Australian military Vietnam veterans (men)	3	5.5 (1.0– > 10.0)
1997a			
Studies Reviewed in *Update 1996*			
Dalager	Female US Vietnam veterans	26	1.0 (0.6–1.8)
et al., 1995			
Studies Reviewed in *VAO*			
Thomas	Female US Vietnam veterans	17	1.2 (0.6–2.5)
et al., 1991			
OCCUPATIONAL			
Studies Reviewed in *Update 2006*			
McLean	IARC cohort of pulp and paper workers		
et al., 2006	Exposure to nonvolatile organochlorine		
	compounds		
	Never	21	0.9 (0.6–1.4)
	Ever	32	0.9 (0.6–1.3)

continued

TABLE 6-22 Continued

Reference	Study Population[a]	Exposed Cases[b]	Estimated Relative Risk (95% CI)[b]
't Mannetje et al., 2005	Phenoxy herbicide producers (men and women)		
	Women	1	1.3 (0.0–7.2)
	Men	1	32 (0.8–175)
	Phenoxy herbicide sprayers (> 99% men)	0	0.0 (nr)
Alavanja et al., 2005	US AHS—incidence		
	Private applicators (men and women)	27	1.1 (0.7–1.6)
	Spouses of private applicators (> 99% women)	474	1.0 (0.9–1.1)
	Commercial applicators (men and women)	1	0.6 (0.1–3.5)
Engel et al., 2005	US AHS, wives of private applicators—incidence		
	Wives' own use of phenoxy herbicides	41	0.8 (0.6–1.1)
	2,4-D	41	0.8 (0.6–1.1)
	Husbands' use of phenoxy herbicides	110	1.1 (0.7–1.8)
	2,4-D	107	0.9 (0.6–1.4)
	2,4,5-T	44	1.3 (0.9–1.9)
	2,4,5-TP	19	2.0 (1.2–3.2)
Blair et al., 2005a	US AHS—mortality		
	Private applicators (men and women)	3	0.9 (0.2–2.7)
	Spouses of private applicators (> 99% women)	54	0.9 (0.7–1.1)
Mills and Yang, 2005	Hispanic agricultural farm workers (women)		
	Cancer diagnosis 1987–1994		
	Low 2,4-D use	12	0.6 (0.2–1.9)
	High 2,4-D use	8	0.6 (0.2–1.7)
	Cancer diagnosis 1995–2001		
	Low 2,4-D use	19	2.2 (1.0–4.9)
	High 2,4-D use	21	2.1 (1.1–4.3)
Studies Reviewed in *Update 2000*			
Duell et al., 2000	Female farm workers, residents in North Carolina		
	Used pesticides in garden	228	2.3 (1.7–3.1)
	Laundered clothes for pesticide user	119	4.1 (2.8–5.9)
Studies Reviewed in *Update 1998*			
Kogevinas et al., 1997	IARC cohort, workers exposed to any phenoxy herbicide or chlorophenol		
	Women (identical with Manz et al. [1991])	12	1.2 (0.6–2.1)
	Exposed to highly chlorinated PCDDs	9	2.2 (1.0–4.1)
	Not exposed to highly chlorinated PCDDs	3	0.5 (0.1–1.6)
	Men	2	1.6 (0.2–5.6)
	Exposed to highly chlorinated PCDDs	2	2.6 (0.3–9.3)
	Not exposed to highly chlorinated PCDDs	0	nr
Studies Reviewed in *Update 1996*			
Blair et al., 1993	US farmers in 23 states		
	Men—white	18	0.7 (0.4–1.2)
	nonwhite	4	1.7 (0.5–4.4)
	Women—white	71	1.0 (0.8–1.3)
	nonwhite	30	0.7 (0.5–1.0)
Kogevinas et al., 1993	IARC cohort—women	7	0.9 (0.4–1.9)

TABLE 6-22 Continued

Reference	Study Population[a]	Exposed Cases[b]	Estimated Relative Risk (95% CI)[b]
Studies Reviewed in *VAO*			
Ronco et al., 1992	Danish, Italian farm workers		
	Male farmers	5	0.5 (nr)
	Female farmers	41	0.9 (nr)
	Female family workers	429	0.8 (p < 0.05)
Manz et al., 1991	German production workers—men, women (included in IARC cohort)		
	Women	9	2.2 (1.0–4.1)
Saracci et al., 1991	IARC cohort—exposed subcohort (men and women)		
	Men	2	3.5 (0.4–12.5)
	Women	1	0.3 (0.0–1.7)
Lynge, 1985	Danish male and female production workers (included in IARC cohort)—incidence		
	Women	13	0.9 (nr)
Wiklund, 1983	Swedish agricultural workers—incidence		99% CI
	Men and women	444	0.8 (0.7–0.9)
	Men only	nr	1.0 (nr)
ENVIRONMENTAL			
New Studies			
Consonni et al., 2008	Seveso residents (men and women)—25-year follow-up		
	Zone A	2	0.6 (0.2–2.4)
	Zone B	13	0.6 (0.3–1.2)
	Zone R	133	0.9 (0.7–1.1)
Teitelbaum et al., 2007	Case–control study in Long Island, New York—incidence		
	Used lawn and garden pesticides		
	Never	240	1.0
	Ever	1,254	1.3 (1.1–1.6)
	Product for weeds	1,109	1.4 (1.2–1.8)
Viel et al., 2008	Case–control study in Besançon, France—incidence		
	Residence in zones of dioxin exposure around solid-waste incinerator		
	Women, 20–59 years old		
	Very low	41	1.0
	Low	81	1.1 (0.7–1.6)
	Intermediate	64	1.3 (0.8–1.9)
	High	11	0.9 (0.4–1.8)
	Women, at least 60 years old		
	Very low	50	1.0
	Low	111	0.9 (0.6–1.3)
	Intermediate	72	1.0 (0.7–1.4)
	High	4	0.3 (0.1–0.9)

continued

TABLE 6-22 Continued

Reference	Study Population[a]	Exposed Cases[b]	Estimated Relative Risk (95% CI)[b]
Studies Reviewed in *Update 2006*			
Reynolds et al., 2005	Total TEQs (pg/g) in adipose breast tissue		
	≤ 14.0	24	1.0
	14.1–20.9	22	0.7 (0.3–1.9)
	≤ 21.0	33	0.3 (0.3–2.0)
			p-trend = 0.99
Reynolds et al., 2004	California Teachers Study cohort		
	Residential proximity to use of "endocrine disruptors" (including 2,4-D, cacodylic acid)		
	Quartiles of use (lb/mi²)		
	< 1	1,027	1.0
	1–21	274	1.0 (0.8–1.1)
	22–323	114	0.9 (0.7–1.1)
	≥ 324	137	1.0 (0.9–1.3)
Studies Reviewed in *Update 2002*			
Holford et al., 2000	Patients at Yale–New Haven hospital with breast-related surgery; dioxin-like congener 156	nr	0.9 (0.8–1.0)
Revich et al., 2001	Residents of Chapaevsk, Russia—women	58	2.1 (1.6–2.7)
Warner et al., 2002	SWHS—981 women who were infants to 40 years old when exposed—incidence		
	With 10-fold increase in TCDD	15	2.1 (1.0–4.6)
Studies Reviewed in *Update 2000*			
Bertazzi et al., 2001	Seseso residents—20-year follow-up		
	Zone A, B—females	14	0.7 (0.4–1.3)
Bagga et al., 2000	Women receiving medical care in Woodland Hills, California	73	nr
Demers et al., 2000	Women in Quebec City—newly diagnosed	314	nr
Høyer et al., 2000			Overall survival relative risk
	Female participants in Copenhagen City Heart Study	195	2.8 (1.4–5.6)
Studies Reviewed in *Update 1998*			
Bertazzi et al. 1997	Seveso residents—15-year follow-up		
	Zone A—women	1	0.6 (0.0–3.1)
	Zone B—women	9	0.8 (0.4–1.5)
	Zone R—women	67	0.8 (0.6–1.0)
Studies Reviewed in *Update 1996*			
Bertazzi et al., 1993	Seveso residents—10-year follow-up—incidence		
	Zone A—women	1	0.5 (0.1–3.3)
	Zone B—women	10	0.7 (0.4–1.4)
	Zone R—women	106	1.1 (0.9–1.3)
	men	1	1.2 (0.1–10.2)

TABLE 6-22 Continued

Reference	Study Population[a]	Exposed Cases[b]	Estimated Relative Risk (95% CI)[b]
Studies Reviewed in *VAO*			
Bertazzi	Seveso residents—10-year follow-up		
et al., 1989b	Zone A—women	1	1.1 (0.1–7.5)
	Zone B—women	5	0.9 (0.4–2.1)
	Zone R—women	28	0.6 (0.4–0.9)

ABBREVIATIONS: 2,4-D, 2,4-dichlorophenoxyacetic acid; 2,4,5-T, 2,4,5-trichlorophenoxyacetic acid; 2,4,5-TP, 2 (2,4,5-trichlorophenoxy) propionic acid; AHS, Agricultural Health Study; CDC, Centers for Disease Control and Prevention; CI, confidence interval; IARC, International Agency for Research on Cancer; nr, not reported; PCDDs, chlorinated dibenzo-*p*-dioxins (highly chlorinated, if four or more chlorines); TCDD, 2,3,7,8-tetrachlorodibenzo-*p*-dioxin; TEQ, toxicity equivalent quotient.
[a]Subjects are female and outcome is mortality unless otherwise noted.
[b]Given when available; results other than estimated risk explained individually.
Studies in italics have been superseded by newer studies of same cohorts.

ties, who served outside Vietnam during the same era. The RR of breast-cancer mortality was 1.00 (95% CI 0.69–1.44). The RR posed by Vietnam service was similar when the analysis was restricted to those serving as nurses (RR = 0.92, 95% CI 0.61–1.41). That study therefore provides no support of an association between Agent Orange exposure and breast-cancer risk. However, although its focus on Vietnam veterans is germane, the analysis did not consider actual exposure to herbicides and was unable to adjust for variables, such as reproductive history, that can confound the relationships of exposures to breast cancer.

Occupational Studies

No occupational studies concerning exposure to the chemicals of interest and breast cancer have been published since *Update 2006.*

Environmental Studies

In a case–control study in France, 434 women who had breast cancer were compared with 2,170 community controls according to the proximity of their residence to emissions from a waste incinerator that generated polychlorinated dibenzodioxins and polychlorinated dibenzofurans (Viel et al., 2008). Four exposure categories were created on the basis of emission data and a wind-dispersion model. Separate analyses were carried out for women 20–59 years old and women at least 60 years old. For the younger women, the OR for the highest exposure relative to the lowest was 0.88 (95% CI 0.43–1.79). In older women, that OR was 0.31 (95% CI 0.08–0.89); however, this was based on only four cases, and there was no evidence of a dose–response trend. Furthermore, the study did not adjust for any potential confounders.

Teitelbaum et al. (2007) reported results of the large case–control study of breast cancer in Long Island, New York. Over 1,500 cases and a similar number of matched controls provided information on their exposure to several categories of household pesticides. The OR for those who reported ever using antiweed chemicals vs those who never used any lawn or garden chemicals was 1.43 (95% CI 1.17–1.75). However, similar ORs were obtained for several other categories of lawn and garden chemicals when those who never used any such chemicals were the referent group. That suggests that recall bias (higher recall of all exposures of cases relative to controls) might have played a role. Although ever vs never use of lawn and garden chemicals was significantly associated with breast-cancer risk, there was no dose–response relationship with respect to number of lifetime applications, and the degree of specificity regarding exposure to the chemicals of interest was rather weak. The relatively low response rate among potential controls (63% of those eligible agreed to participate) further reduces the value of this case–control analysis.

Investigators in Italy completed a 25-year mortality follow-up of people exposed to the industrial accident in Seveso (Consonni et al., 2008). Mortality from breast cancer was compared in residents in three exposure zones—very high (Zone A), high (Zone B), and low (Zone R)—and a nonexposed reference population. There was no evidence of increased breast-cancer mortality in any of the exposure groups. The RRs were 0.60 (95% CI 0.15–2.41) in Zone A, 0.65 (95% CI 0.37–1.12) in Zone B, and 0.87 (95% CI 0.73–1.05) in Zone R. There were two, 13, and 133 breast-cancer deaths during the follow-up period in Zones A, B, and R, respectively. It should be noted that the analysis did not include data on established risk factors for breast cancer and was therefore unable to adjust for potential confounding.

Biologic Plausibility

All the experimental evidence indicates that 2,4-D, 2,4,5-T, and TCDD are at most weakly genotoxic. However, TCDD is a demonstrated carcinogen in animals and is recognized as having carcinogenic potential in humans because of the mechanisms discussed in Chapter 4.

With respect to breast cancer, studies performed in laboratory animals (Sprague-Dawley rats) indicate that the effect of TCDD may depend on the age of the animal. For example, TCDD exposure was found to inhibit mammary-tumor growth in the adult rat (Holcombe and Safe, 1994), but to increase tumor growth in the neonatal rat (21 days old) (Desaulniers et al., 2001). Other studies have failed to demonstrate an effect of TCDD on mammary-tumor incidence or growth (Desaulniers et al., 2004).

Those observations may indicate a close association between the development of mammary cancers and mammary gland differentiation. Agents capable of disrupting the ability of the normal mammary epithelial cell to enter or maintain its appropriate status (a proliferative, differentiated, apoptotic state), to maintain its appropriate architecture, or to conduct normal hormone (estrogen) signaling are likely to act as carcinogenic agents (Fenton, 2006; McGee et al., 2006). In that light, it is interesting that postnatal exposure of pregnant rats to TCDD has been found to alter proliferation and differentiation of the mammary gland (Birnbaum and Fenton, 2003; Vorderstrasse et al., 2004). In a recent publication, Jenkins et al. (2007) used a carcinogen-induced rat mammary-cancer model to show that prenatal exposure to TCDD alters mammary gland differentiation and increases susceptibility to mammary cancer by altering the expression of estrogen-receptor genes and of genes involved in oxidative-stress defense. Thus, the effect of TCDD may depend on the timing of the exposure and on the level of gene expression at the time of exposure; TCDD may affect mammary-tumor development only if exposure to it occurs during a specific window during breast development. The breast is the only human organ that does not fully differentiate until it becomes ready for use; nulliparous women have less-differentiated breast lobules, which are presumably more susceptible to carcinogenesis.

Activation of the AHR by dioxin or by the nondioxin ligand indole-3-carbinol is believed to be protective against breast cancer by mechanisms that disrupt migration and metastasis (Bradlow, 2008; Hsu et al., 2007).

TCDD has been shown to modulate the induction of DNA chain breaks in human breast-cancer cells by regulating the activity of the enzymes responsible for estradiol catabolism and generating more reactive intermediates, which might contribute to TCDD-induced carcinogenesis by altering the ratios of 4-OH-estradiol to 2-OH-estradiol (Lin et al., 2007, 2008). A similar imbalance in metabolite ratios has been observed in pregnant Taiwanese women, in whom the ratio of 4-OH-estradiol to 2-OH-estradiol, a breast-cancer–risk marker, decreased with increasing exposure to TCDD (Wang et al., 2006). Expression of CYP1B1, the cytochrome P450 enzyme responsible for 2-OH-estradiol formation, but not CYP1A1, the one responsible for 4-OH estradiol formation, was found to be highly increased in premalignant and malignant rat mammary tissues in which the AHR was constitutively active in the absence of ligand (Yang et al., 2008). On the basis of recent mechanistic data, it has been proposed that the AHR contributes to mammary-tumor cell growth by inhibiting apoptosis while promoting transition to an invasive, metastatic phenotype (Marlowe et al., 2008; Schlezinger et al., 2006).

Recent evidence has shown that AHR activation by TCDD in human breast and endocervical cell lines induces sustained high concentrations of the IL–6 cytokine, which has tumor-promoting effects in numerous tissues, including breast tissue, so TCDD might promote carcinogenesis in these tissues (Hollingshead et al., 2008).

The biologic plausibility of the carcinogenicity of the chemicals of interest is discussed in general at the beginning of this chapter.

Synthesis

In the early 1990s, it was suggested that exposure to some environmental chemicals, such as organochlorine compounds, might play a role in the etiology of breast cancer through estrogen-related pathways. The relationship between organochlorines and breast-cancer risk has been studied extensively especially in the last decade; TCDD and dioxin-like compounds have been among the organochlorines so investigated. Today there is no clear evidence to support a causal role of most organochlorines in human breast cancer (Salehi et al., 2008).

The committee responsible for *Update 2006* was unable to reach a consensus regarding whether the evidence of an association between the chemicals of interest and breast cancer was suggestive or inadequate. Only a few studies have been published in the interim, but, although each of them has limitations and cannot be considered definitive, they tend to weigh against the conclusion that the herbicides in question cause breast cancer in humans. The study by Cypel and Kang (2008) on mortality in female Vietnam-era veterans, especially nurses, is particularly relevant to the mission of the committee. Even though the study did not include any details of specific chemical exposures or confounding factors, the failure to observe any increase in breast-cancer mortality in women who served in Vietnam is revealing.

Meanwhile, the analysis by Consonni et al. (2008), a long-term mortality follow-up in Seveso, was specific with regard to exposure to dioxin, and it also had null findings. In fact, breast-cancer mortality was lower in exposed residents than in the nonexposed reference population, and the lower risk—although still consistent with a chance finding—begins to approach statistical significance in the Zone B (high-exposure) and Zone R (low-exposure) groups. We note the contrast between that result and the results of an earlier study on Seveso in which a positive association between serum TCDD and breast-cancer risk reached borderline statistical significance (Warner et al., 2002). The study by Viel et al. (2008) of women who lived near a waste incinerator had too few cases and too little control for confounding to provide strong evidence, but it, too, found only inverse associations with breast-cancer risk, especially in older women. The study by Teitelbaum et al. (2007), which reported some increase in risk associated with reports of having used lawn or garden chemicals, may have been affected by the recall bias that is common in case–control studies and also lacked details of specific chemical exposures.

Conclusion

Having considered the new evidence and the results of studies reviewed in previous updates, the present committee concludes that there is inadequate or insufficient evidence to determine whether there is an association (either positive or negative) between exposure to the chemicals of interest and breast cancer.

CANCERS OF THE FEMALE REPRODUCTIVE SYSTEM

This section addresses cancers of the cervix (ICD-9 180), endometrium (also referred to as the corpus uteri; ICD-9 182.0–182.1, 182.8), and ovary (ICD-9 183.0). Other cancers of the female reproductive system that are infrequently reported separately are unspecified cancers of the uterus (ICD-9 179), placenta (ICD-9 181), fallopian tube and other uterine adnexa (ICD-9 183.2–183.9), and other female genital organs (ICD-9 184); findings on these cancers are included in this section. It also presents statistics on other cancers of the female reproductive system. ACS estimates of the numbers of new female reproductive-system cancers in the United States in 2008 are presented in Table 6-23, with genital-system cancers representing roughly 11% of new cancer cases and 10% of cancer deaths in women (Jemal et al., 2008a).

The incidences of and risk factors for those diseases vary (Table 6-24). Cervical cancer occurs more often in blacks than in whites, whereas whites are more likely to develop endometrial and ovarian cancer. The incidence of endometrial and ovarian cancer is increased in older women and in those with positive family histories. Use of unopposed estrogen-hormone therapy and obesity, which increases endogenous concentrations of estrogen, both increase the risk of endometrial cancer. Human papilloma virus (HPV) infection, particularly infection with HPV types 16 and 18, is the most important risk factor for cervical cancer. Use of oral contraceptives is associated with a substantial reduction in the risk of ovarian cancer.

Conclusions from *VAO* and Previous Updates

The committee responsible for *VAO* concluded that there was inadequate or insufficient information to determine whether there is an association between exposure to the chemicals of interest and female reproductive cancers. Additional information available to the committees responsible for *Update 1996*, *Update 1998*, *Update 2000*, *Update 2002*, *Update 2004*, and *Update 2006* did not change that conclusion. Tables 6-25, 6-26, and 6-27 summarize the results of the relevant studies.

Update of the Epidemiologic Literature

Vietnam-Veteran Studies

The long-term mortality study of female Vietnam veterans by Cypel and Kang (2008) found no increase in risk of death from uterine or ovarian cancer in those who served in Vietnam; however, the number of deaths due to these cancers was small, so these estimates lack precision.

TABLE 6-23 Estimates of New Cases of Deaths from Selected Cancers of the Female Reproductive System in the United States in 2008

Site	New Cases	Deaths
Cervix	11,070	3,870
Endometrium	40,100	7,470
Ovary	21,650	15,520
Other female genital	5,670	1,630

SOURCE: Jemal et al., 2008.

Occupational Studies

No occupational studies concerning exposure to the chemicals of interest and cancers of the female reproductive system have been published since *Update 2006*.

Environmental Studies

Consonni et al. (2008) studied mortality of various causes in women exposed to dioxin during the Seveso incident in Italy. Very few deaths from those specific cancers occurred in women in the more heavily exposed areas, so those risk estimates lack precision and are not very informative.

Biologic Plausibility

No animal studies have reported an increased incidence of female reproductive cancer after exposure to the chemicals of interest. One study (Kociba et al., 1978), however, showed a reduced incidence of uterine tumors in rats fed TCDD at 0.1 mg/kg of diet for 2 years.

TABLE 6-24 Average Annual Incidence (per 100,000) of Female Genital System Cancers in United States[a]

	50–54 Years Old			55–59 Years Old			60–64 Years Old		
	All Races	White	Black	All Races	White	Black	All Races	White	Black
All genital sites	84.3	87.6	64.2	119.4	125.5	84.0	148.7	153.2	146.1
Cervix	11.6	10.9	15.2	11.9	10.9	17.5	12.3	10.5	22.8
Endometrium	45.5	48.8	24.6	68.6	73.7	36.6	88.6	93.0	77.1
Ovary	22.3	23.6	15.1	29.9	32.1	19.7	38.3	41.1	29.3
Other genital organs	1.2	1.2	1.0	1.6	1.7	1.1	2.5	2.7	1.6

[a]Surveillance, Epidemiology, and End Results program, nine standard registries, crude age-specific rates, 2000–2005.

TABLE 6-25 Selected Epidemiologic Studies—Cervical Cancer

Reference	Study Population[a]	Exposed Cases[b]	Estimated Relative Risk (95% CI)[b]
VIETNAM VETERANS			
Studies Reviewed in *Update 2002*			
Kang et al., 2000	Female Vietnam veterans	57	1.1 (0.7–1.7)
Studies Reviewed in *Update 2000*			
CDVA, 1998b			Expected number of exposed cases (95% CI)
	Australian Vietnam veterans—self-reported incidence	8	1 (0–5)
OCCUPATIONAL			
Studies Reviewed in *Update 1998*			
Kogevinas et al., 1997	IARC cohort, female workers exposed to any phenoxy herbicide or chlorophenol	3	1.1 (0.2–3.3)
	Exposed to highly chlorinated PCDDs	0	0.0 (0.0–3.8)
	Not exposed to highly chlorinated PCDDs	3	1.8 (0.4–5.2)
Studies Reviewed in *Update 1996*			
Blair et al., 1993	US farmers in 23 states		
	Whites	6	0.9 (0.3–2.0)
	Nonwhites	21	2.0 (1.3–3.1)
Lynge, 1993	Danish phenoxy herbicide workers	7	3.2 (1.3–6.6)
Studies Reviewed in *VAO*			
Ronco et al., 1992	Danish farmers—incidence		
	Self-employed farmers	7	0.5 (p < 0.05)
	Family workers	100	0.5 (p < 0.05)
	Employees	12	0.8 (nr)
Wiklund, 1983			99% CI
	Swedish female agricultural workers—incidence	82	0.6 (0.4–0.8)
ENVIRONMENTAL			
Studies Reviewed in *Update 2002*			
Revich et al., 2001	Residents of Chapaevsk, Russia	13	1.8 (1.0–3.1)

ABBREVIATIONS: CI, confidence interval; IARC, International Agency for Research on Cancer; nr, not reported; PCDDs, chlorinated dibenzo-*p*-dioxins (highly chlorinated, if four or more chlorines).
[a]Subjects are female and outcome is mortality unless otherwise noted.
[b]Given when available; results other than estimated risk explained individually.

Hollingshead et al. (2008) recently showed that TCDD activation of the AHR in human breast and endocervical cell lines induces sustained high concentrations of the IL–6 cytokine, which has tumor-promoting effects in numerous tissues, including ovarian, so TCDD might promote carcinogenesis in these tissue.

The biologic plausibility of the carcinogenicity of the chemicals of interest is discussed in general at the beginning of this chapter.

TABLE 6-26 Selected Epidemiologic Studies—Uterine Cancer

Reference	Study Population[a]	Exposed Cases[b]	Estimated Relative Risk (95% CI)[b]
VIETNAM VETERANS			
New Studies			
Cypel and	US non-Vietnam veterans vs non-Vietnam veterans	5	0.8 (0.2–2.8)
Kang, 2008	Vietnam nurses vs non-Vietnam nurses	5	1.3 (0.3–5.0)
Studies Reviewed in *Update 2002*			
Kang et al., 2000	US Vietnam veterans—incidence	41	1.0 (0.6–1.6)
Studies Reviewed in *Update 2000*			
CDVA, 1998b	Australian Vietnam veterans—self-reported incidence	4	Expected number of exposed cases (95% CI) 1 (0–5)
Studies Reviewed in *Update 1996*			
Dalager et al., 1995	US Vietnam veterans	4	2.1 (0.6–5.4)
OCCUPATIONAL			
Studies Reviewed in *Update 1998*			
Kogevinas et al., 1997	IARC cohort, female workers exposed to any phenoxy herbicide or chlorophenol (includes cancers of endometrium)	3	3.4 (0.7–10.0)
	Exposed to highly chlorinated PCDDs	1	1.2 (0.0–6.5)
	Not exposed to highly chlorinated PCDDs	4	2.3 (0.6–5.9)
Studies Reviewed in *VAO*			
Blair et al., 1993	US farmers in 23 states		
	Whites	15	1.2 (0.7–2.1)
	Nonwhites	17	1.4 (0.8–2.2)
Ronco et al., 1992	Danish farmers—incidence		
	Self-employed farmers	8	0.6 (nr)
	Family workers	103	0.8 (p < 0.05)
	Employees	9	0.9 (nr)
Wiklund, 1983	Swedish female agricultural workers—incidence		99% CI
		135	0.9 (0.7–1.1)
ENVIRONMENTAL			
New Studies			
Consonni et al., 2008	Seseo residents—25-year follow-up		
	Zone A	0	0
	Zone B	2	0.5 (0.1–1.9)
	Zone R	41	1.3 (0.9–1.8)
Studies Reviewed in *Update 2000*			
Bertazzi et al., 2001	Seveso residents—20-year follow-up		
	Zones A, B	2	0.5 (0.1–1.9)
Weiderpass et al., 2000	Swedish women	154	1.0 (0.6–2.0)

continued

TABLE 6-26 Continued

Reference	Study Population[a]	Exposed Cases[b]	Estimated Relative Risk (95% CI)[b]
Bertazzi et al., 1998	Seveso residents—15-year follow-up		
	Zone B	1	0.3 (0.0–2.4)
Studies Reviewed in *Update 1998*			
Bertazzi et al., 1997	Seveso residents—15-year follow-up		
	Zone B	1	0.3 (0.0–1.9)
	Zone R	27	1.1 (0.8–1.7)

ABBREVIATIONS: CI, confidence interval; IARC, International Agency for Research on Cancer; nr = not reported; PCDDs, chlorinated dibenzo-*p*-dioxins (highly chlorinated, if four or more chlorines).
[a]Subjects are female; outcome is mortality unless otherwise noted.
[b]Given when available; results other than estimated risk explained individually.
Studies in italics have been superseded by newer studies of same cohorts.

Synthesis

New information concerning female reproductive cancers since *Update 2006* has been sparse, especially because the two new analyses deal with mortality rather than incidence. Together, they add little weight to the existing body of evidence.

Conclusion

On the basis of the evidence reviewed here and in previous VAO reports, the committee concludes that there is inadequate or insufficient evidence to determine whether there is an association between exposure to the chemicals of interest and uterine, ovarian, or cervical cancer.

TABLE 6-27 Selected Epidemiologic Studies—Ovarian Cancer

Reference	Study Population[a]	Exposed Cases[b]	Estimated Relative Risk (95% CI)[b]
VIETNAM VETERANS			
Studies Reviewed in *Update 2002*			
Kang et al., 2000	Vietnam veterans	16	1.8 (0.7–4.6)
Studies Reviewed in *Update 2000*			
CDVA, 1998b			Expected number of exposed cases (95% CI)
	Australian Vietnam veterans—self-reported incidence	1	0 (0–4)

continued

TABLE 6-27 Continued

Reference	Study Population[a]	Exposed Cases[b]	Estimated Relative Risk (95% CI)[b]
OCCUPATIONAL			
Studies Reviewed in *Update 2006*			
Blair et al.,	US AHS		
2005a	Private applicators (men and women)	4	3.9 (1.1–10.1)
	Spouses of private applicators (> 99% women)	13	0.7 (0.4–1.2)
Alavanja	US AHS—incidence		
et al., 2005	Private applicators (men and women)	8	3.0 (1.3–5.9)
	Spouses of private applicators (> 99% women)	32	0.6 (0.4–0.8)
	Commercial applicators (men and women)	0	0.0 (0.0–16.0)
Studies Reviewed in *Update 1998*			
Kogevinas	IARC cohort, female workers exposed to any		
et al., 1997	phenoxy herbicide or chlorophenol	1	0.3 (0.0–1.5)
	Exposed to highly chlorinated PCDDs	0	0.0 (0.0–2.6)
	Not exposed to highly chlorinated PCDDs	1	0.5 (0.0–2.5)
Studies Reviewed in *Update 1996*			
Kogevinas	IARC cohort		
et al., 1993		1	0.7 (nr)
Studies Reviewed in *VAO*			
Ronco et al.,	Danish farmers—incidence		
1992	Self-employed farmers	12	0.9 (nr)
	Family workers	104	0.8 (p < 0.05)
	Employees	5	0.5 (nr)
Donna	Female residents near Alessandria, Italy	18	4.4 (1.9–16.1)
et al., 1984			
ENVIRONMENTAL			
New Studies			
Consonni	Seveso residents—25-year follow-up		
et al., 2008	Zone A	1	1.2 (0.2–8.5)
	Zone B	2	0.4 (0.1–1.6)
	Zone R	37	1.0 (0.7–1.4)
Studies Reviewed in *Update 2000*			
Bertazzi	Seveso residents—20-year follow-up		
et al., 2001	Zones A, B	3	0.7 (0.2–2.0)
Bertazzi	Seveso residents—15-year follow-up		
et al., 1998	Zone A	1	2.3 (0.3–16.5)
Studies Reviewed in *Update 1998*			
Bertazzi	Seveso residents—15-year follow-up		
et al., 1997	Zone A—women	1	2.3 (0.0–12.8)
	Zone R—women	21	1.0 (0.6–1.6)

ABBREVIATIONS: AHS, Agricultural Health Study; CI, confidence interval; IARC, International Agency for Research on Cancer; nr = not reported; PCDDs, chlorinated dibenzo-*p*-dioxins (highly chlorinated, if four or more chlorines).
[a]Subjects are female and outcome is mortality unless otherwise noted.
[b]Given when available; results other than estimated risk explained individually.
Studies in italics have been superseded by newer studies of same cohorts.

PROSTATE CANCER

ACS estimated that 186,320 new cases of prostate cancer (ICD-9 185) would be diagnosed in the United States in 2008 and that 28,660 men would die from it (Jemal et al., 2008a). That makes prostate cancer the second-most common cancer in men (after nonmelanoma skin cancers); it is expected to account for about 25% of new cancer diagnoses and 10% of cancer deaths in men in 2008. The average annual incidence of prostate cancer is shown in Table 6-28.

The incidence of prostate cancer varies dramatically with age and race. The risk more than doubles between the ages of 50–54 years and 55–59 years, and it nearly doubles again between the ages of 55–59 years and 60–64 years. As a group, American black men have the highest recorded incidence of prostate cancer in the world (Miller et al., 1996); their risk is roughly twice that in whites in the United States, 5 times that in Alaska natives, and nearly 8.5 times that in Korean Americans. Little is known about the causes of prostate cancer. Other than race and age, risk factors include a family history of the disease and possibly some elements of the Western diet, such as high consumption of animal fats. The drug finasteride, which has been widely used to treat benign enlargement of the prostate, was found to decrease the prevalence of prostate cancer substantially in a major randomized trial (Thompson et al., 2003). Finasteride acts by decreasing the formation of potent androgen hormones in the prostate.

The study of the incidence of and mortality from prostate cancer is complicated by trends in screening for the disease. The widespread adoption of serum prostate-specific antigen (PSA) screening in the 1990s led to very large increases in prostate cancer incidence in the United States, which have recently subsided as exposure to screening has become saturated. The long-term influence of better screening on incidence and mortality in any country or population is difficult to predict and will depend on the rapidity with which the screening tool is adopted, its differential use in men of various ages, and the aggressiveness of tumors detected early with this test (Gann, 1997). Because exposure to PSA testing is such a strong determinant of prostate-cancer incidence, epidemiologic studies must be careful to exclude differential PSA testing as an explanation of a difference in risk observed between two populations.

TABLE 6-28 Average Annual Incidence (per 100,000) of Prostate Cancer in United States[a]

50–54 Years Old			55–59 Years Old			60–64 Years Old		
All Races	White	Black	All Races	White	Black	All Races	White	Black
146.7	140.9	269.9	350.5	337.5	633.8	600.6	587.8	1,002.5

[a]Surveillance, Epidemiology, and End Results program, nine standard registries, crude age-specific rates, 2000–2005.

Prostate cancer tends not to be fatal, so mortality studies might miss an increased incidence of the disease. Findings that show an association between an exposure and prostate-cancer mortality should be examined closely to determine whether the exposed group might have had poorer access to treatment that would have increased the likelihood of survival.

Conclusions from *VAO* and Previous Updates

The committee responsible for *VAO* concluded that there was limited or suggestive evidence of an association between exposure to the chemicals of interest and prostate cancer. Additional information available to the committees responsible for *Update 1996*, *Update 1998*, *Update 2000*, *Update 2002*, *Update 2004*, and *Update 2006* did not change that conclusion. Table 6-29 summarizes results of the relevant studies, including both morbidity and mortality studies. The type, quality, and specificity of each study must be considered in the interpretation and weighing of evidence. Because of study heterogeneity, simply examining all the estimated risks in the table together will not yield a good assessment of the risks.

Update of the Epidemiologic Literature

Vietnam-Veteran Studies

Chamie et al. (2008) published a study of prostate cancer incidence in Vietnam-era veterans who were receiving care in the Northern California Veterans Affairs Health System. A total of 6,214 veterans reported having been exposed to Agent Orange while serving in Vietnam, and another 6,930 men served on active duty in Vietnam but reported no exposure. Men categorized as exposed had to have reported it on their initial application to VA for medical benefits. A total of 239 cases of prostate cancer were identified in the exposed group and 124 in the nonexposed group. In Cox proportional-hazards modeling, the hazard ratio was 2.87 (95% CI 2.31–3.57) with a mean time between exposure and diagnosis of 407 months. The proportion of cases with high-grade or advanced cancer at diagnosis was higher in the exposed group. Some 38 cases in the exposed group reported their exposure after receiving a diagnosis of prostate cancer; exclusion of these cases reduces the magnitude of the association, but it remains significant.

Occupational Studies

Investigators in the AHS evaluated the association between exposure to dicamba, a benzoic acid herbicide that is often mixed with 2,4-D when sprayed, and cancer incidence (Samanic et al., 2006). Neither cumulative exposure nor

TABLE 6-29 Selected Epidemiologic Studies—Prostate Cancer

Reference	Study Population[a]	Exposed Cases[b]	Estimated Relative Risk (95% CI)[b]
VIETNAM VETERANS			
New Studies			
Chamie et al., 2008	Vietnam-era veterans in northern California Veterans Affairs Health System—self-reported exposure to Agent Orange	239	2.9 (2.3–3.6)
Studies Reviewed in *Update 2006*			
Leavy et al., 2006	606 prostate cancer cases in Western Australia Vietnam service	25	2.1 (0.9–5.1)
Pavuk et al., 2006	AFHS subjects—incidence		
	20-year cumulative TCDD (ppt-year)		
	Comparison group	81	1.0
	Ranch Hand low (≤ 434 ppt-year)	31	1.0 (0.7–1.6)
	Ranch Hand high (> 434 ppt-year)	28	1.2 (0.8–1.9)
			p-trend = 0.42
	Last tour in SEA before 1969 (heavy spraying)		
	Yes		
	Comparison group	17	1.0
	Ranch Hand low (≤ 434 ppt-year)	9	1.0 (0.4–2.3)
	Ranch Hand high (> 434 ppt-year)	15	2.3 (1.1–4.7)
			p-trend = 0.04
	No		
	Comparison group	64	1.0
	Ranch Hand low (≤ 434 ppt-year)	22	1.1 (0.7–1.8)
	Ranch Hand high (> 434 ppt-year)	13	0.9 (0.5–1.6)
			p-trend = 0.75
	Less than 2 years served in SEA		
	Yes		
	Comparison group	16	1.0
	Ranch Hand low (≤ 434 ppt-year)	20	1.9 (1.0–3.7)
	Ranch Hand high (> 434 ppt-year)	14	2.2 (1.0–4.5)
			p-trend = 0.03
	No		
	Comparison group	65	1.0
	Ranch Hand low (≤ 434 ppt-year)	11	0.8 (0.4–1.5)
	Ranch Hand high (> 434 ppt-year)	14	1.1 (0.6–1.9)
			p-trend = 0.89
Pavuk et al., 2005	White Air Force comparison subjects only—incidence		
	Serum TCDD (pg/g) based on model with exposure variable $\log_e$(TCDD)		
	Per unit increase of $-\log_e$(TCDD)	83	1.1 (0.7–1.5)
	Quartiles (pg/g)		
	0.4–2.6	13	1.0
	2.6–3.8	24	1.7 (0.8–3.3)
	3.8–5.2	24	1.5 (0.7–2.9)
	> 5.2	22	1.2 (0.6–2.4)
	Number of years served in SEA		
	Per year of service	83	1.1 (1.0–1.2)

continued

TABLE 6-29 Continued

Reference	Study Population[a]	Exposed Cases[b]	Estimated Relative Risk (95% CI)[b]
	Quartiles (years in SEA)		
	0.8–1.3	8	1.0
	1.3–2.1	11	1.3 (0.5–3.2)
	2.1–3.7	28	2.2 (1.0–4.9)
	3.7–16.4	36	2.4 (1.1–5.2)
ADVA, 2005a	Australian male Vietnam veterans vs Australian population—incidence	692	1.3 (1.2–1.3)
	Navy	137	1.2 (1.0–1.4)
	Army	451	1.8 (1.2–1.4)
	Air Force	104	1.3 (1.0–1.5)
ADVA, 2005b	Australian male Vietnam veterans vs Australian population—mortality	107	1.2 (1.0–1.5)
	Navy	22	1.3 (0.8–1.8)
	Army	65	1.2 (0.9–1.5)
	Air Force	19	1.4 (0.8–2.1)
ADVA, 2005c	Australian male conscripted Army National Service Vietnam-era veterans—deployed vs nondeployed		
	Incidence	65	1.2 (0.9–1.5)
	Mortality	0	0.0 (0.0–0.7)
Boehmer et al., 2004	Follow-up of CDC Vietnam Experience Cohort	1	0.4 (nr)
Studies Reviewed in *Update 2004*			
Akhtar et al., 2004	AFHS subjects vs national rates		
	White AFHS Ranch Hand veterans		
	Incidence	36	1.5 (1.0–2.0)
	With tours in 1966–1970	34	1.7 (1.2–2.3)
	Mortality	2	0.7 (0.1–2.3)
	White AFHS comparison veterans		
	Incidence	54	1.6 (1.2–2.1)
	With tours between 1966–1970	42	1.6 (1.2–2.2)
	Mortality	3	0.8 (0.2–2.1)
	White AFHS subjects—incidence		
	Who spent at most 2 years in SEA		
	Per unit increase of $-\log_e$(TCDD)	28	1.5 (0.9–2.4)
	Comparison group	7	1.0
	Ranch Hand— < 10 TCDD pg/g in 1987	10	1.5 (0.5–4.4)
	Ranch Hand— < 118.5 TCDD pg/g at end of service	6	2.2 (0.7–6.9)
	Ranch Hand— > 118.5 TCDD pg/g at end of service	5	6.0 (1.4–24.6)
	Only Ranch Hands with 100% service in Vietnam and comparisons with no service in Vietnam		
	Per unit increase of $-\log_e$(TCDD)	20	1.1 (0.6–1.8)
	Comparison group	3	1.0
	Ranch Hand— < 10 TCDD pg/g in 1987	9	2.5 (0.4–16.1)
	Ranch Hand— < 118.5 TCDD pg/g at end of service	4	2.4 (0.4–16.0)

TABLE 6-29 Continued

Reference	Study Population[a]	Exposed Cases[b]	Estimated Relative Risk (95% CI)[b]
	Ranch Hand— > 118.5 TCDD pg/g at end of service	4	4.7 (0.8–29.1)
Giri et al., 2004	Veterans using the VA Medical Center in Ann Arbor, Michigan		
	All cases	11	OR 2.1 (0.8–5.2)
	Cases in white veterans only	nr	OR 2.7 (0.9–8.2)
Studies Reviewed in *Update 2000*			
AFHS, 2000 AIHW, 1999	Air Force Ranch Hand veterans	26	0.7(0.4–1.3) Expected number of exposed cases (95% CI)
	Australian Vietnam veterans—incidence (validation study)	212	147 (123–171)
CDVA, 1998a	Australian Vietnam veterans—self-reported incidence	428	147 (123–171)
Studies Reviewed in *Update 1998*			
Clapp, 1997	Massachusetts Vietnam veterans—incidence	15	0.8 (0.4–1.6)
CDVA, 1997a	Australian military Vietnam veterans	36	1.5 (1.0–2.0)
AFHS, 1996	Air Force Ranch Hand veterans	2	0.6 expected
Watanabe and Kang, 1996	US Army and Marine Corps Vietnam veterans		
	Army Vietnam Service	58	1.1 (nr)
	Non-Vietnam	1	1.2 (nr)[c]
	Marine Vietnam Service	9	1.2 (nr)
	Non-Vietnam	6	1.3 (nr)
Studies Reviewed in *Update 1996*			
Visintainer et al., 1995	PM study of deaths (1974–1989) of Michigan Vietnam-era veterans—deployed vs nondeployed (male genital system)	19	1.1 (0.6–1.7)
Studies Reviewed in *VAO*			
Breslin et al., 1988	Army Vietnam veterans	30	0.9 (0.6–1.2)
	Marine Vietnam veterans	5	1.3 (0.2–10.3)
Anderson et al., 1986	Wisconsin Vietnam veterans	0	nr
OCCUPATIONAL			
New Studies			
Hansen et al., 2007	Danish gardeners (male genital organs, ICD-7 177–178)—incidence		
	10-year follow-up (1975–1984) reported in Hansen et al. (1992)	20	1.2 (0.7–1.8)
	25-year follow-up (1975–2001)		
	Born before 1915 (high exposure)	39	1.3 (1.0–1.8)
	Born 1915–1934 (medium exposure)	35	0.9 (0.6–1.2)
	Born after 1934 (low exposure)	3	0.4 (0.1–1.3)

continued

TABLE 6-29 Continued

Reference	Study Population[a]	Exposed Cases[b]	Estimated Relative Risk (95% CI)[b]
Samanic et al., 2006	Pesticide applicators in AHS—prostate cancer incidence from enrollment through 2002		
	Dicamba—lifetime days exposure		
	None	343	1.0
	1– < 20	106	1.0 (0.8–1.3)
	20– < 56	102	0.9 (0.7–1.2)
	56– < 116	76	1.0 (0.7–1.3)
	≥ 116	67	1.1 (0.8–1.5)
			p-trend = 0.45
Studies Reviewed in *Update 2006*			
McLean et al., 2006	IARC cohort of pulp and paper workers		
	Exposure to nonvolatile organochlorine compounds		
	Never	117	0.9 (0.7–1.0)
	Ever	84	0.9 (0.7–1.2)
't Mannetje et al., 2005	Phenoxy herbicide producers	1	0.4 (0.0–2.1)
	Phenoxy herbicide sprayers (> 99% men)	2	0.6 (0.1–2.2)
Alavanja et al., 2005	US AHS—incidence		
	Private applicators	1,046	1.3 (1.2–1.3)
	Spouses of private applicators (> 99% women)	5	1.2 (0.4–2.8)
	Commercial applicators	41	1.4 (1.0–1.9)
Blair et al., 2005a	US AHS		
	Private applicators	48	0.7 (0.5–0.8)
	Spouses of private applicators (> 99% women)	0	0.0 (0.0–1.6)
Torchio et al., 1994	Italian licensed pesticide users	66	1.0 (0.7–1.2)
Reif et al., 1989	New Zealand forestry workers—nested case–control —incidence	12	0.7 (0.4–1.3)
Studies Reviewed in *Update 2004*			
Alavanja et al., 2003	US AHS—pesticide appliers in Iowa and North Carolina—incidence	566	1.1 (1.1–1.2)
Bodner et al., 2003	Dow chemical production workers (included in IARC cohort, NIOSH Dioxin Registry)	nr	1.7 (1.0–2.6)
Swaen et al., 2004	Dutch licensed herbicide applicators	6	1.0 (0.4–2.2)
Studies Reviewed in *Update 2002*			
Burns et al., 2001	Dow 2,4-D production workers (included in IARC cohort, NIOSH Dioxin Registry)	7	1.3 (0.5–2.8)
Thörn et al., 2000	Swedish lumberjacks exposed to phenoxyacetic herbicides		
	Foremen—incidence	2	4.7 (nr)
	Male lumberjacks—incidence	3	0.9 (nr)

TABLE 6-29 Continued

Reference	Study Population[a]	Exposed Cases[b]	Estimated Relative Risk (95% CI)[b]
Studies Reviewed in *Update 2000*			
Sharma-Wagner et al., 2000	Swedish citizens		
	Agriculture, stock raising	6,080	1.1 (1.0–1.1) (p < 0.01)
	Farmers, foresters, gardeners	5,219	1.1 (1.0–1.1) (p < 0.01)
	Paper-mill workers	304	0.9 (0.8–1.0)
	Pulp grinding	39	1.4 (1.0–1.9) (p < 0.05)
Fleming et al., 1999a	Florida pesticide appliers	353	1.9 (1.7–2.1)
Fleming et al., 1999b	Florida pesticide appliers	64	2.4 (1.8–3.0)
Steenland et al., 1999	US chemical production workers (included in IARC cohort, NIOSH Dioxin Registry)	28	1.2 (0.8–1.7)
Dich and Wiklund, 1998	Swedish pesticide appliers	401	1.1 (1.0–1.2)
	Born 1935 or later	7	2.0 (0.8–4.2)
	Born before 1935	394	1.1 (1.0–1.2)
Studies Reviewed in *Update 1998*			
Gambini et al., 1997	Italian rice growers	19	1.0 (0.6–1.5)
Hertzman et al., 1997	Canadian sawmill workers		
	Morbidity	282	1.0 (0.9–1.1)
	Mortality from male genital tract cancers	116	1.2 (1.0–1.4)
Kogevinas et al., 1997	IARC cohort, workers exposed to any phenoxy herbicide or chlorophenol	68	1.1 (0.9–1.4)
	Exposed to highly chlorinated PCDDs	43	1.1 (0.8–1.5)
	Not exposed to highly chlorinated PCDDs	25	1.1 (0.7–1.6)
Becher et al., 1996	German production workers (included in IARC cohort)	9	1.3 (nr)
Ott and Zober, 1996	BASF employees—incidence		
	TCDD < 0.1 µg/kg of body weight	4	1.1 (0.3–2.8)
	TCDD 0.1–0.99 µg/kg of body weight	1	1.1 (0.0–5.9)
Zhong and Rafnsson, 1996	Icelandic pesticide users	10	0.7 (0.3–1.3)
Studies Reviewed in *Update 1996*			
Asp et al., 1994	Finnish herbicide applicators		
	Incidence	6	0.4 (0.1–0.8)
	Mortality	5	0.8 (0.3–1.8)
Blair et al., 1993	US farmers in 23 states		
	Whites	3,765	1.2 (1.1–1.2)
	Nonwhites	564	1.1 (1.1–1.2)
Bueno de Mesquita et al., 1993	Dutch phenoxy herbicide workers (included in IARC cohort)	3	2.6 (0.5–7.7)

continued

TABLE 6-29 Continued

Reference	Study Population[a]	Exposed Cases[b]	Estimated Relative Risk (95% CI)[b]
Collins et al., 1993	Monsanto Company workers (included in NIOSH cohort)	9	1.6 (0.7–3.0)
Studies Reviewed in *VAO*			
Morrison et al., 1993	Canadian farmers, 45–69 years old, no employees, or custom workers, sprayed ≥ 250 acres	20	2.2 (1.3–3.8)
Ronco et al., 1992	Danish workers—incidence		
	Self-employed	399	0.9 (p < 0.05)
	Employee	63	0.8 (p < 0.05)
Swaen et al., 1992	Dutch licensed herbicide applicators	1	1.3 (0.0–7.3)
Fingerhut et al., 1991	NIOSH—entire cohort	17	1.2 (0.7–2.0)
	≥ 1-year exposure, ≥ 20-year latency	9	1.5 (0.7–2.9)
Manz et al., 1991	German production workers (included in IARC cohort)—men, women	7	1.4 (0.6–2.9)
Saracci et al., 1991	IARC cohort—exposed subcohort	30	1.1 (0.8–1.6)
Zober et al., 1990			90% CI
	BASF employees—basic cohort	0	nr (0.0–6.1)
Alavanja et al., 1989	USDA forest conservationists	nr	1.6 (0.9–3.0)
	Soil conservationists	nr	1.0 (0.6–1.8)
Henneberger et al., 1989	New Hampshire pulp and paper workers	9	1.0 (0.5–1.9)
Solet et al., 1989	US paper and pulp workers	4	1.1 (0.3–2.9)
Alavanja et al., 1988	USDA agricultural extension agents	nr	1.0 (0.7–1.5)
Bond et al., 1988	Dow 2,4-D production workers (included in IARC cohort, NIOSH Dioxin Registry)	1	1.0 (0.0–5.8)
Coggon et al., 1986	British MCPA production workers (included in IARC cohort)	18	1.3 (0.8–2.1)
Robinson et al., 1986	Northwestern US paper and pulp workers	17	90% CI 1.2 (0.7–1.7)
Lynge, 1985	Danish production workers—incidence (included in the IARC cohort)	9	0.8 (nr)
Blair et al., 1983			Expected number of exposed cases (95% CI)
	Florida pesticide applicators	2	3.8 (nr)
Burmeister et al., 1983	Iowa residents—farm exposures	4, 827	1.2 (p < 0.05)
Wiklund, 1983			99% CI
	Swedish male agricultural workers	3,890	1.0 (0.9–1.0)
Burmeister, 1981	Iowa farmers	1,138	1.1 (p < 0.01)

TABLE 6-29 Continued

Reference	Study Population[a]	Exposed Cases[b]	Estimated Relative Risk (95% CI)[b]
ENVIRONMENTAL			
New Studies			
Consonni	Seveso residents—25-year follow-up—men, women		
et al., 2008	Zone A	1	0.9 (0.1–6.2)
	Zone B	8	0.9 (0.4–1.8)
	Zone R	65	1.1 (0.8–1.4)
Studies Reviewed in *Update 2000*			
Bertazzi	Seveso residents—20-year follow-up		
et al., 2001	Zones A, B—men	8	1.1 (0.5–2.2)
Studies Reviewed in *Update 1998*			
Bertazzi	Seveso residents—15-year follow-up		
et al., 1997	Zone B—men	6	1.2 (0.5–2.7)
	Zone R—men	39	1.2 (0.8–1.6)
Svensson	Swedish fishermen—mortality		
et al., 1995	East coast	12	1.0 (0.5–1.8)
	West coast	123	1.1 (0.9–1.3)
	Swedish fishermen—incidence		
	East coast	38	1.1 (0.8–1.5)
	West coast	224	1.0 (0.9–1.1)
Studies Reviewed in *Update 1996*			
Bertazzi	Seveso residents—10-year follow-up—incidence		
et al., 1993	Zone R—men	16	0.9 (0.5–1.5)
Studies Reviewed in *VAO*			
Pesatori	Seveso residents—incidence		
et al., 1992	Zones A, B—men	4	1.4 (0.5–3.9)
	Zone R—men	17	0.9 (0.6–1.5)
Bertazzi	Seveso residents—10-year follow-up		
et al., 1989a	Zones A, B, R—men	19	1.6 (1.0–2.7)
Bertazzi	Seveso residents—10-year follow-up		
et al., 1989b	Zone B—men	3	2.2 (0.7–6.9)
	Zone R—men	16	1.6 (0.9–2.7)

ABBREVIATIONS: 2,4-D, 2,4-dichlorophenoxyacetic acid; AFHS, Air Force Health Study; AHS, Agricultural Health Study; CDC, Centers for Disease Control and Prevention; CI, confidence interval; IARC, International Agency for Research on Cancer; ICD, International Classification of Diseases; MCPA, 2-methyl-4-chlorophenoxyacetic acid; NIOSH, National Institute for Occupational Safety and Health; nr, not reported; OR, odds ratio; PCDDs, chlorinated dibenzo-*p*-dioxins (highly chlorinated, if four or more chlorines); PM, proportionate mortality; SEA, Southeast Asia; TCDD, 2,3,7,8-tetrachlorodibenzo-*p*-dioxin; USDA, US Department of Agriculture; VA, Department of Veterans Affairs.

[a]Subjects are male and outcome is mortality unless otherwise noted.
[b]Given when available; results other than estimated risk explained individually.
[c]Statistically significant with the 95% CI not including 1.0.
Studies in italics have been superseded by newer studies of same cohorts.

intensity-weighted cumulative exposure was associated with prostate-cancer risk.

Hansen et al. (2007) evaluated a cohort consisting of members of a Danish gardeners union, who were followed from 1975 until 2002. Because herbicide and pesticide exposures were reduced over successive calendar periods, year of birth was used as a proxy for magnitude of exposure. Previous analyses had detected an excess of STS in the older workers, which suggested that phenoxy herbicides might have been responsible. Prostate cancers were included in a more general category (male genital organs), and there was some evidence of increased risk compared with that in the general Danish population in the early, most heavily exposed subcohort (SIR = 1.34, 95% CI 0.97–1.81) but no association in the later, less-exposed subcohorts.

Environmental Studies

Consonni et al. (2008) compared prostate cancer mortality over 25 years in men exposed to dioxins in Seveso, Italy, with that in a nearby but nonexposed reference population. The number of deaths due to prostate cancer was too small in residents in the very-high-exposure and high-exposure zones (Zones A and B) to provide informative estimates. There was no evidence of an association in residents in Zone R, the larger, low-exposure area (RR = 1.06, 95% CI 0.81–1.38).

Biologic Plausibility

Prostate cells and prostatic-cancer cell lines are responsive to TCDD in induction of various genes, including those involved in drug metabolism. Simanainen et al. (2004a) used different rat lines (TCDD-resistant Hans/Wistar and TCDD-sensitive Long Evans) and showed that TCDD treatment resulted in a significant decrease in the weight of prostate lobes, but the effect did not appear to be line-specific. In contrast, the TCDD-related reduction in sperm appears to be line-specific and not fully related to the effects of TCDD on serum testosterone (Simanainen et al., 2004b). TCDD effects appear to occur through actions on the urogenital sinus (Lin et al., 2004). In utero and lactational exposure to TCDD appears to retard the aging process in the prostate (Fritz et al., 2005). Progeny mice of a genetic cross between AHR-null mice and the transgenic adenocarcinoma of the mouse prostate (TRAMP) strain that models prostate cancer showed that the presence of the AHR inhibited the formation of prostate tumors that have a neuroendocrine phenotype. In a follow-up, Fritz et al. (2008) used the TRAMP model to show that the presence of the AHR inhibits prostate carcinogenesis. In agreement with a possible potential protective role, negative associations were found in the AFHS between the risk of benign prostate hyperplasia and both TCDD exposure and serum testosterone concentration (Gupta et al., 2006).

The biologic plausibility of the carcinogenicity of the chemicals of interest is discussed in general at the beginning of this chapter.

Synthesis

Among the few studies published since *Update 2006*, the study published by Chamie et al. (2008) stands out because of its direct focus on the relationship between exposure to Agent Orange in Vietnam and prostate cancer risk. The findings support the existence of an association. However, several features of the study limit the strength of its conclusions. First, although exposure was presumably self-reported at the time of application for initial medical benefits, those who reported exposure had more detailed exposure histories taken, and it is not clear how or whether their detailed histories influenced the final exposure categorization. Second, the methods used to control for confounding by PSA testing are unclear. It appears that the groups compared had similar prevalence of ever having received a PSA test, but the frequency of PSA testing during the long follow-up interval and the means used to adjust for PSA-testing differences were not explained in detail. As mentioned above, small differences in the frequency of PSA testing can have a profound effect on prostate-cancer detection rates. There is a particular concern in this case because veterans who reported exposure and therefore entered the Agent Orange medical program were likely to have received additional PSA testing. Third, as acknowledged in the paper, 38 men reported their exposure to Agent Orange after receiving a diagnosis of prostate cancer, although the association appears to have remained significant after exclusion of these cases, further analyses need to be done to determine the extent of any bias that their inclusion might have caused. The study by Chamie et al. offers an important basic blueprint for similar analyses that can be conducted in the VA medical system. However, despite the relatively strong association between Agent Orange and prostate cancer risk in their report on northern California veterans, the committee believes that unresolved questions regarding the methods used in the study warrant caution in interpreting the results.

The existing body of epidemiologic evidence supporting an association between exposure to the chemicals of interest and prostate cancer is robust enough that the committee's judgment that there is limited or suggestive evidence of an association is not reversed by the largely negative results in experimental systems.

Conclusion

On the basis of the evidence reviewed here and in previous VAO reports, the committee concludes that there remains limited or suggestive evidence of an association between exposure to at least one of the chemicals of interest and prostate cancer.

TESTICULAR CANCER

ACS estimated that 8,090 men would receive diagnoses of testicular cancer (ICD-9 186.0–186.9) in the United States in 2008 and that 380 men would die from it (Jemal et al., 2008a). Other cancers of the male reproductive system that are infrequently reported separately are cancers of the penis and other male genital organs (ICD-9 187). The average annual incidence of testicular cancer is shown in Table 6-30.

Testicular cancer occurs more often in men younger than 40 years old than in older men. On a lifetime basis, the risk in white men is about 4 times that in black men. Cryptorchidism (undescended testes) is a major risk factor for testicular cancer. Family history of the disease also appears to be a risk factor. Several other hereditary, medical, and environmental risk factors have been suggested, but the results of research are inconsistent (Bosl and Motzer, 1997).

Conclusions from *VAO* and Previous Updates

The committee responsible for *VAO* concluded that there was inadequate or insufficient information to determine whether there is an association between exposure to the chemicals of interest and testicular cancer. Additional information available to the committees responsible for *Update 1996*, *Update 1998*, *Update 2000*, *Update 2002*, *Update 2004*, and *Update 2006* did not change that conclusion. Table 6-31 summarizes the results of the relevant studies.

Update of the Epidemiologic Literature

No studies concerning exposure to the chemicals of interest and testicular cancer have been published since *Update 2006*.

Biologic Plausibility

No animal studies of the incidence of testicular cancer after exposure to any of the chemicals of interest have been published since *Update 2006*. The biologic plausibility of the carcinogenicity of the chemicals of interest is discussed in general at the beginning of this chapter.

TABLE 6-30 Average Annual Incidence (per 100,000) of Testicular Cancer in United States[a]

50–54 Years Old			55–59 Years Old			60–64 Years Old		
All Races	White	Black	All Races	White	Black	All Races	White	Black
4.0	4.6	1.0	2.4	2.6	1.3	1.5	1.6	0.8

[a]Surveillance, Epidemiology, and End Results program, nine standard registries, crude age-specific rates, 2000–2005.

TABLE 6-31 Selected Epidemiologic Studies—Testicular Cancer

Reference	Study Population[a]	Exposed Cases[b]	Estimated Relative Risk (95% CI)[b]
VIETNAM VETERANS			
Studies Reviewed in *Update 2006*			
ADVA, 2005a	Australian male Vietnam veterans vs Australian population—incidence	54	0.9 (0.6–1.1)
	Navy	17	1.2 (0.7–1.8)
	Army	34	0.8 (0.5–1.0)
	Air Force	3	0.8 (0.2–2.3)
ADVA, 2005b	Australian male Vietnam veterans vs Australian population—mortality	14	0.9 (0.4–1.4)
	Navy	3	0.8 (0.2–2.4)
	Army	10	0.9 (0.4–1.7)
	Air Force	0	0.0 (0.0–3.3)
ADVA, 2005c	Australian male conscripted Army National Service Vietnam-era veterans—deployed vs non-deployed		
	Incidence	17	0.7 (0.4–1.2)
	Mortality	4	0.8 (0.2–2.0)
Studies Reviewed in *Update 2000*			
AFHS, 2000	Air Force Ranch Hand veterans	3	nr
AIHW, 1999	Australian Vietnam veterans—incidence (validation study)		Expected number of exposed cases (95% CI)
		59	110 (89–139)
CDVA, 1998a	Australian Vietnam veterans—self-reported incidence	151	110 (89–131)
Studies Reviewed in *Update 1998*			
Clapp, 1997	Massachusetts Vietnam veterans—incidence	30	1.2 (0.4–3.3)
CDVA, 1997a	Australian military Vietnam veterans	4	ns
CDVA, 1997b	Australian National Service Vietnam veterans	1	1.3
Dalager and Kang, 1997	Army Chemical Corps veterans	2	4.0 (0.5–14.5)
Watanabe and Kang, 1996	Army Vietnam service	114	1.1 (nr)
	Marine Vietnam service	28	1.0 (nr)
Studies Reviewed in *Update 1996*			
Bullman et al., 1994	Navy veterans	12	2.6 (1.1–6.2)
Studies Reviewed in *VAO*			
Tarone et al., 1991	Patients in three Washington, DC, area hospitals	31	2.3 (1.0–5.5)
Watanabe et al., 1991	Army Vietnam veterans	109	1.2 (ns)
	Marine Vietnam veterans	28	0.8 (ns)
Breslin et al., 1988	Army Vietnam veterans	90	1.1 (0.8–1.5)
	Marine Vietnam veterans	26	1.3 (0.5–3.6)

continued

TABLE 6-31 Continued

Reference	Study Population[a]	Exposed Cases[b]	Estimated Relative Risk (95% CI)[b]
Anderson et al., 1986	Wisconsin Vietnam veterans	9	1.0 (0.5–1.9)
OCCUPATIONAL			
Studies Reviewed in *Update 2006*			
McLean et al., 2006	IARC cohort of pulp and paper workers Exposure to nonvolatile organochlorine compounds		
	Never	2	1.1 (0.1–4.1)
	Ever	5	3.6 (1.2–8.4)
Alavanja et al., 2005	US AHS—incidence		
	Private applicators	23	1.1 (0.7–1.6)
	Spouses of private applicators (> 99% women)	nr	0.0 (0.0–50.2)
	Commercial applicators	4	1.2 (0.3–3.2)
Blair et al., 2005a	US AHS		
	Private applicators	0	nr
	Spouses of private applicators (> 99% women)	0	nr
Reif et al., 1989	New Zealand forestry workers—nested case–control —incidence	6	1.0 (0.4–2.6)
Studies Reviewed in *Update 2002*			
Burns et al., 2001	Dow chemical production workers	1	2.2 (0.0–12.5)
Studies Reviewed in *Update 2000*			
Flemming et al., 1999b	Florida pesticide appliers	23	2.5 (1.6–3.7)
Hardell et al., 1998	Swedish workers exposed to herbicides	4	0.3 (0.1–1.0)
Studies Reviewed in *Update 1998*			
Hertzman et al., 1997	British Columbia sawmill workers		
	Mortality (male genital cancers)	116	1.0 (0.8–1.1)
	Incidence	18	1.0 (0.6–1.4)
Kogevinas et al., 1997	IARC cohort, workers exposed to any phenoxy herbicide or chlorophenol	68	1.1 (0.9–1.4)
	Exposed to highly chlorinated PCDDs	43	1.1 (0.8–1.5)
	Not exposed to highly chlorinated PCDDs	25	1.1 (0.3–1.6)
Ramlow et al., 1996	Dow pentachlorophenol production workers (included in IARC cohort, NIOSH Dioxin Registry)	0	nr
Zhong and Rafnsson, 1996	Icelandic pesticide users	2	1.2 (0.1–4.3)
Studies Reviewed in *Update 1996*			
Blair et al., 1993	US farmers in 23 states		
	White men	32	0.8 (0.6–1.2)
	Nonwhite men	6	1.3 (0.5–2.9)

TABLE 6-31 Continued

Reference	Study Population[a]	Exposed Cases[b]	Estimated Relative Risk (95% CI)[b]
Studies Reviewed in *VAO*			
Ronco et al.,	Danish workers—incidence		
1992	Men—self-employed	74	0.9 (nr)
	employee	23	0.6 (p < 0.05)
Saracci et al., 1991	IARC cohort—exposed subcohort	7	2.3 (0.9–4.6)
Bond et al., 1988	Dow 2,4-D production workers (included in IARC cohort, NIOSH Dioxin Registry)	1	4.6 (0.0–25.7)
Coggon et al., 1986	British MCPA production workers (included in IARC cohort)	4	2.2 (0.6–5.7)
Wiklund,			99% CI
1983	Swedish male agricultural workers—incidence	101	1.0 (0.7–1.2)
ENVIRONMENTAL			
Studies Reviewed in *Update 2000*			
Bertazzi et al., 2001	Seveso residents—20-year follow-up		
	Zone A, B—men	17	1.0 (0.6–1.7)
Bertazzi et al., 1998	Seveso residents—15-year follow-up (genitourinary tract)		
	Zone B—men	10	1.0 (0.5–1.8)
	Zone R—men	73	1.0 (0.8–1.3)
Studies Reviewed in *Update 1996*			
Bertazzi et al., 1993	Seveso residents—10-year follow-up—incidence		
	Zone B—men	1	1.0 (0.1–7.5)
	Zone R—men	9	1.4 (0.7–3.0)
Studies Reviewed in *VAO*			
Pesatori et al., 1992	Seveso residents—incidence		
	Zones A, B—men	1	0.9 (0.1–6.7)
	Zone R—men	9	1.5 (0.7–3.0)

ABBREVIATIONS: 2,4-D, 2,4-dichlorophenoxyacetic acid; AHS, Agricultural Health Study; CI, confidence interval; IARC, International Agency for Research on Cancer; MCPA, 2-methyl-4-chlorophenoxyacetic acid; NIOSH, National Institute for Occupational Safety and Health; nr, not reported; ns, not significant; PCDDs, chlorinated dibenzo-*p*-dioxins (highly chlorinated, if four or more chlorines).

[a]Subjects are male and outcome is mortality unless otherwise noted.
[b]Given when available; results other than estimated risk explained individually.
Studies in italics have been superseded by newer studies of the same cohorts.

Synthesis

The evidence from epidemiologic studies is inadequate to link herbicide exposure and testicular cancer. The relative rarity of this cancer makes it difficult to develop risk estimates with any precision. Most cases occur in men 25–35 years old, and men who have received such a diagnosis could be excluded from military service; this could explain the slight reduction in risk observed in some veteran studies.

Conclusion

On the basis of the evidence reviewed here and in previous VAO reports, the committee concludes that there is inadequate or insufficient evidence to determine whether there is an association between exposure to the chemicals of interest and testicular cancer.

BLADDER CANCER

Urinary bladder cancer (ICD-9 188) is the most common urinary tract cancer. Cancers of the urethra, paraurethral glands, and other and unspecified urinary cancers (ICD-9 189.3–189.9) are infrequently reported separately; findings on these cancers would be reported in this section. ACS estimated that 51,230 men and 17,580 women would receive a diagnosis of bladder cancer in the United States in 2008 and that 9,950 men and 4,150 women would die from it (Jemal et al., 2008a). In males, in whom this cancer is about twice as common as it is in females, those numbers represent about 5% of new cancer diagnoses and 3% of cancer deaths. Overall, bladder cancer is fourth in incidence in men in the United States.

Bladder-cancer risk rises rapidly with age. In men in the age groups that characterize most Vietnam veterans, bladder-cancer incidence is about twice as high in whites as in blacks. The average annual incidence of urinary bladder cancer is shown in Table 6-32.

The most important known risk factor for bladder cancer is tobacco use, which accounts for about half the bladder cancers in men and one-third of them in women (Miller et al., 1996). Occupational exposure to aromatic amines (also called arylamines), polycyclic aromatic hydrocarbons (PAHs), and some other organic chemicals used in the rubber, leather, textile, paint-products, and printing industries is associated with higher incidence. In some parts of Africa and Asia, infection with the parasite *Schistosoma haematobium* contributes to the high incidence.

TABLE 6-32 Average Annual Incidence (per 100,000) of Bladder Cancer in United States[a]

	50–54 Years Old			55–59 Years Old			60–64 Years Old		
	All Races	White	Black	All Races	White	Black	All Races	White	Black
Men	23.4	25.6	14.3	46.7	51.3	30.8	81.8	91.1	42.6
Women	6.9	7.6	4.0	13.3	15.1	7.7	22.0	24.7	14.4

[a]Surveillance, Epidemiology, and End Results program. nine standard registries, crude age-specific rates, 2000–2005.

Exposure to inorganic arsenic is also a risk factor for bladder cancer. Although cacodylic acid is a metabolite of inorganic arsenic, as discussed in Chapter 4, the data are insufficient to conclude that studies of inorganic-arsenic exposure are directly relevant to exposure to cacodylic acid, so the literature on inorganic arsenic is not considered in this section.

Conclusions from *VAO* and Previous Updates

The committees responsible for *VAO* and *Update 1996* concluded that there was limited or suggestive evidence of *no* association between exposure to the chemicals of interest and urinary bladder cancer. Additional information available to the committee responsible for *Update 1998* led it to change that conclusion to one of inadequate or insufficient information to determine whether there is an association. The committee responsible for *Update 2000*, *Update 2002*, *Update 2004*, and *Update 2006* did not change that conclusion. Table 6-33 summarizes the results of the relevant studies.

Update of Epidemiologic Literature

Vietnam-Veteran Studies

No Vietnam-veteran studies concerning exposure to the chemicals of interest and bladder cancer have been published since *Update 2006*.

Occupational Studies

Hansen et al. (2007) studied cancer incidence in Danish professional gardeners compared with the general Danish population. For cancer of the urinary system (presumably including bladder cancer and kidney cancer), the RR was 1.07 (95% CI 0.72–1.59) in the older workers with the highest exposure to herbicides. There was evidence of a lower risk in workers in the intermediate and recent birth cohorts, whose exposure to herbicides and pesticides was considered to be lower than that of the older workers. That suggests that there may have been a historical exposure that increased bladder-cancer rates; however, no details of specific chemicals were reported, so it is difficult to attribute the lower risk to any of the chemicals of interest. Samanic et al. (2006) looked at bladder-cancer occurrence in pesticide applicators in the AHS according to their exposure to dicamba, a benzoic acid herbicide often mixed with 2,4-D. There was no evidence of an association between cumulative dicamba exposure and bladder-cancer incidence.

Environmental Studies

Consonni et al. (2008), who compared mortality in residents of Seveso in various zones of exposure to dioxin, found no relationship with bladder-cancer

TABLE 6-33 Selected Epidemiologic Studies—Urinary Bladder Cancer

Reference	Study Population[a]	Exposed Cases[b]	Estimated Relative Risk (95% CI)[b]
VIETNAM VETERANS			
Studies Reviewed in *Update 2006*			
ADVA, 2005a	Australian male Vietnam veterans vs Australian population—incidence	164	1.0 (0.9–1.2)
	Navy	34	1.0 (0.7–1.4)
	Army	104	1.0 (0.8–1.2)
	Air Force	26	1.3 (0.8–1.8)
ADVA, 2005b	Australian male Vietnam veterans vs Australian population—mortality	22	0.7 (0.4–1.0)
	Navy	4	0.6 (0.2–1.6)
	Army	13	0.7 (0.3–1.1)
	Air Force	5	1.1 (0.4–2.5)
ADVA, 2005c	Australian male conscripted Army National Service Vietnam-era veterans: deployed vs nondeployed		
	Incidence	19	0.7 (0.4–1.1)
	Mortality	1	0.3 (0.0–1.7)
Boehmer et al., 2004	Follow-up of CDC Vietnam Experience Cohort	1	nr
Studies Reviewed in *Update 2004*			
Akhtar et al., 2004	AFHS subjects vs national rates		
	White AFHS Ranch Hand veterans		
	Incidence	14	1.1 (0.6–1.7)
	With tours between 1966–1970	14	1.3 (0.7–2.1)
	Mortality	1	0.9 (nr)
	White AFHS comparison veterans		
	Incidence	8	0.4 (0.2–0.8)
	With tours in 1966–1970	4	0.3 (0.1–0.7)
	Mortality	1	0.6 (nr)
Studies Reviewed in *Update 2000*			
AFHS, 2000	Air Force Ranch Hand veterans		
	Bladder, kidney	11	3.1 (0.9–11.0)
Studies Reviewed in *Update 1998*			
Clapp, 1997	Massachusetts Vietnam veterans	80	0.6 (0.2–1.3)
CDVA, 1997a	Australian military Vietnam veterans	11	1.1 (0.6–1.9)
CDVA, 1997b	Australian national service Vietnam veterans	1	0.6 (nr)
Studies Reviewed in *VAO*			
Breslin et al., 1988	Army Vietnam veterans	9	0.6 (0.3–1.2)
	Marine Vietnam veterans	4	2.4 (0.1–66.4)
Anderson et al., 1986	Wisconsin Vietnam veterans	1	nr

TABLE 6-33 Continued

Reference	Study Population[a]	Exposed Cases[b]	Estimated Relative Risk (95% CI)[b]
OCCUPATIONAL			
New Studies			
Hansen et al., 2007	Danish gardeners (urinary system, ICD-7 180–181)—incidence		
	10-year follow-up (1975–1984) reported in Hansen et al. (1992)	18	0.9 (0.7–1.8)
	25-year follow-up (1975–2001)		
	Born before 1915 (high exposure)	25	1.1 (0.7–1.6)
	Born 1915–1934 (medium exposure)	23	0.5 (0.4–0.8)
	Born after 1934 (low exposure)	1	0.2 (0.0–1.1)
Samanic et al., 2006	Pesticide applicators in AHS—bladder-cancer incidence from enrollment through 2002		
	Dicamba—lifetime days exposure		
	None	43	1.0
	1–< 20	6	0.5 (0.2–1.3)
	20–< 56	9	0.7 (0.3–1.4)
	56–< 116	6	0.6 (0.3–1.5)
	≥ 116	8	0.8 (0.4–1.9)
			p-trend = 0.66
Studies Reviewed in *Update 2006*			
McLean et al., 2006	IARC cohort of pulp and paper workers		
	Exposure to nonvolatile organochlorine compounds		
	Never	50	1.0 (0.7–1.3)
	Ever	43	1.1 (0.8–1.5)
Alavanja et al., 2005	US AHS (urinary system)—incidence		
	Private applicators (men and women)	184	0.7 (0.6–0.8)
	Spouses of private applicators (> 99% women)	17	0.7 (0.4–1.1)
	Commercial applicators (men and women)	13	1.1 (0.6–1.8)
't Mannetje et al., 2005	Phenoxy herbicide producers (men and women)	0	nr
	Phenoxy herbicide sprayers (> 99% men)	0	nr
Blair et al., 2005a	US AHS		
	Private applicators (men and women)	7	0.4 (0.1–0.7)
	Spouses of private applicators (> 99% women)	2	0.8 (0.1–2.7)
Torchio et al., 1994	Italian licensed pesticide users	31	0.5 (0.4–0.8)
Reif et al., 1989	New Zealand forestry workers—nested case–control —incidence	4	0.7 (0.3–1.8)
Studies Reviewed in *Update 2004*			
Bodner et al., 2003	Dow chemical production workers (included in IARC cohort, NIOSH Dioxin Registry)	nr	0.7 (0.1–2.0)
Swaen et al., 2004	Dutch licensed herbicide applicators	2	0.7 (0.1–2.4)

continued

TABLE 6-33 Continued

Reference	Study Population[a]	Exposed Cases[b]	Estimated Relative Risk (95% CI)[b]
Studies Reviewed in *Update 2002*			
Burns et al., 2001	Dow 2,4-D production workers (included in IARC cohort, NIOSH Dioxin Registry)	1	0.5 (0.1–2.8)
Studies Reviewed in *Update 2000*			
Steenland et al., 1999	US chemical production workers (included in IARC cohort, NIOSH Dioxin Registry)		
	Total cohort	16	2.0 (1.1–3.2)
	High-exposure cohort	6	3.0 (1.4–8.5)
Hooiveld et al., 1998	Dutch chemical production workers (included in IARC cohort)		
	Total cohort	4	3.7 (1.0–9.5)
	Accidentally exposed subcohort	1	2.8 (0.1–15.5)
Studies Reviewed in *Update 1998*			
Hertzman et al., 1997	Canadian sawmill workers		
	Mortality	33	0.9 (0.7–1.2)
	Incidence	94	1.0 (0.8–1.2)
Kogevinas et al., 1997	IARC cohort, male and female workers exposed to any phenoxy herbicide or chlorophenol	34	1.0 (0.7–1.5)
	Exposed to highly chlorinated PCDDs	24	1.4 (0.9–2.1)
	Not exposed to highly chlorinated PCDDs	10	0.7 (0.3–1.2)
Ott and Zober, 1996	BASF employees (bladder, kidney)—incidence	2	1.4 (0.4–3.2)
Studies Reviewed in *Update 1996*			
Asp et al., 1994	Finnish herbicide applicators—incidence	12	1.6 (0.8–2.8)
Bueno de Mesquita et al., 1993	Dutch phenoxy herbicide workers (included in IARC cohort)	1	1.2 (0.0–6.7)
Collins et al., 1993	Monsanto Company workers (included in IARC cohort) (many also exposed to 4-aminobiphenyl, a known bladder carcinogen)		
	Bladder, other urinary	16	6.8 (3.9–11.1)
Studies Reviewed in *VAO*			
Ronco et al., 1992	Danish workers—incidence		
	Men—self-employed	300	0.6 (p < 0.05)
	employee	70	0.7 (p < 0.05)
	Women—self-employed	1	0.2 (nr)
	employee	2	0.6 (nr)
	family worker	25	0.6 (p < 0.05)
Fingerhut et al., 1991	NIOSH—entire cohort (bladder, other)	9	1.6 (0.7–3.0)
	≥ 1-year exposure, ≥ 20-year latency	4	1.9 (0.5–4.8)
Green, 1991	Herbicide sprayers in Ontario		
	Diseases of genitourinary system	1	1.0 (0.0–5.6)
Saracci et al., 1991	IARC cohort—exposed subcohort (men and women)	13	0.8 (0.4–1.4)

TABLE 6-33 Continued

Reference	Study Population[a]	Exposed Cases[b]	Estimated Relative Risk (95% CI)[b]
Zober et al., 1990	BASF employees—basic cohort	0	90% CI nr (0.0–15.0)
Alavanja et al., 1989	USDA forest, soil conservationists	8	0.8 (0.3–1.6)
Henneberger et al., 1989	New Hampshire pulp and paper workers	4	1.2 (0.3–3.2)
Alavanja et al., 1988	USDA agricultural extension agents	8	0.7 (0.4–1.4)
Bond et al., 1988	Dow 2,4-D production workers (included in IARC cohort, NIOSH Dioxin Registry)	0	nr (0.0–7.2)
Coggon et al., 1986	British MCPA production workers (included in IARC cohort)	8	0.9 (0.4–1.7)
Robinson et al., 1986	Northwestern US paper and pulp workers	8	1.2 (0.6–2.6)
Lynge, 1985	Danish production workers (included in IARC cohort)—incidence	11	0.8 (nr)
Blair et al., 1983	Florida pesticide applicators	3	1.6 (nr)
Burmeister, 1981	Iowa farmers	274	0.9 (nr)

ENVIRONMENTAL
New Studies

Consonni et al., 2008	Seveso residents—25-year follow-up—men and women		
	Zone A	1	1.0 (0.2–7.4)
	Zone B	6	0.9 (0.4–2.0)
	Zone R	42	0.9 (0.6–1.2)

Studies Reviewed in *Update 2002*

Revich et al., 2001	Residents of Chapaevsk, Russia (urinary organs)		
	Men	31	2.6 (1.7–3.6)
	Women	17	0.8 (0.5–1.3)

Studies Reviewed in *Update 2000*

Bertazzi et al., 2001	Seveso residents—20-year follow-up Zone A, B—men	6	1.2 (0.5–2.7)
Bertazzi et al., 1998	Seveso residents—15-year follow-up Zone B—men	1	2.4 (0.3–16.8)
	women	3	0.9 (0.3–3.0)
	Zone R—men	21	0.9 (0.6–1.5)
	women	4	0.6 (0.2–1.8)

Studies Reviewed in *Update 1998*

Gambini et al., 1997	Italian rice growers	12	1.0 (0.5–1.8)

continued

TABLE 6-33 Continued

Reference	Study Population[a]	Exposed Cases[b]	Estimated Relative Risk (95% CI)[b]
Svensson et al., 1995	Swedish fishermen (men and women)—mortality		
	East coast	5	1.3 (0.4–3.1)
	West coast	20	1.0 (0.6–1.6)
	Swedish fishermen (men and women)—incidence		
	East coast	10	0.7 (0.4–1.3)
	West coast	55	0.9 (0.7–1.1)
Studies Reviewed in *VAO*			
Pesatori et al., 1992	Seveso residents—incidence		
	Zones A, B—men	10	1.6 (0.9–3.1)
	women	1	0.9 (0.1–6.8)
	Zone R—men	39	1.0 (0.7–1.4)
	women	4	0.6 (0.2–1.5)
Lampi et al., 1992	Finnish community exposed to chlorophenol contamination (men and women)	14	1.0 (0.6–1.9)

ABBREVIATIONS: 2,4-D, 2,4-dichlorophenoxyacetic acid; AFHS, Air Force Health Study; AHS, Agricultural Health Study; CDC, Centers for Disease Control and Prevention; CI, confidence interval; IARC, International Agency for Research on Cancer; ICD, International Classification of Diseases; MCPA, 2-methyl-4-chlorophenoxyacetic acid; NIOSH, National Institute for Occupational Safety and Health; nr, not reported; PCDDs, chlorinated dibenzo-*p*-dioxins (highly chlorinated, if four or more chlorines); TCDD, 2,3,7,8-tetrachlorodibenzo-*p*-dioxin; USDA, US Department of Agriculture.

[a]Subjects are male and outcome is mortality unless otherwise noted.
[b]Given when available; results other than estimated risk explained individually.
Studies in italics have been superseded by newer studies of same cohorts.

mortality, but the small number of relevant deaths in the highly exposed zone greatly limits the interpretability of this result.

Biologic Plausibility

In laboratory animals, cacodylic acid has been shown to induce primarily bladder tumors (Cohen et al., 2006). In a study of male F344 rats, cacodylic acid administered in drinking water resulted in formation of bladder tumors at the highest concentrations (50 and 200 ppm) (Wei et al., 2002). In another report (Arnold et al., 2006), administration of cacodylic acid in the diet resulted in formation of papillomas and carcinomas in the bladders of female and male F344 rats but not B6C3F1 mice. Experimental work since *Update 2006* has shown that cacodylic acid (dimethyl arsenic acid, DMA) is cytotoxic at very high concentrations in rat urothelial cells in vitro (Nascimento et al., 2008); such concentrations are unlikely to be environmentally relevant. Other recent studies have shown DMA concentrations to be lower in bladder-cancer patients than in matched controls (Pu et al., 2007) and to be associated with a lower incidence of urinary cancer (Huang et al., 2008). In contrast, greater oxidative DNA damage has been found in association with higher DMA concentrations in urothelial-cancer patients (Chung et al., 2008), although this was not the case in primary human hepatocytes (Dopp et al., 2008). In a study that used a rat cancer initiation–promotion model, DMA was found to be a weak cancer-initiator but a tumor-promoter at high dose (Fukushima et al., 2005).

No studies have reported an increased incidence of urinary bladder cancer in TCDD-treated animals.

The biologic plausibility of the carcinogenicity of the chemicals of interest is discussed in general at the beginning of this chapter.

Synthesis

Available analyses of an association between exposure to the chemicals of interest and bladder-cancer risk are characterized by low precision because of the small numbers, low exposure specificity, and lack of ability to control for confounding. The data that have emerged since *Update 2006* suggest that DMA may be a bladder-tumor-promoter and that DMA concentrations are lower in patients with urinary cancer. The evidence in either direction is still too preliminary to alter the conclusion that the cumulative evidence of such an association is inadequate or insufficient.

Conclusion

On the basis of the evidence reviewed here and in previous VAO reports, the committee concludes that there is inadequate or insufficient evidence to determine whether there is an association between exposure to the chemicals of interest and bladder cancer.

RENAL CANCER

Cancers of the kidney (ICD-9 189.0) and renal pelvis (ICD-9 189.1) are often grouped in epidemiologic studies; cancer of the ureter (ICD-9 189.2) is sometimes also included. Although diseases of those organs have different characteristics and could have different risk factors, there is some logic to grouping them: the structures are all exposed to filterable chemicals, such as PAHs, that appear in urine. ACS estimated that 33,130 men and 21,260 women would receive diagnoses of renal cancer (ICD-9 189.0, 189.1) in the United States in 2008 and that 8,100 men and 4,910 women would die from it (Jemal et al., 2008a). Those figures represent 2–4% of all new cancer diagnoses and cancer deaths. The average annual incidence of renal cancer is shown in Table 6-34.

TABLE 6-34 Average Annual Incidence (per 100,000) of Kidney and Renal Pelvis Cancer in United States[a]

	50–54 Years Old			55–59 Years Old			60–64 Years Old		
	All Races	White	Black	All Races	White	Black	All Races	White	Black
Men	23.8	23.2	35.8	36.9	36.4	49.0	55.5	56.2	66.2
Women	12.6	12.8	13.8	18.6	19.1	20.8	24.8	26.0	28.1

[a]Surveillance, Epidemiology, and End Results program, nine standard registries, crude age-specific rates, 2000–2005.

Renal cancer is twice as common in men as in women. In the age groups that include most Vietnam veterans, black men have a higher incidence than white men. With the exception of Wilms' tumor, which is more likely to occur in children, renal cancer is more common in people over 50 years old.

Tobacco use is a well-established risk factor for renal cancer. People with some rare syndromes—notably, von Hippel–Lindau syndrome and tuberous sclerosis—are at higher risk. Other potential risk factors include obesity, heavy acetaminophen use, kidney stones, and occupational exposure to asbestos, cadmium, and organic solvents. Firefighters, who are routinely exposed to numerous pyrolysis products, are in a known higher-risk group.

Conclusions from *VAO* and Previous Updates

The committee responsible for *VAO* concluded that there was inadequate or insufficient information to determine whether there is an association between exposure to the chemicals of interest and renal cancer. Additional information available to the committees responsible for *Update 1996*, *Update 1998*, *Update 2000*, *Update 2002*, *Update 2004*, and *Update 2006* did not change that conclusion. Table 6-35 summarizes the results of the relevant studies.

Update of the Epidemiologic Literature

Vietnam-Veteran Studies

No Vietnam-veteran studies concerning exposure to the chemicals of interest and renal cancer have been published since *Update 2006*.

Occupational Studies

Hansen et al. (2007) reported the results of a follow-up on mortality in an historical cohort of Danish professional gardeners. In the younger workers, the

TABLE 6-35 Selected Epidemiologic Studies—Renal Cancer

Reference	Study Population[a]	Exposed Cases[b]	Estimated Relative Risk (95% CI)[b]
VIETNAM VETERANS			
Studies Reviewed in *Update 2006*			
ADVA, 2005a	Australian male Vietnam veterans vs Australian population—incidence	125	1.0 (0.8–1.2)
	Navy	34	1.3 (0.9–1.7)
	Army	77	0.9 (0.7–1.1)
	Air Force	14	1.1 (0.6–1.8)
ADVA, 2005b	Australian male Vietnam veterans vs Australian population—mortality	50	1.0 (0.7–1.2)
	Navy	12	1.1 (0.6–1.9)
	Army	33	0.9 (0.6–1.3)
	Air Force	5	0.8 (0.3–1.8)
ADVA, 2005c	Australian male conscripted Army National Service Vietnam-era veterans—deployed vs nondeployed		
	Incidence	19	0.7 (0.4–1.0)
	Mortality	4	0.4 (0.1–1.1)
Boehmer et al., 2004	Follow-up of CDC Vietnam Experience Cohort	1	nr
Studies Reviewed in *Update 2000*			
AFHS, 2000	Air Force Ranch Hand veterans	11	3.1 (0.9–11.0)
Studies Reviewed in *Update 1998*			
CDVA, 1997a	Australian military Vietnam veterans	22	1.2 (0.7–1.8)
CDVA, 1997b	Australian National Service Vietnam veterans	3	3.9 (nr)
Studies Reviewed in *Update 1996*			
Visintainer et al., 1995	PM study of deaths (1974–1989) of Michigan Vietnam-era veterans—deployed vs nondeployed	21	1.4 (0.9–2.2)
Studies Reviewed in *VAO*			
Breslin et al., 1988	Army Vietnam veterans	55	0.9 (0.5–1.5)
	Marine Vietnam veterans	13	0.9 (0.5–1.5)
Kogan and Clapp, 1988	Massachusetts Vietnam veterans	9	1.8 (1.0–3.5)
Anderson et al., 1986	Wisconsin Vietnam veterans	2	nr
OCCUPATIONAL			
New Studies			
Hansen et al., 2007	Danish gardeners—incidence (urinary system, ICD-7 180–181)		
	10-year follow-up (1975–1984) reported in Hansen et al. (1992)	18	0.9 (0.7–1.8)
	25-year follow-up (1975–2001)		
	Born before 1915 (high exposure)	25	1.1 (0.7–1.6)
	Born 1915–1934 (medium exposure)	23	0.5 (0.4–0.8)
	Born after 1934 (low exposure)	1	0.2 (0.0–1.1)

continued

TABLE 6-35 Continued

Reference	Study Population[a]	Exposed Cases[b]	Estimated Relative Risk (95% CI)[b]
Studies Reviewed in *Update 2006*			
McLean	Exposure to nonvolatile organochlorine compounds		
et al., 2006	Never	41	0.9 (0.7–1.3)
	Ever	18	0.5 (0.3–0.8)
't Mannetje	Phenoxy herbicide producers (men and women)	1	1.2 (0.0–6.6)
et al., 2006	Phenoxy herbicide sprayers (> 99% men)	3	2.7 (0.6–8.0)
Torchio	Italian licensed pesticide users	16	0.6 (0.4–1.0)
et al., 1994			
Reif et al.,	New Zealand forestry workers—nested case–control		
1989	—incidence	2	0.6 (0.2–2.3)
Magnani	UK case–control		
et al., 1987	Herbicides	nr	1.3 (0.6–3.1)
	Chlorophenols	nr	0.9 (0.4–1.9)
Studies Reviewed in *Update 2004*			
Swaen et al.,	Dutch licensed herbicide applicators	4	1.3 (0.4–3.4)
2004			
Studies Reviewed in *Update 2002*			
Burns et al.,	Dow 2,4-D production workers (included in IARC		
2001	cohort, NIOSH Dioxin Registry)	2	0.9 (0.1–3.3)
Studies Reviewed in *Update 2000*			
Steenland	US chemical workers (included in IARC cohort,		
et al., 1999	NIOSH Dioxin Registry)	13	1.6 (0.8–2.7)
Hooiveld	Dutch chemical production workers (included in		
et al., 1998	IARC cohort)		
	Total cohort—kidney cancer	4	4.1 (1.1–10.4)
	Total cohort—"urinary organs"	8	3.9 (1.7–7.6)
Studies Reviewed in *Update 1998*			
Kogevinas	IARC cohort, male and female workers exposed to		
et al., 1997	any phenoxy herbicide or chlorophenol	29	1.1 (0.7–1.6)
	Exposed to highly chlorinated PCDDs	26	1.6 (1.1–2.4)
	Not exposed to highly chlorinated PCDDs	3	0.3 (0.1–0.9)
Studies Reviewed in *Update 1996*			
Mellemgaard	Danish Cancer Registry patients		
et al., 1994	Occupational herbicide exposure, men	13	1.7 (0.7–4.3)
	Occupational herbicide exposure, women	3	5.7 (0.6–58.0)
Blair et al.,	US farmers in 23 states		
1993	White men	522	1.1 (1.0–1.2)
	White women	6	0.8 (0.3–1.7)
Studies Reviewed in *VAO*			
Ronco et al.,	Danish workers—incidence		
1992	Men—self-employed	141	0.6 (p < 0.05)
	employee	18	0.4 (p < 0.05)
	Women—self-employed	4	0.9 (nr)
	employee	3	1.0 (nr)
	family worker	30	0.8 (nr)

TABLE 6-35 Continued

Reference	Study Population[a]	Exposed Cases[b]	Estimated Relative Risk (95% CI)[b]
Fingerhut	NIOSH cohort—entire cohort	8	1.4 (0.6–2.8)
et al., 1991	≥ 1-year exposure, ≥ 20-year latency	2	1.1 (0.1–3.8)
Manz et al.,	German production workers—men, women		
1991	(included in IARC cohort)	3	1.6 (0.3–4.6)
Saracci	IARC cohort—exposed subcohort (men and women)	11	1.0 (0.5–1.7)
et al., 1991			
Alavanja	USDA forest conservationists	nr	1.7 (0.5–5.5)
et al., 1989	Soil conservationists	nr	2.4 (1.0–5.9)
Henneberger	New Hampshire paper and pulp workers		
et al., 1989		3	1.5 (0.3–4.4)
Alavanja	USDA agricultural extension agents		
et al., 1988		nr	1.7 (0.9–3.3)
Bond et al.,	Dow 2,4-D production workers (included in IARC		
1988	cohort, NIOSH Dioxin Registry)	0	nr (0.0–6.2)
Robinson	Northwestern US paper and pulp workers		
et al., 1986		6	1.2 (0.5–3.0)
Coggon	British MCPA production workers (included in the		
et al., 1986	IARC cohort)	5	1.0 (0.3–2.3)
Lynge, 1985	Danish production workers—incidence	3	0.6 (nr)
Wiklund,	Swedish male and female agricultural		99% CI
1983	workers—incidence	775	0.8 (0.7–0.9)
Blair et al.,	Florida pesticide applicators	1	0.5 (nr)
1983			
Burmeister,	Iowa farmers	178	1.1 (ns)
1981			

ENVIRONMENTAL
New Studies

Consonni	Seveso residents—25-year follow-up—men, women		
et al., 2008	Zone A	0	nr
	Zone B	3	0.6 (0.2–2.0)
	Zone R	39	1.2 (0.8–1.6)

Studies Reviewed in *Update 2000*

Bertazzi	Seveso residents—20-year follow-up		
et al., 2001	Zone A, B—men	3	0.8 (0.3–2.6)
	women	3	1.8 (0.6–5.8)

Studies Reviewed in *Update 1996*

Bertazzi	Seveso residents—10-year follow-up (kidney, other		
et al., 1993	urinary organs)—incidence		
	Zone R—men	10	0.9 (0.4–1.7)
	women	7	1.2 (0.5–2.7)

continued

TABLE 6-35 Continued

Reference	Study Population[a]	Exposed Cases[b]	Estimated Relative Risk (95% CI)[b]
Studies Reviewed in *VAO*			
Pesatori	Seveso residents—incidence		
et al., 1992	Zones A, B—men	0	nr
	women	1	1.1 (0.2–8.1)
	Zone R—men	11	0.9 (0.5–1.7)
	women	7	1.2 (0.5–2.6)

ABBREVIATIONS: 2,4-D, 2,4-dichlorophenoxyacetic acid; CDC, Centers for Disease Control and Prevention; CI, confidence interval; IARC, International Agency for Research on Cancer; ICD, International Classification of Diseases; MCPA, 2-methyl-4-chlorophenoxyacetic acid; NIOSH, National Institute for Occupational Safety and Health; nr, not reported; ns, not significant; PCDDs, chlorinated dibenzo-*p*-dioxins (highly chlorinated, if four or more chlorines); PM, proportionate mortality; TCDD, 2,3,7,8-tetrachlorodibenzo-*p*-dioxin; USDA, US Department of Agriculture.
[a]Subjects are male and outcome is mortality unless otherwise noted.
[b]Given when available; results other than estimated risk explained individually.
Studies in italics have been superseded by newer studies of same cohorts.

incidence of those cancers was significantly lower than the general population, which probably represents a healthy worker effect. In older workers (who may have been exposed to higher concentrations of pesticides than younger workers), however, the incidence of urinary system cancers (presumably including bladder and kidney cancer) was comparable to that in the general population. That provides a weak suggestion that older workers may have been exposed to some chemicals that increased renal-cancer risk. The Danish National Environmental Board reports that 2,4-D and other chlorophenoxy acids were used during the periods when the older members of the cohort were working, but the study contained no details regarding specific chemical exposures, so relevance to the chemicals of interest here is limited.

Environmental Studies

Consonni et al. (2008) reported on mortality from kidney cancer in residents of Seveso who were exposed to dioxin at various concentrations. The number of deaths due to kidney cancer in residents in the highly exposed areas was too small to permit useful conclusions regarding any association.

Biologic Plausibility

No animal studies have reported an increased incidence of renal cancer after exposure to the chemicals of interest. The biologic plausibility of the carcinogenicity of the chemicals of interest is discussed in general at the beginning of this chapter.

Synthesis

Available analyses of an association between exposure to the chemicals of interest and renal-cancer risk are limited by the small number of cases and lack of exposure specificity. No data have emerged since *Update 2006* to alter the committee's conclusion that the evidence is inadequate or insufficient to determine whether there is an association.

Conclusion

On the basis of the evidence reviewed here and in previous VAO reports, the committee concludes that there is inadequate or insufficient evidence to determine whether there is an association between exposure to the chemicals of interest and renal cancer.

BRAIN CANCER

Brain and other nervous system cancers (ICD-9 191–192) involve the central nervous system (CNS) and include tumors of the brain and spinal cord, the cranial nerves, and the meninges (the outer coverings of the brain and spinal cord). Any of the cell types in the CNS can produce cancer. Tumors of the peripheral nerves and autonomic nervous system are considered soft-tissue tumors (ICD-9 171). Most cancers in the CNS originate in other parts of the body, such as the lung or breast, but have metastasized to the brain or spinal cord. This section focuses on cancers that originate in the CNS.

Cancer of the eye (ICD-9 190) was considered retrospectively in *Update 2006*, but the present committee decided that findings concerning cancer of the eye would be tracked with results on brain cancer because, when it is reported, it is often grouped with brain cancer.

The average annual incidence of CNS cancer is shown in Table 6-36. About 95% of cases derive from the brain, cranial nerves, and cranial meninges. In people over 45 years old, about 90% of tumors that originate in the brain are gliomas—astrocytoma, ependymoma, oligodendroglioma, or glioblastoma multiforme. Astrocytoma is the most common; glioblastoma multiforme has the worst prognosis. Meningioma accounts for 20–40% of CNS cancers. It tends to occur in middle age and more commonly in women. Most meningiomas are benign and can be removed surgically. ACS estimated that about 11,780 men and 10,030 women would receive diagnoses of brain and other nervous system cancers in the United States in 2008 and that 7,420 men and 5,650 women would die from them (Jemal et al., 2008a). Those numbers represent about 1.5% of new cancer

TABLE 6-36 Average Annual Incidence (per 100,000) of Brain and Other Nervous System Cancers in United States[a]

	50–54 Years Old			55–59 Years Old			60–64 Years Old		
	All Races	White	Black	All Races	White	Black	All Races	White	Black
Men	9.1	10.1	4.9	13.1	14.5	8.2	16.3	18.6	6.6
Women	6.4	7.2	3.5	8.6	9.2	6.6	10.6	11.4	5.9

[a]Surveillance, Epidemiology, and End Results program, nine standard registries, crude age-specific rates, 2000–2005.

diagnoses and 2.3% of cancer deaths. ACS estimated that 1,340 men and 1,050 women would receive diagnoses of cancers of the eye and orbit in the United States in 2008 and that 130 men and 110 women would die from them (Jemal et al., 2008a).

In reviewing the descriptive epidemiology of these cancers, it is important to recognize the variation with which specific cancers are included in published reports, many of which distinguish between benign and malignant cancers. Another variation is whether cancer derived from related tissues (such as the pituitary or the eye) is included. Various types of cancer are usually grouped; although this may bias results in unpredictable ways, the most likely consequence is dilution of risk estimates toward the null.

The only well-established environmental risk factor for brain tumors is exposure to high doses of ionizing radiation (ACS, 2007d; Wrensch et al., 2002). Other environmental exposures—such as to vinyl chloride, petroleum products, and electromagnetic fields—are unproved as risk factors. The causes of most cancers of the brain and other portions of the nervous system are not known.

Conclusions from *VAO* and Previous Updates

The committee responsible for *VAO* concluded that there was limited or suggestive evidence of *no* association between exposure to the chemicals of interest and brain cancer. The committees responsible for *Update 1996*, *Update 1998*, *Update 2000*, *Update 2002*, and *Update 2004* did not change that conclusion. The committee responsible for *Update 2006* changed the classification for brain cancer (formally expanded to include cancers of the eye and orbit) to inadequate or insufficient information to determine an association between exposure to the chemicals of interest and brain cancer. That committee considered one study that suggested a relationship between adult gliomas and phenoxy acid herbicides (Lee et al., 2005), studies that reported slightly but not statistically significantly higher risks of brain cancer in deployed than in nondeployed Australian Vietnam-era veterans (ADVA, 2005a,b) and in pesticide applicators in the AHS (Alavanja et al.,

2005), and several studies with essentially neutral findings (Carreon et al., 2005; Magnani et al., 1987; McLean et al., 2006; Ruder et al., 2004; Torchio et al., 1994). Overall, the studies discussed in *Update 2006* suggested that a conclusion of *no* association between exposure to the chemicals of interest and brain cancer was too definitive. Table 6-37 summarizes the results of the relevant studies.

Update of Epidemiologic Literature

Vietnam-Veteran Studies

Since *Update 2006*, Cypel and Kang (2008) have evaluated mortality from all causes among female Vietnam veterans. The vital status through 2004 of the 4,390 veterans who had been alive in 1991 was assessed; overall, mortality from cancer was not higher than that in a control group of era veterans or the general population. Eight deaths attributed to cancer of the brain and CNS were observed in the Vietnam veterans (crude rate, 0.54 per 10,000) and seven in the era-veteran cohort, giving an adjusted RR of 1.97 (95% CI 0.67–5.86). In a comparison of Vietnam nurses with non-Vietnam nurses, there were eight and three deaths, respectively (RR = 3.55, 95% CI 0.87–14.53).

Occupational Studies

Samanic et al. (2008) conducted a case–control study of 462 patients with gliomas (43.5% in women) and 195 patients with meningiomas (76.4% in women) diagnosed at three major cancer-referral centers in 1994–1998 and 765 controls treated for nonneoplastic conditions in the same hospitals. Cumulative lifetime exposure to insecticides and herbicides was estimated by applying a job–exposure matrix to the occupational histories reported in interviews with the subjects or proxies for 15.2% of the gliomas, 7.2% of the meningiomas, and 2.4% of the controls. There was no relationship between herbicide exposure and incidence of gliomas in men or women. For the meningiomas, only the number of cases in women was adequate to perform the analysis. Among the cases, the women had a significantly increased risk of meningiomas in association with herbicide exposure (OR = 2.4, 95% CI 1.4–4.3); risk increased with estimated cumulative dose (p < 0.01) and years of exposure (p < 0.01). The increase in meningioma risk in women exposed to herbicides is of concern, given the apparent dose–response relationship, but there was no specification of the herbicides to which subjects were exposed.

Environmental Studies

Consonni et al. (2008) evaluated mortality in a follow-up period of 1997–2001 in 278,108 people exposed to TCDD as a result of the industrial accident in

TABLE 6-37 Selected Epidemiologic Studies—Brain Tumors

Reference	Study Population[a]	Exposed Cases[b]	Estimated Relative Risk (95% CI)[b]
VIETNAM VETERANS			
New Studies			
Cypel and	US Vietnam veterans (brain and CNS)—women	8	2.0 (0.7–5.9)
Kang, 2008	Vietnam veteran nurses	8	3.6 (0.9–14.5)
Studies Reviewed in *Update 2006*			
ADVA,	Australian male Vietnam veterans vs Australian		
2005a	population (brain)—incidence	97	1.1 (0.9–1.2)
	Navy	24	1.2 (0.7–1.7)
	Army	63	1.0 (0.8–1.3)
	Air Force	10	1.1 (0.6–2.1)
ADVA,	Australian male Vietnam veterans vs Australian		
2005b	population (brain, CNS)—mortality	99	1.0 (0.8–1.1)
	Navy	23	1.0 (0.6–1.4)
	Army	66	0.9 (0.7–1.2)
	Air Force	9	0.9 (0.4–1.6)
ADVA,	Australian male conscripted Army National Service		
2005c	Vietnam-era veterans—deployed vs nondeployed		
	(brain, CNS)		
	Incidence (1982–2000)	23	1.4 (0.7–2.6)
	Mortality (1966–2001)	27	1.6 (0.9–3.1)
Boehmer	Follow-up of CDC Vietnam Experience Cohort		
et al., 2004	(meninges, brain, other CNS)	9	1.2 (0.4–3.2)
Studies Reviewed in *Update 2004*			
Akhtar	White AFHS subjects vs national rates		
et al., 2004	Ranch Hand veterans		
	Incidence (brain and nervous system)	5	1.8 (0.7–4.1)
	With tours in 1966–1970	5	2.2 (0.8–4.8)
	Mortality (CNS)	3	1.3 (0.3–3.6)
	Comparison veterans		
	Incidence (brain and nervous system)	2	0.5 (0.1–1.8)
	With tours in 1966–1970	2	0.7 (0.1–2.3)
	Mortality (CNS)	1	0.3 (nr)
Studies Reviewed in *Update 1998*			
CDVA,	Australian military Vietnam veterans	39	1.1 (0.7–1.4)
1997a			
CDVA,	Australian National Service Vietnam veterans	13	1.4 (nr)
1997b			
Dalager and	Army Chemical Corps veterans (crude rate ratio vs		
Kang, 1997	nondeployed)	2	1.9 (nr)
Studies Reviewed in *Update 1996*			
Dalager	US Vietnam veterans—women	4	1.4 (0.4–3.7)
et al., 1995			
Visintainer	PM study of deaths (1974–1989) of Michigan		
et al., 1995	Vietnam-era veterans—deployed vs nondeployed	36	1.1 (0.8–1.5)
Boyle et al.,	Vietnam Experience Study	3	nr
1987			

TABLE 6-37 Continued

Reference	Study Population[a]	Exposed Cases[b]	Estimated Relative Risk (95% CI)[b]
Studies Reviewed in *VAO*			
Thomas and Kang, 1990	Army Chemical Corps Vietnam veterans	2	nr
Breslin et al., 1988	Army Vietnam veterans	116	1.0 (0.3–3.2)
	Marine Vietnam veterans	25	1.1 (0.2–7.1)
Anderson et al., 1986	Wisconsin Vietnam veterans	8	0.8 (0.3–1.5)
Lawrence et al., 1985	New York Vietnam veterans (brain and CNS)	4	0.5 (0.2–1.5)
OCCUPATIONAL			
New Studies			
Samanic et al., 2008	US hospital-based case–control study		
	Cumulative lifetime occupational exposure to herbicides vs unexposed		
	Gliomas		
	Men	65	0.9 (0.6–1.3)
	Low quartile	20	1.0 (0.5–1.9)
	Second quartile	16	1.0 (0.5–2.1)
	Third quartile	12	0.6 (0.3–1.3)
	Fourth quartile	17	0.8 (0.4–1.6)
			p-trend = 0.50
	Women	35	1.3 (0.8–2.0)
	Below median	23	1.5 (0.8–2.7)
	Above median	12	1.0 (0.5–2.1)
			p-trend = 0.91
	Meningiomas (women only)	33	2.4 (1.4–4.3)
	Below median	16	2.1 (1.0–4.4)
	Above median	17	2.9 (1.3–6.2)
			p-trend = 0.01
Studies Reviewed in *Update 2006*			
McLean et al., 2006	IARC cohort of pulp and paper workers		
	Exposure to nonvolatile organochlorine compounds		
	Never	44	1.0 (0.7–1.4)
	Ever	28	0.8 (0.5–1.2)
't Mannetje et al., 2005	New Zealand phenoxy herbicide workers		
	Phenoxy herbicide producers (men and women)	1	0.8 (0.0–4.6)
	Phenoxy herbicide sprayers (> 99% men)	1	0.6 (0.0–3.4)
Alavanja et al., 2005	US AHS—incidence		
	Private applicators (men and women)	33	0.8 (0.6–0.8)
	Spouses of private applicators (> 99% women)	15	0.9 (0.5–1.4)
	Commercial applicators (men and women)	5	1.9 (0.6–4.3)

continued

TABLE 6-37 Continued

Reference	Study Population[a]	Exposed Cases[b]	Estimated Relative Risk (95% CI)[b]
Blair et al., 2005a	US AHS		
	Private applicators (men and women)	19	0.7 (0.4–1.1)
	Years handled pesticides		
	≤ 10 years	5	0.9 (ns)
	> 10 years	12	0.6 (ns)
	Spouses of private applicators (> 99% women)	11	1.1 (0.5–1.8)
Torchio et al., 1994	Italian licensed pesticide users		
	Brain, nervous system	15	0.5 (0.3–0.9)
	Eye	4	2.4 (0.7–6.1)
Lee et al., 2005	Nebraska case–control study (gliomas)—incidence		
	Phenoxy herbicides—combined reports		
	(identical with results for 2,4-D specifically)	32	1.8 (1.0–3.3)
	By self	7	0.6 (0.2–1.6)
	By proxy	25	3.3 (1.5–7.2)
	2,4,5-T—combined reports	7	1.3 (0.5–3.6)
	By self	2	0.4 (0.1–2.3)
	By proxy	5	2.7 (0.7–9.8)
Carreon et al., 2005	NIOSH UMHS—case–control		
	Women		
	Arsenicals	13	1.0 (0.5–1.9)
	Phenoxy herbicides	25	0.9 (0.5–1.5)
	2,4-D	24	0.9 (0.5–1.6)
Ruder et al., 2004	Men		
	Arsenicals	15	0.7 (0.4–1.4)
	Phenoxy herbicides	67	0.9 (0.6–1.2)
	2,4-D	nr	nr
Reif et al., 1989	Case–control study, all men with occupation entered into New Zealand Cancer Registry 1980–1984 (brain, CNS cancers)		
	Forestry workers	4	1.2 (0.4–3.3)
Magnani et al., 1987	UK case–control, JEM used on occupation given on death certificate		
	Herbicides	nr	1.2 (0.7–2.1)
	Chlorophenols	nr	1.1 (0.7–1.8)
Studies Reviewed in *Update 2004*			
Bodner et al., 2003	Dow chemical production workers (included in IARC cohort, NIOSH Dioxin Registry) (brain and CNS)	nr	0.6 (0.1–1.8)
Swaen et al., 2004	Dutch licensed herbicide applicators	4	1.6 (0.4–4.1)
Studies Reviewed in *Update 2002*			
Burns et al., 2001	Dow 2,4-D production workers (included in IARC cohort, NIOSH Dioxin Registry)	3	1.1 (0.2–3.2)
Thörn et al., 2000	Swedish lumberjacks exposed to phenoxy acetic herbicides		
	Foreman—incidence	0	nr

TABLE 6-37 Continued

Reference	Study Population[a]	Exposed Cases[b]	Estimated Relative Risk (95% CI)[b]
Studies Reviewed in *Update 2000*			
Steenland et al., 1999	US chemical workers (included in IARC cohort, NIOSH Dioxin Registry) (brain and CNS)	8	0.8 (0.4–1.6)
Studies Reviewed in *Update 1998*			
Gambini et al., 1997	Italian rice growers (brain and CNS)	4	0.9 (0.2–2.3)
Kogevinas et al., 1997	IARC cohort, male and female workers exposed to any phenoxy herbicide or chlorophenol	22	0.7 (0.4–1.0)
	Exposed to highly chlorinated PCDDs	12	0.6 (0.3–1.1)
	Not exposed to highly chlorinated PCDDs	10	0.8 (0.4–1.5)
Becher et al., 1996	German production workers (included in IARC cohort)—cohort I	3	2.3 (0.5–6.8)
Ramlow et al., 1996	Dow pentachlorophenol production workers (included in IARC cohort, NIOSH Dioxin Registry) (brain and CNS)		
	0-year latency	1	nr
	15-year latency	1	nr
Studies Reviewed in *Update 1996*			
Asp et al., 1994	Finnish herbicide applicators (eye, brain)		
	Incidence	3	0.7 (0.1–2.0)
	Mortality	3	1.2 (0.3–3.6)
Dean, 1994	Irish farmers, farm workers		
	Men	195	nr
	Women	72	nr
Blair et al., 1993	US farmers in 23 states		
	White men	447	1.2 (1.1–1.3)
	White women	9	1.1 (0.5–2.1)
Studies Reviewed in *VAO*			
Morrison et al., 1992	Farmers in Canadian prairie province		
	250+ acres sprayed with herbicides	24	0.8 (0.5–1.2)
Ronco et al., 1992	Danish farmers (brain and CNS)—incidence		
	Men	194	1.1 (nr)
	Women	5	1.0 (nr)
Swaen et al., 1992	Dutch licensed herbicide applicators	3	3.2 (0.6–9.3)
Fingerhut et al., 1991	NIOSH cohort—entire cohort (brain and CNS)		
	≥ 1-year exposure, ≥ 20-year latency	2	1.1 (0.1–3.8)
Saracci et al., 1991	IARC cohort (men and women)—exposed subcohort	6	0.4 (0.1–0.8)
Wigle et al., 1990	Canadian farmers	96	1.0 (0.8–1.3)
Alavanja et al., 1989	USDA forest, soil conservationists	6	1.7 (0.6–3.7)
Henneberger et al., 1989	New Hampshire pulp and paper workers	2	1.2 (0.1–4.2)

continued

TABLE 6-37 Continued

Reference	Study Population[a]	Exposed Cases[b]	Estimated Relative Risk (95% CI)[b]
Alavanja et al., 1988	USDA agricultural extension agents	nr	1.0 (0.4–2.4)
Bond et al., 1988	Dow 2,4-D production workers (included in IARC cohort, NIOSH Dioxin Registry)		
	Brain, other system tissues	0	nr (0.0–4.1)
Musicco et al., 1988	Brain-tumor patients in Milan, Italy (male, female farmers)	61	1.6 (1.1–2.4)
Coggon et al., 1986	British MCPA chemical workers (included in IARC cohort) (brain and CNS)	11	1.2 (0.6–2.2)
Robinson et al., 1986	Northwestern US paper and pulp workers	4	0.6 (0.2–2.1)
Lynge, 1985	Danish production workers (included in IARC cohort)—incidence	4	0.7 (nr)
Blair et al., 1983	Florida pesticide applicators	5	2.0 (nr)
Burmeister, 1981	Iowa farmers	111	1.1 (ns)

ENVIRONMENTAL
New Studies

Consonni et al., 2008	Seveso residents—25-year follow-up—men, women		
	Zone A	0	nr
	Zone B	3	0.7 (0.2–2.1)
	Zone R	34	1.1 (0.8–1.6)
Studies Reviewed in *Update 2000*			
Bertazzi et al., 2001	Seveso residents—20-year follow-up		
	Zone A, B—men	1	0.4 (0.1–3.0)
	women	3	1.9 (0.6–6.0)
Bertazzi et al., 1998	Seveso residents—15-year follow-up		
	Zone B—men	1	0.8 (0.1–5.5)
	women	3	3.2 (1.0–10.3)
	Zone R—men	12	1.3 (0.7–2.5)
	women	8	1.1 (0.5–2.4)
Studies Reviewed in *Update 1998*			
Svensson et al., 1995	Swedish fishermen (men and women)—mortality		
	East coast	2	0.6 (0.1–2.1)
	West coast	15	1.1 (0.6–1.7)
	Swedish fishermen (men and women)—incidence		
	East coast	3	0.5 (0.1–1.5)
	West coast	24	0.9 (0.6–1.4)
Studies Reviewed in *Update 1996*			
Bertazzi et al., 1993	Seveso residents—10-year follow-up—incidence		
	Zone R—men	6	0.6 (0.3–1.4)
	women	6	1.4 (0.6–3.4)

TABLE 6-37 Continued

Reference	Study Population[a]	Exposed Cases[b]	Estimated Relative Risk (95% CI)[b]
Studies Reviewed in *VAO*			
Pesatori	Seveso residents—incidence		
et al., 1992	Zones A, B—women	1	1.5 (0.2–11.3)
	Zone R—men	6	0.6 (0.3–1.4)
	women	5	1.2 (0.4–3.0)
Bertazzi	Seveso residents—10-year follow-up		
et al., 1989a	Zones A, B, R—men	5	1.2 (0.4–3.1)
	women	5	2.1 (0.8–5.9)

ABBREVIATIONS: 2,4-D, 2,4-dichlorophenoxyacetic acid; 2,4,5-T, 2,4,5-trichlorophenoxyacetic acid; AFHS, Air Force Health Study; AHS, Agricultural Health Study; CDC, Centers for Disease Control and Prevention; CI, confidence interval; CNS, central nervous system; IARC, International Agency for Research on Cancer; JEM, job–exposure matrix; MCPA, 2-methyl-4-chlorophenoxyacetic acid; NIOSH, National Institute for Occupational Safety and Health; nr, not reported; ns, not significant; PCDDs, chlorinated dibenzo-*p*-dioxins (highly chlorinated, if four or more chlorines); PM, proportionate mortality; TCDD, 2,3,7,8-tetrachlorodibenzo-*p*-dioxin; UMHS, Upper Midwest Health Study; USDA, US Department of Agriculture.
[a]Subjects are male and outcome is mortality unless otherwise noted.
[b]Given when available; results other than estimated risk explained individually.
Studies in italics have been superseded by newer studies of same cohorts.

Seveso, Italy, in 1976. Compared with that in residents in a nonexposed adjacent area, there was no increase in mortality from brain cancer in any of the three exposed zones with increasing exposure and no indication of a dose–response relationship.

Biologic Plausibility

No animal studies have reported an association between exposure to the chemicals of interest and brain cancer. The biologic plausibility of the carcinogenicity of the chemicals of interest is discussed in general at the beginning of this chapter.

Synthesis

Since *Update 2006*, several studies relevant to the possibility of an association between the chemicals of interest and brain cancer have been identified, including cohort and case–control studies. All recent studies are consistent in identifying no relationship between exposure to the chemicals of interest and the development of gliomas. Samanic et al. (2008) did identify a possible relationship between herbicide exposure and meningiomas in women, but lack of identification of specific chemicals of interest makes the interpretation of this result uncertain.

Conclusion

On the basis of the epidemiologic evidence from new and previously reported studies of populations with potential exposure to the chemicals of interest, the committee concludes that there is inadequate or insufficient evidence to determine whether there is an association between exposure to the chemicals of interest and brain cancer and other nervous system cancers.

ENDOCRINE CANCERS

Cancers of the endocrine system as grouped by the SEER program (see Table B-2 in Appendix B) make up a disparate group of ICD codes: thymus cancer (ICD-9 164.0), thyroid cancer (ICD-9 193), and other endocrine cancer (ICD-9 194).

ACS estimated that 8,930 men and 28,410 women would receive diagnoses of thyroid cancer in the United States in 2008 and that 680 men and 910 women would die from it and estimated that 1,100 men and 1,070 women would receive diagnoses of other endocrine cancers in 2008 and that 430 men and 410 women would die from them (Jemal et al., 2008a). Incidence data on cancers of the endocrine system are presented in Table 6-38.

Thyroid cancer is the most prevalent of the endocrine cancers. Many types of tumors can develop in the thyroid gland; most are benign. The thyroid gland contains two main types of cells: follicular cells, which make and store thyroid hormones and that make thyroglobulin, and C cells, which make the hormone calcitonin, which helps to regulate calcium metabolism. Different cancers can develop from each kind of cell, and the classification of thyroid cancer is still evolving (Liu et al., 2006). The several types into which thyroid cancer is currently

TABLE 6-38 Average Annual Incidence (per 100,000) of Endocrine System Cancer in United States[a]

	50–54 Years Old			55–59 Years Old			60–64 Years Old		
	All Races	White	Black	All Races	White	Black	All Races	White	Black
Men	6.7	9.3	7.2	11.1	11.4	7.2	12.5	12.7	7.0
Women	23.5	24.4	14.1	22.2	22.1	18.3	21.7	22.5	15.0

[a]Surveillance, Epidemiology, and End Results program, nine standard registries, crude age-specific rates, 2000–2005.

classified differ in their seriousness. Papillary carcinoma is the most common and usually affects women of childbearing age; it metastasizes slowly and is the least malignant type of thyroid cancer. Follicular carcinoma accounts for about 30% of all cases and has a greater rate of recurrence and metastasis. Medullary carcinoma is a cancer of nonthyroid cells in the thyroid gland and tends to occur in families; it requires treatment different from other types of thyroid cancer. Anaplastic carcinoma (also called giant-cell cancer and spindle-cell cancer) is rare but is the most malignant form of thyroid cancer; it does not respond to radioiodine therapy and metastasizes quickly, invading such nearby structures as the trachea and causing compression and breathing difficulties.

Thyroid cancer can occur in all age groups. People who have had radiation therapy directed at the neck are at higher risk. That therapy was commonly used in the 1950s in treatment for enlarged thymus glands, adenoids, and tonsils and for skin disorders. People who received radiation therapy as children have a higher incidence of thyroid cancer. Other risk factors are a family history of thyroid cancer and chronic goiter.

Conclusions from *VAO* and Previous Updates

The committees responsible for *VAO*, *Update 1996*, *Update 1998*, *Update 2000*, *Update 2002*, and *Update 2004* did not consider endocrine cancers separately and therefore reached no conclusion as to whether there was an association between exposure to the chemicals of interest and endocrine cancers. The committee responsible for *Update 2006* considered endocrine cancers separately and concluded that there was inadequate or insufficient evidence to determine whether there was an association between the chemicals of interest and endocrine cancers. Table 6-39 summarizes the pertinent results of the relevant studies.

Update of the Epidemiologic Literature

No studies concerning exposure to the chemicals of interest and thyroid or other endocrine cancers have been published since *Update 2006*.

Biologic Plausibility

The National Toxicology Program (NTP) conducted carcinogenesis bioassays in Osborne-Mendel rats and B6C3F1 mice exposed to TCDD by gavage (NTP, 1982a). The incidence of follicular-cell adenoma, but not of carcinoma, increased with increasing TCDD dose in male and female rats; the increase was significant in male but not female rats. There was a significant increase in follicular-cell adenoma in female but not male mice. The NTP carried out a similar study in female Sprague-Dawley rats more recently (NTP, 2006), and Walker et al. (2006) compared the data from that study and the results of the Dow

TABLE 6-39 Selected Epidemiologic Studies—Endocrine Cancers (Thyroid, Thymus, and Other)

Reference	Study Population[a]	Exposed Cases[b]	Estimated Relative Risk (95% CI)[b]
VIETNAM VETERANS			
ADVA, 2005a	Australian male Vietnam veterans vs Australian population (thyroid)—incidence	17	0.6 (0.3–0.9)
	Navy	3	0.5 (0.1–1.3)
	Army	11	0.5 (0.3–1.0)
	Air Force	3	1.2 (0.2–3.5)
ADVA, 2005b	Australian male Vietnam veterans vs Australian population (thyroid)—mortality	2	0.5 (0.0–1.8)
	Navy	1	1.2 (0.0–6.5)
	Army	1	0.4 (0.0–2.0)
	Air Force	0	0.0 (0.0–7.8)
ADVA, 2005c	Australian male conscripted Army National Service Vietnam-era veterans—deployed vs nondeployed		
	Thyroid—incidence	4	0.6 (0.1–2.2)
	Thyroid—mortality	1	1.2 (0.0–91.7)
Breslin et al., 1988	Veterans with service in Vietnam vs. era veterans (thyroid and other endocrine, ICD-9 193–194)		
	Army	15	0.6 (0.3–1.2)
	Marine Corps	4	0.6 (0.1–3.4)
Clapp, 1997	Massachusetts male Vietnam veterans vs era veterans (thyroid)—incidence 1988–1993	4	1.2 (0.3–4.5)
OCCUPATIONAL			
Alavanja et al., 2005	US AHS (thyroid, other endocrine)—incidence		
	Private applicators (men and women)	29	1.3 (0.8–1.8)
	Spouses of private applicators (> 99% women)	24	0.9 (0.5–1.4)
	Commercial applicators (men and women)	3	1.6 (0.3–5.0)
't Mannetje et al., 2005	Phenoxy herbicide producers (men and women)	0	nr
	Phenoxy herbicide sprayers (> 99% men)	0	nr
Blair et al., 2005a	US AHS (thyroid)—mortality		
	Private applicators (men and women)	3	1.8 (0.4–5.3)
	Spouses of private applicators (> 99% women)	0	0.0 (0.0–2.2)
Kogevinas et al., 1997	IARC cohort, male and female workers exposed to any phenoxy herbicide or chlorophenol		
	Thyroid (ICD-9 193)	4	1.7 (0.5–4.3)
	Exposed to highly chlorinated PCDDs	2	1.4 (0.2–4.9)
	Not exposed to highly chlorinated PCDDs	2	2.2 (0.3–7.9)
	Other endocrine organs (ICD-9 194)	5	3.6 (1.2–8.4)
	Exposed to highly chlorinated PCDDs	2	2.3 (0.3–8.1)
	Not exposed to highly chlorinated PCDDs	3	6.4 (1.3–18.7)
Zhong and Rafnsson, 1996	Icelandic men, women exposed to agricultural pesticides, primarily 2,4-D (other endocrine organs, ICD-9 194)—incidence	2	1.3 (0.1–4.7)
Ramlow et al., 1996	Dow cohort of pentachlorophenol factory workers employed in 1940–1989 in Michigan Division	0	nr

TABLE 6-39 Continued

Reference	Study Population[a]	Exposed Cases[b]	Estimated Relative Risk (95% CI)[b]
Asp et al., 1994	Finnish phenoxy herbicide applicators (thyroid, other endocrine)—incidence		
	No latency	2	1.9 (0.3–7.0)
	10-year latency	2	2.4 (0.3–8.6)
	15-year latency	2	3.4 (0.4–12.2)
	Mortality (thyroid)		
	No latency	1	3.8 (0.1–21.3)
	10-year latency	1	4.7 (0.1–26.4)
	15-year latency	1	6.5 (0.2–36.2)
Hallquist et al., 1993	Case–control study of male, female thyroid cancers from Swedish Cancer Registry, 1980–1989		
	Phenoxy herbicide exposure	3	0.5 (0.0–2.0)
	Chlorophenol exposure	4	2.8 (0.5–18)
Blair et al., 1993	US farmers in 23 states (thyroid)		
	White men	39	1.3 (1.0–1.8)
	White women	1	0.8 (0.0–4.4)
Ronco et al., 1992	Danish workers—incidence		
	Men—self-employed	13	0.7 (nr)
	employee	5	1.1 (nr)
	Women—self-employed	1	1.3 (nr)
	employee	1	1.4 (nr)
	family worker	15	1.7 (p < 0.05)
Green, 1991	Cohort mortality study of forestry workers exposed to phenoxy acid herbicides	1	nr
Wiklund et al., 1989a	Cancer risk in licensed pesticide applicators in Sweden	6	1.1 (0.4–2.4)
Bond et al., 1988	Workers engaged in manufacture of phenoxy herbicides	0	nr
Coggon et al., 1986	British MCPA procuction workers (thyroid) (included in IARC cohort)	1	1.8 (0.4–9.8)
Wiklund, 1983	Swedish male and female agricultural workers—incidence		99% CI
	Thyroid	126	0.9 (0.7–1.1)
	Other endocrine gland	117	0.7 (0.5–0.9)
ENVIRONMENTAL			
Bertazzi et al., 1998	Cancer mortality after Seveso incident		
	Zone A	nr	nr
	Zone B—men	1	4.9 (0.6–39.0)
	women	1	3.2 (0.4–24.5)
	Zone R—men	0	nr
	women	2	0.8 (0.2–3.6)

ABBREVIATIONS: 2,4-D, 2,4-dichlorophenoxyacetic acid; AHS, Agricultural Health Study; CI, confidence interval; IARC, International Agency for Research on Cancer; ICD, International Classification of Diseases; MCPA, 2-methyl-4-chlorophenoxyacetic acid; nr, not reported; PCDDs, chlorinated dibenzo-p-dioxins (highly chlorinated, if four or more chlorines).
[a]Subjects are male and outcome is mortality unless otherwise noted.
[b]Given when available; results other than estimated risk explained individually.

Chemical assessment of TCDD carcinogenicity (Kociba et al., 1978). In the NTP and Dow studies, the incidence of thyroid cancer (C-cell adenoma and carcinoma) decreased with increasing dose of TCDD. However, an increased incidence of minimal thyroid follicular-cell hypertrophy was noted in rats given TCDD at 22 ng/kg of body weight or more.

As indicated in Chapter 4, 2,4-D and 2,4,5-T are at most only weakly mutagenic or carcinogenic. No studies that addressed a possible association between exposure to those herbicides and thyroid cancer in animal models have been identified.

The biologic plausibility of the carcinogenicity of the chemicals of interest is discussed in general at the beginning of this chapter.

Synthesis

The studies reviewed previously did not provide sufficient evidence to determine whether there is an association between exposure to the chemicals of interest and thyroid cancer or other endocrine cancers, and no new additional information was found by the present committee.

Conclusion

On the basis of the epidemiologic evidence reviewed here, the committee concludes that there is insufficient evidence to determine whether there is an association between exposure to the chemicals of interest and thyroid or other endocrine cancers.

LYMPHOHEMATOPOIETIC CANCERS (LYMPHOMAS AND LEUKEMIAS)

As in the case of other cancers that are subject to idiosyncratic grouping in the results reported from epidemiologic studies (notably, head and neck cancers and gastrointestinal cancers), the conclusions that the VAO committees have been able to draw about associations between herbicide exposure and specific lymphohematopoietic cancers are complicated and curtailed by the lack of specificity and the occasional inconsistency of groupings in the available evidence. Categorization of cancers of the lymphatic and hematopoietic systems continues to evolve on the basis of increasing insight into the lineage of the clonal cancer cells that characterize each of a broad spectrum of neoplasms arising in these tissues.

Stem cells in the bone marrow generate two major lineages of leukocytes: myeloid and lymphoid. Myeloid cells include monocytes and three types of granulocytes (neutrophils, eosinophils, and basophils). Lymphoid cells include T and B lymphocytes and a smaller subset of cells called natural killer cells. All those cells circulate in the blood and are collectively referred to as white blood cells. Monocytes move out of the bloodstream into inflamed tissues, where they differentiate into macrophages or dendritic cells. Stem cells that are destined to become T lymphocytes migrate from the bone marrow to the thymus, where they acquire antigen-specific receptors. Antigen stimulation induces the T cells to differentiate into the several types involved in cell-mediated immunity. Pre-B cells mature in the bone marrow into antigen-specific B cells. On encountering their cognate antigens, B cells differentiate into antibody-secreting plasma cells involved in humoral immunity.

Lymphoma is a general term for cancers that arise from B or T lymphocytes. As stem cells mature into B or T cells, they pass through several developmental stages, each with unique functions. The developmental stage at which a cell becomes malignant defines the kind of lymphoma. About 85% of lymphomas are of B-cell origin, and 15% of T-cell origin. Lymphomas grow as circumscribed solid tumors in the lymph nodes.

If a cell that becomes cancerous resides in the bone marrow, its daughter cells may crowd normal cells in the bone marrow or be released from the bone marrow and circulate in the blood. Such cancers are called leukemias. Leukemias are generally classified as myeloid or lymphoid, depending on the differentiation pathway of the original mutated cell. If the original mutated cell of a cancer of the blood arises in a lymphocytic cell line, the cancer is called lymphocytic leukemia; lymphocytic leukemias are further partitioned into acute (ALL) forms if they are derived from precursor B or T lymphoid cells and chronic (CLL) forms derived from more mature lymphoid cells, which tend to replicate less rapidly. Similarly, myeloid leukemias are portioned into acute and chronic forms, AML and CML, respectively.

B lymphocytes (B cells) give rise to a number of types of neoplasms that are given names based on the stage at which B-cell development was arrested when the cells became cancerous. Follicular, large-cell, and immunoblastic lymphomas result when a malignancy develops *after* a B cell has been exposed to antigens (such as bacteria and viruses). CLL is now believed to be a tumor of antigen-experienced (memory) B cells, not naive B cells (Chiorazzi et al., 2005); small lymphocytic lymphoma (SLL), which presents primarily in lymph nodes rather than in the bone marrow and blood, is now considered to be the same disease as CLL at a different stage (Jaffe et al., 2008). (Although some may now prefer to designate the two closely related entities as CLL/SLL, the committee has opted to continue using the abbreviation CLL to refer to this condition in its more inclusive sense.) Some of those stages are more common than others and therefore have been subclassified for diagnostic purposes. However, why one stage of B-cell development rather than another is affected by a cancerous mutation is not known; it may reflect individual genetic predispositions or other environmental exposures.

The more common cancers of the hematopoietic system are described in the sections below on Hodgkin's disease; non-Hodgkin's lymphomas; multiple myeloma, followed by a separate section on the related condition, AL amyloidosis; and leukemias. An additional section on CLL has been included in light of VA's request that it be considered separately for *Update 2002*. The introduction to the CLL section includes an explanation of why the committee accepts the epidemiologic and toxicologic data on CLL to be applicable to hairy-cell leukemia (HCL).

Hodgkin's Disease

Hodgkin's disease (HD) (ICD-9 201) is now often designated as Hodgkin's lymphoma, but the present committee continues its use of *disease* to maintain consistency throughout the VAO reports. HD is distinguished from non-Hodgkin's lymphoma (NHL) primarily on the basis of its neoplastic cells, mononucleated Hodgkin cells and multinucleated Reed–Sternberg cells originating in germinal center B cells (Kuppers et al., 2002). HD's demographics and genetics are also characteristic. ACS estimated that 4,400 men and 3,820 women would receive diagnoses of HD in the United States in 2008 and that 700 men and 650 women would die from it (Jemal et al., 2008a). The average annual incidence is shown in Table 6-40.

The possibility that HD has an infectious etiology has been a topic of discussion since its earliest description. An increased incidence in people with a history of infectious mononucleosis has been observed in some studies, and a link with Epstein–Barr virus has been proposed. In addition to the occupational associations discussed below, higher rates of the disease have been observed in people who have suppressed or compromised immune systems.

Conclusions from *VAO* and Previous Updates

The committee responsible for *VAO* determined that there were sufficient epidemiologic data to support an association between exposure to the chemicals of interest and HD. Additional studies available to the committees responsible for *Update 1996*, *Update 1998*, *Update 2000*, *Update 2002*, *Update 2004*, and *Update 2006* did not change that conclusion. Table 6-41 summarizes the results of the relevant studies.

TABLE 6-40 Average Annual Incidence (per 100,000) of Hodgkin's Disease in United States[a]

| | 50–54 Years Old | | | 55–59 Years Old | | | 60–64 Years Old | | |
	All Races	White	Black	All Races	White	Black	All Races	White	Black
Men	3.3	3.4	4.3	2.8	2.9	2.4	3.3	3.5	4.3
Women	1.7	1.7	1.6	1.6	1.7	1.8	2.0	2.2	0.3

[a]Surveillance, Epidemiology, and End Results program, nine standard registries, crude age-specific rates, 2000–2005.

TABLE 6-41 Selected Epidemiologic Studies—Hodgkin's Disease

Reference	Study Population[a]	Exposed Cases[b]	Estimated Relative Risk (95% CI)[b]
VIETNAM VETERANS			
New Studies			
Cypel and Kang, 2008	US Vietnam veterans (lymphopoietic cancers[c])—women	18	0.7 (0.4–1.3)
	Vietnam-veteran nurses	14	0.7 (0.3–1.3)
Studies Reviewed in *Update 2006*			
ADVA, 2005a	Australian male Vietnam veterans vs Australian population—incidence	51	2.1 (1.5–2.6)
	Navy	7	1.3 (0.5–2.6)
	Army	40	2.3 (1.6–3.0)
	Air Force	4	2.1 (0.6–5.3)
ADVA, 2005b	Australian male Vietnam veterans vs Australian population—mortality	13	0.9 (0.5–1.5)
	Navy	2	0.6 (0.1–2.1)
	Army	11	1.1 (0.5–1.9)
	Air Force	0	0.0 (0.0–2.9)
ADVA, 2005c	Australian male conscripted Army National Service Vietnam era veterans: deployed vs non-deployed		
	Incidence	12	0.9 (0.4–2.0)
	Mortality	4	1.7 (0.3–11.8)
Boehmer et al., 2004	Vietnam Experience Cohort	2	0.9 (nr)
Studies Reviewed in *Update 2004*			
Akhtar et al., 2004	White Air Force Ranch Hand veterans vs national rates (lymphopoietic cancer[c])—incidence		
	Ranch Hand veterans	10	0.9 (0.4–1.5)
	Comparison Air Force veterans	9	0.6 (0.3–1.0)
Studies Reviewed in *Update 2000*			
AFHS, 2000	Air Force Ranch Hand veterans	1	0.3 (0.0–3.2)
Studies Reviewed in *Update 1998*			
Watanabe and Kang, 1996	Marine Vietnam veterans	25	1.9 (1.2–2.7)
Studies Reviewed in *Update 1996*			
Visintainer et al., 1995	PM study of deaths (1974–1989) of Michigan Vietnam-era veterans—deployed vs nondeployed	20	1.1 (0.7–1.8)
Studies Reviewed in *VAO*			
Watanabe et al., 1991	Army Vietnam veterans		
	Vs Army non-Vietnam veterans	116	1.0 (nr)
	Vs all non-Vietnam veterans	116	1.1 (nr)
	Marine Vietnam veterans		
	Vs Marine non-Vietnam veterans	25	1.9 (nr)
	Vs all non-Vietnam veterans	25	1.0 (nr)
CDC, 1990a	US men born 1921–1953		
	Vietnam veterans	28	1.2 (0.7–2.4)
	Army	12	1.0 (0.5–2.0)
	Marine Corps	4	1.7 (0.5–5.9)
	Air Force	5	1.7 (0.6–4.9)
	Navy	7	1.1 (0.4–2.6)

continued

TABLE 6-41 Continued

Reference	Study Population[a]	Exposed Cases[b]	Estimated Relative Risk (95% CI)[b]
Michalek et al., 1990; Wolfe et al., 1990	Air Force Ranch Hand veteran	0	nr
Breslin et al., 1988	Vietnam-era veterans—deployed vs nondeployed		
	Army	92	1.2 (0.7–1.9)
	Marine Corps	22	1.3 (0.7–2.6)
Boyle et al., 1987	Vietnam Experience Study	0	nr
Fett et al., 1987	Australian Vietnam veterans	0	nr
Anderson et al., 1986	Wisconsin Vietnam veterans	4	nr
Holmes et al., 1986	West Virginia Vietnam veterans compared with West Virginia Vietnam-era veterans	5	8.3 (2.7–19.5)
Lawrence et al., 1985	New York Vietnam veterans compared with New York Vietnam-era veterans (lymphoma and HD)	10	99% CI 1.0 (0.4–2.2)

OCCUPATIONAL
Studies Reviewed in *Update 2006*

McLean et al., 2006	IARC cohort of pulp and paper workers Exposure to nonvolatile organochlorine compounds		
	Never	7	0.6 (0.2–1.2)
	Ever	17	1.8 (1.0–2.8)
't Mannetje et al., 2006	Phenoxy herbicide producers (men and women)	1	5.6 (0.1–31.0)
	Phenoxy herbicide sprayers (> 99% men)	0	0.0 (0.0–16.1)
Alavanja et al., 2005	US AHS—incidence		
	Private applicators (men and women)	11	0.9 (0.4–1.6)
	Spouses of private applicators (> 99% women)	4	0.7 (0.2–1.9)
	Commercial applicators (men and women)	1	0.8 (0.1–4.2)
Blair et al., 2005a	US AHS	3	1.1 (0.2–3.3)
	Private applicators (men and women)	3	1.7 (0.3–4.8)
	Spouses of private applicators (> 99% women)	0	0.0 (0.0–2.5)
Torchio et al., 1994	Italian licensed pesticide users	11	1.0 (0.5–1.7)

Studies Reviewed in *Update 2004*

Swaen et al., 2004	Dutch licensed herbicide applicators	0	nr

Studies Reviewed in *Update 2002*

Burns et al., 2001	Dow 2,4-D production workers (included in IARC cohort, NIOSH Dioxin Registry)	1	1.5 (0.0–8.6)

Studies Reviewed in *Update 2000*

Steenland et al., 1999	US chemical production workers (included in IARC cohort, NIOSH Dioxin Registry)	3	1.1 (0.2–3.2)
Hooiveld et al., 1998	Dutch chemical production workers (included in IARC cohort)	1	3.2 (0.1–17.6)
Rix et al., 1998	Danish paper mill workers—incidence		
	Men	18	2.0 (1.2–3.2)
	Women	2	1.1 (0.1–3.8)

TABLE 6-41 Continued

Reference	Study Population[a]	Exposed Cases[b]	Estimated Relative Risk (95% CI)[b]
Studies Reviewed in *Update 1998*			
Gambini et al., 1997	Italian rice growers	1	0.7 (0.0–3.6)
Kogevinas et al., 1997	IARC cohort, male and female workers exposed to any phenoxy herbicide or chlorophenol	10	1.0 (0.5–1.8)
	Exposed to highly chlorinated PCDDs	8	1.3 (0.6–2.5)
	Not exposed to highly chlorinated PCDDs	1	0.3 (0.0–1.5)
Becher et al., 1996	German production workers (included in IARC cohort)	0	nr
Ramlow et al., 1996	Dow pentachlorophenol production workers (included in IARC cohort, NIOSH Dioxin Registry)	0	nr
Waterhouse et al., 1996	Residents of Tecumseh, Michigan	13	2.0 (1.1–3.4)
Studies Reviewed in *Update 1996*			
Asp et al., 1994	Finnish herbicide applicators	2	1.7 (0.2–6.0)
Blair et al., 1993	US farmers in 23 states	56	1.0 (0.8–1.3)
Kogevinas et al., 1993	IARC cohort—females—incidence	1	nr
Persson et al., 1993	Swedish NHL patients—exposure to phenoxy herbicides	5	90% CI 7.4 (1.4–40.0)
Kogevinas et al., 1992	IARC cohort (men and women)	3	0.6 (0.1–1.7)
Studies Reviewed in *VAO*			
Eriksson et al., 1992	Swedish Cancer Registry patients (men and women)		
	Male sawmill workers	10	2.2 (nr)
	Male farmers	97	1.2 (nr)
	Male forestry workers	35	1.2 (nr)
	Male horticulture workers	11	1.2 (nr)
Ronco et al., 1992	Danish workers—incidence		
	Men—self-employed	27	0.6 (p < 0.05)
	employee	13	1.0 (nr)
	Female—self-employed	1	1.1 (nr)
	employee	1	1.2 (nr)
	family worker	9	0.9 (nr)
Swaen et al., 1992	Dutch licensed herbicide applicators	1	3.3 (0.04–18.6)
Fingerhut et al., 1991	NIOSH cohort—entire cohort	3	1.2 (0.3–3.5)
	≥ 1-year exposure, ≥ 20-year latency	1	2.8 (0.1–15.3)
Green, 1991	Ontario herbicide sprayers	0	nr
Saracci et al., 1991	IARC cohort—exposed subcohort (men and women)	2	0.4 (0.1–1.4)
Zober et al., 1990	BASF employees—basic cohort	0	nr

continued

TABLE 6-41 Continued

Reference	Study Population[a]	Exposed Cases[b]	Estimated Relative Risk (95% CI)[b]
Alavanja et al., 1989	USDA forest, soil conservationists	4	2.2 (0.6–5.6)
LaVecchia et al., 1989	Residents of the Milan, Italy, area (men and women)		
	Agricultural occupations	nr	2.1(1.0–3.8)
	Chemical-industry occupations	nr	4.3 (1.4–10.2)
Persson et al., 1989	Orebro (Sweden) Hospital patients (men and women)		90% CI
	Farming	6	1.2 (0.4–3.5)
	Exposed to phenoxy acids	4	3.8 (0.7–21.0)
Wiklund et al., 1989b	Swedish pesticide applicators	15	1.5 (0.8–2.4)
Alavanja et al., 1988	USDA agricultural extension agents		
	PM analysis	6	2.7 (1.2–6.3)
	Case–control analysis	6	1.1 (0.3–3.5)
Bond et al., 1988	Dow 2,4-D production workers (included in IARC cohort, NIOSH Dioxin Registry)	1	2.7 (0.0–14.7)
Dubrow et al., 1988	Hancock County, Ohio, residents—farmers	3	2.7 (nr)
Wiklund et al., 1988	Swedish agricultural and forestry workers (men and women)		
	Workers in land or in animal husbandry	242	1.0 (0.9–1.2)
	Workers in silviculture	15	2.3 (1.3–3.7)
Hoar et al., 1986	Kansas residents		
	All farmers	71	0.8 (0.5–1.2)
	Farm use of herbicides (phenoxy acids and others)	28	0.9 (0.5–1.5)
	Farmers using herbicides > 20 days/year	3	1.0 (0.2–4.1)
	Farmers using herbicides > 15 years	10	1.2 (0.5–2.6)
Pearce et al., 1985	New Zealand residents with agricultural occupations, 20–64 years old	107	1.1 (0.6–2.0)
Hardell and Bengtsson, 1983	Umea (Sweden) Hospital patients—incidence		
	Exposed to phenoxy acids	14	5.0 (2.4–10.2)
	Exposed to high-grade chlorophenols	6	6.5 (2.2–19.0)
	Exposed to low-grade chlorophenols	5	2.4 (0.9–6.5)
Riihimaki et al., 1982	Finnish herbicide applicators	0	nr
Wiklund, 1983	Swedish male and female agricultural workers—incidence	226	99% CI 1.0 (0.9–1.2)
Burmeister, 1981	Iowa farmers	47	1.2 (ns)
Hardell et al., 1981	Umea (Sweden) Hospital patients (all lymphomas)—incidence		
	Exposed to phenoxy acids	41	4.8 (2.9–8.1)
	Exposed to chlorophenols	50	4.3 (2.7–6.9)

TABLE 6-41 Continued

Reference	Study Population[a]	Exposed Cases[b]	Estimated Relative Risk (95% CI)[b]
ENVIRONMENTAL			
New Studies			
Consonni et al., 2008	Seveso residents (men and women)—25-year follow-up		
	Zone A	0	nr
	Zone B (Bertazzi et al. [2001, 1997] reported 4 HD cases in Zone B)	3	2.2 (0.7–6.9)
	Zone R	9	0.9 (0.5–1.9)
Miligi et al., 2006	Italian case–control study—herbicide exposure in men, women with diagnosis of HD	6	0.4 (0.2–1.2)
Read et al., 2007	Residents of New Plymouth Territorial Authority, New Zealand near plant manufacturing 2,4,5-T (1962–1987)		
	Incidence	49	1.1 (0.8–1.5)[d]
	1970–1974	9	1.2 (0.6–2.3)
	1975–1979	9	1.1 (0.5–2.2)
	1980–1984	8	1.1 (0.5–2.1)
	1985–1989	9	1.3 (0.6–2.5)
	1990–1994	7	1.3 (0.5–2.7)
	1995–1999	4	0.7 (0.2–1.7)
	2000–2001	3	1.0 (0.2–3.1)
	Mortality	22	1.3 (0.8–2.0)[d]
	1970–1974	7	1.6 (0.7–3.3)
	1975–1979	4	1.2 (0.3–3.0)
	1980–1984	6	2.1 (0.8–4.5)
	1985–1989	3	1.2 (0.2–3.5)
	1990–1994	1	0.6 (0.0–3.5)
	1995–1999	1	0.6 (0.0–3.6)
	2000–2001	0	nr
Studies Reviewed in *Update 2006*			
Pahwa et al., 2006	Canadian men (at least 19 years old) in any of 6 provinces		
	Any phenoxy herbicide	65	1.0 (0.7–1.4)
	2,4-D	57	1.0 (0.7–1.4)
	Mecoprop	20	1.3 (0.7–2.2)
	MCPA	11	1.2 (0.6–2.6)
Studies Reviewed in *Update 2000*			
Bertazzi et al., 2001	Seveso residents—20-year follow-up		
	Zone A, B—men	2	2.6 (0.6–10.9)
	women	2	3.7 (0.9–16.0)
Viel et al., 2000	Residents around French municipal solid-waste incinerator—incidence	9	1.5 (nr)
Studies Reviewed in *Update 1998*			
Bertazzi et al., 1997	Seveso residents—15-year follow-up		
	Zone B—men	2	3.3 (0.4–11.9)
	women	2	6.5 (0.7–23.5)
	Zone R—women	4	1.9 (0.5–4.9)

continued

TABLE 6-41 Continued

Reference	Study Population[a]	Exposed Cases[b]	Estimated Relative Risk (95% CI)[b]
Studies Reviewed in *Update 1996*			
Bertazzi	Seveso residents—10-year follow-up—incidence		
et al., 1993	Zone B—men	1	1.7 (0.2–12.8)
	women	1	2.1 (0.3–15.7)
	Zone R—men	4	1.1 (0.4–3.1)
	women	3	1.0 (0.3–3.2)

ABBREVIATIONS: 2,4-D, 2,4-dichlorophenoxyacetic acid; AHS, Agricultural Health Study; CI, confidence interval; HD, Hodgkin's disease; IARC, International Agency for Research on Cancer; MCPA, 2-methyl-4-chlorophenoxyacetic acid; NHL, non-Hodgkin's lymphoma; NIOSH, National Institute for Occupational Safety and Health; nr, not reported; ns, not significant; PCDDs, chlorinated dibenzo-*p*-dioxins (highly chlorinated, if four or more chlorines); PM, proportionate mortality; TCDD, 2,3,7,8-tetrachlorodibenzo-*p*-dioxin; USDA, US Department of Agriculture.
[a]Subjects are male and outcome is mortality unless otherwise noted.
[b]Given when available; results other than estimated risk explained individually.
[c]Lymphopoietic cancers comprise all forms of lymphoma (including Hodgkin's disease and non-Hodgkin's lymphoma) and leukemia (ALL, AML, CLL, CML).
[d]Committee computed total SMR and SIR by dividing sum of observed values by sum of expected values over all years, 95% CIs on these total ratios were computed with exact methods.
Studies in italics have been superseded by newer studies of same cohorts.

Update of the Epidemiologic Literature

Vietnam-Veteran Studies   Cypel and Kang (2008) compiled and analyzed the data on two cohorts of female veterans who served in Vietnam (the Vietnam-veteran cohort, n = 4,586) or served elsewhere during the Vietnam War (the era-veteran cohort, n = 5,325). All-cause mortality and cause-specific mortality in the Vietnam-veteran cohort, the era-veteran cohort, the US population, and earlier research were compared. Similar analyses were performed for nurses only. Eighteen deaths attributed to lymphopoietic cancer were observed in the Vietnam veterans (crude rate, 1.22/10,000), and 29 in the era-veterans, for an adjusted RR of 0.68 (95% CI 0.37–1.25). No excess risk was observed in the nurses-only analysis (RR = 0.65, 95% CI 0.32–1.30).

Occupational Studies   Hansen et al. (2007) conducted a historical-cohort study of 3,156 male gardeners who were members of a Danish union and reported their findings in terms of lymphohematopoietic cancers (ICD-7 200–2005), which include HD. In the 10-year follow-up (Hansen et al., 1992), the 15 cases of lymphohematopoietic cancers observed had included no cases of HD. The 25-year follow-up did not specify the breakdown of the lymphohematopoietic cancers, so it is not certain whether the additional 27 cases observed in the last 15 years included any cases of HD. The statistics on NHL in Table 8-43 are not repeated here in Table 8-41, because if any cases of HD did occur, it is not known how they were distributed over the three birth periods that were used as surrogates for potential exposure to pesticides and herbicides in the more recent analysis.

Environmental Studies   Consonni et al. (2008) reported on a mortality follow-up of the Seveso cohort of 273,108 subjects who were resident at the time of the accident or immigrated or were born in the 10 years thereafter. Analyses were performed according to three zones with increasing soil TCDD contamination. In the overall sample, no statistically significant increases in deaths from HD were observed. No deaths from HD were observed in Zone A, the zone with very high TCDD contamination. Zone B, the high-contamination zone, had three HD deaths (RR = 2.15, 95% CI 0.67–6.86), and Zone R, the low contamination zone, had nine HD deaths (RR = 0.94, 95% CI 0.46–1.89).

Miligi et al. (2006) reported further results of a population-based case–control study carried out in 11 areas of Italy that was included in *Update 2004* (Miligi et al., 2003). Newly diagnosed cases of hematolymphopoietic malignancies (NHL, CLL, leukemia, HD, and multiple myeloma) were identified during 1991–1993. The control group comprised a random sample of the residents of each area. No significant association was found between exposure to herbicides and HD in men (OR = 0.4, 95% CI 0.1–1.3), in women (OR = 0.5, 95% CI 0.1–4.0), or in men and women combined (OR = 0.4, 95% CI 0.2–1.2).

Read et al. (2007) conducted a follow-up of residents of the coastal community of Paritutu, New Plymouth, near the Ivon Watkins–Dow Limited plant in which 2,4,5-T was manufactured. They reported that the body burden of TCDD was comparable with that in residents of Zone B in the Seveso area. Incidence and mortality were ascertained for the period 1970–2001, and increased risks were found especially for mortality (SMR = 1.3, 95% CI 0.8–2.0), but the confidence intervals were wide and included the null. There was also a weaker, positive association with incidence (SIR = 1.11, 95% CI 0.8–1.5).

Biologic Plausibility

HD arises from the malignant transformation of a germinal center B cell and is characterized by malignant cells that have a distinctive structure and phenotype; these binucleate cells are known as Reed–Sternberg cells (Jaffe et al., 2008). No animal studies have shown an increase in HD after exposure to the chemicals of interest. Reed–Sternberg cells have not been demonstrated in mice or rats, so there is no good animal model of HD. Thus, there are no specific animal data to support the biologic plausibility of the development of HD after exposure to the chemicals of interest.

The biologic plausibility of the carcinogenicity of the chemicals of interest is discussed in general at the beginning of this chapter.

Synthesis

The relative rarity of HD complicates the evaluation of epidemiologic studies because their statistical power is generally quite low. Earlier studies (Eriksson et al., 1992; Hardell et al., 1981; Holmes et al., 1986; LaVecchia et al., 1989; Persson et al., 1993; Rix et al., 1998; Waterhouse et al., 1996; Wiklund et al., 1988) were generally well conducted and included excellent characterization of exposure, and they formed the basis of previous committees' conclusions. The present committee believes that the small amount of additional information available to it does not contradict those findings, especially given that most studies had low statistical power. Although it has not been demonstrated as clearly as for NHL, a positive association between the chemicals of interest and the development of HD is biologically plausible because of the common lymphoreticular origin of HD and NHL and their common risk factors.

Conclusion

On the basis of the evidence reviewed here and in previous VAO reports, the committee concludes that there is sufficient evidence of an association between exposure to at least one of the chemicals of interest and HD.

Non-Hodgkin's Lymphoma

NHL (ICD-9 200.0–200.8, 202.0–202.2, 202.8–202.9) is a general name for cancers of the lymphatic system other than HD. NHL comprises a large group of lymphomas that can be partitioned into acute, aggressive (fast-growing) or chronic, indolent (slow-growing) types of either B-cell or T-cell origin. B-cell NHL includes Burkitt lymphoma, diffuse large B-cell lymphoma, follicular lymphoma, large-cell lymphoma, precursor B-lymphoblastic lymphoma, and mantle-cell lymphoma. T-cell NHL includes mycosis fungoides, anaplastic large-cell lymphoma, and precursor T-lymphoblastic lymphoma. Although CLL and HCL share many traits with NHL (including B-cell origin and immunohistochemical properties) and may progress to an acute aggressive form of NHL, they have usually been classified with leukemias; in response to requests from VA, CLL and HCL are discussed separately after the general section on leukemia.

ACS estimated that 35,450 men and 30,670 women would receive diagnoses of NHL in the United States in 2008 and that 9,790 men and 9,370 women would die from it (Jemal et al., 2008a). The incidence of NHL is uniformly higher in men than in women and typically higher in whites than in blacks. In the groups

TABLE 6-42 Average Annual Incidence (per 100,000) of Non-Hodgkin's Lymphoma in United States[a]

	50–54 Years Old			55–59 Years Old			60–64 Years Old		
	All Races	White	Black	All Races	White	Black	All Races	White	Black
Men	27.2	27.9	29.6	38.0	39.3	38.4	53.1	56.1	38.7
Women	19.1	19.5	18.9	28.3	29.2	23.6	38.4	41.1	30.0

[a]Surveillance, Epidemiology, and End Results program, nine standard registries, crude age-specific rates, 2000–2005.

that characterize most Vietnam veterans, incidence increases with age. Average annual incidences are shown in Table 6-42.

The causes of NHL are poorly understood. People with suppressed or compromised immune systems are known to be at higher risk, and some studies show an increased incidence in people who have HIV, human T-cell leukemia virus type I, Epstein–Barr virus, and gastric *Helicobacter pylori* infections. Behavioral, occupational, and environmental risk factors also have been proposed (Blair et al., 1997).

Conclusions from *VAO* and Previous Updates

The committee responsible for *VAO* concluded that there was sufficient evidence to support an association between exposure to at least one of the chemicals of interest and NHL. Additional information available to the committees responsible for *Update 1996*, *Update 1998*, *Update 2000*, *Update 2002*, *Update 2004*, and *Update 2006* did not change that conclusion. Table 6-43 summarizes the results of the relevant studies.

Update of the Epidemiologic Literature

Vietnam-Veteran Studies Cypel and Kang (2008) compiled and analyzed the data on two cohorts of female veterans who served in Vietnam (the Vietnam-veteran cohort, n = 4,586) or served elsewhere during the Vietnam War (the era-veteran cohort, n = 5,325). All-causes mortality and cause-specific mortality in the Vietnam-veteran and era-veteran cohorts, the US population, and earlier research were compared. Similar analyses were performed for nurses only. Eighteen deaths attributed to lymphopoietic cancer were observed in the Vietnam veterans (crude rate, 1.22/10,000) and 29 deaths in the era-veterans, for an adjusted RR of 0.68 (95% CI 0.37–1.25). No excess risk was observed in the nurses-only analysis (RR = 0.65, 95% CI 0.32–1.30).

TABLE 6-43 Selected Epidemiologic Studies—Non-Hodgkin's Lymphoma

Reference	Study Population[a]	Exposed Cases[b]	Estimated Relative Risk (95% CI)[b]
VIETNAM VETERANS			
New Studies			
Cypel and Kang, 2008	US Vietnam veterans—women (lymphopoietic cancers[c])	18	0.7 (0.4–1.3)
	Vietnam-veteran nurses	14	0.7 (0.3–1.3)
Studies Reviewed in *Update 2006*			
ADVA, 2005a	Australian male Vietnam veterans vs Australian population—incidence	126	0.7 (0.6–0.8)
	Navy	31	0.8 (0.5–1.0)
	Army	86	0.7 (0.5–0.8)
	Air Force	9	0.5 (0.2–0.9)
ADVA, 2005b	Australian male Vietnam veterans vs Australian population—mortality	70	0.8 (0.6–1.0)
	Navy	10	0.5 (0.3–0.9)
	Army	52	0.9 (0.6–1.1)
	Air Force	8	0.9 (0.4–1.6)
ADVA, 2005c	Australian male conscripted Army National Service Vietnam-era veterans: deployed vs nondeployed		
	Incidence	35	1.1 (0.7–1.9)
	Mortality	21	1.4 (0.7–2.8)
Boehmer et al., 2004	Vietnam Experience Cohort	6	0.9 (0.3–2.9)
Studies Reviewed in *Update 2004*			
Akhtar et al., 2004	White Air Force Ranch Hand veterans (lymphopoietic cancer[c])—incidence		
	Ranch Hand veterans	10	0.9 (0.4–1.5)
	Comparison Air Force veterans	9	0.6 (0.3–1.0)
Studies Reviewed in *Update 2000*			
AFHS, 2000	Air Force Ranch Hand veterans—incidence	1	0.2 (0.0–2.6)
AIHW, 1999			Expected number of exposed cases (95% CI)
	Australian Vietnam veterans—incidence (validation study)	62	48 (34–62)
CDVA, 1998a	Australian Vietnam veterans—self-reported incidence	137	48 (34–62)
CDVA, 1998b	Australian Vietnam veterans (women)—self-reported incidence	2	0 (0–4)
Studies Reviewed in *Update 1998*			
CDVA, 1997a	Australian military Vietnam veterans NHL deaths, 1980–1994	33	0.9 (0.6–1.2)
Watanabe and Kang, 1996	Marine Vietnam veterans (ICDA-8 200, 202)	46	1.7 (1.2–2.2)
Studies Reviewed in *Update 1996*			
Visintainer et al., 1995	PM study of deaths (1974–1989) of Michigan Vietnam-era veterans—deployed vs nondeployed	32	1.5 (1.0–2.1)

TABLE 6-43 Continued

Reference	Study Population[a]	Exposed Cases[b]	Estimated Relative Risk (95% CI)[b]
Studies Reviewed in *VAO*			
Clapp et al., 1991	Massachusetts Vietnam veterans		1.2 (0.6–2.4)
Dalager et al., 1991	US Vietnam veterans—incidence	100	1.0 (0.7–1.5)
O'Brien et al., 1991	Army enlisted Vietnam veterans (all lymphomas)	7	1.8 (nr)
Thomas et al., 1991	US Vietnam veterans—women (NHL, ICD-8 200, 200–203, 208)	3	1.3 (0.3–1.8)
Watanabe et al., 1991	Army Vietnam veterans vs non-Vietnam veterans (ICD-8 200, 202)	140	0.8 (nr)
	Army Vietnam veterans vs combined Army and Marine Vietnam-era veterans (ICD-8 200, 202)	140	0.9 (nr)
	Marine Vietnam veterans vs non-Vietnam veterans (ICD-8 200, 202)	42	1.8 (1.3–2.4)
	Marine Vietnam veterans vs combined Army and Marine Vietnam-era veterans (ICDA-8 200, 202)	42	1.2 (nr)
CDC, 1990b	US Vietnam veterans born 1921–1953—incidence	99	1.5 (1.1–2.0)
	Army Vietnam veterans	45	1.2 (0.8–1.8)
	Marine Vietnam veterans	10	1.8 (0.8–4.3)
	Air Force Vietnam veterans	12	1.0 (0.5–2.2)
	Navy Vietnam veterans	32	1.9 (1.1–3.2)
	Blue Water Navy Vietnam veterans	28	2.2 (1.2–3.9)
Michalek et al., 1990	Air Force Ranch Hand veterans—mortality Lymphatic and hematopoietic tissue	0	nr
Wolfe et al., 1990	Air Force Ranch Hand veterans—incidence	1	nr
Breslin et al., 1988	Army Vietnam veterans (ICDA-8 200, 202)	108	0.8 (0.6–1.0)
	Marine Vietnam veterans (ICDA-8 200, 202)	35	2.1 (1.2–3.8)
Garland et al., 1988	Navy enlisted personnel (white males, 1974–1983)—incidence	68	0.7 (0.5–0.9)
Burt et al., 1987	Army combat Vietnam veterans	39	1.1 (0.7–1.5)
	Marine combat Vietnam veterans	17	3.2 (1.4–7.4)
	Army Vietnam veterans (service 1967–1969)	64	0.9 (0.7–1.3)
	Marine Vietnam veterans (service 1967–1969)	17	2.5 (1.1–5.8)
Fett et al., 1987	Australian Vietnam veterans (ICD-8 200, 202)	4	1.8 (0.4–8.0)
Anderson et al., 1986	Wisconsin Vietnam veterans (includes lymphosarcoma, reticulosarcoma)	4	nr
Holmes et al., 1986	West Virginia Vietnam veterans vs West Virginia Vietnam-era veterans	2	1.1 (nr)
Lawrence et al., 1985	New York Vietnam veterans vs New York Vietnam-era veterans (all lymphomas)	10	1.0 (0.4–2.2)

continued

TABLE 6-43 Continued

Reference	Study Population[a]	Exposed Cases[b]	Estimated Relative Risk (95% CI)[b]
OCCUPATIONAL			
New Studies			
Hansen et al., 2007	Danish gardeners (lymphohematopoietic, ICD-7 200–205)—incidence		
	10-year follow-up (1975–1984) reported in		
	Hansen et al. (1992)	15	1.4 (0.8–2.4)
	NHL (ICD-7 200, 202, 205)	6	1.7 (0.6–3.8)
	HD (ICD-7 201)	0	nr
	Multiple myeloma (ICD-7 203)	0	nr
	CLL (ICD-7 204.0)	6	2.8 (1.0–6.0)
	Other leukemias (ICD-7 204.1–204.4)	3	1.4 (0.3–4.2)
	25-year follow-up (1975–2001)		
	Born before 1915 (high exposure)	16	1.4 (0.9–2.3)
	Born 1915–1934 (medium exposure)	25	1.2 (0.8–1.8)
	Born after 1934 (low exposure)	1	0.2 (0.0–1.0)
Richardson et al., 2008	German case–control study, occupational factors associated with NHL		
	Chlorophenols		
	NHL—high-grade malignancy	61	2.0 (1.3–2.9)
	NHL—low-grade malignancy	77	1.3 (1.0–1.8)
	CLL	44	0.9 (0.6–1.3)
	Herbicides		
	NHL—high-grade malignancy	56	2.2 (1.4–3.3)
	NHL—low-grade malignancy	79	1.4 (1.0–1.9)
	CLL	43	1.2 (0.8–1.7)
Samanic et al., 2006	Pesticide applicators in AHS—NHL incidence from enrollment through 2002		
	Dicamba—lifetime days exposure		
	None	39	1.0
	1– < 20	18	1.8 (1.0–3.2)
	20– < 56	14	1.3 (0.7–2.5)
	56– < 116	7	0.9 (0.4–2.2)
	≥ 116	7	1.2 (0.5–2.9)
			p-trend = 0.92
Studies Reviewed in *Update 2006*			
Chiu et al., 2006 (based on Zahm et al., 1990, 1993)	Nebraska residents (men and women), NHL reclassified according to specific chromosomal translocation (t(14;18)(q32;q21))—incidence		
	Translocation present in cases		
	Herbicides	25	2.9 (1.1–7.9)
	Translocation absent in cases		
	Herbicides	22	0.7 (0.3–1.2)

TABLE 6-43 Continued

Reference	Study Population[a]	Exposed Cases[b]	Estimated Relative Risk (95% CI)[b]
McLean et al., 2006	IARC cohort of pulp and paper workers—men, women (ICD-9 200, 202)		
	Exposure to nonvolatile organochlorine compounds		
	Never	35	0.9 (0.7–1.3)
	Ever	25	0.9 (0.6–1.3)
't Mannetje et al., 2005	Phenoxy herbicide producers (men and women)	1	0.9 (0.0–4.9)
	Phenoxy herbicide sprayers (> 99% men)	1	0.7 (0.0–3.8)
Alavanja et al., 2005	US AHS—incidence		
	Private applicators (men and women)	114	1.0 (0.8–1.2)
	Spouses of private applicators (> 99% women)	42	0.9 (0.6–1.2)
	Commercial applicators (men and women)	6	1.0 (0.4–2.1)
Blair et al., 2005a	US AHS		
	Private applicators (men and women)	33	0.9 (0.6–1.2)
	Spouses of private applicators (> 99% women)	16	1.2 (0.7–2.0)
Fritschi et al., 2005	Population-based case–control study in New South Wales, Australia, 2000–2001		
	Phenoxy herbicides		
	Nonsubstantial exposure	10	0.7 (0.3–1.7)
	Substantial exposure	5	1.8 (0.4–7.4)
Mills et al., 2005	Nested case–control analyses of Hispanic workers in cohort of 139,000 California United Farm Workers		
	Ever used 2,4-D	nr	3.8 (1.9–7.8)
Chiu et al., 2004	Herbicide use—incidence		
	Farmers (no herbicide use)	294	1.2 (1.0–1.5)
	Farmers (herbicide use)	273	1.0 (0.8–1.2)
Lee et al., 2004b	Asthmatics—incidence		
	Herbicide exposure—phenoxyacetic acid	17	1.3 (0.7–2.4)
	Exposures among farmers		
	2,4-D	17	1.3 (0.7–2.5)
	2,4,5-T	7	2.2 (0.8–6.1)
	Nonasthmatics—incidence		
	Herbicide exposure—phenoxyacetic acid	176	1.0 (0.8–1.3)
	Exposures among farmers		
	2,4-D	172	1.0 (0.8–1.3)
	2,4,5-T	36	1.1 (0.7–1.8)
Hardell et al., 2002	Pooled analysis of Swedish case–control studies of NHL, hairy-cell leukemia		
	Herbicide exposure	77	1.8 (1.3–2.4)
	Phenoxyacetic acids	64	1.7 (1.2–2.3)
	MCPA	21	2.6 (1.4–4.9)
	2,4-D, 2,4,5-T	48	1.5 (1.0–2.2)
	Other	15	2.9 (1.3–6.4)
Torchio et al., 1994	Italian licensed pesticide users (ICD-8 202.0–202.9)	15	0.9 (0.5–1.5)

continued

TABLE 6-43 Continued

Reference	Study Population[a]	Exposed Cases[b]	Estimated Relative Risk (95% CI)[b]
Reif et al., 1989	New Zealand forestry workers—nested case–control (ICD-9 200, 202)—incidence	7	1.8 (0.9–4.0)
Studies Reviewed in *Update 2004*			
Miligi et al., 2003	Residents of 11 areas in Italy (NHL other than lymphosarcoma and reticulosarcoma)—incidence		
	Phenoxy acid herbicides exposure		
	Men	18	1.0 (0.5–2.0)
	Women	11	1.3 (0.5–3.7)
	2,4-D exposure		
	Men	6	0.7 (0.3–1.9)
	Women	7	1.5 (0.4–5.7)
Bodner et al., 2003	Dow chemical production workers (included in IARC cohort, NIOSH Dioxin Registry)	nr	1.4 (0.6–2.7)
Studies Reviewed in *Update 2002*			
Burns et al., 2001	Dow 2,4-D production workers (included in IARC cohort, NIOSH Dioxin Registry)	3	1.0 (0.2–2.9)
Thörn et al., 2000	Swedish lumberjacks exposed to phenoxyacetic herbicides—incidence	2	2.3 (0.3–8.5)
Studies Reviewed in *Update 2000*			
Steenland et al., 1999	US chemical production workers (included in IARC cohort, NIOSH Dioxin Registry)	12	1.1 (0.6–1.9)
Hooiveld et al., 1998	Dutch phenoxy herbicide workers (included in IARC cohort)	3	3.8 (0.8–11.0)
Studies Reviewed in *Update 1998*			
Gambini et al., 1997	Italian rice growers	4	1.3 (0.3–3.3)
Keller-Byrne et al., 1997	Farmers in central United States	nr	1.3 (1.2–1.6)
Kogevinas et al., 1997	IARC cohort, male and female workers exposed to any phenoxy herbicide or chlorophenol	34	1.3 (0.9–1.8)
	Exposed to highly chlorinated PCDDs	24	1.4 (0.9–2.1)
	Not exposed to highly chlorinated PCDDs	9	1.0 (0.5–1.9)
Becher et al., 1996	German production workers (included in IARC cohort)	6	3.3 (1.2–7.1)
Nanni et al., 1996	Italian farming and animal-breeding workers (men and women) (NHL other than lymphosarcoma and reticulosarcoma)—incidence		
	Exposure to herbicides	3	1.4 (0.4–5.7)
Ramlow et al., 1996	Dow pentachlorophenol production workers (included in IARC cohort, NIOSH Dioxin Registry)		
	All lymphopoietic cancer (ICDA-8 200–209)		
	0-year latency	7	1.4 (0.6–2.9)
	15-year latency	5	1.3 (0.4–3.1)
	Other, unspecified lymphopoietic cancer (ICDA-8 200, 202–203, 209)		
	0-year latency	5	2.0 (0.7–4.7)
	15-year latency	4	2.0 (0.5–5.1)

TABLE 6-43 Continued

Reference	Study Population[a]	Exposed Cases[b]	Estimated Relative Risk (95% CI)[b]
Amadori et al., 1995	Italian farming, animal-breeding workers (men and women)—incidence		
	NHL, CLL combined	164	1.8 (1.2–2.6)
Studies Reviewed in *Update 1996*			
Kogevinas et al., 1995	IARC cohort (men and women)—incidence		
	Exposed to 2,4,5-T	10	1.9 (0.7–4.8)
	Exposed to TCDD	11	1.9 (0.7–5.1)
Asp et al., 1994	Finnish herbicide applicators—incidence		
	No latency	1	0.4 (0.0–2.0)
	10-year latency	1	0.4 (0.0–2.4)
Dean, 1994	Irish farmers and farm workers		
	Other malignant neoplasms of lymphoid and histiocytic tissue (including some types of NHL) (ICD–9 202)		
	Men	244	nr
	Women	84	nr
Hardell et al., 1994	Umea (Sweden) Hospital patients—incidence		
	Exposure to phenoxy herbicides	25	5.5 (2.7–11.0)
	Exposure to chlorophenols	35	4.8 (2.7–8.8)
Morrison et al., 1994	Farm operators in three Canadian provinces		
	All farm operators	nr	0.8 (0.7–0.9)
	Highest quartile of herbicides sprayed	19	2.1 (1.1–3.9)
	Highest quartile of herbicides sprayed relative to no spraying	6	3.0 (1.1–8.1)
Blair et al., 1993	US farmers in 23 states (white men)	843	1.2 (1.1–1.3)
Bloemen et al., 1993	Dow 2,4-D production workers (included in IARC cohort, NIOSH Dioxin Registry)	2	2.0 (0.2–7.1)
Bueno de Mesquita et al., 1993	Dutch phenoxy herbicide workers (included in IARC cohort)	2	3.0 (0.4–10.8)
Lynge, 1993	Danish male and female production workers (included in IARC cohort)—updated incidence		
	Exposure to phenoxy herbicides (men)	10	1.7 (0.5–4.5)
Persson et al., 1993	Swedish NHL patients		
	Exposure to phenoxy herbicides	10	2.3 (0.7–7.2)
	Occupation as lumberjack	9	6.0 (1.1–31.0)
Zahm et al., 1993	Females on eastern Nebraska farms	119	1.0 (0.7–1.4)
Kogevinas et al., 1992	IARC cohort (men and women)		
	Workers exposed to any phenoxy herbicide or chlorophenol	11	1.0 (0.5–1.7)
Studies Reviewed in *VAO*			
Ronco et al., 1992	Danish farm workers—incidence	147	1.0 (nr)
	Italian farm workers—mortality	14	1.3 (nr)

continued

TABLE 6-43 Continued

Reference	Study Population[a]	Exposed Cases[b]	Estimated Relative Risk (95% CI)[b]
Smith and	Australian residents		
Christophers,	Exposure > 1 day	15	1.5 (0.6–3.7)
1992	Exposure > 30 days	7	2.7 (0.7–9.6)
Swaen et al., 1992	Dutch herbicide applicators	0	nr
Vineis et al.,	Residents of selected Italian provinces		
1991	Male residents of contaminated areas	nr	2.2 (1.4–3.5)
Wigle et al.,	Canadian farmers		
1990	All farmers	103	0.9 (0.8–1.1)
	Spraying herbicides on 250+ acres	10	2.2 (1.0–4.6)
Zahm et al.,	Eastern Nebraska residents—incidence		
1990	Ever done farm work	147	0.9 (0.6–1.4)
	Ever mixed or applied 2,4-D	43	1.5 (0.9–2.5)
Alavanja et al., 1989	USDA forest, soil conservationists	22	2.4 (1.5–3.6)
Corrao et al.,	Italian farmers licensed to apply pesticides		
1989	Lymphatic tissue (ICD-8 200–202.9)		
	Licensed pesticide users and nonusers	45	1.4 (1.0–1.9)
	Farmers in arable land areas	31	1.8 (1.2–2.5)
LaVecchia et al., 1989	Residents of Milan, Italy, area (men and women)—incidence		
	Agricultural occupations	nr	2.1 (1.3–3.4)
Persson et al., 1989	Örebro (Sweden) Hospital (men and women)—incidence		
	Exposed to phenoxy acids	6	4.9 (1.0–27.0)
Wiklund et al., 1989b	Swedish pesticide applicators (men and women)—incidence	27	1.1 (0.7–1.6)
Alavanja et al., 1988	USDA agricultural extension agents	nr	1.2 (0.7–2.3)
Dubrow et al., 1988	Hancock County, Ohio, residents—farmers	15	1.6 (0.8–3.4)
Olsson and	Lund (Sweden) Hospital patients—incidence		
Brandt, 1988	Exposed to herbicides	nr	1.3 (0.8–2.1)
	Exposed to chlorophenols	nr	1.2 (0.7–2.0)
Wiklund et al., 1988	Swedish agricultural, forestry workers (men and women)		
	Workers in land, animal husbandry		1.0 (0.9–1.1)
	Timber cutters		0.9 (0.7–1.1)
Pearce et al.,	New Zealand residents—incidence		
1987	Farming occupations	33	1.0 (0.7–1.5)
	Fencing work	68	1.4 (1.0–2.0)
Woods et al.,	Washington state residents—incidence		
1987	Phenoxy herbicide use	nr	1.1 (0.8–1.4)
	Chlorophenol use	nr	1.0 (0.8–1.2)
	Farming occupations	nr	1.3 (1.0–1.7)
	Forestry herbicide appliers	nr	4.8 (1.2–19.4)

TABLE 6-43 Continued

Reference	Study Population[a]	Exposed Cases[b]	Estimated Relative Risk (95% CI)[b]
Hoar et al., 1986	Kansas residents—incidence		
	Farmers compared with nonfarmers	133	1.4 (0.9–2.1)
	Farmers using herbicides at least 21 days/year	7	6.0 (1.9–19.5)
Pearce et al., 1986	New Zealand residents (ICD-9 202 only)—incidence		
	Agricultural sprayers (phenoxy herbicides)	19	1.5 (0.7–3.3)
Pearce et al., 1985	New Zealand residents with agricultural occupations, 20–64 years old—incidence	224	1.4 (0.9–2.0)
Burmeister et al., 1983	Iowa residents—farming exposures	1,101	1.3 (nr)
Riihimaki et al., 1982	Finnish herbicide applicators	0	nr
Wiklund, 1983	Swedish male and female agricultural workers—incidence	476	99% CI 1.1 (0.9–1.2)
Cantor, 1982	Wisconsin residents—farmers (ICD-8 200.0, 200.1, 202.2)	175	1.2 (1.0–1.5)
Hardell et al., 1981	Umea (Sweden) Hospital patients (lymphoma and HD)—incidence		
	Exposed to phenoxy acids	41	4.8 (2.9–8.1)
	Exposed to chlorophenols	50	4.3 (2.7–6.9)
ENVIRONMENTAL			
New Studies			
Consonni et al., 2008	Seveso residents—25-year follow-up—men, women		
	Zone A	3	3.4 (1.1–10.5)
	Zone B	7	1.2 (0.6–2.6)
	Zone R	40	1.0 (0.7–1.4)
Eriksson et al., 2008	NHL case–control study of exposure to pesticides in Sweden (men and women)—incidence		
	Herbicides, total	74	1.7 (1.2–2.5)
	≤ 20 days	36	1.6 (1.0–2.7)
	> 20 days	38	1.9 (1.1–3.2)
	Phenoxyacetic acids	47	2.0 (1.2–3.4)
	≤ 45 days	32	2.8 (1.5–5.5)
	> 45 days	15	1.3 (0.6–2.7)
	MCPA	21	2.8 (1.3–6.2)
	≤ 32 days	15	3.8 (1.4–10.5)
	> 32 days	6	1.7 (0.5–6.0)
	2,4,5-T, 2,4-D	33	1.6 (0.9–3.0)
	≤ 29 days	21	2.1 (1.0–4.4)
	> 29 days	12	1.3 (0.6–3.1)

continued

TABLE 6-43 Continued

Reference	Study Population[a]	Exposed Cases[b]	Estimated Relative Risk (95% CI)[b]
Miligi et al., 2006	Italian case–control study of hematolymphopoietic malignancies		
	NHL or CLL—ever exposed to herbicides		
	Men and women	73	1.0 (0.7–1.4)
	Men	49	0.8 (0.5–1.3)
	Women	24	1.3 (0.7–2.5)
	NHL (men and women)		
	Phenoxy herbicides—ever	32	1.1 (0.6–1.8)
	Probability of use more than "low," lack of protective equipment	13	2.4 (0.9–7.6)
	2,4-D—ever	17	0.9 (0.5–1.8)
	Probability of use more than "low," lack of protective equipment	9	4.4 (1.1–29.1)
	MCPA—ever	18	0.9 (0.4–1.8)
	Probability of use more than "low," lack of protective equipment	7	3.4 (0.8–23.2)
Read et al., 2007	Residents of New Plymouth Territorial Authority, New Zealand near plant manufacturing 2,4,5-T (1962–1987)		
	Incidence	223	1.0 (0.9–1.1)[d]
	1970–1974	33	1.8 (1.2–2.5)
	1975–1979	29	1.3 (0.9–1.9)
	1980–1984	22	0.8 (0.5–1.3)
	1985–1989	24	0.7 (0.5–1.1)
	1990–1994	35	0.8 (0.6–1.1)
	1995–1999	61	1.1 (0.8–1.4)
	2000–2001	19	0.8 (0.5–1.3)
	Mortality	138	1.1 (0.9–1.3)[d]
	1970–1974	19	1.6 (0.9–2.4)
	1975–1979	24	1.6 (1.0–2.4)
	1980–1984	14	1.0 (0.5–1.6)
	1985–1989	25	1.3 (0.9–2.0)
	1990–1994	23	0.9 (0.6–1.4)
	1995–1999	21	0.7 (0.4–1.1)
	2000–2001	12	1.0 (0.5–1.8)
Spinelli et al., 2007	Case–control study in British Columbia, Canada		
	Total dioxin-like PCBs		
	Lowest quartile	82	1.0
	Second quartile	96	1.4 (0.9–2.2)
	Third quartile	82	1.6 (1.0–2.5)
	Highest quartile	143	2.4 (1.5–3.7)
			p-trend < 0.001

TABLE 6-43 Continued

Reference	Study Population[a]	Exposed Cases[b]	Estimated Relative Risk (95% CI)[b]
Xu et al., 2007	Case–control study of nasal NK/T-cell lymphomas in East Asia (men and women)—incidence		
	Pesticide use	23	4.0 (2.0–8.1)
	Herbicide	13	3.2 (1.4–7.4)
	Insecticide	20	3.5 (1.7–7.1)
	Fungicide	10	6.1 (2.0–18.5)
Studies Reviewed in *Update 2006*			
Hartge et al., 2005	NCI SEER case–control study (Iowa, Los Angeles County, Detroit, Seattle) 1998–2000		
	Exposures to 2,4-D in carpet dust (ng/g)		
	Under detection limit	147	1.0
	< 500	257	1.1 (0.8–1.6)
	500–999	86	0.9 (0.6–1.5)
	1,000–9,999	165	0.7 (0.5–1.0)
	> 10,000	24	0.8 (0.4–1.7)
Kato et al., 2004	Population-based case–control study in upstate New York, women, 20–79 years old, 1995–1998		
	Home use only of herbicides, pesticides (times)		
	0	231	1.0
	1–4	33	0.9 (0.5–1.5)
	5–17	30	0.7 (0.4–1.3)
	18–39	27	1.0 (0.6–1.7)
	≥ 40	40	0.9 (0.5–1.5)
Studies Reviewed in *Update 2004*			
Floret et al., 2003	Residents near French municipal solid-waste incinerator—incidence		
	High exposure category	31	2.3 (1.4–3.8)
Studies Reviewed in *Update 2002*			
Hardell et al., 2001	Case–control study of NHL—TEQ > 27.8, EA > 80	8	2.8 (0.5–18.0)
McDuffie et al., 2001	Case–control study of NHL in Canada		
	Exposed to phenoxy herbicides	131	1.4 (1.1–1.8)
	2,4-D	111	1.3 (1.0–1.7)
	Mecoprop	53	2.3 (1.6–3.4)
Studies Reviewed in *Update 2000*			
Bertazzi et al., 2001	Seveso residents—20-year follow-up		
	Zone A, B—men	3	1.2 (0.4–3.9)
	women	4	1.8 (0.7–4.9)
Viel et al., 2000	Residents near French solid-waste incinerator—incidence		
	Spatial cluster	286	1.3 (p = 0.00003)
	1991–1994	109	1.8 (p = 0.00003)

continued

TABLE 6-43 Continued

Reference	Study Population[a]	Exposed Cases[b]	Estimated Relative Risk (95% CI)[b]
Studies Reviewed in Update 1998			
Bertazzi	Seveso residents—15-year follow-up		
et al., 1997	Zone B—men	2	1.5 (0.2–5.3)
	Zone R—men	10	1.1 (0.5–2.0)
	women	8	0.9 (0.4–1.7)
Studies Reviewed in Update 1996			
Bertazzi	Seveso residents—10-year follow-up—incidence		
et al., 1993	Zone B—men	3	2.3 (0.7–7.4)
	women	1	0.9 (0.1–6.4)
	Zone R—men	12	1.3 (0.7–2.5)
	women	10	1.2 (0.6–2.3)
Studies Reviewed in VAO			
Lampi et al., 1992	Finnish community exposed to chlorophenol contamination (men and women)—incidence	16	2.8 (1.4–5.6)
Pesatori	Seveso residents—incidence		
et al., 1992	Zones A, B—men	3	1.9 (0.6–6.1)
	women	1	0.8 (0.1–5.5)
	Zone R—men	13	1.4 (0.7–2.5)
	women	10	1.1 (0.6–2.2)
Bertazzi	Seveso residents—10-year follow-up		
et al., 1989b	Zone B—women (ICD-9 200–208)	2	1.0 (0.3–4.2)
	Zone R—men (ICD-9 202)	3	1.0 (0.3–3.4)
	women (ICD-9 202)	4	1.6 (0.5–4.7)

ABBREVIATIONS: 2,4-D, 2,4-dichlorophenoxyacetic acid; 2,4,5-T, 2,4,5-trichlorophenoxyacetic acid; AHS, Agricultural Health Study; CI, confidence interval; CLL, chronic lymphocytic leukemia; EA, Epstein-Barr virus early antigen; HD, Hodgkin's disease; IARC, International Agency for Research on Cancer; ICD, International Classification of Diseases; ICDA, International Classification of Diseases, Adapted for Use in the United States; MCPA, 2-methyl-4-chlorophenoxyacetic acid; NCI, National Cancer Institute; NHL, non-Hodgkin's lymphoma; NIOSH, National Institute for Occupational Safety and Health; nr, not reported; PCB, polychlorinated biphenyl; PCDDs, chlorinated dibenzo-*p*-dioxins (highly chlorinated, if four or more chlorines); PM, proportionate mortality; SEER, Surveillance, Epidemiology, and End Results; SIR, standard incidence ratio; TEQ, toxicity equivalent quotient; USDA, US Department of Agriculture.

[a]Subjects are male and outcome is mortality unless otherwise noted.
[b]Given when available; results other than estimated risk explained individually.
[c]Lymphopoietic cancers comprise all of forms of lymphoma (including Hodgkin's disease and non-Hodgkin's lymphoma) and leukemia (ALL, AML, CLL, CML).
[d]Committee computed total SMR and SIR by dividing sum of observed values by sum of expected values over all years; 95% CIs on these total ratios were computed with exact methods.
Studies in italics have been superseded by newer studies of same cohorts.

Occupational Studies   Hansen et al. (2007) conducted a historical-cohort study of 3,156 male gardeners who were members of a Danish union (the study was first reported in *VAO* as Hansen et al., 1992). Subjects were then followed up by using population and cancer registries, and the incidence of cancer from 1975 until the end of 2001 was ascertained. Birth date served as a surrogate for potential exposure to pesticides and herbicides; earlier cohorts represented higher potential exposures. An association in those born before 1915 (presumptive high exposure) was found for cancers of the lymphatic and hematopoietic tissue (ICD 200–205) (RR = 1.40, 95% CI 0.86–2.28).

Richardson et al. (2008) conducted a population-based case–control study of incident NHL and CLL in men and women 15–75 years old who lived in six German counties during 1986–1998. Control subjects were selected randomly from German population registries and were matched individually to cases by sex, age, and region; two controls per case were recruited. The job–exposure matrix developed by Pannett and co-workers in the middle 1990s was used to assign exposures to chemicals that subjects were presumably exposed to occupationally. NHL was classified as "high" or "low" grade by using the Kiel classification. On the basis of an analysis whereby cumulative exposure (the sum across jobs of the product of the number of hours exposed, intensity, and probability of exposure) was categorized in three levels, there was some evidence that risk increased with increasing cumulative exposure. This metric of cumulative exposure is difficult to interpret because it combines duration of exposure (continuous) with rank-ordered scales of intensity and probability; for example, an intensity coded as 2 and a probability coded as 1 yield the same product as an intensity coded as 1 and a probability coded as 2. Moreover, simple categorization of exposure can obscure trends in the data that can be seen with other techniques that make use of the continuous nature of the data (such as natural cubic spline functions).

In a report on the AHS, Samanic et al. (2006) conducted an analysis of the incidence of NHL and exposure to dicamba in male pesticide applicators. With a metric defined as a lifetime exposure days, the rate ratios comparing subjects exposed to dicamba with those not exposed, a 75% excess risk was observed in the lowest quintile (less than 20 exposure days) (RR = 1.75, 95% CI 0.96–3.21), but the rate ratios declined with higher exposures (p for linear trend = 0.92). Similar results were obtained by using a metric defined as "intensity-weighted lifetime exposure days" (data not shown; p for linear trend = 0.68).

Environmental Studies   Consonni et al. (2008) reported on a 25-year follow-up through 2001 conducted on the population in the area of the accident that occurred in Seveso in 1976. The number of deaths from NHL in Zones A (very high TCDD contamination) and B (high TCDD contamination) had increased to 10 from the seven reported in the 20-year follow-up (Bertazzi et al., 2001), and the excess mortality from NHL in men and women combined in the zone closest to the accident (SMR = 3.4, 95% CI 1.1–10.5) was now statistically significant but was based on only three deaths.

Eriksson et al. (2008) conducted a population-based case–control study of histologically confirmed NHL in men and women 18–74 years old who lived in Sweden during 1999–2002. Controls were selected randomly from the Swedish population registry and were frequency-matched to cases by age and sex. Information was obtained from subjects with self-administered questionnaires and was followed up with interviews if information was lacking; thus, exposure to herbicides was based on self-reports. Positive associations were found between all herbicides combined, phenoxyacetic acid, and 2-methyl-4-chlorophenoxyacetic acid (MCPA) and NHL, but there was no discernable gradient by duration of exposure.

Miligi et al. (2006) reported further results of a population-based case–control study carried out in 11 areas of Italy that was included in *Update 2004* (Miligi et al., 2003). Newly diagnosed cases of hematolymphopoietic malignancies that occurred (NHL, CLL, leukemia, HD, and multiple myeloma) were identified during 1991–1993. The control group comprised a random sample of the population of each area. The reported results combined NHL and CLL and showed an association with exposure (medium or high probability of use) to phenoxy herbicides (OR = 2.4, 95% CI 0.9–7.6), 2,4-D (OR = 4.4, 95% CI 1.1–29.1), and MCPA (OR = 3.4, 95% CI 0.8–23.2). Those associations are stronger than the ones reported in the author's previous paper.

Read et al. (2007) conducted a follow-up of residents of the coastal community of Paritutu, New Plymouth, near the Ivon Watkins–Dow Limited plant in which 2,4,5-T was manufactured. It was reported that the body burden of TCDD was comparable with that in residents of Zone B of the Seveso area. Incidence and mortality were ascertained for the period 1970–2001, and RRs were no more than 10% greater than expected.

Spinelli et al. (2007) conducted a population-based case–control study of histologically confirmed NHL in men and women 20–79 years old who lived in the greater metropolitan areas of Vancouver and Victoria, British Columbia, during 2000–2004. Population controls, frequency-matched to cases by 5-year age groups and area, were identified from the client registry of the provincial healthcare system. A random subset of controls was included in the analyses. The analyses were based on serum concentrations of organochlorines and related chemicals obtained from controls at the time of interview and from cases before chemotherapy. Cases who lost weight rapidly were excluded. Strong monotonic increases in risk by serum concentrations were found individually for two of the dioxin-like polychlorinated biphenyls (PCBs)—PCB-118 (p = 0.004) and PCB-156 (p = 0.004)—and for all three measured dioxin-like congeners combined (p < 0.001), but not for PCB-105 alone.

Xu et al. (2007) conducted a hospital-based, incident case–control study of sinonasal NK/T-cell lymphoma, a lethal granuloma infrequently observed in

Western populations, in 2000–2005 in selected cities in Japan, Korea, and China. They identified 126 cases and matched 305 control subjects who had a variety of other conditions (inflammatory diseases, hearing problems, benign cystic diseases, or otolaryngologic problems) by hospital. Subjects completed a self-administered questionnaire on a variety of possible risk factors. Little information was provided on the type of questions asked or on their validity or reliability. Increases in risks were found in association with ever using pesticides (OR = 4.0, 95% CI 2.0–8.1) and more specifically for any use of herbicides (OR = 3.2, 95% CI 1.4–7.4), but the risks associated with insecticide use (OR = 3.5, 95% CI 1.7–7.1) or fungicide use (OR = 6.1, 95% CI 2.0–18.5) were at least as high.

Biologic Plausibility

The diagnosis of NHL encompasses a wide variety of lymphoma subtypes. In humans, about 85% are of B-cell origin and 15% of T-cell origin. In commonly used laboratory mice, the lifetime incidence of spontaneous B-cell lymphomas is about 30% in females and about 10% in males. Although researchers seldom note the subtypes of B lymphomas observed, lymphoblastic, lymphocytic, follicular, and plasma-cell lymphomas are seen in mice and are similar to types of NHL seen in humans. Laboratory rats are less prone to develop lymphomas, but Fisher 344 rats have an increased incidence of spontaneous mononuclear cell leukemia of nonspecific origin. The lifetime incidence of leukemia is about 50% in male rats and about 20% in female rats. Neither mice nor rats develop T-cell lymphomas spontaneously at a predictable incidence, but T-cell–derived tumors can be induced by exposure to some carcinogens.

Several long-term feeding studies of various strains of mice and rats have been conducted over the last 30 years to determine the effects of TCDD on cancer incidence. Few of them have shown effects of TCDD on lymphoma or leukemia incidence. The NTP (1982a) reported no increase in overall incidence of lymphoma in female B6C3F1 mice exposed to TCDD at 0.04, 0.2, or 2.0 μg/kg per week for 104 weeks but found that histiocytic lymphomas (now considered to be equivalent to large B-cell lymphomas) were more common in the high-dose group. No effects on lymphoma incidence were seen in Osborne–Mendel rats treated with TCDD at 0.01, 0.05, or 0.5 μg/kg per week. Sprague–Dawley rats treated with TCDD at 0.003, 0.010, 0.022, 0.046, or 0.100 μg/kg per day showed no change in the development of malignant lymphomas. Long-term exposure to phenoxy herbicides or cacodylic acid also has not resulted in an increased incidence of lymphomas in laboratory animals. Thus, there are few laboratory animal data to support the biologic plausibility of promotion of NHL by TCDD or other chemicals of interest.

In contrast, recent studies indicate that activation of the AHR by TCDD inhibits apoptosis, a mechanism of cell death that controls the growth of cancer cells. Vogel et al. (2007) studied human cancer cells in tissue culture and showed that addition of TCDD inhibited apoptosis in histiocytic-lymphoma cells, Burkitt-lymphoma cells, and NHL cell lines. The reduced apoptosis was associated with an increase in the expression of Cox-2, C/EBP β, and Bcl-xL mRNA in the cells. Those expressed genes code for proteins that protect cells from apoptosis. The effects of TCDD on apoptosis were blocked when an AHR antagonist or a Cox-2 inhibitor was added to the culture, this demonstrated the underlying AHR-dependent mechanism of the effects. More important, when C57Bl/10J mice were given multiple doses of TCDD over a period of 140 days, premalignant lymphoproliferation of B cells was induced in the TCDD-treated mice before the appearance of any spontaneous lymphomas in the control mice. When the B cells were examined, they were found to manifest changes in gene expression similar to those induced by TCDD in the human cell lines, providing support for this mechanism of lymphoma promotion by TCDD.

Recent evidence has shown that AHR activation by TCDD in human breast and endocervical cell lines induces sustained high levels of the IL–6 cytokine, which has tumor promotional effects in numerous tissues (Hollingshead et al., 2008). IL–6 plays a role in B-cell maturation and induces a transcriptional inflammatory response. It is known to be elevated in B-cell neoplasms, including multiple myeloma and various lymphomas, especially diffuse large B-cell lymphoma (Hussein et al., 2002; Kato et al., 1998; Kovacs, 2006).

An alternative link that could help to explain the association between TCDD and NHL has been explored in human studies. Chromosomal rearrangements, with consequent expression dysregulation of various genes, are very prevelant in B-cell lymphomas, and the t(14;18) reciprocal translocation, which juxtaposes the BCL2 with the locus of the immunoglobin heavy chain, found in the tumor cells in most cases of follicular lymphoma.

Roulland et al. (2004) investigated the prevalence of the t(14;18) translocation characteristic of most cases of follicular lymphoma among a subset of 53 never-smoking and pesticide-using men from a cohort of French farmers whose pesticides exposures and confounding information had been previously well characterized; for 21 blood samples had been gathered during periods of high pesticide use, while for the other 32 the samples were drawn during a period of low pesticide use. They found a higher prevalence of cells carrying this translocation among the farmers whose blood had been drawn during a period of high pesticide use than among those with samples drawn during a low-use period.

Baccarelli et al. (2006) reported an increase in t(14;18) chromosomal translocations in lymphocytes from humans exposed to TCDD in the Seveso explosion. In most cases of follicular lymphoma, the tumor cells carry the t(14;18) chromosomal translocation, and there is evidence to suggest that an increased frequency of lymphocytes from the peripheral blood carrying this tumor marker may be a necessary but not sufficient step toward development of follicular lymphoma (Roulland et al., 2006).

Synthesis

Previous VAO committees found the evidence to be sufficient to support an association between exposure to at least one of the chemicals of interest and NHL. The evidence was drawn from occupational and other studies in which subjects were exposed to a variety of herbicides and herbicide components. New data generally strengthen the conclusion that there is an association with the chemicals of interest. Xu et al. (2007) reported an excess risk of nasal NK/T-cell lymphomas after uncharacterized herbicide exposure, and Miligi et al. (2006) found an increased risk in Italy after frequent and unprotected use of phenoxy herbicides. Much of the earlier epidemiologic evidence suggests that 2,4-D or 2,4,5-T, rather than TCDD, might be responsible for the associations observed in occupational cohorts, but the strongest new data available to the present committee are related to TCDD exposure: a continuing increase in lymphoma mortality in the most highly exposed zone in Seveso (Consonni et al., 2008), increased risks with higher serum concentrations of dioxin-like congeners in British Columbia (Spinelli et al., 2007), and excess risks after occupational chlorophenol exposure in a German case–control study (Richardson et al., 2008).

Conclusions

On the basis of the evidence reviewed here and in previous VAO reports, the committee concludes that there is sufficient evidence of an association between exposure to at least one of the chemicals of interest and NHL.

Multiple Myeloma

Multiple myeloma (ICD-9 203.0) is characterized by proliferation of bone marrow stem cells that results in an excess of neoplastic plasma cells and in the production of excess abnormal proteins, usually fragments of immunoglobulins. Multiple myeloma is sometimes grouped with other immunoproliferative neoplasms (ICD-9 203.8). ACS estimated that 11,190 men and 8,730 women would receive diagnoses of multiple myeloma in the United States in 2008 and that 5,640 men and 5,050 women would die from it (Jemal et al., 2008a). The average annual incidence of multiple myeloma is shown in Table 6-44.

The incidence of multiple myeloma is highly age-dependent, with a relatively low rate in people under 40 years old. The incidence is slightly higher in men than in women, and the difference becomes more pronounced with age.

An increased incidence of multiple myeloma has been observed in several occupational groups, including farmers and other agricultural workers and those with workplace exposure to rubber, leather, paint, and petroleum (Riedel et al., 1991). People with high exposure to ionizing radiation and those who suffer

TABLE 6-44 Average Annual Incidence (per 100,000) of Multiple Myeloma in United States[a]

	50–54 Years Old			55–59 Years Old			60–64 Years Old		
	All Races	White	Black	All Races	White	Black	All Races	White	Black
Men	7.2	6.2	17.2	11.9	11.0	23.6	18.9	18.2	33.3
Women	5.2	4.3	13.3	8.0	7.3	13.9	12.3	10.1	30.9

[a]Surveillance, Epidemiology, and End Results program, nine standard registries, crude age-specific rates, 2000–2005.

from other plasma-cell diseases, such as monoclonal gammopathy of unknown significance or solitary plasmacytoma, are also at greater risk.

Conclusions from *VAO* and Previous Updates

The committee responsible for *VAO* concluded that there was limited or suggestive evidence of an association between exposure to the chemicals of interest and multiple myeloma. Additional information available to the committees responsible for *Update 1996*, *Update 1998*, *Update 2000*, *Update 2002*, *Update 2004*, and *Update 2006* did not change that conclusion. Table 6-45 summarizes the results of the relevant studies.

Update of the Epidemiologic Literature

Vietnam-Veteran Studies   Cypel and Kang (2008) compiled and analyzed the data on two cohorts of female veterans who served in Vietnam (the Vietnam-veteran cohort, n = 4,586) or served elsewhere during the Vietnam War (the era-veteran cohort, n = 5,325). All causes mortality and cause-specific mortality in the Vietnam-veteran and era-veteran cohorts, the US population, and earlier research were compared. Similar analyses were performed for nurses only. Although no separate analysis examined multiple myeloma mortality specifically, 18 deaths attributed to lymphopoietic cancer were observed in the Vietnam veterans (crude rate, 1.22/10,000) and 29 deaths in the era veterans, for an adjusted RR of 0.68 (95% CI 0.37–1.25). No excess risk was observed in the nurses-only analysis (RR = 0.65, 95% CI 0.32–1.30).

Occupational Studies   Hansen et al. (2007) conducted a historical-cohort study of 3,156 male gardeners who were members of a Danish union and reported their findings in terms of lymphohematopoietic cancers (ICD-7 200–2005), which include multiple myeloma. In the 10-year follow-up (Hansen et al., 1992), the 15 cases of lymphohematopoietic cancers observed included no cases of multiple myeloma. The 25-year follow-up did not specify a breakdown of the lymphohematopoietic cancers, so it is not certain whether the additional 27 cases observed in the last 15 years included any cases of multiple myeloma. The statistics for NHL in Table 6-43 are not repeated in Table 6-45, because if any cases of multiple myeloma did occur, it is not known how they were distributed over the three birth periods that were used as surrogates for potential exposure to pesticides and herbicides in the more recent analysis.

Environmental Studies Consonni et al. (2008) conducted a follow-up of the population of the accident that occurred in Seveso in 1976. The follow-up was extended to 2001, and an association in the most highly exposed zone (Zone A) was found (RR = 4.3, 95% CI 1.1–17.5), but it was based on only two deaths from multiple myeloma.

Miligi et al. (2006) reported further results of a population-based case–control study carried out in 11 areas of Italy that was included in *Update 2004* (Miligi et al., 2003). Newly diagnosed cases of lymphohematopoietic cancers (NHL, CLL, leukemia, HD, and multiple myeloma) were identified during 1991–1993. The control group comprised a random sample of the population of each area. A nonsignificantly increased OR was seen in men and women who had multiple myeloma and were exposed to herbicides (OR = 1.6, 95% CI 0.8–3.5).

Biologic Plausibility

No animal studies have reported an association between exposure to the chemicals of interest and multiple myeloma. Thus, there are no specific animal data to support the biologic plausibility of an association between exposure to the chemicals of interest and multiple myeloma.

Recent evidence has shown that AHR activation by TCDD in human breast and endocervical cell lines induces sustained high levels of the IL–6 cytokine, which has tumor promotional effects in numerous tissues (Hollingshead et al., 2008). IL–6 plays a role in B-cell maturation and induces a transcriptional inflammatory response. It is known to be elevated in B-cell neoplasms, including multiple myeloma and various lymphomas (Hussein et al., 2002; Kovacs, 2006).

The biologic plausibility of the carcinogenicity of the chemicals of interest is discussed in general at the beginning of this chapter.

Synthesis

Only one study provided updated information on the risk of dying from multiple myeloma, and it was the most recent analysis of the Seveso incident (Consonni et al., 2008). The main limitation of the study is the small number of deaths, which is always an issue for such a rare cancer.

TABLE 6-45 Selected Epidemiologic Studies—Multiple Myeloma

Reference	Study Population[a]	Exposed Cases[b]	Estimated Relative Risk (95% CI)[b]
VIETNAM VETERANS			
New Studies			
Cypel and Kang, 2008	US Vietnam veterans—women (lymphopoietic cancers) vs nondeployed	18	0.7 (0.4–1.3)
	Vietnam-veteran nurses only	14	0.7 (0.3–1.3)
Studies Reviewed in *Update 2006*			
Boehmer et al., 2004	Vietnam Experience Cohort	1	0.4 (nr)
ADVA, 2005a	Australian male Vietnam veterans vs Australian population—incidence	31	0.7 (0.4–0.9)
	Navy	4	0.4 (0.1–1.0)
	Army	21	0.7 (0.4–1.0)
	Air Force	6	1.1 (0.4–2.4)
ADVA, 2005b	Australian male Vietnam veterans vs Australian population—mortality	24	0.9 (0.5–1.2)
	Navy	3	0.5 (0.1–1.5)
	Army	15	0.8 (0.4–1.3)
	Air Force	6	1.7 (0.6–3.6)
ADVA, 2005c	Australian male conscripted Army National Service Vietnam-era veterans—deployed vs nondeployed		
	Incidence	8	2.1 (0.7–6.0)
	Mortality	5	0.9 (0.2–3.4)
Studies Reviewed in *Update 2004*			
Akhtar et al., 2004	White Air Force Vietnam veterans (lymphopoietic cancers)—incidence		
	Ranch Hand veterans—incidence	10	0.9 (0.4–1.5)
	Comparison Air Force veterans—incidence	9	0.6 (0.3–1.0)
Studies Reviewed in *Update 2000*			
AFHS, 2000	Air Force Ranch Hand veterans	2	0.7 (0.1–5.0)
Studies Reviewed in *Update 1998*			
CDVA, 1997a	Australian military Vietnam veterans	6	0.6 (0.2–1.3)
CDVA, 1997b	Australian military Vietnam veterans	0	
Watanabe and Kang, 1996	Army Vietnam veterans	36	0.9 (nr)
	Marine Vietnam veterans	4	0.6 (nr)
Studies Reviewed in *VAO*			
Breslin et al., 1988	Army Vietnam veterans	18	0.8 (0.2–2.5)
	Marine Vietnam veterans	2	0.5 (0.0–17.1)
OCCUPATIONAL			
Studies Reviewed in *Update 2006*			
McLean et al., 2006	IARC cohort of pulp and paper workers Exposure to nonvolatile organochlorine compounds		
	Never	21	0.8 (0.5–1.3)
	Ever	20	1.1 (0.7–1.7)

TABLE 6-45 Continued

Reference	Study Population[a]	Exposed Cases[b]	Estimated Relative Risk (95% CI)[b]
't Mannetje et al., 2005	Phenoxy herbicide producers (men and women)	3	5.5 (1.1–16.1)
	Phenoxy herbicide sprayers (> 99% men)	0	0.0 (0.0–5.3)
Alavanja et al., 2005	US AHS—incidence		
	Private applicators (men and women)	43	1.3 (1.0–1.8)
	Spouses of private applicators (> 99% women)	13	1.1 (0.6–1.9)
	Commercial applicators (men and women)	0	0.0 (0.0–2.7)
Blair et al., 2005a	US AHS		
	Private applicators (men and women)	11	0.6 (0.3–1.2)
	Spouses of private applicators (> 99% women)	5	0.9 (0.3–2.1)
Torchio et al., 1994	Italian licensed pesticide users	5	0.4 (0.1–1.0)
Reif et al., 1989	New Zealand forestry workers—nested case–control—incidence	1	0.5 (0.1–3.7)
Studies Reviewed in *Update 2004*			
Swaen et al., 2004	Dow chemical production workers (included in IARC cohort, NIOSH Dioxin Registry)	3	2.1 (0.4–6.1)
Studies Reviewed in *Update 2002*			
Burns et al., 2001	Dow 2,4-D production workers (included in IARC cohort, NIOSH Dioxin Registry)	1	0.8 (0.0–4.5)
Thörn et al., 2000	Swedish lumberjacks exposed to phenoxyacetic herbicides—incidence	0	nr
Studies Reviewed in *Update 2000*			
Steenland et al., 1999	US chemical production workers (included in IARC cohort, NIOSH Dioxin Registry)	10	2.1 (1.0–3.8)
Hooiveld et al., 1998	Dutch phenoxy herbicide workers (included in IARC cohort)	0	0.0 (nr)
Studies Reviewed in *Update 1998*			
Gambini et al., 1997	Italian rice growers	0	nr
Kogevinas et al., 1997	IARC cohort, male and female workers exposed to any phenoxy herbicide or chlorophenol	17	1.3 (0.8–2.1)
	Exposed to highly chlorinated PCDDs	9	1.2 (0.6–2.3)
	Not exposed to highly chlorinated PCDDs	8	1.6 (0.7–3.1)
Becher et al., 1996	German production workers (included in IARC cohort)		
	Plant I	3	5.4 (1.1–15.9)
Studies Reviewed in *Update 1996*			
Asp et al., 1994	Finnish herbicide applicators		
	Incidence	2	1.5 (0.2–5.2)
	Mortality	3	2.6 (0.5–7.7)
Dean, 1994	Irish farmers and farm workers (men and women)		
	Men	171	1.0 (nr)
Semenciw et al., 1994	Farmers in Canadian prairie provinces	160	0.8 (0.7–1.0)
Blair et al., 1993	US farmers in 23 states	413	1.2 (1.0–1.3)

continued

TABLE 6-45 Continued

Reference	Study Population[a]	Exposed Cases[b]	Estimated Relative Risk (95% CI)[b]
Brown et al., 1993	Iowa residents who used pesticides or herbicides	111	1.2 (0.8–1.7)
Lynge, 1993	Danish production workers (included in IARC cohort)—updated incidence		
	Men	0	nr
	Women	2	12.5 (1.5–45.1)
Zahm et al., 1992	Eastern Nebraska users of herbicides		
	Men	8	0.6 (0.2–1.7)
	Women	10	2.3 (0.8–7.0)
	Eastern Nebraska users of insecticides		
	Men	11	0.6 (0.2–1.4)
	Women	21	2.8 (1.1–7.3)
Studies Reviewed in *VAO*			
Eriksson and			90% CI
Karlsson, 1992	Residents of northern Sweden	20	2.2 (1.2–4.7)
Swaen et al., 1992	Dutch herbicide applicators	3	8.2 (1.6–23.8)
Fingerhut	NIOSH cohort—entire cohort	5	1.6 (0.5–3.9)
et al., 1991	≥ 1-year exposure, ≥ 20-year latency	3	2.6 (0.5–7.7)
Saracci et al., 1991	IARC cohort (men and women)—exposed subcohort	4	0.7 (0.2–1.8)
Alavanja et al., 1989	USDA forest, soil conservationists	6	1.3 (0.5–2.8)
Boffetta et al., 1989	ACS Prevention Study II subjects	12	2.1 (1.0–4.2)
	Farmers using herbicides, pesticides	8	4.3 (1.7–10.9)
LaVecchia et al., 1989	Residents (men and women) of Milan, Italy, area		
	Agricultural occupations	nr	2.0 (1.1–3.5)
Morris et al., 1986	Residents of four SEER program areas		2.9 (1.5–5.5)
Pearce et al., 1986	New Zealand residents—agricultural sprayers		
	Use of agricultural spray	16	1.3 (0.7–2.5)
	Likely sprayed 2,4,5-T	14	1.6 (0.8–3.1)
Cantor and Blair, 1984	Wisconsin residents—farmers in counties with highest herbicide use	nr	1.4 (0.8–2.3)
Burmeister et al., 1983	Iowa residents—farming exposures		
	Born 1890–1900	nr	2.7 (p < 0.05)
	Born after 1900	nr	2.4 (p < 0.05)
Riihimaki et al., 1982	Finnish herbicide applicators		Expected number of exposed cases
		1	0.2 (nr)
ENVIRONMENTAL			
New Studies			
Consonni et al., 2008	Seveso residents—25-year follow-up—men, women		
	Zone A	2	4.3 (1.1–17.5)

TABLE 6-45 Continued

Reference	Study Population[a]	Exposed Cases[b]	Estimated Relative Risk (95% CI)[b]
	Zone B	5	1.7 (0.7–4.1)
	Zone R	24	1.1 (0.7–1.7)
Miligi et al., 2006	Italian case–control study—herbicide exposure among men, women with diagnosis of multiple myeloma	11	1.6 (0.8–3.5)
Studies Reviewed in *Update 2006*			
Pahwa et al., 2006	Canadian men (at least 19 years old) in any of 6 provinces		
	Any phenoxy herbicide	62	1.2 (0.8–1.8)
	2,4-D	59	1.3 (0.9–1.9)
	Mecoprop	16	1.2 (0.7–2.8)
	MCPA	7	0.5 (0.2–1.2)
Studies Reviewed in *Update 2000*			
Bertazzi et al., 2001	Seveso residents—20-year follow-up		
	Zone A, B—men	1	0.6 (0.1–4.3)
	women	4	3.2 (1.2–8.8)
Studies Reviewed in *Update 1998*			
Bertazzi et al., 1997	Seveso residents—15-year follow-up		
	Zone B—men	1	1.1 (0.0–6.2)
	women	4	6.6 (1.8–16.8)
	Zone R—men	5	0.8 (0.3–1.9)
	women	5	1.0 (0.3–2.3)
Studies Reviewed in *Update 1996*			
Bertazzi et al., 1993	Seveso residents—10-year follow-up—incidence		
	Zone B—men	2	3.2 (0.8–13.3)
	women	2	5.3 (1.2–22.6)
	Zone R—men	1	0.2 (0.0–1.6)
	women	2	0.6 (0.2–2.8)
Studies Reviewed in *VAO*			
Pesatori et al., 1992	Seveso residents—incidence		
	Zones A, B—men	2	2.7 (0.6–11.3)
	women	2	4.4 (1.0–18.7)
	Zone R—men	1	0.2 (0.0–1.5)
	women	3	0.9 (0.3–3.1)

ABBREVIATIONS: 2,4-D, 2,4-dichlorophenoxyacetic acid; 2,4,5-T, 2,4,5-trichlorophenoxyacetic acid; ACS, American Cancer Society; AHS, Agricultural Health Study; CI, confidence interval; IARC, International Agency for Research on Cancer; MCPA, 2-methyl-4-chlorophenoxyacetic acid; NIOSH, National Institute for Occupational Safety and Health; nr, not reported; PCDDs, chlorinated dibenzo-*p*-dioxins (highly chlorinated, if four or more chlorines); SEER, Surveillance, Epidemiology, and End Results; USDA, US Department of Agriculture.

[a]Subjects are male and outcome is mortality unless otherwise noted.

[b]Given when available; results other than estimated risk explained individually.

Studies in italics have been superseded by newer studies of same cohorts.

Conclusion

On the basis of the evidence reviewed here and in previous VAO reports, the committee concludes that there is limited or suggestive evidence of an association between exposure to at least one of the chemicals of interest and multiple myeloma.

AL Amyloidosis

The committee responsible for *Update 2006* moved the discussion of AL amyloidosis from the chapter on miscellaneous nonneoplastic health conditions to the cancer chapter to put it closer to related neoplastic conditions, such as multiple myeloma and some types of B-cell lymphoma. The conditions share several biologic features, most notably clonal hyperproliferation of B-cell-derived plasma cells and production of abnormal amounts of immunoglobulins.

The primary feature of amyloidosis (ICD-9 277.3) is the accumulation and deposition in various tissues of insoluble proteins historically denoted by the generic term "amyloid." Amyloid protein accumulates in the extracellular spaces of various tissues. The pattern of organ involvement depends on the nature of the protein; some amyloid proteins are more fibrillogenic than others. Amyloidosis is classified according to the biochemical properties of the fibril-forming protein. Excessive amyloid protein can have limited clinical consequences or can produce severe, rapidly progressive multiple–organ-system dysfunction. The annual incidence is estimated at 1/100,000; there are about 2,000 new cases each year in the United States. Amyloidosis occurs mainly in people 50–70 years old and occurs more often in males than in females.

AL amyloidosis is the most common form of systemic amyloidosis; the *A* stands for amyloid, and the *L* indicates that the amyloid protein is derived from immunoglobin light chains. That links AL amyloidosis with other B-cell disorders that involve overproduction of immunoglobin, such as multiple myeloma and some types of B-cell lymphomas. AL amyloidosis results from the abnormal overproduction of immunoglobulin light-chain protein from a monoclonal population of plasma cells. Clinical findings can include excessive AL protein or immunoglobulin fragments in the urine or serum, renal failure with nephrotic syndrome, liver failure with hepatomegaly, heart failure with cardiomegaly, marcroglossia, carpal tunnel syndrome, and peripheral neuropathy. Bone marrow biopsies commonly show an increased density of plasma cells, suggesting a premalignant state. Historically, that test emphasized routine histochemical analysis, but modern immunocytochemistry and flow cytometry now commonly identify monoclonal populations of plasma cells with molecular techniques. AL amyloidosis can progress rapidly and is often far advanced by the time it is diagnosed (Buxbaum, 2004).

Conclusions from *VAO* and Previous Updates

VA identified AL amyloidoisis as of concern after the publication of *Update 1998*. The committees responsible for *Update 2000*, *Update 2002*, and *Update 2004* concluded that there was inadequate or insufficient evidence to determine whether there is an association between exposure to the chemicals of interest and AL amyloidosis. Although there are few epidemiologic data specifically on AL amyloidosis, the committee responsible for *Update 2006* changed the categorization to limited or suggestive evidence of an association on the basis of commonalities in its cellular lineage with multiple myeloma and B-cell lymphomas.

Update of the Epidemiologic Literature

No studies concerning exposure to the chemicals of interest and amyloidosis of any sort have been published since *Update 2006*.

Biologic Plausibility

A 1979 study reported the dose-dependent development of a "generalized lethal amyloidosis" in Swiss mice that were treated with TCDD for 1 year (Toth et al., 1979). That finding has not been validated in 2-year carcinogenicity studies of TCDD in mice or rats. Thus, there are few animal data to support an association between TCDD exposure and AL amyloidosis in humans. And there are no animal data to support an association between the other chemicals of interest and AL amyloidosis.

It is known, however, that AL amyloidosis is associated with B-cell diseases and 15–20% of cases of AL amyloidosis occur with multiple myeloma. Other diagnoses associated with AL amyloidosis include B-cell lymphomas (Cohen et al., 2004), monoclonal gammopathies, and agammaglobulinemia (Rajkumar et al., 2006). Thus, AL amyloidosis can occur with such medical conditions as multiple myeloma and B-cell lymphomas.

Synthesis

AL amyloidosis is very rare and it is not likely that population-based epidemiology will ever provide substantial direct evidence regarding its causation. However, the biologic and pathophysiologic features linking AL amyloidosis, multiple myeloma, and some types of B-cell lymphomas—especially clonal hyperproliferation of plasma cells and abnormal immunoglobulin production—indicate that AL amyloidosis is pathophysiologically related to those conditions.

Conclusion

On the basis of the evidence reviewed here and in previous VAO reports, the committee concludes that there is limited or suggestive evidence of an association between exposure to the chemicals of interest and AL amyloidosis.

Leukemia

There are four primary types of leukemia (ICD-9 202.4, 203.1, 204.0–204.9, 205.0–205.9, 206.0–206.9, 207.0–207.2, 207.8, 208.0–208.9): acute and chronic lymphocytic leukemia and acute and chronic myelogenous (or granulocytic) leukemia. AML (ICD-9 205) is also commonly called acute myeloid leukemia or acute nonlymphocytic leukemia. There are numerous subtypes of AML; for consistency, the present report uses *acute myelogenous leukemia*, regardless of designations in the source materials.

ACS estimated that 25,180 men and 19,090 women would receive diagnoses of some form of leukemia in the United States in 2008 and that 12,460 men and 9,250 women would die from it (Jemal et al., 2008a). Collectively, leukemia was expected to account for 3.1% of all new diagnoses of cancer and 3.8% of deaths from cancer in 2008. The different forms of leukemia have different patterns of incidence and in some cases different risk factors. The incidences of the various forms of leukemia are presented in Table 6-46.

In adults, acute leukemia is nearly always in the form of AML (ICD-9 205.0, 207.0, 207.2). ACS estimated that about 7,200 men and 6,090 women would receive new diagnoses of AML in the United States in 2008 and that 5,100 men and 3,720 women would die from it (Jemal et al., 2008a). In the age groups that include most Vietnam veterans, AML makes up roughly one-fourth of cases of leukemia in men and one-third in women. Overall, AML is slightly more common in men than in women. Risk factors associated with AML include high doses of ionizing radiation, occupational exposure to benzene, and exposure to some medications used in cancer chemotherapy (such as melphalan). Fanconi anemia and Down syndrome are associated with an increased risk of AML, and tobacco use is thought to account for about 20% of AML cases.

ALL is a disease of the young and of people over 70 years old. It is relatively uncommon in the age groups that include most Vietnam veterans. The lifetime incidence of ALL is slightly higher in whites than in blacks and higher in men than in women. Exposure to high doses of ionizing radiation is a known risk factor for ALL, but there is little consistent evidence on other factors.

CLL shares many traits with lymphomas (such as immunohistochemistry, B-cell origin, and progression to an acute, aggressive form of NHL), so the committee reviews it below separately from the other leukemias.

The incidence of CML increases steadily with age in people over 30 years old. Its lifetime incidence is roughly equal in whites and blacks and is slightly

TABLE 6-46 Average Annual Incidence (per 100,000) of Leukemias in United States[a]

	50–54 Years Old			55–59 Years Old			60–64 Years Old		
	All Races	White	Black	All Races	White	Black	All Races	White	Black
All leukemias:									
Men	13.2	13.6	12.1	20.7	21.7	18.0	32.7	34.0	30.2
Women	8.0	8.0	7.6	12.2	12.6	10.2	17.4	18.2	14.7
Acute lymphocytic leukemia:									
Men	0.9	0.9	0.8	0.9	0.8	0.8	1.2	1.3	0.7
Women	0.6	0.5	1.1	1.1	1.2	0.4	0.7	0.6	0.6
Acute myelogenous leukemia:									
Men	3.1	3.1	2.7	5.2	5.3	5.3	8.3	8.5	7.5
Women	2.8	2.4	2.4	4.4	4.4	3.8	5.4	5.3	6.2
Chronic lymphocytic leukemia:									
Men	5.2	5.7	5.3	9.4	10.1	6.1	15.7	16.8	12.4
Women	2.3	2.4	2.0	4.2	4.7	2.4	7.0	8.0	3.1
Chronic myelogenous leukemia:									
Men	1.9	2.0	0.9	2.3	2.3	2.7	3.6	3.6	4.3
Women	1.1	1.1	0.6	1.2	1.2	1.1	2.3	2.1	2.5
All other leukemia:[b]									
Men	0.5	0.4	0.8	0.7	0.5	2.1	1.2	1.2	1.6
Women	0.3	0.3	0.2	0.6	0.5	0.4	0.8	0.8	0.9

[a]Surveillance, Epidemiology, and End Results program, nine standard registries, crude age-specific rates, 2000–2005.
[b]Includes leukemic reticuloendotheliosis (hairy cell leukemia), plasma-cell leukemia, monocytic leukemia, and acute and chronic erythremia and erythroleukemia.

higher in men than in women. CML accounts for about one-fifth of the cases of leukemia in people in the age groups that include most Vietnam veterans. It is associated with an acquired chromosomal abnormality known as the Philadelphia chromosome, for which exposure to high doses of ionizing radiation is a known risk factor.

Little is known about the risk factors associated with other forms of leukemia. However, two human retroviruses have been linked to human leukemias: HTLV-1 causes adult T-cell leukemia or lymphoma, but early reports that HTLV-2 might play a role in the etiology of hairy cell leukemia (HCL) have not been substantiated.

Conclusions from VAO and Previous Updates

The committee responsible for VAO concluded that there was inadequate or insufficient information to determine whether there is an association between exposure to the chemicals of interest and all types of leukemia. Additional information available to the committees responsible for *Update 1996, Update 1998, Update 2000, Update 2002, Update 2004*, and *Update 2006* did not change that conclusion. The committee responsible for *Update 2002*, however, considered CLL separately and judged that there was sufficient evidence of an association with the herbicides used in Vietnam and CLL alone. The committee responsible for *Update 2006* considered AML individually but did not find evidence to suggest that its occurrence is associated with exposure to the chemicals of interest, so it was retained with other non-CLL leukemias in the category of inadequate and insufficient evidence. Table 6-47 summarizes the results of the relevant studies.

Update of the Epidemiologic Literature

Vietnam-Veteran Studies   Cypel and Kang (2008) compiled and analyzed the data on two cohorts of female veterans who served in Vietnam (the Vietnam-veteran cohort, n = 4,586) or served elsewhere during the Vietnam War (the era-veteran cohort, n = 5,325). All-cause mortality and cause-specific mortality in the Vietnam-veteran and era-veteran cohorts, the US population, and earlier research were compared. Similar analyses were performed for nurses only. Although no separate analysis examined leukemia specifically, 18 deaths attributed to lymphopoietic cancer were observed in the Vietnam veterans (crude rate, 1.22/10,000) and 29 in the era-veteran cohort, for an adjusted RR of 0.68 (95% CI 0.37–1.25). No excess risk was observed in the nurses-only analysis (RR = 0.65, 95% CI 0.32–1.30).

Occupational Studies   Hansen et al. (2007) conducted a historical-cohort study of 3,156 male gardeners who were members of a Danish union (the study was first reported in *VAO* as Hansen et al., 1992). Subjects were then followed up by using population and cancer registries, and the incidence of cancer was ascertained from 1975 until the end of 2001. Birth date served as a surrogate for potential exposure to pesticides and herbicides; earlier cohorts represented higher potential exposure. After the 25-year follow-up, no associations were found with pesticide and herbicide exposures and all lymphatic and hematopoietic tumors (ICD-7 200–205) (SIR = 1.1), but a positive association was observed for all leukemias (SIR = 1.4, 95% CI 0.9–2.1), especially in the presumptive high-exposure subcohort (SIR = 2.3, 95% CI 1.3–4.1).

Environmental Studies   Consonni et al. (2008) conducted a follow-up of the population of the area of the accident that occurred in Seveso in 1976. The follow-up was extended until 2001, and an association was found in Zone B (high TCDD contamination) with mortality from all leukemias combined (RR = 1.7, 95% CI 1.0–3.0), myeloid leukemia (RR = 2.0, 95% CI 0.9–4.5), and unspecific leukemias (RR = 2.4, 95% CI 0.9–6.5). In addition, an association in Zone R was found for mortality from lymphatic leukemia (RR = 1.4, 95% CI 0.9–2.2).

TABLE 6-47 Selected Epidemiologic Studies—Leukemia

Reference	Study Population[a]	Exposed Cases[b]	Estimated Relative Risk (95% CI)[b]
VIETNAM VETERANS			
New Studies			
Cypel and Kang, 2008	US Vietnam veterans (women)—lymphopoietic cancers[c]		
	Deployed vs nondeployed	18	0.7 (0.4–1.3)
	Nurses only	14	0.7 (0.3–1.3)
Studies Reviewed in *Update 2006*			
ADVA, 2005a	Australian Vietnam veterans vs Australian population—incidence		
	All branches	130	1.1 (1.0–1.4)
	Lymphocytic leukemia	72	1.4 (1.1–1.7)
	Myelogenous leukemia	54	1.0 (0.8–1.3)
	Navy	35	1.5 (1.0–2.0)
	Lymphocytic leukemia	14	1.3 (0.7–2.1)
	Myelogenous leukemia	19	1.7 (1.0–2.6)
	Army	80	1.1 (0.8–1.3)
	Lymphocytic leukemia	50	1.4 (1.0–1.8)
	Myelogenous leukemia	28	0.8 (0.5–1.1)
	Air Force	15	1.2 (0.7–2.0)
	Lymphocytic leukemia	8	1.4 (0.6–2.7)
	Myelogenous leukemia	7	1.3 (0.5–2.6)
ADVA, 2005b	Australian Vietnam veterans vs Australian population—mortality		
	All branches	84	1.0 (0.8–1.3)
	Lymphocytic leukemia	24	1.2 (0.7–1.7)
	Myelogenous leukemia	55	1.1 (0.8–1.3)
	Navy	17	1.3 (0.8–1.8)
	Lymphocytic leukemia	4	0.2 (0.0–1.2)
	Myelogenous leukemia	11	1.6 (0.9–2.5)
	Army	48	0.1 (0.7–1.2)
	Lymphocytic leukemia	17	1.3 (0.7–2.0)
	Myelogenous leukemia	30	0.8 (0.5–1.1)
	Air Force	14	1.6 (0.8–2.6)
	Lymphocytic leukemia	6	2.7 (1.0–5.8)
	Myelogenous leukemia	8	1.3 (0.5–2.5)
ADVA, 2005c	Australian male conscripted Army National Service Vietnam-era veterans: deployed vs nondeployed		
	Incidence	16	0.6 (0.3–1.1)
	Lymphocytic leukemia	9	0.8 (0.3–2.0)
	Myelogenous leukemia	7	0.5 (0.2–1.3)
	Mortality	11	0.6 (0.3–1.3)
	Lymphocytic leukemia	2	0.4 (0.0–2.4)
	Myelogenous leukemia	8	0.7 (0.3–1.7)
Boehmer et al., 2004	Vietnam Experience Cohort	8	1.0 (0.4–2.5)

continued

TABLE 6-47 Continued

Reference	Study Population[a]	Exposed Cases[b]	Estimated Relative Risk (95% CI)[b]
Studies Reviewed in *Update 2004*			
Akhtar et al., 2004	White Air Force Ranch Hand veterans— lymphopoietic cancers[c]		
	All Ranch Hand veterans		
	Incidence	10	0.9 (0.4–1.5)
	Mortality	6	1.0 (0.4–2.0)
	Veterans with tours in 1966–1970—incidence	7	0.7 (0.3–1.4)
	White Air Force Comparison veterans— lymphopoietic cancers[c]		
	All comparison veterans		
	Incidence	9	0.6 (0.3–1.0)
	Mortality	5	0.6 (0.2–1.2)
	Veterans with tours in 1966–1970—incidence	4	0.3 (0.1–0.8)
Studies Reviewed in *Update 2000*			
AFHS, 2000	Air Force Ranch Hand veterans	2	0.7 (0.1–5.0)
AIHW, 1999			Expected number of exposed cases (95% CI)
	Australian Vietnam veterans—incidence (validation study)	27	26 (16–36)
CDVA, 1998a	Australian Vietnam veterans (men)— self-reported incidence	64	26 (16–36)
CDVA, 1998b	Australian Vietnam veterans (women)— self-reported incidence	1	0 (0–4)
Studies Reviewed in *Update 1998*			
Dalager and Kang, 1997	Army Chemical Corps veterans		1.0 (0.1–3.8)
CDVA, 1997a	Australian military Vietnam veterans	33	1.3 (0.8–1.7)
Studies Reviewed in *VAO*			
Visintainer et al., 1995	PM study of deaths (1974–1989) of Michigan Vietnam-era veterans—deployed vs nondeployed	30	1.0 (0.7–1.5)
OCCUPATIONAL			
New Studies			
Hansen et al., 2007	Danish gardeners (all hematopoietic, ICD-7 200–205—incidence)		
	10-year follow-up (1975–1984) reported in		
	Hansen et al. (1992)	15	1.4 (0.8–2.4)
	NHL (ICD-7 200, 202, 205)	6	1.7 (0.6–3.8)
	HD (ICD-7 201)	0	nr
	Multiple myeloma (ICD-7 203)	0	nr
	CLL (ICD-7 204.0)	6	2.8 (1.0–6.0)
	Other leukemias (204.1–204.4)	3	1.4 (0.3–4.2)

TABLE 6-47 Continued

Reference	Study Population[a]	Exposed Cases[b]	Estimated Relative Risk (95% CI)[b]
	25-year follow-up (1975–2001)	42	1.1 (0.8–1.4)
	Leukemia (ICD-7 204)	22	1.4 (0.9–2.1)
	Born before 1915 (high exposure)	16	1.4 (0.9–2.3)
	Leukemia (ICD-7 204)	12	2.3 (1.3–4.1)
	Born 1915–1934 (medium exposure)	25	1.2 (0.8–1.8)
	Leukemia (ICD-7 204)	9	1.0 (0.5–2.0)
	Born after 1934 (low exposure)	1	0.2 (0.0–1.0)
	Leukemia (ICD-7 204)	1	0.5 (0.0–3.4)
Studies Reviewed in *Update 2006*			
McLean et al., 2006	IARC cohort of pulp and paper workers Exposure to nonvolatile organochlorine compounds		
	Never	49	1.0 (0.7–1.3)
	Ever	35	0.9 (0.6–1.2)
't Mannetje et al., 2005	Phenoxy herbicide producers (men and women)	0	0.0 (0.0–5.3)
	Phenoxy herbicide sprayers (> 99% men) (myelogenous leukemia)	1	1.2 (0.0–6.4)
Alavanja et al., 2005	US AHS—incidence		
	Private applicators (men and women)	70	0.9 (0.7–1.2)
	Spouses of private applicators (> 99% women)	17	0.7 (0.4–1.2)
	Commercial applicators (men and women)	4	0.9 (0.3–2.4)
Blair et al., 2005a	US AHS		
	Private applicators (men and women)	27	0.8 (0.5–1.1)
	Spouses of private applicators (> 99% women)	14	1.4 (0.8–2.4)
Mills et al., 2005	Cohort study of 139,000 United Farm Workers, with nested case–control analyses restricted to Hispanic workers in California Ever used 2,4-D		
	Total leukemia	nr	1.0 (0.4–2.6)
	Lymphocytic leukemia	nr	1.5 (0.3–6.6)
	Granulocytic (myelogenous) leukemia	nr	1.3 (0.3–5.4)
Hertzman et al., 1997	British Columbia sawmill workers with chlorophenate process (more hexa-, hepta-, octa-chlorinated dibenzodioxins than TCDD), all leukemias—incidence	47	1.2 (0.9–1.5)
	ALL	2	1.0 (0.2–3.1)
	CLL	24	1.7 (1.2–2.4)
	AML	5	0.8 (0.3–1.7)
	CML	7	1.1 (0.5–2.0)
	Other, unspecified	5	0.5 (0.2–1.0)
Torchio et al., 1994	Italian licensed pesticide users	27	0.8 (0.5–1.1)

continued

TABLE 6-47 Continued

Reference	Study Population[a]	Exposed Cases[b]	Estimated Relative Risk (95% CI)[b]
Reif et al., 1989	Case–control study of all men with occupation indicated entered into New Zealand Cancer Registry 1980–1984 (all leukemias)		
	Forestry workers	4	1.0 (0.4–2.6)
	AML	3	2.2 (nr)
Studies Reviewed in *Update 2004*			
Miligi et al., 2003	Case–control study of residents of 11 areas in Italy—incidence of leukemia excluding CLL		
	Exposure to phenoxy herbicides		2.1 (0.7–6.2)
Swaen et al., 2004	Dutch licensed herbicide applicators—mortality	3	1.3 (0.3–3.7)
Studies Reviewed in *Update 2002*			
Burns et al., 2001	Dow 2,4-D production workers (included in IARC cohort, NIOSH Dioxin Registry)		
	Lymphopoietic mortality in workers with high 2,4-D exposure	4	1.3 (0.4–3.3)
Thörn et al., 2000	Swedish lumberjacks exposed to phenoxyacetic herbicides	0	nr
Studies Reviewed in *Update 2000*			
Steenland et al., 1999	US chemical production workers (included in IARC cohort, NIOSH Dioxin Registry)	10	0.8 (0.4–1.5)
Hooiveld et al., 1998	Dutch chemical production workers (included in IARC cohort)	1	1.0 (0.0–5.7)
Rix et al., 1998	Danish paper mill workers—incidence		
	Men	20	0.8 (0.5–1.2)
	Women	7	1.3 (0.5–2.7)
Studies Reviewed in *Update 1998*			
Gambini et al., 1997	Italian rice growers	4	0.6 (0.2–1.6)
Kogevinas et al., 1997	IARC cohort, male and female workers exposed to any phenoxy herbicide or chlorophenol	34	1.0 (0.7–1.4)
	Exposed to highly chlorinated PCDDs	16	0.7 (0.4–1.2)
	Not exposed to highly chlorinated PCDDs	17	1.4 (0.8–2.3)
Becher et al., 1996	German chemical production workers (included in IARC cohort)—Cohort I	4	1.8 (0.5–4.7)
Ramlow et al., 1996	Dow pentachlorophenol production workers (included in IARC cohort, NIOSH Dioxin Registry)		
	0-year latency	2	1.0 (0.1–3.6)
	15-year latency	1	nr
Waterhouse et al., 1996	Residents of Tecumseh, Michigan—incidence		
	All leukemias		
	Men	42	1.4 (1.0–1.9)
	Women	32	1.2 (0.9–1.8)
	CLL	10	1.4 (1.0–1.9)

TABLE 6-47 Continued

Reference	Study Population[a]	Exposed Cases[b]	Estimated Relative Risk (95% CI)[b]
Amadori et al.,	Italian farming, animal-breeding workers—CLL	15	2.3 (0.9–5.8)
1995	Farmers	5	1.6 (0.5–5.2)
	Breeders	10	3.1 (1.1–8.3)
Studies Reviewed in *Update 1996*			
Asp et al., 1994	Finnish herbicide applicators		
	Mortality	2	nr
	Lymphatic	1	0.9 (0.0–5.1)
	Myelogenous	1	0.7 (0.0–3.7)
	Incidence		
	Lymphatic	3	1.0 (0.2–3.0)
Semenciw	Farmers in Canadian prairie provinces	357	0.9 (0.8–1.0)
et al., 1994	Lymphatic	132	0.9 (0.8–1.1)
	Myelogenous	127	0.8 (0.7–0.9)
Blair et al.,	US farmers in 23 states		
1993	White men	1,072	1.3 (1.2–1.4)
	White women	24	1.5 (0.9–2.2)
Kogevinas	IARC cohort (women only, myelogenous		
et al., 1993	leukemia)	1	2.0 (0.2–7.1)
Studies Reviewed in *VAO*			
Bueno de	Dutch phenoxy herbicide workers (included in		
Mesquita et al.,	IARC cohort)		
1993	Leukemia, aleukemia (ICD-9 204–207)	2	2.2 (0.3–7.9)
	Myelogenous leukemia (ICD-8 205)	2	4.2 (0.5–15.1)
Hansen et al.,	Danish gardeners—incidence		
1992	All gardeners—CLL	6	2.5 (0.9–5.5)
	all other types of leukemia	3	1.2 (0.3–3.6)
	Men—CLL	6	2.8 (1.0–6.0)
	all other types of leukemia	3	1.4 (0.3–4.2)
Ronco et al.,	Danish workers—incidence		
1992	Men—self-employed	145	0.9 (nr)
	employee	33	1.0 (nr)
	Women—self-employed	8	2.2 (p < 0.05)
	employee	3	1.3 (nr)
	family worker	27	0.9 (nr)
Fingerhut et al.,	NIOSH—entire cohort	6	0.7 (0.2–1.5)
1991			
Saracci et al.,	IARC cohort—exposed subcohort (men and		
1991	women)	18	1.2 (0.7–1.9)
Brown et al.,	Case–control study on white men in Iowa,		
1990	Minnesota, all types of leukemia—incidence	578	
	Ever farmed	335	1.2 (1.0–1.5)
	AML	81	1.2 (0.8–1.8)
	CML	27	1.1 (0.6–2.0)
	CLL	156	1.4 (1.1–1.9)
	ALL	7	0.9 (0.3–2.5)
	Myelodysplasias	32	0.8 (0.5–1.4)

continued

TABLE 6-47 Continued

Reference	Study Population[a]	Exposed Cases[b]	Estimated Relative Risk (95% CI)[b]
	Any herbicide use	157	1.2 (0.9–1.6)
	AML	39	1.3 (0.8–2.0)
	CML	16	1.3 (0.7–2.6)
	CLL	74	1.4 (1.0–2.0)
	ALL	2	0.5 (0.1–2.2)
	Myelodysplasias	10	0.7 (0.3–1.5)
	Phenoxy acid use	120	1.2 (0.9–1.6)
	2,4-D use	98	1.2 (0.9–1.6)
	2,4,5-T use	22	1.3 (0.7–2.2)
	First use > 20 years before	11	1.8 (0.8–4.0)
	MCPA	11	1.9 (0.8–4.3)
	First use > 20 years before	5	2.4 (0.7–8.2)
Wigle et al., 1990	Canadian farmers	138	0.9 (0.7–1.0)
Zober et al., 1990	BASF employees at plant with 1953 explosion		90% CI
	All 3 cohorts (n = 247)	1	1.7 (nr)
	Cohort 3	1	5.2 (0.4–63.1)
	Incident case of AML in Cohort 1		
Alavanja et al., 1988	USDA agricultural extension agents	23	1.9 (1.0–3.5)
	Lymphatic	nr	2.1 (0.7–6.4)
	Trend over years worked		(p < 0.01)
	Myelogenous	nr	2.8 (1.1–7.2)
	Trend over years worked		(p < 0.01)
Bond et al., 1988	Dow 2,4-D production workers (included in IARC cohort, NIOSH Dioxin Registry)	2	3.6 (0.4–13.2)
Blair and White, 1985	1,084 leukemia deaths in Nebraska in 1957–1974		
	Farmer—usual occupation on death certificate		1.3 (p < 0.05)
	99 ALL cases	nr	1.3 (nr)
	248 CLL cases	nr	1.7 (p < 0.05)
	105 unspecified lymphatic cases	nr	0.9 (nr)
	235 AML cases	nr	1.2 (nr)
	96 CML cases	nr	1.1 (nr)
	39 unspecified myelogenous cases	nr	1.0 (nr)
	39 acute monocytic cases	nr	1.9 (nr)
	52 acute unspecified leukemia cases	nr	2.4 (nr)
	65 unspecified leukemia cases	nr	1.2 (nr)
Burmeister et al., 1982	1,675 leukemia deaths in Iowa 1968–1978		
	Farmer—usual occupation on death certificate		1.2 (p < 0.05)
	ALL	28	0.7 (0.4–1.2)
	CLL	132	1.7 (1.2–2.4)
	Lived in one of 33 counties with highest herbicide use	nr	1.9 (1.2–3.1)
	Unspecified lymphatic	64	1.7 (1.0–2.7)
	AML	86	1.0 (0.8–1.5)
	CML	46	1.0 (0.7–1.7)

TABLE 6-47 Continued

Reference	Study Population[a]	Exposed Cases[b]	Estimated Relative Risk (95% CI)[b]
	Unspecified myelogenous	36	0.8 (0.5–1.4)
	Acute monocytic	10	1.1 (0.4–2.6)
	Unspecified leukemia	31	1.1 (0.6–2.0)
ENVIRONMENTAL			
New Studies			
Consonni et al., 2008	Seveso residents—25-year follow-up—men, women		
	Leukemia (ICD-9 204–208)		
	Zone A	1	0.9 (0.1–6.3)
	Zone B	13	1.7 (1.0–3.0)
	Zone R	51	1.0 (0.7–1.3)
	Lymphatic leukemia (ICD-9 204)		
	Zone A	0	nr
	Zone B	3	1.3 (0.4–4.1)
	Zone R	23	1.4 (0.9–2.2)
	Myeloid leukemia (ICD-9 205)		
	Zone A	1	2.1 (0.3–15.2)
	Zone B	6	2.0 (0.9–4.5)
	Zone R	16	0.7 (0.4–1.2)
	Monoccytic leukemia (ICD-9 206)	0	nr
	Leukemia, unspecified (ICD-9 208)		
	Zone A	0	nr
	Zone B	4	2.4 (0.9–6.5)
	Zone R	10	0.8 (0.4–1.6)
Studies Reviewed in *Update 2002*			
Revich et al., 2001	Residents of Chapaevsk, Russia		
	Mortality standardized to Samara Region		
	Men	11	1.5 (0.8–2.7)
	Women	15	1.5 (0.8–2.4)
Studies Reviewed in *Update 2000*			
Bertazzi et al., 2001	Seveso residents—20-year follow-up		
	Zones A, B—men	9	2.1 (1.1–4.1)
	women	3	1.0 (0.3–3.0)
Bertazzi et al., 1998	Seveso residents—15-year follow-up		
	Zone B—men	7	3.1 (1.4–6.7)
	women	1	0.6 (0.1–4.0)
	Zone R—males	12	0.8 (0.4–1.5)
	women	12	0.9 (0.5–1.6)
Studies Reviewed in *Update 1998*			
Bertazzi et al., 1997	Seveso residents—15-year follow-up		
	Zone B—men	7	3.1 (1.3–6.4)
	women	1	0.6 (0.0–3.1)
	Zone R—men	12	0.8 (0.4–1.4)
	women	12	0.9 (0.4–1.5)

continued

TABLE 6-47 Continued

Reference	Study Population[a]	Exposed Cases[b]	Estimated Relative Risk (95% CI)[b]
Studies Reviewed in *Update 1996*			
Swensson et al.,	Swedish fishermen		
1995	All leukemias—mortality		
	East coast (higher serum TEQs)	5	1.4 (0.5–3.2)
	West coast (lower serum TEQs)	24	1.0 (0.6–1.5)
	Lymphocytic—incidence		
	East coast (higher serum TEQs)	4	1.2 (0.3–3.3)
	West coast (lower serum TEQs)	16	1.3 (0.8–2.2)
	Myelogenous—incidence		
	East coast (higher serum TEQs)	2	0.9 (0.1–3.1)
	West coast (lower serum TEQs)	6	0.5 (0.2–1.1)
Bertazzi et al.,	Seveso residents—10-year follow-up—incidence		
1993	Zone B—men	2	1.6 (0.4–6.5)
	Myelogenous leukemia (ICD-9 205)	1	2.0 (0.3–14.6)
	women	2	1.8 (0.4–7.3)
	Myelogenous leukemia (ICD-9 205)	2	3.7 (0.9–15.7)
	Zone R—men	8	0.9 (0.4–1.9)
	Myelogenous leukemia (ICD-9 205)	5	1.4 (0.5–3.8)
	women	3	0.4 (0.1–1.2)
	Myelogenous leukemia (ICD-9 205)	2	0.5 (0.1–2.1)
Studies Reviewed in *VAO*			
Bertazzi et al.,	Seveso residents—10-year follow-up		
1992	Zones A, B, R—men	4	2.1 (0.7–6.9)
	women	1	2.5 (0.2–27.0)

ABBREVIATIONS: 2,4-D, 2,4-dichlorophenoxyacetic acid; 2,4,5-T, 2,4,5-trichlorophenoxyacetic acid; AHS, Agricultural Health Study; ALL, acute lymphocytic leukemia; AML, acute myelogenous leukemia; CI, confidence interval; CLL, chronic lymphocytic leukemia; CML, chronic myelogenous leukemia; HD, Hodgkin's disease; IARC, International Agency for Research on Cancer; ICD, International Classification of Diseases; MCPA, 2-methyl-4-chlorophenoxyacetic acid; NHL, non-Hodgkin's lymphoma; NIOSH, National Institute for Occupational Safety and Health; nr = not reported; PCDDs, chlorinated dibenzo-*p*-dioxins (highly chlorinated, if four or more chlorines); PM, proportionate mortality; TCDD, 2,3,7,8-tetrachlorodibenzo-*p*-dioxin; TEQ, toxicity equivalent quotient; USDA, US Department of Agriculture.
[a]Subjects are male and outcome is mortality unless otherwise noted.
[b]Given when available; results other than estimated risk explained individually.
[c]Lymphopoietic cancers comprise all forms of lymphoma (including Hodgkin's disease and non-Hodgkin's lymphoma) and leukemia (ALL, AML, CLL, CML).
Studies in italics have been superseded by newer studies of same cohorts.

For leukemia, the results presented by Miligi et al. (2006) on the Italian case–control study of lymphohematopoietic malignancies were not as informative for the purposes of the VAO series as those presented by Miligi et al. in 2003, as considered in *Update 2004*. The later publication reported estimated risk of all types of leukemia (ICD-9 204–208) in men and women who were exposed to any herbicide (OR = 1.4, 95% CI 0.8–2.3), whereas the earlier one had given findings on exposure to phenoxy herbicides specifically for leukemias excluding CLL (OR = 2.1, 95% CI 0.7–6.2).

Biologic Plausibility

Leukemia is a relatively rare spontaneous tumor in mice, but it is less rare in some strains of rats. A small study reported that five of 10 male rats fed TCDD at 1 ng/kg per week for 78 weeks showed an increased incidence of various cancers, one of which was lymphocytic leukemia (Van Miller et al., 1977). Later studies of TCDD's carcinogenicity have not shown an increased incidence of lymphocytic leukemia in mice or rats.

Two recent studies using cells in tissue culture suggest that TCDD exposure does not promote leukemia. Proliferation of cultured human bone marrow stem cells (the source of leukemic cells) was not influenced by addition of TCDD to the culture medium (van Grevenynghe et al., 2006). Likewise, Mulero-Navarro et al. (2006) reported that the AHR promoter is silenced in ALL—an effect that could lead to reduced expression of the receptor, which binds TCDD and mediates its toxicity. No reports of animal studies have noted an increased incidence of leukemia after exposure to the phenoxy herbicides or other chemicals of interest.

The biologic plausibility of the carcinogenicity of the chemicals of interest is discussed in general at the beginning of this chapter.

Synthesis

The positive associations found in the most recent analyses of the Seveso accident (Consonni et al., 2008) suggest an association between residence in the high TCDD exposure zone and all types of leukemia combined. For lymphatic and myeloid leukemias, the committee is concerned about misclassification of causes of death of the few people whose deaths were attributed to lymphatic leukemia (three in Zone B), myeloid leukemia (six in Zone B), and unspecified types of leukemia (four in Zone B). The findings from the study of Danish gardeners (Hansen et al., 2007) were consistent with a previous report (Hansen et al., 1992). The committee does not believe that the negative findings from Kang and Cypel are robust.

Conclusion

On the basis of the evidence reviewed here and in previous VAO reports, the committee concludes that there is inadequate or insufficient evidence to determine whether there is an association between exposure to the chemicals of interest and leukemias in general. An exception is made for the specific leukemia subtypes of chronic B-cell hematoproliferative diseases, including CLL and HCL; the rationale for this exception is discussed in the following section.

Chronic Lymphocytic Leukemia and Hairy Cell Leukemia

The proposed World Health Organization classification of NHL notes that CLL (ICD-9 204.1) and its lymphomatous form, small lymphocytic lymphoma, are both derived from mature B cells (Chiorazzi et al., 2005; IARC, 2001). (The committee has opted to continue using the abbreviation CLL to refer to this condition, although some now favor CLL/SLL.) ACS estimated that about 8,750 men and 6,360 women would receive diagnoses of CLL in the United States in 2008 and that 2,600 men and 1,790 women would die from it (Jemal et al., 2008a). Nearly all cases occur after the age of 50 years. For average annual incidence, see Table 6-46.

The requirements for diagnosis of CLL include an absolute peripheral-blood count of more than 5×10^9 clonal lymphocytes per liter, a predominant population of mature-looking lymphocytes, and hypercellular or normal cellular bone marrow that contains more than 30% lymphocytes. The malignant cells in CLL exhibit a characteristic membrane phenotype with coexpression of pan-B-cell antigens—including CD19, CD20, and CD23—with CD5. However, the cell-surface membranes express only weak surface-membrane immunoglobulin (Hallek et al., 2008).

Although it is now regarded as a different manifestation of the same disease, diffuse small lymphocytic lymphoma (SLL) is the term that has been used for the condition of patients who have lymphomatous CLL. Patients seek medical attention for painless generalized lymphadenopathy that in many cases has lasted for several years. Unlike the situation in other CLLs, the peripheral blood may be normal or reveal only mild lymphocytosis (fewer than 5×10^9 clonal lymphocytes per liter). However, the bone marrow has abnormal cells in 75–95% of cases. Both SLL and CLL can transform into aggressive NHL, known as Richter's syndrome (Omati and Omati, 2008). Richter's syndrome is characterized by diffuse large-cell lymphoma or its immunoblastic variant. It is resistant to current therapies, and the median survival is about 6 months.

For the present update, VA specifically asked that the committee address whether HCL should be considered to be in the group of neoplasms on which the evidence supports an association with herbicide exposure. As noted in *Update 2004* and *Update 2006*, HCL has been classified as a rare form of CLL (AJCC, 2002). The committee's response to VA's request is based on considerations of the biology of HCL rather than its diagnosis because it is far too uncommon to be reported and analyzed individually in the cohort studies considered in the VAO series and has not been the subject of case–control investigations considering exposures to the chemicals of interest.

HCL is a chronic B-cell lymphoproliferative disorder characterized by pancytopenia, splenomegaly, and the absence of lymphadenopathy. A leukemic blood profile is rare, occurring in about 8–10% of all cases. HCL is unique among the low-grade lymphomas not only because of its peculiar biologic properties but because treatment responses differ basically from those of all the other forms of NHL (König et al., 2000). The B–cell-derived tumor cells in the blood show many projections on their surface, hence the reference to "hairy"; the significance of the projections is not known.

No studies have specifically described HCL in animals exposed to the chemicals of interest. Thus, in addition to there being no epidemiologic results on HCL and the chemicals of interest, no animal data support the biological plausibility of an association between the chemicals of interest and this rare cancer. The committee sees no reason to exclude HCL or any other chronic hematoproliferative diseases of B-cell origin lacking their own specific epidemiologic evidence from the overaching broader groupings on which positive epidemiologic evidence is available. Because HCL is related to CLL, the committee explicitly includes it in the discussion and conclusions on CLL that follows.

Conclusions from *VAO* and Previous Updates   *Update 2002* was the first to discuss CLL separately from other leukemias. The epidemiologic studies indicated that farming, especially with exposure to 2,4-D and 2,4,5-T, is associated with significant mortality from CLL. Many more studies support the hypothesis that herbicide exposure can contribute to NHL risk. Most cases of CLL and NHL reflect malignant transformation of B-lymphocyte germinal center B cells, so these diseases could have a common etiology. Studies reviewed in *Update 2002*, *Update 2004*, *Update 2006*, and the present update are summarized in Table 6-48.

Update of the Epidemiologic Literature

Vietnam-Veteran Studies   No Vietnam-veteran studies addressing exposure to the chemicals of interest and CLL have been published since *Update 2006*.

Occupational Studies   Richardson et al. (2008) conducted a population-based case–control study of incident NHL and CLL in men and women 15–75 years old and living in six German counties in 1986–1998. Control subjects were selected randomly from German population registries and were matched individually to cases by sex, age, and region; two controls per case were recruited. The job–exposure matrix developed by Pannett and co-workers in the middle 1990s was used to assign chemicals that subjects were presumably exposed to occupationally. On the basis of an analysis whereby cumulative exposure (the sum across jobs of the product of the number of hours exposed, intensity, and probability of exposure) was categorized in three levels, there was no evidence that risks of CLL increased with increasing cumulative exposure (all ORs were less than 1; p for

TABLE 6-48 Selected Epidemiologic Studies—Chronic Lymphocytic Leukemia

Reference	Study Population[a]	Exposed Cases[b]	Estimated Relative Risk (95% CI)[b]
VIETNAM VETERANS			
Studies Reviewed in *Update 2006*			
ADVA, 2005a	Australian Vietnam veterans vs Australian population—incidence		
	All branches	58	1.2 (0.7–1.7)
	Navy	12	1.5 (0.8–2.6
	Army	42	1.6 (1.2–2.2)
	Air Force	4	0.9 (0.2–2.2)
OCCUPATIONAL			
New Studies			
Richardson et al., 2008	German residents, occupational factors associated with CLL—incidence		
	Chlorophenols	44	0.9 (0.6–1.3)
	Lowest tertile cumulative exposure	12	0.9 (0.4–1.8)
	Middle tertile	15	0.9 (0.5–1.8)
	Highest tertile	17	0.9 (0.5–1.6)
			p-trend = 0.770
	Herbicides	43	1.2 (0.8–1.7)
	Lowest tertile cumulative exposure	13	1.3 (0.7–2.7)
	Middle tertile	15	1.3 (0.7–2.5)
	Highest tertile	15	1.0 (0.5–1.9)
			p-trend = 0.755
Studies Reviewed in *Update 2006*			
Hertzman et al., 1997	British Columbia sawmill worker with chlorophenate process (more hexa-, hepta-, and octa-chlorinated dibenzo-*p*-dioxins than TCDD), all leukemias—incidence	47	1.2 (0.9–1.5)
	ALL	2	1.0 (0.2–3.1)
	CLL	24	1.7 (1.2–2.4)
	AML	5	0.8 (0.3–1.7)
	CML	7	1.1 (0.5–2.0)
	Other, unspecified	5	0.5 (0.2–1.0)
Studies Reviewed in *Update 1998*			
Waterhouse et al., 1996	Residents of Tecumseh, Michigan (men and women)—incidence	10	1.8 (0.8–3.2)
Amadori et al., 1995	Workers in northeast Italy (men and women)	15	2.3 (0.9–5.8)
	Farming workers only	5	1.6 (0.5–5.2)
	Breeding workers only	10	3.1 (1.1–8.3)

TABLE 6-48 Continued

Reference	Study Population[a]	Exposed Cases[b]	Estimated Relative Risk (95% CI)[b]
Studies Reviewed in *VAO*			
Hansen et al., 1992	Danish gardeners (men and women)		
	All gardeners	6	2.5 (0.9–5.5)
	Male gardeners	6	2.8 (1.0–6.0)
Brown et al., 1990	Residents of Iowa, Minnesota		
	Ever farmed	156	1.4 (1.1–1.9)
	Any herbicide use	74	1.4 (1.0–2.0)
	Ever used 2,4,5-T	10	1.6 (0.7–3.4)
	Use at least 20 years before interview	7	3.3 (1.2–8.7)
Blair and White, 1985	1,084 leukemia deaths in Nebraska 1957–1974		
	Farmer usual occupation on death certificate	nr	1.3 (p < 0.05)
	248 CLL cases	nr	1.7 (p < 0.05)
Burmeister et al., 1982	1,675 leukemia deaths in Iowa 1968–1978		
	Farmer usual occupation on death certificate		1.2 (p < 0.05)
	CLL	132	1.7 (1.2–2.4)
	Lived in 33 counties with highest herbicide use	nr	1.9 (1.2–3.1)
ENVIRONMENTAL			
New Studies			
Consonni et al., 2008	Seveso residents (men and women)— 25-year follow-up		
	Lymphatic leukemia (ICD-9 204)		
	Zone A	0	nr
	Zone B	3	1.3 (0.4–4.1)
	Zone R	23	1.4 (0.9–2.2)
Read et al., 2007	Residents of New Plymouth Territorial Authority, New Zealand near plant manufacturing 2,4,5-T (1962–1987)		
	Incidence	104	1.3 (1.1–1.6)[c]
	1970–1974	16	2.5 (1.4–4.1)
	1975–1979	7	0.9 (0.4–1.8)
	1980–1984	21	2.6 (1.6–3.9)
	1985–1989	16	1.4 (0.8–2.3)
	1990–1994	13	0.9 (0.5–1.6)
	1995–1999	19	0.9 (0.5–1.4)
	2000–2001	12	1.1 (0.6–1.9)
	Mortality	40	1.3 (0.9–1.8)[c]
	1970–1974	7	1.7 (0.7–3.5)
	1975–1979	7	1.8 (0.7–3.6)
	1980–1984	6	1.4 (0.5–3.0)
	1985–1989	4	0.8 (0.2–2.2)

continued

TABLE 6-48 Continued

Reference	Study Population[a]	Exposed Cases[b]	Estimated Relative Risk (95% CI)[b]
	1990–1994	6	1.1 (0.4–2.5)
	1995–1999	8	1.3 (0.6–2.6)
	2000–2001	2	0.8 (0.1–2.8)
Studies Reviewed in *Update 2000*			
Bertazzi et al., 2001	Seveso residents—20-year follow-up		
	Lymphatic leukemia		
	Zones A, B—men	2	1.6 (0.4–6.8)
	women	0	nr

ABBREVIATIONS: 2,4,5-T, 2,4,5-trichlorophenoxyacetic acid; ALL, acute lymphocytic leukemia; AML, acute myelogenous leukemia; CI, confidence interval; CLL, chronic lymphocytic leukemia; CML, chronic myelogenous leukemia; ICD, International Classification of Diseases; nr, not reported; TCDD, 2,3,7,8-tetrachlorodibenzo-*p*-dioxin; USDA, US Department of Agriculture.
[a]Subjects are male and outcome is mortality unless otherwise noted.
[b]Given when available; results other than estimated risk explained individually.
[c]The total SMR/SIR were computed by dividing sum of observed values by sum of expected values over all years; 95% CIs on these total ratios were computed with exact methods.
Studies in italics have been superseded by newer studies of same cohort.

linear trend = 0.77). This metric of cumulative exposure is difficult to interpret because it combines duration of exposure (continuous) with rank-ordered scales of intensity and probability; for example, an intensity coded as 2 and a probability coded as 1 yield the same product as an intensity coded as 1 and a probability coded as 2. Moreover, simple categorization of exposure can obscure trends in the data that can be seen with other techniques that make use of the continuous nature of the data (such as natural cubic spline functions).

Environmental Studies Consonni et al. (2008) reported on a mortality follow-up of the Seveso, Italy, cohort exposed to large amounts of environmental contamination with TCDD. The study cohort of 273,108 subjects who were resident at the time of the incident or immigrated or were born in the 10 years thereafter were analyzed according to three zones with increasing levels of soil TCDD. Mortality from leukemia was reported according to type of leukemia—lymphatic, myelocytic, and not reported—with no indication of acute or chronic subtypes. No deaths from lymphocytic leukemia were found in Zone A (the most highly exposed area), and no association with lymphocytic leukemia mortality was found in Zone B (RR = 1.3, 95% CI 0.4–4.1); however, an association was found in Zone R (RR = 1.4, 95% CI 0.9–2.2), the area with the lowest exposure. Although CLL is considerably less aggressive, it is considerable more prevalent than ALL, so it is not possible to infer that the statistics on mortality refer primarily to either of the two leukemia types.

Read et al. (2007) studied residents of a community where a plant had manufactured 2,4,5-T from 1962–1987. They reported that the body burden of TCDD was comparable with that in residents of Zone B of the Seveso area. Cancer incidence and mortality for the period 1970–2001 in the surrounding New Plymouth Territorial Authority were compared to those of the general population of New Zealand. Allowing for a latency period of about 10 years from the start of production, relative risks for incidence and mortality from CLL in this area were reported for five-year intervals starting in 1970. There was considerable fluctuation in the estimated risks, but significant increases in the incidence of CLL were noted during two intervals while production continued. The committee computed overall risks for the full 32-year observation period by dividing the sum of the observed values by the sum of the expected values over all years and derived 95% CIs on these total ratios by exact methods (SIR = 1.3, 95% CI 1.1–1.6; SMR = 1.3, 95% CI 0.9–1.8).

Biologic Plausibility   No animal studies have reported on the occurrence specifically of CLL after exposure to the chemicals of interest, but the information reported above in the biologic-plausibility section on all types of leukemias is relevant here. Given the similarities between CLL and B-cell lymphomas, a similar argument for biologic plausibility can be made for them. An increased incidence of lymphoma was reported in female B6C3F mice exposed to TCDD at 1 µg/kg of body weight via gavage twice a week for 2 years (NTP, 1982a). The finding was confirmed and extended in recent NTP studies in which a dose-related increase in the incidence of lymphoma was observed in female mice given TCDD orally at 0.04, 0.2, or 2.0 µg/kg twice a week for 104 weeks. Laboratory-animal studies of 2,4-D found no induction of lymphomas.

The biologic plausibility of the carcinogenicity of the chemicals of interest is discussed in general at the beginning of this chapter.

Synthesis   The study by Read et al. (2007) suggested an association between 2.4.5-T and CLL in people who lived near a plant in which 2,4,5-T was manufactured (RR = 1.3). In contrast, no excess risks of lymphatic leukemia in the two zones closest to the epicenter of the Seveso incident or of CLL in the German case–control study (Richardson et al., 2008) were found.

Although considerably more studies support the hypothesis that herbicide exposure can contribute to the development of NHL, some high-quality studies show that exposure to 2,4-D and 2,4,5-T appears to be associated with the occurrence of CLL, including the incidence study of Australian veterans (ADVA, 2005a), the high-quality case–control study by Hertzman et al. (1997) of British Columbia sawmill workers exposed to chlorophenates, the Danish-gardener study (Hansen et al., 1992), and the population-based case–control study in two US states by Brown et al. (1990) that showed increased risks associated with any herbicide use and use of 2,4,5-T at least 20 years before interview. Other studies that showed positive associations but do not contribute greatly to the overall conclusion include the population-based case–control study by Amadori et al. (1995) that made use of occupational titles but did not include specific assessments of exposure to the chemicals; the cancer-incidence study in Tecumseh County, Michigan, in which no exposure assessments were available (Waterhouse et al., 1996); and proportionate-mortality studies by Blair and White (1985) and Burmeister et al. (1982).

Malignant transformation of B-lymphocyte germinal center B is apparent in most cases of CLL and NHL, so it is plausible that these diseases could have a common etiology.

Conclusion   On the basis of the evidence reviewed here and in previous VAO reports, the committee concludes that there is sufficient evidence of an association between exposure to the chemicals of interest and CLL, including HCL and all other chronic B-cell hematoproliferative diseases.

SUMMARY

The committee had four categories available to classify the strength of the evidence from the veteran, occupational, and environmental studies reviewed regarding an association between exposure to the chemicals of interest and each kind of cancer. In categorizing diseases according to the strength of the evidence, the committee applied the same criteria (discussed in Chapter 2) that were used in *VAO*, *Update 1996*, *Update 1998*, *Update 2000*, *Update 2002*, *Update 2004*, and *Update 2006*. To be consistent with the charge to the committee from the Secretary of Veterans Affairs in Public Law 102-4 and with accepted standards of scientific reviews, the committee distinguished among the four categories on the basis of statistical association, not causality.

Health Outcomes with Sufficient Evidence of an Association

For outcomes in this category, a positive association with at least one of the chemicals of interest must be observed in studies in which chance, bias, and confounding can be ruled out with reasonable confidence. The committee regarded evidence from several small studies that were free of bias and confounding and that showed an association that was consistent in magnitude and direction as sufficient evidence of an association.

Previous VAO committees found sufficient evidence of an association between exposure to at least one of the chemicals of interest and four kinds of cancer: soft-tissue sarcoma, non-Hodgkin's lymphoma, Hodgkin's disease, and chronic lymphocytic leukemia. The scientific literature continues to support the classification of those four kinds of cancers in the category of sufficient evidence. The current committee agreed with the findings of previous VAO committees but broadened the categorization of chronic lymphocytic leukemia to include hairy-cell leukemia and other chronic B-cell leukemias.

Health Outcomes with Limited or Suggestive Evidence of an Association

For outcomes in this category, the evidence must suggest an association with at least one of the chemicals of interest that could be limited because chance, bias, or confounding could not be ruled out with confidence. A high-quality study may have demonstrated a strong positive association amid a field of less convincing positive findings, or, more often, several studies yielded positive results, but the results of other studies were inconsistent.

Previous VAO committees found limited or suggestive evidence of an association between exposure to at least one of the chemicals of interest and laryngeal cancer; cancer of the lung, bronchus, or trachea; prostatic cancer; multiple myeloma; and AL amyloidosis. The literature continues to support the classification of those diseases in the category of limited or suggestive evidence.

Health Outcomes with Inadequate or Insufficient Evidence to Determine Whether There Is an Association

This is the default category for any disease outcome for which there is not enough information upon which to base a discussion. For many of the kinds of cancer reviewed by the committee, some scientific data were available, but they were inadequate or insufficient in quality, consistency, or statistical power to support a conclusion as to the presence or absence of an association. Some studies fail to control for confounding or fail to provide adequate exposure assessment. In addition to any specific kinds of cancer that have not been directly addressed in the present report, this category includes hepatobiliary cancer (cancer of the liver, gallbladder, and bile ducts); cancer of the oral cavity, pharynx, and nose; cancer of the pleura, mediastinum, and other unspecified sites in the respiratory system and intrathoracic organs; cancer of the colon, rectum, esophagus, stomach, and pancreas; bone and joint cancer; melanoma and nonmelanoma skin cancer (including basal-cell carcinoma and squamous-cell carcinoma); breast cancer; cancer of the male and female reproductive systems (excluding prostate cancer); urinary bladder cancer; renal cancer (cancer of the kidney and renal pelvis); cancer of the brain and nervous system (including eye); and the various forms of leukemia other than chronic B-cell leukemias, including chronic lymphocytic leukemia and hairy cell leukemia.

Health Outcomes with Limited or Suggestive Evidence of No Association

For outcomes in this category, several adequate studies covering the full known range of human exposure are consistent in *not* showing a positive association with exposure to one of the chemicals of interest. The studies have relatively narrow confidence intervals. A conclusion of *no* association is inevitably limited to the conditions, magnitude of exposure, and length of observation of the available studies. The possibility of a very small increase in risk associated with a given exposure can never be excluded. Inclusion in this category does, however, presume evidence of a lack of association between each of the chemicals of interest and a particular health outcome, but there have been virtually no cancer-epidemiologic studies specifically evaluating the consequences of exposure to picloram or cacodylic acid.

On the basis of evaluation of the scientific literature, no kinds of cancer satisfy the criteria for inclusion in this category.

REFERENCES[1]

ACS (American Cancer Society). 2006. Cancer Facts and Figures 2006. Atlanta: American Cancer Society. http://www.cancer.org/downloads/STT/CAFF2006PWSecured.pdf (Accessed March 6, 2007).

ACS. 2007a. What are the risk factors for . . . http://www.cancer.org/docroot/CRI/content/CRI_2_4_2X_What_are_the_risk_factors_for . . . (Accessed September 18).

ACS. 2007b. What are the risk factors for . . . http://www.cancer.org/docroot/CRI/content/CRI_2_2_2X_What_causes_laryngeal_and_hypopharyngeal_cancers . . . (Accessed September 18).

ACS. 2007c. What are the risk factors for . . . http://www.cancer.org/docroot/CRI/content/CRI_2_2_2x_What_Causes . . . (Accessed September 18).

ACS. 2007d. What are the risk factors for . . . . http://www.cancer.org/docroot/CRI/content/CRI_2_4_2X_What_are_the_risk_factors_for_brain . . . (Accessed September 18).

ADVA (Australia Department of Veterans' Affairs). 2005a. *Cancer Incidence in Australian Vietnam Veteran Study 2005.* Canberra, Australia: Department of Veterans' Affairs.

ADVA. 2005b. *The Third Australian Vietnam Veterans Mortality Study 2005.* Canberra, Australia: Department of Veterans' Affairs.

ADVA. 2005c. *Australian National Service Vietnam Veterans: Mortality and Cancer Incidence 2005.* Canberra, Australia: Department of Veterans' Affairs.

AFHS (Air Force Health Study). 1996. *An Epidemiologic Investigation of Health Effects in Air Force Personnel Following Exposure to Herbicides. Mortality Update 1996.* Brooks AFB, TX: Epidemiologic Research Division. Armstrong Laboratory. AL/AO-TR-1996-0068. 31 pp.

AFHS. 2000. *An Epidemiologic Investigation of Health Effects in Air Force Personnel Following Exposure to Herbicides. 1997 Follow-up Examination and Results.* Reston, VA: Science Application International Corporation. F41624–96–C1012.

---

[1]Throughout the report the same alphabetic indicator following year of publication is used consistently for the same article when there were multiple citations by the same first author in a given year. The convention of assigning the alphabetic indicator in order of citation in a given chapter is not followed.

AIHW (Australian Institute of Health and Welfare). 1999. *Morbidity of Vietnam Veterans: A Study of the Health of Australia's Vietnam Veteran Community, Volume 3: Validation Study.* Canberra, Australia.

AJCC (American Joint Committee on Cancer). 2002. *Lymphoid Neoplasms. AJCC Cancer Staging Manual, 6th Edition.* New York: Springer-Verlag, pp. 393–406.

Akhtar FZ, Garabrant DH, Ketchum NS, Michalek JE. 2004. Cancer in US Air Force veterans of the Vietnam War. *Journal of Occupational and Environmental Medicine* 46(2):123–136.

Alavanja MC, Blair A, Merkle S, Teske J, Eaton B. 1988. Mortality among agricultural extension agents. *American Journal of Industrial Medicine* 14(2):167–176.

Alavanja MC, Blair A, Merkle S, Teske J, Eaton B, Reed B. 1989. Mortality among forest and soil conservationists. *Archives of Environmental Health* 44:94–101.

Alavanja MC, Samanic C, Dosemeci M, Lubin J, Tarone R, Lynch CF, Knott C, Thomas K, Hoppin JA, Barker J, Coble J, Sandler DP, Blair A. 2003. Use of agricultural pesticides and prostate cancer risk in the Agricultural Health Study cohort. *American Journal of Epidemiology* 157(9):800–814.

Alavanja MCR, Sandler DP, Lynch CF, Knott C, Lubin JH, Tarone R, Thomas K, Dosemeci M, Barker J, Hoppin JA, Blair A. 2005. Cancer incidence in the Agricultural Health Study. *Scandinavian Journal of Work, Environment and Health* 31(Suppl 1):39–45.

Allen JR, Barsotti DA, Van MJP, Abrahamson LJ, Lalich JJ. 1977. Morphological changes in monkeys consuming a diet containing low levels of 2,3,7,8-tetrachlorodibenzo-*p*-dioxin. *Food and Cosmetics Toxicology* 15:401–410.

Amadori D, Nanni O, Falcini F, Saragoni A, Tison V, Callea A, Scarpi E, Ricci M, Riva N, Buiatti E. 1995. Chronic lymphocytic leukaemias and non-Hodgkin's lymphomas by histological type in farming-animal breeding workers: A population case–control study based on job titles. *Occupational and Environmental Medicine* 52(6):374–379.

Anderson HA, Hanrahan LP, Jensen M, Laurin D, Yick W-Y, Wiegman P. 1986. *Wisconsin Vietnam Veteran Mortality Study: Final Report.* Madison: Wisconsin Division of Health.

Andersson P, McGuire J, Rubioi C, Gradin K, Whitelaw ML, Pettersson S, Hanberg A, Poellinger L. 2002a. A constitutively active dioxin/aryl hydrocarbon receptor induces stomach tumors. *Proceedings of the National Academy of Sciences of the United States* 99(15):9990–9995.

Andersson P, Rubio C, Poellinger L, Hanberg A. 2005. Gastric hamartomatous tumours in a transgenic mouse model expressing an activated dioxin/Ah receptor. *Anticancer Research* 25(2A): 903–911.

Arnold LL, Eldan M, Nyska A, van Gemert M, Cohen SM. 2006. Dimethylarsinic acid: Results of chronic toxicity/oncogenicity studies in F344 rats and in B6C3F1 mice. *Toxicology* 223(1-2): 82–100.

Asp S, Riihimaki V, Hernberg S, Pukkala E. 1994. Mortality and cancer morbidity of Finnish chlorophenoxy herbicide applicators: An 18-year prospective follow-up. *American Journal of Industrial Medicine* 26(2):243–253.

Axelson O, Sundell L. 1974. Herbicide exposure, mortality and tumor incidence. An epidemiological investigation on Swedish railroad workers. *Scandinavian Journal of Work, Environment and Health* 11:21–28.

Axelson O, Sundell L, Andersson K, Edling C, Hogstedt C, Kling H. 1980. Herbicide exposure and tumor mortality. An updated epidemiologic investigation on Swedish railroad workers. *Scandinavian Journal of Work, Environment, and Health* 6(1):73–79.

Baccarelli A, Hirt C, Pesatori AC, Consonni D, Patterson DG Jr, Bertazzi PA, Dolken G, Landi MT. 2006. t(14;18) translocations in lymphocytes of healthy dioxin-exposed individuals from Seveso, Italy. *Carcinogenesis* 27(10):2001–2007.

Bagga D, Anders KH, Wang HJ, Roberts E, Glaspy JA. 2000. Organochlorine pesticide content of breast adipose tissue from women with breast cancer and control subjects. *Journal of the National Cancer Institute* 92(9):750–753.

Balarajan R, Acheson ED. 1984. Soft tissue sarcomas in agriculture and forestry workers. *Journal of Epidemiology and Community Health* 38(2):113–116.

Becher H, Flesch-Janys D, Kauppinen T, Kogevinas M, Steindorf K, Manz A, Wahrendorf J. 1996. Cancer mortality in German male workers exposed to phenoxy herbicides and dioxins. *Cancer Causes and Control* 7(3):312–321.

Beebe LE, Fornwald LW, Diwan BA, Anver MR, Anderson LM. 1995. Promotion of N-nitrosodiethylamine-initiated hepatocellular tumors and hepatoblastomas by 2,3,7,8-tetrachlorodibenzo-*p*-dioxin or Aroclor 1254 in C57BL/6, DBA/2, and B6D2F1 mice. *Cancer Research* 55(21):4875–4880.

Bender AP, Parker DL, Johnson RA, Scharber WK, Williams AN, Marbury MC, Mandel JS. 1989. Minnesota highway maintenance worker study: Cancer mortality. *American Journal of Industrial Medicine* 15(5):545–556.

Bertazzi PA, Zocchetti C, Pesatori AC, Guercilena S, Sanarico M, Radice L. 1989a. Mortality in an area contaminated by TCDD following an industrial incident. *Medicina Del Lavoro* 80(4):316–329.

Bertazzi PA, Zocchetti C, Pesatori AC, Guercilena S, Sanarico M, Radice L. 1989b. Ten-year mortality study of the population involved in the Seveso incident in 1976. *American Journal of Epidemiology* 129(6):1187–1200.

Bertazzi PA, Zocchetti C, Pesatori AC, Guercilena S, Consonni D, Tironi A, Landi MT. 1992. Mortality of a young population after accidental exposure to 2,3,7,8-tetrachlorodibenzodioxin. *International Journal of Epidemiology* 21(1):118–123.

Bertazzi A, Pesatori AC, Consonni D, Tironi A, Landi MT, Zocchetti C. 1993. Cancer incidence in a population accidentally exposed to 2,3,7,8-tetrachlorodibenzo-*para*-dioxin. *Epidemiology* 4(5): 398–406.

Bertazzi PA, Zochetti C, Guercilena S, Consonni D, Tironi A, Landi MT, Pesatori AC. 1997. Dioxin exposure and cancer risk: A 15-year mortality study after the "Seveso accident." *Epidemiology* 8(6):646–652.

Bertazzi PA, Bernucci I, Brambilla G, Consonni D, Pesatori AC. 1998. The Seveso studies on early and long-term effects of dioxin exposure: A review. *Environmental Health Perspectives* 106(Suppl 2):625–633.

Bertazzi PA, Consonni D, Bachetti S, Rubagotti M, Baccarelli A, Zocchetti C, Pesatori AC. 2001. Health effects of dioxin exposure: A 20-year mortality study. *American Journal of Epidemiology* 153(11):1031–1044.

Birnbaum LS, Fenton SE. 2003. Cancer and developmental exposure to endocrine disruptors. *Environmental Health Perspectives* 111(4):389–394.

Blair A, Kazerouni N. 1997. Reactive chemicals and cancer. *Cancer Causes and Control* 8(3): 473–490.

Blair A, White DW. 1985. Leukemia cell types and agricultural practices in Nebraska. *Archives of Environmental Health* 40(4):211–214.

Blair A, Grauman DJ, Lubin JH, Fraumeni JF Jr. 1983. Lung cancer and other causes of death among licensed pesticide applicators. *Journal of the National Cancer Institute* 71(1):31–37.

Blair A, Dosemeci M, Heineman EF. 1993. Cancer and other causes of death among male and female farmers from twenty-three states. *American Journal of Industrial Medicine* 23(5):729–742.

Blair A, Zahm SH, Cantor KP, Ward MH. 1997. Occupational and environmental risk factors for chronic lymphocytic leukemia and non-Hodgkin's lymphoma. In: Marti GE, Vogt RF, Zenger VE, eds. *Proceedings of the USPHS Workshop on Laboratory and Epidemiologic Approaches to Determining the Role of Environmental Exposures as Risk Factors for B-Cell Chronic Lymphocytic and Other B-Cell Lymphoproliferative Disorders.* US Department of Health and Human Services, Public Health Service.

Blair A, Sandler DP, Tarone R, Lubin J, Thomas K, Hoppin JA, Samanic C, Coble J, Kamel F, Knott C, Dosemeci M, Zahm SH, Lynch CF, Rothman N, Alavanja MC. 2005a. Mortality among participants in the Agricultural Health Study. *Annals of Epidemiology* 15(4):279–285.

Blair A, Sandler D, Thomas K, Hoppin JA, Kamel F, Coble J, Lee WJ, Rusiecki J, Knott C, Dosemeci M, Lynch CF, Lubin J, Alavanja M. 2005b. Disease and injury among participants in the Agricultural Health Study. *Journal of Agricultural Safety and Health* 11(2):141–150.

Bloemen LJ, Mandel JS, Bond GG, Pollock AF, Vitek RP, Cook RR. 1993. An update of mortality among chemical workers potentially exposed to the herbicide 2,4-dichlorophenoxyacetic acid and its derivatives. *Journal of Occupational Medicine* 35(12):1208–1212.

Blot WJ, McLaughlin JK. 1999. The changing epidemiology of esophageal cancer. *Seminars in Oncology* 26(5 Supplement 15):2–8.

Bodner KM, Collins JJ, Bloemen LJ, Carson ML. 2003. Cancer risk for chemical workers exposed to 2,3,7,8-tetrachlorodibenzo-*p*-dioxin. *Occupational and Environmental Medicine* 60(9): 672–675.

Boehmer TK, Flanders WD, McGeehin MA, Boyle C, Barrett DH. 2004. Postservice mortality in Vietnam veterans: 30-year follow-up. *Archives of Internal Medicine* 164(17):1908–1916.

Boffetta P, Stellman SD, Garfinkel L. 1989. A case–control study of multiple myeloma nested in the American Cancer Society prospective study. *International Journal of Cancer* 43(4):554–559.

Bond GG, Wetterstroem NH, Roush GJ, McLaren EA, Lipps TE, Cook RR. 1988. Cause specific mortality among employees engaged in the manufacture, formulation, or packaging of 2,4-dichlorophenoxyacetic acid and related salts. *British Journal of Industrial Medicine* 45(2): 98–105.

Bosl GJ, Motzer RJ. 1997. Testicular germ-cell cancer. *New England Journal of Medicine* 337(4): 242–253.

Boyle C, Decoufle P, Delaney RJ, DeStefano F, Flock ML, Hunter MI, Joesoef MR, Karon JM, Kirk ML, Layde PM, McGee DL, Moyer LA, Pollock DA, Rhodes P, Scally MJ, Worth RM. 1987. *Postservice Mortality Among Vietnam Veterans.* Atlanta, GA: Centers for Disease Control. CEH 86-0076. 143 pp.

Bradlow H. 2008. Review. Indole-3-carbinol as a chemoprotective agent in breast and prostate cancer. *In Vivo* 22(4):441–445.

Brenner J, Rothenbacher D, Arndt V. 2009. Epidemiology of stomach cancer. *Methods in Molecular Biology* 472:467–477.

Breslin P, Lee Y, Kang H, Burt V, Shepard BM. 1986. *A Preliminary Report: The Vietnam Veterans Mortality Study.* Washington, DC: Veterans Administration, Office of Environmental Epidemiology.

Breslin P, Kang H, Lee Y, Burt V, Shepard BM. 1988. Proportionate mortality study of US Army and US Marine Corps veterans of the Vietnam War. *Journal of Occupational Medicine* 30(5): 412–419.

Brown LM, Blair A, Gibson R, Everett GD, Cantor KP, Schuman LM, Burmeister LF, Van Lier SF, Dick F. 1990. Pesticide exposures and other agricultural risk factors for leukemia among men in Iowa and Minnesota. *Cancer Research* 50(20):6585–6591.

Brown LM, Burmeister LF, Everett GD, Blair A. 1993. Pesticide exposures and multiple myeloma in Iowa men. *Cancer Causes and Control* 4(2):153–156.

Brunnberg S, Andersson P, Lindstam M, Paulson I, Poellinger L, Hanberg A. 2006. The constitutively active Ah receptor (CA-Ahr) mouse as a potential model for dioxin exposure—effects in vital organs. *Toxicology* 224(3):191–201.

Bueno de Mesquita HB, Doornbos G, Van der Kuip DA, Kogevinas M, Winkelmann R. 1993. Occupational exposure to phenoxy herbicides and chlorophenols and cancer mortality in the Netherlands. *American Journal of Industrial Medicine* 23(2):289–300.

Bullman TA, Kang HK, Watanabe KK. 1990. Proportionate mortality among US Army Vietnam veterans who served in Military Region I. *American Journal of Epidemiology* 132(4):670–674.

Bullman TA, Watanabe KK, Kang HK. 1994. Risk of testicular cancer associated with surrogate measures of Agent Orange exposure among Vietnam veterans on the Agent Orange Registry. *Annals of Epidemiology* 4(1):11–16.

Burmeister LF. 1981. Cancer mortality in Iowa farmers, 1971–1978. *Journal of the National Cancer Institute* 66(3):461–464.

Burmeister LF, Van Lier SF, Isacson P. 1982. Leukemia and farm practices in Iowa. *American Journal of Epidemiology* 115(5):720–728.

Burmeister LF, Everett GD, Van Lier SF, Isacson P. 1983. Selected cancer mortality and farm practices in Iowa. *American Journal of Epidemiology* 118(1):72–77.

Burns CJ, Beard KK, Cartmill JB. 2001. Mortality in chemical workers potentially exposed to 2,4-dichlorophenoxyacetic acid (2,4-D) 1945–1994: An update. *Occupational and Environmental Medicine* 58(1):24–30.

Burt VL, Breslin PP, Kang HK, Lee Y. 1987. *Non-Hodgkin's Lymphoma in Vietnam Veterans.* Department of Medicine and Surgery, Veterans Administration, 33 pp.

Buxbaum JN. 2004. The systemic amyloidoses. *Current Opinion in Rheumatology* 16(1):67–75.

Cantor KP. 1982. Farming and mortality from non-Hodgkin's lymphoma: A case–control study. *International Journal of Cancer* 29(3):239–247.

Cantor KP, Blair A. 1984. Farming and mortality from multiple myeloma: A case control study with the use of death certificates. *Journal of the National Cancer Institute* 72(2):251–255.

Caplan LS, Hall HI, Levine RS, Zhu K. 2000. Preventable risk factors for nasal cancer. *Annals of Epidemiology* 10(3):186–191.

Carreon T, Butler MA, Ruder AM, Waters MA, Davis-King KE, Calvert GM, Schulte PA, Connally B, Ward EM, Sanderson WT, Heineman EF, Mandel JS, Morton RF, Reding DJ, Rosenman KD, Talaska G, Cancer B. 2005. Gliomas and farm pesticide exposure in women: The Upper Midwest Health Study. *Environmental Health Perspectives* 113(5):546–551.

CDC (Centers for Disease Control and Prevention). 1990a. The association of selected cancers with service in the US military in Vietnam. III. Hodgkin's disease, nasal cancer, nasopharyngeal cancer, and primary liver cancer. The Selected Cancers Cooperative Study Group. *Archives of Internal Medicine* 150(12):2495–2505.

CDC. 1990b. The association of selected cancers with service in the US military in Vietnam. I. Non-Hodgkin's lymphoma. *Archives of Internal Medicine* 150:2473–2483.

CDVA (Commonwealth Department of Veterans' Affairs). 1997a. *Mortality of Vietnam Veterans: The Veteran Cohort Study. A Report of the 1996 Retrospective Cohort Study of Australian Vietnam Veterans.* Canberra, Australia: Department of Veterans' Affairs.

CDVA. 1997b. *Mortality of National Service Vietnam Veterans: A Report of the 1996 Retrospective Cohort Study of Australian Vietnam Veterans.* Canberra, Australia: Department of Veterans' Affairs.

CDVA. 1998a. *Morbidity of Vietnam Veterans: A Study of the Health of Australia's Vietnam Veteran Community. Volume 1: Male Vietnam Veterans Survey and Community Comparison Outcomes.* Canberra, Australia: Department of Veterans' Affairs.

CDVA. 1998b. *Morbidity of Vietnam Veterans: A Study of the Health of Australia's Vietnam Veteran Community. Volume 2: Female Vietnam Veterans Survey and Community Comparison Outcomes.* Canberra, Australia: Department of Veterans' Affairs.

Chamie K, deVere White R, Volpp B, Lee D, Ok J, Ellison L. 2008. Agent Orange Exposure, Vietnam War Veterans, and the Risk of Prostate Cancer. *Cancer* 113(9):2464–2470.

Charles JM, Bond DM, Jeffries TK, Yano BL, Stott WT, Johnson KA, Cunny HC, Wilson RD, Bus JS. 1996. Chronic dietary toxicity/oncogenicity studies on 2,4-dichlorophenoxyacetic acid in rodents. *Fundamental and Applied Toxicology* 33:166–172.

Chiorazzi N, Rai KR, Ferrarini M. 2005. Mechanisms of disease: Chronic lymphocytic leukemia. *The New England Journal of Medicine* 352(8):804–815.

Chiu BC, Weisenburger DD, Zahm SH, Cantor KP, Gapstur SM, Holmes F, Burmeister LF, Blair A. 2004. Agricultural pesticide use, familial cancer, and risk of non-Hodgkin lymphoma. *Cancer Epidemiology, Biomarkers and Prevention* 13(4):525–531.

Chiu BC, Dave BJ, Blair A, Gapstur SM, Zahm SH, Weisenburger DD. 2006. Agricultural pesticide use and risk of t(14;18)-defined subtypes of non-Hodgkin lymphoma. *Blood* 108(4):1363–1369.

Chlebowski RT, Hendrix SL, Langer RD, Stefanick ML, Gass M, Lane D, Rodabough RJ, Gilligan MA, Cyr MG, Thomson CA, Khandekar J, Petrovitch H, McTiernan A, WHI Investigators. 2003. Influence of estrogen plus progestin on breast cancer and mammography in healthy postmenopausal women: The Women's Health Initiative Randomized Trial. *Journal of the American Medical Association* 289(24):3243–3253.

Chung CJ, Huang CJ, Pu YS, Su CT, Huang YK, Chen YT, Hsueh YM. 2008. Urinary 8-hydroxy-deoxyguanosine and urothelial carcinoma risk in low arsenic exposure area. *Toxicology and Applied Pharmacology* 226(1):14–21.

Clapp RW. 1997. Update of cancer surveillance of veterans in Massachusetts, USA. *International Journal of Epidemiology* 26(3):679–681.

Clapp RW, Cupples LA, Colton T, Ozonoff DM. 1991. Cancer surveillance of veterans in Massachusetts, 1982–1988. *International Journal of Epidemiology* 20(1):7–12.

Cocco P, Heineman EF, Dosemeci M. 1999. Occupational risk factors for cancer of the central nervous system (CNS) among US women. *American Journal of Industrial Medicine* 36(1):70–74.

Coggon D, Pannett B, Winter PD, Acheson ED, Bonsall J. 1986. Mortality of workers exposed to 2-methyl-4-chlorophenoxyacetic acid. *Scandinavian Journal of Work, Environment, and Health* 12(5):448–454.

Coggon D, Pannett B, Winter P. 1991. Mortality and incidence of cancer at four factories making phenoxy herbicides. *British Journal of Industrial Medicine* 48(3):173–178.

Cohen AD, Zhou P, Xiao Q, Fleisher M, Kalakonda N, Akhurst T, Chitale DA, Moscowitz MV, Dhodapkar J, Teruya-Feldstein D, Filippa D, Comenzo RL. 2004. Systemic AL amyloidosis due to non-Hodgkin's lymphoma: An unusual clinicopathologic association. *British Journal of Haematology* 124:309–314.

Cohen SM, Arnold LL, Eldan M, Lewis AS, Beck BD. 2006. Methylated arsenicals: The implications of metabolism and carcinogenicity studies in rodents to human risk assessment. *Critical Reviews in Toxicology* 36(2):99–133.

Collins JJ, Strauss ME, Levinskas GJ, Conner PR. 1993. The mortality experience of workers exposed to 2,3,7,8-tetrachlorodibenzo-*p*-dioxin in a trichlorophenol process accident. *Epidemiology* 4(1):7–13.

Comba P, Ascoli V, Belli S, Benedetti M, Gatti L, Ricci P, Tieghi A. 2003. Risk of soft tissue sarcomas and residence in the neighbourhood of an incinerator of industrial wastes. *Occupational and Environmental Medicine* 60(9):680–683.

Consonni D, Pesatori AC, Zocchetti C, Sindaco R, D'Oro LC, Rubagotti M, Bertazzi PA. 2008. Mortality in a population exposed to dioxin after the Seveso, Italy, accident in 1976: 25 years of follow-up. *American Journal of Epidemiology* 167(7):847–858.

Cordier S, Le TB, Verger P, Bard D, Le CD, Larouze B, Dazza MC, Hoang TQ, Abenhaim L. 1993. Viral infections and chemical exposures as risk factors for hepatocellular carcinoma in Vietnam. *International Journal of Cancer* 55(2):196–201.

Corrao G, Caller M, Carle F, Russo R, Bosia S, Piccioni P. 1989. Cancer risk in a cohort of licensed pesticide users. *Scandinavian Journal of Work, Environment, and Health* 15(3):203–209.

Costani G, Rabitti P, Mambrini A, Bai E, Berrino F. 2000. Soft tissue sarcomas in the general population living near a chemical plant in northern Italy. *Tumori* 86(5):381–383.

Cypel Y, Kang H. 2008. Mortality patterns among women Vietnam-era veterans: Results of a retrospective cohort study. *Annals of Epidemiology* 18(3):244–252.

Dalager NA, Kang HK. 1997. Mortality among Army Chemical Corps Vietnam veterans. *American Journal of Industrial Medicine* 31(6):719–726.

Dalager NA, Kang HK, Burt VL, Weatherbee L. 1991. Non-Hodgkin's lymphoma among Vietnam veterans. *Journal of Occupational Medicine* 33(7):774–779.

Dalager NA, Kang HK, Thomas TL. 1995. Cancer mortality patterns among women who served in the military: The Vietnam experience. *Journal of Occupational and Environmental Medicine* 37(3):298–305.

Davis BJ, McCurdy EA, Miller BD, Lucier GW, Tritscher AM. 2000. Ovarian tumors in rats induced by chronic 2,3,7,8-tetrachlorodibenzo-*p*-dioxin treatment. *Cancer Research* 60(19):5414–5419.

Dean G. 1994. Deaths from primary brain cancers, lymphatic and haematopoietic cancers in agricultural workers in the Republic of Ireland. *Journal of Epidemiology and Community Health* 48(4):364–368.

Demers A, Ayotte P, Brisson J, Dodin S, Robert J, Dewailly E. 2000. Risk and aggressiveness of breast cancer in relation to plasma organochlorine concentrations. *Cancer Epidemiology, Biomarkers and Prevention* 9(2):161–166.

Demers PA, Boffetta P, Kogevinas M, Blair A, Miller BA, Robinson CF, Roscoe RJ, Winter PD, Colin D, Matos E, et al. 1995. Pooled reanalysis of cancer mortality among five cohorts of workers in wood-related industries. *Scandinavian Journal of Work, Environment and Health* 21(3):179–190.

Desaulniers D, Leingartner K, Russo J, Perkins G, Chittim BG, Archer MC, Wade M, Yang J. 2001. Modulatory effects of neonatal exposure to TCDD or a mixture of PCBs, p,p′-DDT, and p-p′-DDE on methylnitrosourea-induced mammary tumor development in the rat. *Environmental Health Perspectives* 109:739–747.

Desaulniers D, Leingartner K, Musicki B, Cole J, Li M, Charboneau M, Tsang BK. 2004. Lack of effects of postnatal exposure to a mixture of aryl hydrocarbon-receptor agonists on the development of methylnitrosourea-induced mammary tumors in Sprague-Dawley rats. *Journal of Toxicology and Environmental Health, Part A* 67(18):1457–1475.

Dich J, Wiklund K. 1998. Prostate cancer in pesticide applicators in Swedish agriculture. *Prostate* 34(2):100–112.

Donna A, Betta P-G, Robutti F, Crosignani P, Berrino F, Bellingeri D. 1984. Ovarian mesothelial tumors and herbicides: A case–control study. *Carcinogenesis* 5(7):941–942.

Dopp E, Von Recklinghausen U, Hartmann LM, Stueckradt I, Pollok I, Rabieh S, Hao L, Nussler A, Katier C, Hirner AV, Rettenmeier AW. 2008. Subcellular distribution of inorganic and methylated arsenic compounds in human urothelial cells and human hepatocytes. *Drug Metabolism and Disposition* 36(5):971–979.

Dubrow R, Paulson JO, Indian RW. 1988. Farming and malignant lymphoma in Hancock County, Ohio. *British Journal of Industrial Medicine* 45(1):25–28.

Duell EJ, Millikan RC, Savitz DA, Newman B, Smith JC, Schell MJ, Sandler DP. 2000. A population-based case–control study of farming and breast cancer in North Carolina. *Epidemiology* 11(5):523–531.

Ekström AM, Eriksson M, Hansson L-E, Lindgren A, Signorello LB, Nyrén O, Hardell L. 1999. Occupational exposures and risk of gastric cancer in a population-based case–control study. *Cancer Research* 59:5932–5937.

Engel LS, Hill DA, Hoppin JA, Lubin JH, Lynch CF, Pierce J, Samanic C, Sandler DP, Blair A, Alavanja MC. 2005. Pesticide use and breast cancer risk among farmers' wives in the Agricultural Health Study. *American Journal of Epidemiology* 161(2):121–135.

Eriksson M, Karlsson M. 1992. Occupational and other environmental factors and multiple myeloma: A population based case–control study. *British Journal of Industrial Medicine* 49(2):95–103.

Eriksson M, Hardell L, Berg NO, Moller T, Axelson O. 1979. Case–control study on malignant mesenchymal tumor of the soft tissue and exposure to chemical substances. *Lakartidningen* 76(44):3872–3875.

Eriksson M, Hardell L, Berg NO, Moller T, Axelson O. 1981. Soft-tissue sarcomas and exposure to chemical substances: A case-referent study. *British Journal of Industrial Medicine* 38(1):27–33.

Eriksson M, Hardell L, Malker H, Weiner J. 1992. Malignant lymphoproliferative diseases in occupations with potential exposure to phenoxyacetic acids or dioxins: A register-based study. *American Journal of Industrial Medicine* 22:305–312.

Eriksson M, Hardell L, Carlberg M, Akerman M. 2008. Pesticide exposure as risk factor for non-Hodgkin lymphoma including histopathological subgroup analysis. *International Journal of Cancer* 123(7):1657–1663.

Fenton SE. 2006. Endocrine-disrupting compounds and mammary gland development: Early exposure and later life consequences. *Endocrinology* 147(6):S18–S24.

Fett MJ, Nairn JR, Cobbin DM, Adena MA. 1987. Mortality among Australian conscripts of the Vietnam conflict era. II. Causes of death. *American Journal of Epidemiology* 125(15):878–884.

Fingerhut MA, Halperin WE, Marlow DA, Piacitelli LA, Honchar PA, Sweeney MH, Greife AL, Dill PA, Steenland K, Suruda AJ. 1991. Cancer mortality in workers exposed to 2,3,7,8-tetrachlorodibenzo-*p*-dioxin. *New England Journal of Medicine* 324(4):212–218.

Fleming LE, Bean JA, Rudolph M, Hamilton K. 1999a. Mortality in a cohort of licensed pesticide applicators in Florida. *Journal of Occupational and Environmental Medicine* 56(1):14–21.

Fleming LE, Bean JA, Rudolph M, Hamilton K. 1999b. Cancer incidence in a cohort of licensed pesticide applicators in Florida. *Journal of Occupational and Environmental Medicine* 41(4): 279–288.

Floret N, Mauny F, Challier B, Arveux P, Cahn J-Y, Viel J-F. 2003. Dioxin emissions from a solid waste incinerator and risk of non-Hodgkin lymphoma. *Epidemiology* 14(4):392–398.

Fortes C, Mastroeni S, Melchi F, Pilla MA, Alotto M, Antonelli G, Camaione D, Bolli S, Luchetti E, Pasquini P. 2007. The association between residential pesticide use and cutaneous melanoma. *European Journal of Cancer* 43(6):1066–1075.

Fritschi L, Benke G, Hughes AM, Kricker A, Turner J, Vajdic CM, Grulich A, Milliken S, Kaldor J, Armstrong BK. 2005. Occupational exposure to pesticides and risk of non-Hodgkin's lymphoma. *American Journal of Epidemiology* 162(9):849–857.

Fritz WA, Lin TM, Moore RW, Cooke PS, Peterson RE. 2005. In utero and lactational 2,3,7,8-tetrachlorodibenzo-*p*-dioxin exposure: Effects on the prostate and its response to castration in senescent C57BL/6J mice. *Toxicological Sciences* 86(2):387–395.

Fritz WA, Lin T-M, Peterson RE. 2008. The aryl hydrocarbon receptor (AhR) inhibits vanadate-induced vascular endothelial growth factor (VEGF) production in TRAMP prostates. *Carcinogenesis* 29(5):1077–1082.

Fukuda Y, Nakamura K, Takano T. 2003. Dioxins released from incineration plants and mortality from major diseases: An analysis of statistical data by municipalities. *Journal of Medical and Dental Sciences* 50(4):249–255.

Fukushima S, Morimura K, Wanibuchi H, Kinoshita A, Salim EI. 2005. Current and emerging challenges in toxicopathology: Carcinogenic threshold of phenobarbital and proof of arsenic carcinogenicity using rat medium-term bioassays for carcinogens. *Toxicology and Applied Pharmacology* 207(2 Suppl):225–229.

Gallagher RP, Bajdik CD, Fincham S, Hill GB, Keefe AR, Coldman A, McLean DI. 1996. Chemical exposures, medical history, and risk of squamous and basal cell carcinoma of the skin. *Cancer Epidemiology, Biomarkers and Prevention* 5(6):419–424.

Gambini GF, Mantovani C, Pira E, Piolatto PG, Negri E. 1997. Cancer mortality among rice growers in Novara Province, northern Italy. *American Journal of Industrial Medicine* 31(4):435–441.

Gann PH. 1997. Interpreting recent trends in prostate cancer incidence and mortality. *Epidemiology* 8(2):117–120.

Garland FC, Gorham ED, Garland CF, Ferns JA. 1988. Non-Hodgkin's lymphoma in US Navy personnel. *Archives of Environmental Health* 43(6):425–429.

Giri VN, Cassidy AE, Beebe-Dimmer J, Smith DC, Bock CH, Cooney KA. 2004. Association between Agent Orange and prostate cancer: A pilot case–control study. *Urology* 63(4):757–760; discussion 760–761.

Green LM. 1991. A cohort mortality study of forestry workers exposed to phenoxy acid herbicides. *British Journal of Industrial Medicine* 48(4):234–238.

Greenwald P, Kovasznay B, Collins DN, Therriault G. 1984. Sarcomas of soft tissues after Vietnam service. *Journal of the National Cancer Institute* 73(5):1107–1109.

Gupta A, Ketchum N, Roehrborn CG, Schecter A, Aragaki CC, Michalek JE. 2006. Serum dioxin, testosterone, and subsequent risk of benign prostatic hyperplasia: A prospective cohort study of Air Force veterans. *Environmental Health Perspectives* 114(11):1649–1654.

Hahn WC, Weinberg RA. 2002. Rules for making human tumor cells. *New England Journal of Medicine* 347(20):1593–1603.

Hallek M, Cheson B, Catovsky D, Caligaris-Cappio F, Dighiero G, Döhner H, Hillmen P, Keating MJ, Montserrat E, Rai K, Kipps TJ. 2008. Guidelines for the diagnosis and treatment of chronic lymphocytic leukemia: A report from the International Workshop on Chronic Lymphocytic Leukemia updating the National Cancer Institute Working Group 1996 guidelines. *Blood* 111(12):5446–5456.

Hallquist A, Hardell L, Degerman A, Boquist L. 1993. Occupational exposures and thyroid cancer: Results of a case–control study. *European Journal of Cancer Prevention* 2(4):345–349.

Hansen ES, Hasle H, Lander F. 1992. A cohort study on cancer incidence among Danish gardeners. *American Journal of Industrial Medicine* 21(5):651–660.

Hansen ES, Lander F, Lauritsen JM. 2007. Time trends in cancer risk and pesticide exposure, a long-term follow-up of Danish gardeners. *Scandinavian Journal of Work, Environment and Health* 33(6):465–469.

Hardell L. 1981. Relation of soft-tissue sarcoma, malignant lymphoma and colon cancer to phenoxy acids, chlorophenols and other agents. *Scandinavian Journal of Work, Environment, and Health* 7(2):119–130.

Hardell L, Bengtsson NO. 1983. Epidemiological study of socioeconomic factors and clinical findings in Hodgkin's disease, and reanalysis of previous data regarding chemical exposure. *British Journal of Cancer* 48(2):217–225.

Hardell L, Eriksson M, Lenner P, Lundgren E. 1981. Malignant lymphoma and exposure to chemicals, especially organic solvents, chlorophenols and phenoxy acids: A case–control study. *British Journal of Cancer* 43:169–176.

Hardell L, Johansson B, Axelson O. 1982. Epidemiological study of nasal and nasopharyngeal cancer and their relation to phenoxy acid or chlorophenol exposure. *American Journal of Industrial Medicine* 3(3):247–257.

Hardell L, Bengtsson NO, Jonsson U, Eriksson S, Larsson LG. 1984. Aetiological aspects on primary liver cancer with special regard to alcohol, organic solvents and acute intermittent porphyria: An epidemiological investigation. *British Journal of Cancer* 50(3):389–397.

Hardell L, Eriksson M, Degerman A. 1994. Exposure to phenoxyacetic acids, chlorophenols, or organic solvents in relation to histopathology, stage, and anatomical localization of non-Hodgkin's lymphoma. *Cancer Research* 54(9):2386–2389.

Hardell L, Nasman A, Ohlson CG, Fredrikson M. 1998. Case–control study on risk factors for testicular cancer. *International Journal of Oncology* 13(6):1299–1303.

Hardell L, Lindström G, van Bavel B, Hardell K, Linde A, Carlberg M, Liljegren G. 2001. Adipose tissue concentrations of dioxins and dibenzofurans, titers of antibodies to Epstein-Barr virus early antigen and the risk for non-Hodgkin's lymphoma. *Environmental Research* 87(2):99–107.

Hardell L, Eriksson M, Nordstrom M. 2002. Exposure to pesticides as risk factor for non-Hodgkin's lymphoma and hairy cell leukemia: Pooled analysis of two Swedish case–control studies. *Leukemia and Lymphoma* 43(5):1043–1049.

Hartge P, Colt JS, Severson RK, Cerhan JR, Cozen W, Camann D, Zahm SH, Davis S. 2005. Residential herbicide use and risk of non-Hodgkin lymphoma. *Cancer Epidemiology, Biomarkers and Prevention* 14(4):934–937.

Hayashi H, Kanisawa M, Yamanaka K, Ito T, Udaka N, Ohji H, Okudela K, Okada S, Kitamura H. 1998. Dimethylarsinic acid, a main metabolite of inorganic arsenics, has tumorigenicity and progression effects in the pulmonary tumors of A/J mice. *Cancer Letters* 125(1-2):83–88.

Hayes RB. 1997. The carcinogenicity of metals in humans. *Cancer Causes and Control* 8(3): 371–385.

Hebert CD, Harris MW, Elwell MR. Birnbaum LS. 1990. Relative toxicity and tumor-promoting ability of 2,3,7,8-tetrachlorodibenzo-*p*-dioxin (TCDD), 2,3,4,7,8-pentachlorodibenzofuran (PCDF), and 1,2,3,4,7,8-hexachlorodibenzofuran (HCDF) in hairless mice. *Toxicology and Applied Pharmacology* 102(2):362–377.

Henneberger PK, Ferris BG Jr, Monson RR. 1989. Mortality among pulp and paper workers in Berlin, New Hampshire. *British Journal of Industrial Medicine* 46(9):658–664.

Heron M, Hoyert D, Murphy S, Xu J, Kochanek K, Tejada-Vera B. 2009. Deaths: Final data for 2006. *National Vital Statistics Reports* 57(14):1–80.

Hertzman C, Teschke K, Ostry A, Hershler R, Dimich-Ward H, Kelly S, Spinelli JJ, Gallagher RP, McBride M, Marion SA. 1997. Mortality and cancer incidence among sawmill workers exposed to chlorophenate wood preservatives. *American Journal of Public Health* 87(1):71–79.

Hoar SK, Blair A, Holmes FF, Boysen CD, Robel RJ, Hoover R, Fraumeni JF. 1986. Agricultural herbicide use and risk of lymphoma and soft-tissue sarcoma. *Journal of the American Medical Association* 256(9):1141–1147.

Hobbs CG, Birchall MA. 2004. Human papillomavirus infection in the etiology of laryngeal carcinoma. *Current Opinion in Otolaryngology and Head and Neck Surgery* 12(2):88–92.

Hoffman RE, Stehr-Green PA, Webb KB, Evans RG, Knutsen AP, Schramm WF, Staake JL, Gibson BB, Steinberg KK. 1986. Health effects of long-term exposure to 2,3,7,8-tetrachlorodibenzo-*p*-dioxin. *Journal of the American Medical Association* 255(15):2031–2038.

Holcombe M, Safe S. 1994. Inhibition of 7,12-dimethylbenzanthracene-induced rat mammary tumor growth by 2,3,7,8-tetrachlorodibenzo-*p*-dioxin. *Cancer Letters* 82(1):43–47.

Holford TR, Zheng T, Mayne ST, Zahm SH, Tessari JD, Boyle P. 2000. Joint effects of nine polychlorinated biphenyl (PCB) congeners on breast cancer risk. *International Journal of Epidemiology* 29(6):975–982.

Hollingshead BD, Beischlag TV, Dinatale BC, Ramadoss P, Perdew GH. 2008. Inflammatory signaling and aryl hydrocarbon receptor mediate synergistic induction of interleukin 6 in MCF-7 cells. *Cancer Research* 68(10):3609–3617.

Holmes AP, Bailey C, Baron RC, Bosanac E, Brough J, Conroy C, Haddy L. 1986. *West Virginia Department of Health Vietnam-Era Veterans Mortality Study: Preliminary Report.* Charlestown: West Virginia Health Department.

Hooiveld M, Heederik DJ, Kogevinas M, Boffetta P, Needham LL, Patterson DG Jr, Bueno de Mesquita HB. 1998. Second follow-up of a Dutch cohort occupationally exposed to phenoxy herbicides, chlorophenols, and contaminants. *American Journal of Epidemiology* 147(9):891–901.

Høyer AP, Jørgensen T, Brock JW, Grandjean P. 2000. Organochlorine exposure and breast cancer survival. *Journal of Clinical Epidemiology* 53(3):323–330.

Hsu EL, Yoon D, Choi HH, Wang F, Taylor RT, Chen N, Zhang R, Hankinson O. 2007. A proposed mechanism for the protective effect of dioxin against breast cancer. *Toxicological Sciences* 98(2):436–444.

Huang YK, Pu YS, Chung CJ, Shiue HS, Yang MH, Chen CJ, Hsueh YM. 2008. Plasma folate level, urinary arsenic methylation profiles, and urothelial carcinoma susceptibility. *Food and Chemical Toxicology* 46(3):929–938.

Hussein MA, Juturi JV, Lieberman I. 2002. Multiple myeloma: Present and future. *Current Opinions in Oncology* 14(1):31–35.

IARC (International Agency for Research on Cancer). 2001. Pathology and genetics of tumours of the haemopoietic and lymphoid tissues. In: Jaffe NL, Harris H, Stein, Vardiman JW, eds. *World Health Organization*, IARC.

IOM (Institute of Medicine). 1994. *Veterans and Agent Orange: Health Effects of Herbicides Used in Vietnam.* Washington, DC: National Academy Press.

IOM. 1996. *Veterans and Agent Orange: Update 1996.* Washington, DC: National Academy Press.
IOM. 1999. *Veterans and Agent Orange: Update 1998.* Washington, DC: National Academy Press.
IOM. 2001.*Veterans and Agent Orange: Update 2000.* Washington, DC: National Academy Press.
IOM. 2003. *Veterans and Agent Orange: Update 2002.* Washington, DC: The National Academies Press.
IOM. 2005. *Veterans and Agent Orange: Update 2004.* Washington, DC: The National Academies Press.
IOM. 2006. *Asbestos: Selected Cancers.* Washington, DC: The National Academies Press.
IOM. 2007. *Veterans and Agent Orange: Update 2006.* Washington, DC: The National Academies Press.
Jemal A, Siegel R, Ward E, Hao Y, Xu J, Murray T, Thun M. 2008a. Cancer Statistics, 2008. *CA: A Cancer Journal for Clinicians* 58(2):71–96.
Jemal A, Thun MJ, Ries L, Howe H, Weir HK, Center MM, Ward E, Wu X-C, Eheman C, Anderson R, Ajani UA, Kohler B, Edwards BK. 2008b. Annual report to the nation on the status of cancer, 1975–2005, featuring trends in lung cancer, tobacco use, and tobacco control. *Journal of the National Cancer Institute* 100(23):1672–1694.
Jenkins S, Rowell C, Wang J, Lamartiniere CA. 2007. Prenatal TCDD exposure predisposes for mammary cancer in rats. *Reproductive Toxicology* 23(3):391–396.
Kang HK, Weatherbee L, Breslin PP, Lee Y, Shepard BM. 1986. Soft tissue sarcomas and military service in Vietnam: A case comparison group analysis of hospital patients. *Journal of Occupational Medicine* 28(12):1215–1218.
Kang HK, Mahan CM, Lee KY, Magee CA, Selvin S. 2000. Prevalence of gynecologic cancers among female Vietnam veterans. *Journal of Occupational and Environmental Medicine* 42(11): 1121–1127.
Kato H, Kinshita T, Suzuki S, Nagasaka T, Hatano S, Murate T, Saito H, Hotta T. 1998. Production and effects of interleukin–6 and other cytokines in patients with non-Hodgkin's lymphoma. *Leukemia and Lmphoma* 29(1–2):71–79.
Kato I, Watanabe-Meserve H, Koenig KL, Baptiste MS, Lillquist PP, Frizzera G, Burke JS, Moseson M, Shore RE. 2004. Pesticide product use and risk of non-Hodgkin lymphoma in women. *Environmental Health Perspectives* 112(13):1275–1281.
Keller-Byrne JE, Khuder SA, Schaub EA, McAfee O. 1997. A meta-analysis of non-Hodgkin's lymphoma among farmers in the central United States. *American Journal of Industrial Medicine* 31(4):442–444.
Ketchum NS, Michalek JE, Burton JE. 1999. Serum dioxin and cancer in veterans of Operation Ranch Hand. *American Journal of Epidemiology* 149(7):630–639.
Key TJ, Schatzkin A, Willett WC, Allen NE, Spencer EA, Travis RC. 2004. Diet, nutrition and the prevention of cancer. *Public Health Nutrition* 7(1A):187–200.
Knerr S, Schrenk D. 2006. Carcinogenicity of 2,3,7,8-tetrachlorodibenzo-*p*-dioxin in experimental models. *Molecular Nutrition and Food Research* 50(10):897–907.
Kociba RJ, Keys DG, Beyer JE, Careon RM, Wade CE, Dittenber DA, Kalnins RP, Frauson LE, Park CN, Barnar SD, Hummel RA, Humiston CG. 1978. Results of a two-year chronic toxicity and oncogenicity study of 2,3,7,8-tetrachlorodibenzo-*p*-dioxin in rats. *Toxicology and Applied Pharmacology* 46:279–303.
Kogan MD, Clapp RW. 1988. Soft tissue sarcoma mortality among Vietnam veterans in Massachusetts, 1972 to 1983. *International Journal of Epidemiology* 17(1):39–43.
Kogevinas M, Saracci R, Bertazzi PA, Bueno de Mesquita BH, Coggon D, Green LM, Kauppinen T, Littorin M, Lynge E, Mathews JD, Neuberger M, Osman J, Pearce N, Winkelmann R. 1992. Cancer mortality from soft-tissue sarcoma and malignant lymphomas in an international cohort of workers exposed to chlorophenoxy herbicides and chlorophenols. *Chemosphere* 25: 1071–1076.

Kogevinas M, Saracci R, Winkelmann R, Johnson ES, Bertazzi PA, Bueno de Mesquita BH, Kauppinen T, Littorin M, Lynge E, Neuberger M. 1993. Cancer incidence and mortality in women occupationally exposed to chlorophenoxy herbicides, chlorophenols, and dioxins. *Cancer Causes and Control* 4(6):547–553.

Kogevinas M, Kauppinen T, Winkelmann R, Becher H, Bertazzi PA, Bas B, Coggon D, Green L, Johnson E, Littorin M, Lynge E, Marlow DA, Mathews JD, Neuberger M, Benn T, Pannett B, Pearce N, Saracci R. 1995. Soft tissue sarcoma and non-Hodgkin's lymphoma in workers exposed to phenoxy herbicides, chlorophenols and dioxins: Two nested case–control studies. *Epidemiology* 6(4):396–402.

Kogevinas M, Becher H, Benn T, Bertazzi PA, Boffetta P, Bueno de Mesquita HB, Coggon D, Colin D, Flesch-Janys D, Fingerhut M, Green L, Kauppinen T, Littorin M, Lynge E, Mathews JD, Neuberger M, Pearce N, Saracci R. 1997. Cancer mortality in workers exposed to phenoxy herbicides, chlorophenols, and dioxins. An expanded and updated international cohort study. *American Journal of Epidemiology* 145(12):1061–1075.

Korenaga T, Fukusato T, Ohta M, Asaoka K, Murata N, Arima A, Kubota S. 2007. Long-term effects of subcutaneously injected 2,3,7,8-tetrachlorodibenzo-*p*-dioxin on the liver of rhesus monkeys. *Chemosphere* 67(9):S399–S404.

Kovacs E. 2006. Multiple myeloma and B cell lymphoma: Investigation of IL–6, IL–6 receptor antagonist (IL–6RA), and GP130 antagonist (GP130A) using various parameters in an in vitro model. *The Scientific World Journal* 6:888–898.

Küppers R, Schwering I, Bräuninger A, Rajewsky K, Hansmann M. 2002. Biology of Hodgkin's lymphoma. *Annals of Oncology* 13 (Supplement 1):11–18.

Lampi P, Hakulinen T, Luostarinen T, Pukkala E, Teppo L. 1992. Cancer incidence following chlorophenol exposure in a community in southern Finland. *Archives of Environmental Health* 47(3):167–175.

LaVecchia C, Negri E, D'Avanzo B, Franceschi S. 1989. Occupation and lymphoid neoplasms. *British Journal of Cancer* 60(3):385–388.

Lawrence CE, Reilly AA, Quickenton P, Greenwald P, Page WF, Kuntz AJ. 1985. Mortality patterns of New York State Vietnam veterans. *American Journal of Public Health* 75(3):277–279.

Leavy J, Ambrosini G, Fritschi L. 2006. Vietnam military service history and prostate cancer. *BMC Public Health* 6:75.

Lee WJ, Lijinsky W, Heineman EF, Markin RS, Weisenburger DD, Ward MH. 2004a. Agricultural pesticide use and adenocarcinomas of the stomach and oesophagus. *Occupational and Environmental Medicine* 61(9):743–749.

Lee WJ, Cantor KP, Berzofsky JA, Zahm SH, Blair A. 2004b. Non-Hodgkin's lymphoma among asthmatics exposed to pesticides. *International Journal of Cancer* 111(2):298–302.

Lee WJ, Colt JS, Heineman EF, McComb R, Weisenburger DD, Lijinsky W, Ward MH. 2005. Agricultural pesticide use and risk of glioma in Nebraska, United States. *Occupational and Environmental Medicine* 62(11):786–792.

Lee WJ, Sandler DP, Blair A, Samanic C, Cross AJ, Alavanja MC. 2007. Pesticide use and colorectal cancer risk in the Agricultural Health Study. *International Journal of Cancer* 121(2):339–346.

Lin PH, Lin CH, Huang CC, Chuang MC, Lin P. 2007. 2,3,7,8-tetrachlorodibenzo-*p*-dioxin (TCDD) induces oxidative stress, DNA strand breaks, and poly(ADP-ribose) polymerase-1 activation in human breast carcinoma cell lines. *Toxicology Letters* 172(3):146–158.

Lin PH, Lin CH, Huang CC, Fang JP, Chuang MC. 2008. 2,3,7,8-tetrachlorodibenzo-*p*-dioxin modulates the induction of DNA strand breaks and poly(ADP-ribose) polymerase-1 activation by 17beta-estradiol in human breast carcinoma cells through alteration of CYP1A1 and CYP1B1 expression. *Chemical Research in Toxicology* 21(7):1337–1347.

Lin TM, Rasmussen NT, Moore RW, Albrecht RM, Peterson RE. 2004. 2,3,7,8-tetrachlorodibenzo-*p*-dioxin inhibits prostatic epithelial bud formation by acting directly on the urogenital sinus. *Journal of Urology* 172(1):365–368.

Liu J, Singh B, Tallini G, Carlson DL, Katabi N, Shaha A, Tuttle RM, Ghossein RA. 2006. Follicular variant of papillary thyroid carcinoma: A clinicopathologic study of a problematic entity. *Cancer* 107:1255–1264.

Lynge E. 1985. A follow-up study of cancer incidence among workers in manufacture of phenoxy herbicides in Denmark. *British Journal of Cancer* 52(2):259–270.

Lynge E. 1993. Cancer in phenoxy herbicide manufacturing workers in Denmark, 1947–87—an update. *Cancer Causes and Control* 4(3):261–272.

Mack TM. 1995. Sarcomas and other malignancies of soft tissue, retroperitoneum, peritoneum, pleura, heart, mediastinum, and spleen. *Cancer* 75(1):211–244.

Magnani C, Coggon D, Osmond C, Acheson ED. 1987. Occupation and five cancers: A case–control study using death certificates. *British Journal of Industrial Medicine* 44(11):769–776.

Mahan CM, Bullman TA, Kang HK, Selvin S. 1997. A case–control study of lung cancer among Vietnam veterans. *Journal of Occupational and Environmental Medicine* 39(8):740–747.

Mantovani A, Allavena P, Sica A, Balkwill F. 2008. Cancer-related inflammation. *Nature* 454: 436–444.

Manz A, Berger J, Dwyer JH, Flesch-Janys D, Nagel S, Waltsgott H. 1991. Cancer mortality among workers in chemical plant contaminated with dioxin. *Lancet* 338(8773):959–964.

Marlowe JL, Fan Y, Chang X, Peng L, Knudsen ES, Xia Y, Puga A. 2008. The aryl hydrocarbon receptor binds to E2F1 and inhibits E2F1-induced apoptosis. *Molecular Biology of the Cell* 19:3263–3271.

McDuffie HH, Klaassen DJ, Dosman JA. 1990. Is pesticide use related to the risk of primary lung cancer in Saskatchewan? *Journal of Occupational Medicine* 32(10):996–1002.

McDuffie HH, Pahwa P, McLaughlin JR, Spinelli JJ, Fincham S, Dosman JA, Robson D, Skinnider LF, Choi NW. 2001. Non-Hodgkin's lymphoma and specific pesticide exposures in men: Cross-Canada study of pesticides and health. *Cancer Epidemiology, Biomarkers and Prevention* 10(11): 1155–1163.

McGee SF, Lanigan F, Gilligan E, Groner B. 2006. Mammary gland biology and breast cancer. Conference on Common Molecular Mechanisms of Mammary Gland Development and Breast Cancer Progression. *EMBO Reports* 7(11):1084–1088.

McLean D, Pearce N, Langseth H, Jäppinen P, Szadkowska-Stanczyk I, Person B, Wild P, Kishi R, Lynge E, Henneberger P, Sala M, Teschke K, Kauppinen T, Colin D, Kogevinas M, Boffetta P. 2006. Cancer mortality in workers exposed to organochlorine compounds in the pulp and paper industry: An international collaborative study. *Environmental Health Perspectives* 114(7):1007–1012.

Mellemgaard A, Engholm G, McLaughlin JK, Olsen JH. 1994. Occupational risk factors for renal-cell carcinoma in Denmark. *Scandinavian Journal of Work, Environment, and Health* 20(3): 160–165.

Merletti F, Richiardi L, Bertoni F, Ahrens W, Buemi A, Costa-Santos C, Eriksson M, Guenel P, Kaerlev L, Jockel K-H, Llopis-Gonzalez A, Merler E, Miranda A, Morales-Suarez-Varela, MM, Olsson H, Fletcher T, Olsen J. 2006. Occupational factors and risk of adult bone sarcomas: A multicentric case–control study in Europe. *International Journal of Cancer* 118(3):721–727.

Michalek JE, Pavuk M. 2008. Diabetes and cancer in Veterans of Operation Ranch Hand after adjustment for calendar period, days of sprayings, and time spent in Southeast Asia. *Journal of Occupational and Environmental Medicine* 50(3):330–340.

Michalek JE, Wolfe WH, Miner JC. 1990. Health status of Air Force veterans occupationally exposed to herbicides in Vietnam. II. Mortality. *Journal of the American Medical Association* 264(14):1832–1836.

Miligi L, Costantini AS, Bolejack V, Veraldi A, Benvenuti A, Nanni O, Ramazzotti V, Tumino R, Stagnaro E, Rodella S, Fontana A, Vindigni C, Vineis P. 2003. Non-Hodgkin's lymphoma, leukemia, and exposures in agriculture: Results from the Italian Multicenter Case–Control Study. *American Journal of Industrial Medicine* 44:627–636.

Miligi L, Costantini AS, Veraldi A, Benvenuti A, Will, Vineis P. 2006. Cancer and pesticides: An overview and some results of the Italian multicenter case–control study on hematolymphopoietic malignancies. *Annals of the New York Academy of Sciences* 1076:366–377.

Miller BA, Kolonel LN, Bernstein L, Young JL Jr, Swanson GM, West D, Key CR, Liff JM, Glover CS, Alexander GA, et al. (eds). 1996. *Racial/Ethnic Patterns of Cancer in the United States 1988–1992.* Bethesda, MD: National Cancer Institute. NIH Pub. No. 96-4104.

Mills PK, Yang R. 2005. Breast cancer risk in Hispanic agricultural workers in California. *International Journal of Occupational and Environmental Health* 11(2):123–131.

Mills PK, Yang RC. 2007. Agricultural exposures and gastric cancer risk in Hispanic farm workers in California. *Environmental Research* 104(2):282–289.

Mills PK, Yang R, Riordan D. 2005. Lymphohematopoietic cancers in the United Farm Workers of America (UFW), 1988–2001. *Cancer Causes and Control* 16(7):823–830.

Morris PD, Koepsell TD, Daling JR, Taylor JW, Lyon JL, Swanson GM, Child M, Weiss NS. 1986. Toxic substance exposure and multiple myeloma: A case–control study. *Journal of the National Cancer Institute* 76(6):987–994.

Morrison H, Semenciw RM, Morison D, Magwood S, Mao Y. 1992. Brain cancer and farming in western Canada. *Neuroepidemiology* 11(4-6):267–276.

Morrison H, Savitz D, Semenciw RM, Hulka B, Mao Y, Morison D, Wigle D. 1993. Farming and prostate cancer mortality. *American Journal of Epidemiology* 137(3):270–280.

Morrison HI, Semenciw RM, Wilkins K, Mao Y, Wigle DT. 1994. Non-Hodgkin's lymphoma and agricultural practices in the prairie provinces of Canada. *Scandinavian Journal of Work, Environment, and Health* 20(1):42–47.

Mulero-Navarro S, Carvajal-Gonzalez JM, Herranz M, Ballestar E, Fraga MF, Ropero S, Esteller M, Fernandez-Salguero PM. 2006. The dioxin receptor is silenced by promoter hypermethylation in human acute lymphoblastic leukemia through inhibition of Sp1 binding. *Carcinogenesis* 27(5):1099–1104.

Musicco M, Sant M, Molinari S, Filippini G, Gatta G, Berrino F. 1988. A case–control study of brain gliomas and occupational exposure to chemical carcinogens: The risks to farmers. *American Journal of Epidemiology* 128:778–785.

Nanni O, Amadori D, Lugaresi C, Falcini F, Scarpi E, Saragoni A, Buiatti E. 1996. Chronic lymphocytic leukaemias and non-Hodgkin's lymphomas by histological type in farming-animal breeding workers: A population case–control study based on a priori exposure matrices. *Occupational and Environmental Medicine* 53(10):652–657.

Nascimento MG, Suzuki S, Wei M, Tiwari A, Arnold LL, Lu X, Le XC, Cohen SM. 2008. Cytotoxicity of combinations of arsenicals on rat urinary bladder urothelial cells in vitro. *Toxicology* 249(1):69–74.

NCI (National Cancer Institute). 2008. *Surveillance, Epidemiology, and End Results (SEER) Incidence and US Mortality Statistics: SEER Incidence—Crude Rates for White/Black/Other 2000–2005.* http://www.seer.cancer.gov/canques/incidence.html (Accessed February 2, 2009).

Nordby KC, Andersen A, Kristensen P. 2004. Incidence of lip cancer in the male Norwegian agricultural population. *Cancer Causes and Control* 15(6):619–626.

NTP (National Toxicology Program). 1982a. *Technical Report Series No. 209. Carcinogenesis Bioassay of 2,3,7,8-Tetrachlorodibenzo-p-dioxin (CAS No. 1746-01-6) in Osborne-Mendel Rats and B6c3F1 Mice (Gavage Study).* NIH Publication No. 82-1765. 195 pp. National Toxicology Program, Research Triangle Park, NC, and Bethesda, MD.

NTP. 1982b. *Technical Report Series No. 201. Carcinogenesis Bioassay of 2,3,7,8-Tetrachlorodibenzo-p-dioxin (CAS No. 1746-01-6) in Swiss-Webster Mice (Dermal Study).* National Toxicology Program, Research Triangle Park, NC, and Bethesda, MD.

NTP. 2006. *NTP Technical Report on the Toxicology and Carcinogenesis Studies of 2,3,7,8-Tetrachlorodibenzo-p-dioxin (TCDD) (CAS No. 1746-01-6) in Female Harlan Sprague-Dawley Rats (Gavage Studies).* Issue 521:4–232. National Toxicology Program, Research Triangle Park, NC, and Bethesda, MD.

Nyska A, Jokinen MP, Brix AE, Sells DM, Wyde ME, Orzech D, Haseman JK, Flake G, Walker NJ. 2004. Exocrine pancreatic pathology in female Harlan Sprague-Dawley rats after chronic treatment with 2,3,7,8-tetrachlorodibenzo-*p*-dioxin and dioxin-like compounds. *Environmental Health Perspectives* 112(8):903–909.

Nyska A, Yoshizawa K, Jokinen MP, Brix AE, Sells DM, Wyde ME, Orzech DP, Kissling GE, Walker NJ. 2005. Olfactory epithelial metaplasia and hyperplasia in female Harlan Sprague-Dawley rats following chronic treatment with polychlorinated biphenyls. *Toxicologic Pathology* 33(3):371–377.

O'Brien TR, Decoufle P, Boyle CA.1991. Non-Hodgkin's lymphoma in a cohort of Vietnam veterans. *American Journal of Public Health* 81:758–760.

Ojajärvi IA, Partanen TJ, Ahlbom A, Boffetta P, Hakulinen T, Jourenkova N, Kauppinen TP, Kogevinas M, Porta M, Vainio HU, Weiderpass E, Wesseling CH. 2000. Occupational exposures and pancreatic cancer: A meta-analysis. *Occupational and Environmental Medicine* 57:316–324.

Olsson H, Brandt L. 1988. Risk of non-Hodgkin's lymphoma among men occupationally exposed to organic solvents. *Scandinavian Journal of Work, Environment, and Health* 14:246–251.

Omoti C, Omoti A. 2008. Richter syndrome: A review of clinical, ocular, neurological and other manifestations. *British Journal of Haematology* 142:709–716.

Ott MG, Zober A. 1996. Cause specific mortality and cancer incidence among employees exposed to 2,3,7,8-TCDD after a 1953 reactor accident. *Occupational and Environmental Medicine* 53:606–612.

Pahwa P, McDuffie HH, Dosman JA, McLaughlin JR, Spinelli JJ, Robson D, Fincham S. 2006. Hodgkin lymphoma, multiple myeloma, soft tissue sarcomas, insect repellents, and phenoxyherbicides. *Journal of Occupational and Environmental Medicine* 48(3):264–274.

Park JY, Shigenaga MK, Ames BN. 1996. Induction of cytochrome P4501A1 by 2,3,7,8-tetrachlorodibenzo-*p*-dioxin or indolo(3,2-b)carbazole is associated with oxidative DNA damage. *Proceedings of the National Academy of Sciences of the United States of America* 93(6):2322–2327.

Pavuk M, Michalek JE, Schecter A, Ketchum NS, Akhtar FZ, Fox KA. 2005. Did TCDD exposure or service in Southeast Asia increase the risk of cancer in Air Force Vietnam veterans who did not spray Agent Orange? *Journal of Occupational and Environmental Medicine* 47(4):335–342.

Pavuk M, Michalek JE, Ketchum NS. 2006. Prostate cancer in US Air Force veterans of the Vietnam War. *Journal of Exposure Science and Environmental Epidemiology* 16(2):184–190.

Pearce NE, Smith AH, Fisher DO. 1985. Malignant lymphoma and multiple myeloma linked with agricultural occupations in a New Zealand cancer registry-based sudy. *American Journal of Epidemiology* 121:225–237.

Pearce NE, Smith AH, Howard JK, Sheppard RA, Giles HJ, Teague CA. 1986. Non-Hodgkin's lymphoma and exposure to phenoxyherbicides, chlorophenols, fencing work, and meat works employment: A case control study. *British Journal of Industrial Medicine* 43:75–83.

Pearce NE, Sheppard RA, Smith AH, Teague CA. 1987. Non-Hodgkin's lymphoma and farming: An expanded case–control study. *International Journal of Cancer* 39:155–161.

Percy C, Ries GL, Van Holten VD. 1990. The accuracy of liver cancer as the underlying cause of death on death certificates. *Public Health Reports* 105:361–368.

Persson B, Dahlander AM, Fredriksson M, Brage HN, Ohlson CG, Axelson O. 1989. Malignant lymphomas and occupational exposures. *British Journal of Industrial Medicine* 46:516–520.

Persson B, Fredriksson M, Olsen K, Boeryd B, Axelson O. 1993. Some occupational exposures as risk factors for malignant lymphomas. *Cancer* 72:1773–1778.

Pesatori AC, Consonni D, Tironi A, Landi MT, Zocchetti C, Bertazzi PA. 1992. Cancer morbidity in the Seveso area, 1976–1986. *Chemosphere* 25:209–212.

Poland A, Palen D, Glover E. 1982. Tumour promotion by TCDD in skin of HRS/J hairless mice. *Nature* 300(5889):271–273.

Pu YS, Yang SM, Huang YK, Chung CJ, Huang SK, Chiu AW, Yang MH, Chen CJ, Hsueh YM. 2007. Urinary arsenic profile affects the risk of urothelial carcinoma even at low arsenic exposure. *Toxicology and Applied Pharmacology* 218(2):99–106.

Rajkumar SV, Dispenzieri A, Kyle RA. 2006. Monoclonal gammopathy of undetermined significance, Waldenstrom macroglobulinemia, AL amyloidosis, and related plasma cell disorders: Diagnosis and treatment. *Mayo Clinic Proceedings* 81(5):693–703.

Ramlow JM, Spadacene NW, Hoag SR, Stafford BA, Cartmill JB, Lerner PJ. 1996. Mortality in a cohort of pentachlorophenol manufacturing workers, 1940–1989. *American Journal of Industrial Medicine* 30:180–194.

Read D, Wright C, Weinstein P, Borman B. 2007. Cancer incidence and mortality in a New Zealand community potentially exposed to 2,3,7,8-tetrachlorodibenzo-*p*-dioxin from 2,4,5-trichlorophenoxyacetic acid manufacture. *Australian and New Zealand Journal of Public Health* 31(1):13–18.

Reif JS, Pearce N, Fraser J. 1989. Occupational risks of brain cancer: A New Zealand cancer registry-based study. *Journal of Occupational Medicine* 31(10):863–867.

Revich B, Aksel E, Ushakova T, Ivanova I, Zhuchenko N, Klyuev N, Brodsky B, Sotskov Y. 2001. Dioxin exposure and public health in Chapaevsk, Russia. *Chemosphere* 243(4-7):951–966.

Reynolds P, Hurley SE, Goldberg DE, Anton-Culver H, Bernstein L, Deapen D, Horn-Ross PL, Peel D, Pinder R, Ross RK, West D, Wright WE, Ziogas A. 2004. Residential proximity to agricultural pesticide use and incidence of breast cancer in the California Teachers Study cohort. *Environmental Research* 96(2):206–218.

Reynolds P, Hurley SE, Petreas M, Goldberg DE, Smith D, Gilliss D, Mahoney ME, Jeffrey SS. 2005a. Adipose levels of dioxins and risk of breast cancer. *Cancer Causes and Control* 16(5): 525–535.

Richardson DB, Terschuren C, Hoffmann W. 2008. Occupational risk factors for non-Hodgkin's lymphoma: A population-based case–control study in Northern Germany. *American Journal of Industrial Medicine* 51(4):258–268.

Riedel D, Pottern LM, Blattner WA. 1991. Etiology and epidemiology of multiple myeloma. In: Wiernick PH, Camellos G, Kyle RA, Schiffer CA, eds. *Neoplastic Disease of the Blood and Blood Forming Organs.* New York: Churchill Livingstone.

Riihimaki V, Asp S, Hernberg S. 1982. Mortality of 2,4-dichlorophenoxyacetic acid and 2,4,5-trichlorophenoxyacetic acid herbicide applicators in Finland: First report of an ongoing prospective cohort study. *Scandinavian Journal of Work, Environment, and Health* 8:37–42.

Rix BA, Villadsen E, Engholm G, Lynge E. 1998. Hodgkin's disease, pharyngeal cancer, and soft tissue sarcomas in Danish paper mill workers. *Journal of Occupational and Environmental Medicine* 40(1):55–62.

Robinson CF, Waxweiler RJ, Fowler DP. 1986. Mortality among production workers in pulp and paper mills. *Scandinavian Journal of Work, Environment, and Health* 12:552–560.

Ronco G, Costa G, Lynge E. 1992. Cancer risk among Danish and Italian farmers. *British Journal of Industrial Medicine* 49:220–225.

Roulland S, Navarro J-M, Grenot P, Milili M, Agopian J, et al. 2006. Follicular lymphoma-like B cell in healthy individuals: A novel intermediate step in early lymphomagenesis. *The Journal of Experimental Medicine* 203(11):2425–2431.

Rowland RE, Edwards LA, Podd JV. 2007. Elevated sister chromatid exchange frequencies in New Zealand Vietnam War veterans. *Cytogenetic and Genome Research* 116(4):248–251.

Ruder AM, Waters MA, Butler MA, Carreon T, Calvert GM, Davis-King KE, Schulte PA, Sanderson WT, Ward EM, Connally LB, Heineman EF, Mandel JS, Morton RF, Reding DJ, Rosenman KD, Talaska G. 2004. Gliomas and farm pesticide exposure in men: The Upper Midwest Health Study. *Archives of Environmental Health* 59(12):650–657.

Salehi F, Turner MC, Phillips KP, Wigle DT, Krewski D, Aronson KJ. 2008. Review of the etiology of breast cancer with special attention to organochlorines as potential endocrine disruptors. *Journal of Toxicology and Environmental Health—Part B: Critical Reviews* 11(3–4):276–300.

Samanic C, Rusiecki J, Dosemeci M, Hou L, Hoppin JA, Sandler DP, Lubin J, Blair A, Alavanja MC. 2006. Cancer incidence among pesticide applicators exposed to dicamba in the agricultural health study. *Environmental Health Perspectives* 114(10):1521–1526.

Samanic CM, De Roos AJ, Stewart PA, Rajaraman P, Waters MA, Inskip PD. 2008. Occupational exposure to pesticides and risk of adult brain tumors. *American Journal of Epidemiology* 167(8):976–985.

Saracci R, Kogevinas M, Bertazzi PA, Bueno de Mesquita BH, Coggon D, Green LM, Kauppinen T, L'Abbe KA, Littorin M, Lynge E, Mathews JD, Neuberger M, Osman J, Pearce N, Winkelmann R. 1991. Cancer mortality in workers exposed to chlorophenoxy herbicides and chlorophenols. *Lancet* 338:1027–1032.

Schlezinger JJ, Liu D, Farago M, Seldin DC, Belguise K, Sonenshein GE, Sherr DH. 2006. A role for the aryl hydrocarbon receptor in mammary gland tumorigenesis. *Biological Chemistry* 387(9):1175–1187.

Semenciw RM, Morrison HI, Morison D, Mao Y. 1994. Leukemia mortality and farming in the prairie provinces of Canada. *Canadian Journal of Public Health* 85:208–211.

Senft AP, Dalton TP, Nebert DW, Genter MB, Puga A, Hutchinson RJ, Kerzee JK, Uno S, Shertzer HG. 2002. Mitochondrial reactive oxygen production is dependent on the aromatic hydrocarbon receptor. *Free Radical Biology and Medicine* 33(9):1268–1278.

Sharma-Wagner S, Chokkalingam AP, Malker HS, Stone BJ, McLaughlin JK, Hsing AW. 2000. Occupation and prostate cancer risk in Sweden. *Journal of Occupational and Environmental Medicine* 42(5):517–525.

Shertzer HG, Nebert DW, Puga A, Ary M, Sonntag D, Dixon K, Robinson LJ, Cianciolo E, Dalton TP. 1998. Dioxin causes a sustained oxidative stress response in the mouse. *Biochemical and Biophysical Research Communications* 253(1):44–48.

Siemiatycki J, Wacholder S, Dewar R, Wald L, Bégin D, Richardson L, Rosenman K, Gérin M. 1988. Smoking and degree of occupational exposure: Are internal analyses in cohort studies likely to be confounded by smoking status? *American Journal of Industrial Medicine* 13(1):59–69.

Simanainen U, Haavisto T, Tuomisto JT, Paranko J, Toppari J, Tuomisto J, Peterson RE, Viluksela M. 2004a. Pattern of male reproductive system effects after in utero and lactational 2,3,7,8-tetrachlorodibenzo-*p*-dioxin (TCDD) exposure in three differentially TCDD-sensitive rat lines. *Toxicological Sciences* 80(1):101–108.

Simanainen U, Adamsson A, Tuomisto JT, Miettinen HM, Toppari J, Tuomisto J, Viluksela M. 2004b. Adult 2,3,7,8-tetrachlorodibenzo-*p*-dioxin (TCDD) exposure and effects on male reproductive organs in three differentially TCDD-susceptible rat lines. *Toxicological Sciences* 81(2):401–407.

Smith AH, Pearce NE. 1986. Update on soft tissue sarcoma and phenoxyherbicides in New Zealand. *Chemosphere* 15:1795–1798.

Smith AH, Fisher DO, Giles HJ, Pearce NE. 1983. The New Zealand soft tissue sarcoma case–control study: Interview findings concerning phenoxyacetic acid exposure. *Chemosphere* 12:565–571.

Smith AH, Pearce NE, Fisher DO, Giles HJ, Teague CA, Howard JK. 1984. Soft tissue sarcoma and exposure to phenoxyherbicides and chlorophenols in New Zealand. *Journal of the National Cancer Institute* 73:1111–1117.

Smith JG, Christophers AJ. 1992. Phenoxy herbicides and chlorophenols: A case control study on soft tissue sarcoma and malignant lymphoma. *British Journal of Cancer* 65:442–448.

Smith-Warner SA, Spiegelman D, Yaun SS, van den Brandt PA, Folsom AR, Goldbohm RA, Graham S, Holmberg L, Howe GR, Marshall JR, Miller AB, Potter JD, Speizer FE, Willett WC, Wolk A, Hunter DJ. 1998. Alcohol and breast cancer in women: A pooled analysis of cohort studies. *Journal of the American Medical Association* 279(7):535–540.

Solet D, Zoloth SR, Sullivan C, Jewett J, Michaels DM. 1989. Patterns of mortality in pulp and paper workers. *Journal of Occupational Medicine* 31:627–630.

Spinelli JJ, Ng CH, Weber JP, Connors JM, Gascoyne RD, Lai AS, Brooks-Wilson AR, Le ND, Berry BR, Gallagher RP. 2007. Organochlorines and risk of non-Hodgkin lymphoma. *International Journal of Cancer* 121(12):2767–2775.

Steenland K, Piacitelli L, Deddens J, Fingerhut M, Chang LI. 1999. Cancer, heart disease, and diabetes in workers exposed to 2,3,7,8-tetrachlorodibenzo-*p*-dioxin. *Journal of the National Cancer Institute* 91(9):779–786.

Stott WT, Johnson KA, Landry TD, Gorzinski SJ, Cieszlak FS. 1990. Chronic toxicity and oncogenicity of picloram in Fischer 344 rats. *Journal of Toxicology and Environmental Health* 30:91–104.

Svensson BG, Mikoczy Z, Stromberg U, Hagmar L. 1995. Mortality and cancer incidence among Swedish fishermen with a high dietary intake of persistent organochlorine compounds. *Scandinavian Journal of Work, Environmental, and Health* 21(2):106–115.

Swaen GMH, van Vliet C, Slangen JJM, Sturmans F. 1992. Cancer mortality among licensed herbicide applicators. *Scandinavian Journal of Work, Environment, and Health* 18:201–204.

Swaen GM, van Amelsvoort LG, Slangen JJ, Mohren DC. 2004. Cancer mortality in a cohort of licensed herbicide applicators. *International Archives of Occupational and Environmental Health* 77(4):293–295.

't Mannetje A, McLean D, Cheng S, Boffetta P, Colin D, Pearce N. 2005. Mortality in New Zealand workers exposed to phenoxy herbicides and dioxins. *Occupational and Environmental Medicine* 62(1):34–40.

Tarone RE, Hayes HM, Hoover RN, Rosenthal JF, Brown LM, Pottern LM, Javadpour N, O'Connell KJ, Stutzman RE. 1991. Service in Vietnam and risk of testicular cancer. *Journal of the National Cancer Institute* 83:1497–1499.

Teitelbaum SL, Gammon MD, Britton JA, Neugut AI, Levin B, Stellman SD. 2007. Reported residential pesticide use and breast cancer risk on Long Island, New York. *American Journal of Epidemiology* 165(6):643–651.

Thiess AM, Frentzel-Beyme R, Link R. 1982. Mortality study of persons exposed to dioxin in a trichlorophenol-process accident that occurred in the BASF AG on November 17, 1953. *American Journal of Industrial Medicine* 3:179–189.

Thomas TL. 1987. Mortality among flavour and fragrance chemical plant workers in the United States. *British Journal of Industrial Medicine* 44:733–737.

Thomas TL, Kang HK. 1990. Mortality and morbidity among Army Chemical Corps Vietnam veterans: A preliminary report. *American Journal of Industrial Medicine* 18:665–673.

Thomas TL, Kang H, Dalager N. 1991. Mortality among women Vietnam veterans, 1973–1987. *American Journal of Epidemiology* 134:973–980.

Thompson IM, Goodman PJ, Tangen CM, Lucia MS, Miller GJ, Ford LG, Lieber MM, Cespedes RD, Atkins JN, Lippman SM, Carlin SM, Ryan A, Szczepanek CM, Crowley JJ, Coltman CA Jr. 2003. The influence of finasteride on the development of prostate cancer. *New England Journal of Medicine* 349(3):215–224.

Thörn Å, Gustavsson P, Sadigh J, Westerlund-Hännerstrand B, Hogstedt C. 2000. Mortality and cancer incidence among Swedish lumberjacks exposed to phenoxy herbicides. *Occupational and Environmental Medicine* 57:718–720.

Torchio P, Lepore AR, Corrao G, Comba P, Settimi L, Belli S, Magnani C, di Orio F. 1994. Mortality study on a cohort of Italian licensed pesticide users. *The Science of the Total Environment* 149(3):183–191.

Toth K, Somfai-Relle S, Sugar J, Bence J. 1979. Carcinogenicity testing of herbicide 2,4,5-trichlorophenoxyethanol containing dioxin and of pure dioxin in Swiss mice. *Nature* 278(5704): 548–549.

Tuomisto JT, Pekkanen J, Kiviranta H, Tukiainen E, Vartiainen T, Tuomisto J. 2004. Soft-tissue sarcoma and dioxin: A case–control study. *International Journal of Cancer* 108(6):893–900.

van Grevenynghe J, Bernard M, Langouet S, Le Berre C, Fest T, Fardel O. 2005. Human CD34-positive hematopoietic stem cells constitute targets for carcinogenic polycyclic aromatic hydrocarbons. *Journal of Pharmacology and Experimental Therapeutics* 314(2):693–702.

Van Miller JP, Lalich JJ, Allen JR. 1977. Increased incidence of neoplasms in rats exposed to low levels of 2,3,7,8-tetrachlorodibenzo-*p*-dioxin. *Chemosphere* 9:537–544.

Viel JF, Arveux P, Baverel J, Cahn JY. 2000. Soft-tissue sarcoma and non-Hodgkin's lymphoma clusters around a municipal solid waste incinerator with high dioxin emission levels. *American Journal of Epidemiology* 152(1):13–19.

Viel JF, Clement MC, Hagi M, Grandjean S, Challier B, Danzon A. 2008. Dioxin emissions from a municipal solid waste incinerator and risk of invasive breast cancer: A population-based case–control study with GIS-derived exposure. *International Journal of Health Geographics [Electronic Resource]* 7:4.

Vineis P, Terracini B, Ciccone G, Cignetti A, Colombo E, Donna A, Maffi L, Pisa R, Ricci P, Zanini E, Comba P. 1986. Phenoxy herbicides and soft-tissue sarcomas in female rice weeders. A population-based case-referent study. *Scandinavian Journal of Work, Environment, and Health* 13:9–17.

Vineis P, Faggiano F, Tedeschi M, Ciccone G. 1991. Incidence rates of lymphomas and soft-tissue sarcomas and environmental measurements of phenoxy herbicides. *Journal of the National Cancer Institute* 83:362–363.

Visintainer PF, Barone M, McGee H, Peterson EL. 1995. Proportionate mortality study of Vietnam-era veterans of Michigan. *Journal of Occupational and Environmental Medicine* 37(4):423–428.

Vorderstrasse BA, Fenton SE, Bohn AA, Cundiff JA, Lawrence BP. 2004. A novel effect of dioxin: Exposure during pregnancy severely impairs mammary gland differentiation. *Toxicological Sciences* 78(2):248–257.

Walker NJ, Wyde ME, Fischer LJ, Nyska A, Bucher JR. 2006. Comparison of chronic toxicity and carcinogenicity of 2,3,7,8-tetrachlorodibenzo-*p*-dioxin (TCDD) in 2-year bioassays in female Sprague-Dawley rats. *Molecular Nutrition and Food Research* 50(10):934–944.

Wang S-L, Chang Y-C, Chao H-R, Li C-M, Li L-A, Lin L-Y, Papke O. 2006. Body burdens of polychlorinated dibenzo-*p*-dioxins, dibenzofurans, and biphenyls and their relations to estrogen metabolism in pregnant women. *Environmental Health Perspectives* 114(5):740–745.

Wanibuchi H, Salim E, Kinoshita A, Shen J, Wei M, Morimura K, Yoshida K, Kuroda K, Endo G, Fukushima S. 2004. Understanding arsenic carcinogenicity by the use of animal models. *Toxicology and Applied Pharmacology* 198(3):366–376.

Warner M, Eskenazi B, Mocarelli P, Gerthoux PM, Samuels S, Needham L, Patterson D, Brambilla P. 2002. Serum dioxin concentrations and breast cancer risk in the Seveso Women's Health Study. *Environmental Health Perspectives* 110(7):625–628.

Watanabe KK, Kang HK. 1995. Military service in Vietnam and the risk of death from trauma and selected cancers. *Annals of Epidemiology* 5:407–412.

Watanabe KK, Kang HK. 1996. Mortality patterns among Vietnam veterans: A 24-year retrospective analysis. *Journal of Occupational and Environmental Medicine* 38(3):272–278.

Watanabe KK, Kang HK, Thomas TL. 1991. Mortality among Vietnam veterans: With methodological considerations. *Journal of Occupational Medicine* 33:780–785.

Waterhouse D, Carman WJ, Schottenfeld D, Gridley G, McLean S. 1996. Cancer incidence in the rural community of Tecumseh, Michigan: A pattern of increased lymphopoietic neoplasms. *Cancer* 77(4):763–770.

Wei M, Wanibuchi H, Morimura K, Iwai S, Yoshida K, Endo G, Nakae D, Fukushima S. 2002. Carcinogenicity of dimethylarsinic acid in make F344 rats and genetic alterations in incuded urinary bladder tumors. *Carcinogenesis* 23(8):1387–1397.

Weiderpass E, Adami HO, Baron JA, Wicklund-Glynn A, Aune M, Atuma S, Persson I. 2000. Organochlorines and endometrial cancer risk. *Cancer Epidemiology, Biomarkers and Prevention* 9:487–493.

Weinberg RA. 2008. Twisted epithelial-mesenchymal transition blocks senescence. *Nature Cell Biology* 10(9):1021–1023.

Wen S, Yang FX, Gong Y, Zhang XL, Hui Y, Li JG, Liu AIL, Wu YN, Lu WQ, Xu Y. 2008. Elevated levels of urinary 8-hydroxyl-2'-deoxyguanosine in male electrical and electronic equipment dismantling workers exposed to high concentrations of polychlorinated dibenzo-*p*-dioxins and dibenzofurans, polybrominated diphenyl ethers, and polychlorinated biphenyls. *Environmental Science and Technology* 42(11):4202–4207.

Wigle DT, Semenciw RB, Wilkins K, Riedel D, Ritter L, Morrison HI, Mao Y. 1990. Mortality study of Canadian male farm operators: Non-Hodgkin's lymphoma mortality and agricultural practices in Saskatchewan. *Journal of the National Cancer Institute* 82:575–582.

Wiklund K. 1983. Swedish agricultural workers: A group with a decreased risk of cancer. *Cancer* 51:566–568.

Wiklund K, Lindefors BM, Holm LE. 1988. Risk of malignant lymphoma in Swedish agricultural and forestry workers. *British Journal of Industrial Medicine* 45:19–24.

Wiklund K, Dich J, Holm LE, Eklund G. 1989a. Risk of cancer in pesticide applicators in Swedish agriculture. *British Journal of Industrial Medicine* 46:809–814.

Wiklund K, Dich J, Holm LE. 1989b. Risk of soft tissue sarcoma, Hodgkin's disease and non-Hodgkin's lymphoma among Swedish licensed pesticide applicators. *Chemosphere* 18:395–400.

Wolfe WH, Michalek JE, Miner JC, Rahe A, Silva J, Thomas WF, Grubbs WD, Lustik MB, Karrison TG, Roegner RH, Williams DE. 1990. Health status of Air Force veterans occupationally exposed to herbicides in Vietnam. I. Physical health. *Journal of the American Medical Association* 264:1824–1831.

Woods JS, Polissar L, Severson RK, Heuser LS, Kulander BG. 1987. Soft tissue sarcoma and non-Hodgkin's lymphoma in relation to phenoxy herbicide and chlorinated phenol exposure in western Washington. *Journal of the National Cancer Institute* 78:899–910.

Wrensch M, Minn Y, Chew T, Bondy M, Berger MS. 2002. Epidemiology of primary brain tumors: Current concepts and review of the literature. *Neuro-Oncology* 4(4):278–299.

Wu CH, Chen HL, Su HJ, Lee CC, Shen KT, Ho WL, Ho SY, Ho YS, Wang YJ. 2004. The topical application of 2,3,7,8-tetrachlorodibenzo-*p*-dioxin lacks skin tumor-promoting potency but induces hepatic injury and tumor necrosis factor-alpha expression in ICR male mice. *Food and Chemical Toxicology* 42(8):1217–1225.

Wyde ME, Braen AP, Hejtmancik M, Johnson JD, Toft JD, Blake JC, Cooper SD, Mahler J, Vallant M, Bucher JR, Walker NJ. 2004. Oral and dermal exposure to 2,3,7,8-tetrachlorodibenzo-*p*-dioxin (TCDD) induces cutaneous papillomas and squamous cell carcinomas in female hemizygous Tg.AC transgenic mice. *Toxicological Sciences* 82(1):34–45.

Xu JX, Hoshida Y, Yang WI, Inohara H, Kubo T, Kim GE, Yoon JH, Kojya S, Bandoh N, Harabuchi Y, Tsutsumi K, Koizuka I, Jia XS, Kirihata M, Tsukuma H, Aozasa K. 2007. Life-style and environmental factors in the development of nasal NK/T-cell lymphoma: A case–control study in East Asia. *International Journal of Cancer* 120(2):406–410.

Yamamoto S, Konishi Y, Matsuda T, Murai T, Shibata MA, Matsui-Yuasa I, Otani S, Kuroda K, Endo G, Fukushima S. 1995. Cancer incidence by an organic arsenic compound, dimethylarsinic acid (cacodylic acid), in F344/DuCrj rats after pretreatment with five carcinogens. *Cancer Research* 55(6):1271–1276.

Yamanaka K, Ohtsubo K, Hasegawa A, Hayashi H, Ohji H, Kanisawa M, Okada S. 1996. Exposure to dimethylarsinic acid, a main metabolite of inorganic arsenics, strongly promotes tumorigenesis initiated by 4-nitroquinoline 1-oxide in the lungs of mice. *Carcinogenesis* 17(4):767–770.

Yang X, Solomon S, Fraser LR, Trombino AF, Liu D, Sonenshein GE, Hestermann EV, Sherr DH. 2008. Constitutive regulation of CYP1B1 by the aryl hydrocarbon receptor (AhR) in pre-malignant and malignant mammary tissue. *Journal of Cellular Biochemistry* 104(2):402–417.

Yoshizawa K, Walker NJ, Jokinen MP, Brix AE, Sells DM, Marsh T, Wyde ME, Orzech D, Haseman JK, Nyska A. 2005a. Gingival carcinogenicity in female Harlan Sprague-Dawley rats following two-year oral treatment with 2,3,7,8-tetrachlorodibenzo-*p*-dioxin and dioxin-like compounds. *Toxicological Sciences* 83(1):64–77. [erratum appears in *Toxicological Sciences* 2005; 83(2):405–406].

Yoshizawa K, Marsh T, Foley JF, Cai B, Peddada S, Walker NJ, Nyska A. 2005b. Mechanisms of exocrine pancreatic toxicity induced by oral treatment with 2,3,7,8-tetrachlorodibenzo-*p*-dioxin in female Harlan Sprague-Dawley rats. *Toxicological Sciences* 85(1):594–606.

Yoshizawa K, Heatherly A, Malarkey DE, Walker NJ, Nyska A. 2007. A critical comparison of murine pathology and epidemiological data of TCDD, PCB126, and PeCDF. *Toxicologic Pathology* 35(7):865–879.

Zack JA, Suskind RR. 1980. The mortality experience of workers exposed to tetrachlorodibenzo-dioxin in a trichlorophenol process accident. *Journal of Occupational Medicine* 22:11–14.

Zahm SH, Fraumeni JF Jr. 1997. The epidemiology of soft tissue sarcoma. *Seminars in Oncology* 24(5):504–514.

Zahm SH, Weisenburger DD, Babbitt PA, Saal RC, Vaught JB, Cantor KP, Blair A. 1990. A case–control study of non-Hodgkin's lymphoma and the herbicide 2,4-dichlorophenoxyacetic acid (2,4-D) in eastern Nebraska. *Epidemiology* 1:349–356.

Zahm SH, Blair A, Weisenburger DD. 1992. Sex differences in the risk of multiple myeloma associated with agriculture (2). *British Journal of Industrial Medicine* 49:815–816.

Zahm SH, Weisenburger DD, Saal RC, Vaught JB, Babbitt PA, Blair A. 1993. The role of agricultural pesticide use in the development of non-Hodgkin's lymphoma in women. *Archives of Environmental Health* 48:353–358.

Zambon P, Ricci P, Bovo E, Casula A, Gattolin M, Fiore AR, Chiosi F, Guzzinati S. 2007. Sarcoma risk and dioxin emissions from incinerators and industrial plants: A population-based case–control study (Italy). *Environmental Health: A Global Access Science Source* 6:19.

Zhong Y, Rafnsson V. 1996. Cancer incidence among Icelandic pesticide users. *International Journal of Epidemiology* 25(6):1117–1124.

Zober A, Messerer P, Huber P. 1990. Thirty-four-year mortality follow-up of BASF employees exposed to 2,3,7,8-TCDD after the 1953 accident. *International Archives of Occupational and Environmental Health* 62:139–157.

7

Reproductive Effects and Impacts on Future Generations

This chapter summarizes the scientific literature published since *Veterans and Agent Orange: Update 2006*, hereafter referred to as *Update 2006* (IOM, 2007), on the association between exposure to herbicides and adverse reproductive or developmental effects. (Analogous shortened names are used to refer to the updates for 1996, 1998, 2000, 2002, and 2004 [IOM, 1996, 1999, 2001, 2003, 2005].) The categories of association and the approach to categorizing the health outcomes are discussed in Chapters 1 and 2. The literature considered in this chapter includes studies of a broad spectrum of reproductive effects in Vietnam veterans or other populations occupationally or environmentally exposed to the herbicides sprayed in Vietnam or to 2,3,7,8-tetrachlorodibenzo-*p*-dioxin (TCDD). Because some polychlorinated biphenyls (PCBs) and polychlorodibenzofurans (PCDFs) have dioxin-like biologic activity, studies of populations exposed to PCBs or PCDFs were reviewed if their results were presented in terms of toxicity equivalence quotients (TEQs).

As in previous updates, the adverse outcomes evaluated include impaired fertility (in which endometriosis or declines in sperm quality may be involved), increased fetal loss (spontaneous abortion and stillbirth) or neonatal and infant mortality, and other adverse birth outcomes (including low birth weight, preterm birth, and birth defects). In addition to the more delayed problem of childhood cancer in their offspring, this update also addresses the concern of Vietnam veterans that their military exposures may contribute to other problems that their children experience later in life or are manifested in later generations.

To reduce repetition throughout the report, Chapter 5 presented design information on new studies that report findings on multiple health outcomes. To provide context for publications that present new results on study populations that were addressed in publications reviewed in earlier updates, Chapter 5 also discussed the overall characteristics of those populations with details about design and analysis relevant to individual papers. For new studies that report only reproductive health outcomes and that are not revisiting previously studied populations, design information is summarized in this chapter with results.

This chapter's primary emphasis is on the potential adverse reproductive effects of herbicide exposure of men because the vast majority of Vietnam veterans are men. However, about 8,000 women served in Vietnam (H. Kang, US Department of Veterans Affairs, personal communication, December 14, 2000), so findings relevant to female reproductive health are also included. Whenever the information was available, an attempt was made to evaluate the effects of maternal and paternal exposure separately. Exposure scenarios in human populations and experimental animals studied differ in their applicability to our population of concern according to whether the exposed parent was a male or female veteran. In addition, for published epidemiologic or experimental results to be fully relevant to evaluation of the plausibility of reproductive effects in Vietnam veterans, female as well as male, the timing of exposure needs to correspond to the veterans' experience (that is, occur only prior to conception). With the possible exception of female veterans who became pregnant while serving in Vietnam, pregnancies that might have been affected occurred after deployment, when primary exposure had ceased.

BIOLOGIC PLAUSIBILITY OF REPRODUCTIVE EFFECTS

This chapter opens with a general discussion of factors that influence the plausibility that TCDD and the four herbicides used in Vietnam could produce adverse reproductive effects. There have been very few reproductive studies of the four herbicides in question, particularly picloram and cacodylic acid, and those studies generally have shown toxicity only at very high doses, so the preponderance of the following discussion concerns TCDD.

Because dioxin is stored in fat tissue and has a very long biologic half-life, internal exposure at generally constant concentrations may continue after episodic, high-level exposure to external sources has ceased. If a person had high exposure, there may still be high amounts of dioxin stored in fat tissue, which may be mobilized, particularly at times of weight loss. That would not be expected to be the case for nonlipophilic chemicals, such as cacodylic acid.

The paternal contribution to a pregnancy is limited to the contents of the sperm that fertilizes an egg, any damage would be conveyed as DNA mutations or epigenetic effects (that is, heritable changes in genome function that occur without a change in primary DNA sequences). Dioxins have not been shown to alter DNA sequences (they do not produce mutations), so the potential effects in offspring are limited to epigenetic effects. Two possible mechanisms could theoretically produce affected children: if sperm stem cells are altered by exposure, they could continue to produce altered sperm; and mobilization of dioxin from storage in adipose tissue (for example, due to weight loss) could continue to damage a man's developing sperm, and thus interfere with conception and conceptuses. In any case, any exposure of the father that could affect his children must occur before their conception.

Although ova, the maternal contribution to a conceptus, do not undergo the repeated 90-day cycles of spermatogenesis, they might be damaged by modes of exposure analogous to those affecting male gametes. In addition, at critical periods of gestation and even postnatally through breast milk, the female can mediate exposure to the offspring as it develops. Such exposure can interfere with cell replication, differentiation, and migration; with formation of tissues, organs, and systems; and with structure. Dioxin in her bloodstream, whether from external sources or released from fat stores, can cross the placenta and expose the developing embryo and fetus. Mobilization of dioxin during pregnancy or lactation may be increased because the body is drawing on fat stores to supply nutrients to the developing fetus or nursing infant. Breast milk has a high fat content, and the concentration of dioxin in breast milk is about 100 times that in a mother's blood. In animal studies, TCDD crosses the placenta and is transferred via breast milk. In humans, TCDD has been measured in circulating maternal blood, cord blood, placenta, and breast milk (Suzuki et al., 2005), and it is estimated that an infant breastfed for 1 year accumulates a dose of TCDD that is 6 times as high as that in an infant not breastfed (Lorber and Phillips, 2002). Thus, the exposure of human infants to TCDD in utero and via lactation has been demonstrated.

Toxicologists often distinguish between reproductive effects, which concern the reproductive process itself, and developmental effects, which involve differentiation of fetal tissues and maturation of the offspring. A connection between TCDD exposure and human reproductive and developmental effects is, in general, biologically plausible. However, more definitive conclusions about the potential for such TCDD toxicity in humans are complicated by differences in sensitivity and susceptibility among individual animals, strains, and species; by the lack of strong evidence of organ-specific effects among species; by differences in route, dose, duration, and timing of exposure; and by substantial differences in the toxicokinetics of TCDD between laboratory animals and humans. Experiments with 2,4-dichlorophenoxyacetic acid (2,4-D) and 2,4,5-trichlorophenoxyacetic acid (2,4,5-T) indicate that they have subcellular effects that could constitute a biologically plausible mechanism for reproductive and developmental effects. Evidence from animals, however, indicates that they do not have reproductive effects and that they have developmental effects only at very high doses. There is insufficient information on picloram and cacodylic acid to assess the biologic plausibility of those compounds' reproductive or developmental effects.

The biologic plausibility portions of sections on the specific outcomes considered in this chapter present more detailed toxicologic findings that are of particular relevance to the outcomes discussed.

ENDOMETRIOSIS

Endometriosis (*International Classification of Diseases, 9th revision* [ICD-9], code 617) affects 5.5 million women in the United States and Canada at any given time (NICHD, 2007). The endometrium is the tissue that lines the inside of the uterus and is built up and shed each month during menstruation. In endometriosis, endometrial cells are found outside the uterus—usually in other parts of the reproductive system, in the abdomen, or on surfaces near the reproductive organs. That misplaced tissue develops into growths or lesions that continue to respond to hormonal changes in the body and break down and bleed each month in concert with the menstrual cycle. Unlike blood released during normal shedding of the endometrium lining the uterus, blood released in endometriosis has no way to leave the body, and the results are inflammation, internal bleeding, and degeneration of blood and tissue that can cause scarring, pain, infertility, adhesions, and intestinal problems.

There are several theories of the etiology of endometriosis, including a genetic contribution, but the cause remains unknown. Estrogen dependence and immune modulation are established features of endometriosis but do not adequately explain the cause of this disorder. It has been proposed that endometrium is distributed through the body via blood or the lymphatic system; that menstrual tissue backs up into the fallopian tubes, implants in the abdomen, and grows; and that all women experience some form of tissue backup during menstruation but only those with immune-system or hormonal problems experience the tissue growth associated with endometriosis. Despite numerous symptoms that can indicate endometriosis, diagnosis is possible only through laparoscopy or a more invasive surgical technique. Several treatments for endometriosis are available, but there is no cure.

Conclusions from *VAO* and Updates

Endometriosis was first reviewed in this series of reports in *Update 2002*, which identified two relevant environmental studies, and *Update 2004* examined three environmental studies. Two additional environmental studies considered in *Update 2006* did not change the conclusion that the evidence was inadequate or insufficient to support an association with herbicide exposure. Table 7-1 provides a summary of relevant studies that have been reviewed.

Update of the Epidemiologic Literature

No new Vietnam-veteran or occupational studies addressing endometriosis have been published since *Update 2006*.

439

TABLE 7-1 Selected Epidemiologic Studies—Endometriosis

Reference	Study Population	Study Results
ENVIRONMENTAL		
New Studies		
Heilier et al., 2006	Serum DLC and aromatase activity in endometriotic tissue from 47 patients in Belgium	No association between TEQs of DLCs in serum and aromatase activity by regression analyses. p-values = 0.37–0.90 for different endometriosis subgroups.
Heilier et al., 2007	88 matched triads (264 total); patients with deep endometriotic nodules, pelvic endometriosis, controls matched for age, gynecologic practice in Belgium; routes of exposure to DLCs examined	Results for pelvic endometriosis vs controls Dietary fat: OR = 1.0 (95% CI 1.0–1.0) BMI: OR = 1.0 (95% CI 0.9–1.0) Occupation: OR = 0.5 (95% CI 0.2–1.1) Traffic: OR = 1.0 (95% CI 0.3–2.8) Incinerator: OR = 1.0 (95% CI 1.0–1.1)
Tsuchiya et al., 2007	138 infertility patients in Japan; laproscopically confirmed case–control status, serum dioxin, PCB TEQ; P450 genetic polymorphism	Results for advanced endometriosis Total TEQ: OR = 0.5 (95% CI 0.2–1.7) Genotype-specific: ORs = 0.3–0.6 No significant interaction between genotype, dioxin TEQ
Studies Reviewed in *Update 2006*		
Heilier et al., 2005	Endometriosis in Belgian women with overnight fasting serum levels of PCDD, PCDF, PCB	50 exposed cases, risk of increase of 10 pg/p lipid of TEQ compounds: OR = 2.6 (95% CI 1.3–5.3)
Porpora et al., 2006	Case–control study of Italian women with endometriosis, measured serum PCBs	Mean total PCBs (ng/g) Cases, 410 ng/g Control, 250 ng/g All PCB congeners: OR = 4.0 (95% CI 1.3–13)
Studies Review in *Update 2004*		
De Felip et al., 2004	Pilot study of Italian, Belgian women of reproductive age; compared concentrations of TCDD, total TEQ in pooled blood samples from women who had diagnosis endometriosis with controls	Mean concentration of TCDD (ppt of lipid) Italy: Controls (10 pooled samples), 1.6 Cases (two sets of six pooled samples), 2.1, 1.3 Belgium: Controls (seven pooled samples), 2.5 Cases (Set I, five pooled samples; Set II, six pooled samples), 2.3, 2.3 Mean concentration of TEQ (ppt of lipid) Italy: Controls (10 pooled samples), 8.9 ± 1.3 (99% CI 7.2–11) Cases (two sets of six pooled samples), 10.7 ± 1.6; 10.1 ± 1.5 Belgium: Controls (seven pooled samples), 24.7 ± 3.7 (99% CI 20–29) Cases (Set I, five pooled samples; Set II, six pooled samples), 18.1 ± 2.7; 27.1 ± 4 .0

continued

TABLE 7-1 Continued

Reference	Study Population	Study Results
Fierens et al., 2003	Belgian women with environmental exposure to PCDDs, PCDFs; compared analyte concentrations in cases vs controls	Mean concentration of TEQ a (ppt of lipid) Cases (n = 10), 26.2 (95% CI 18.2–37.7) Controls (n = 132), 25.6 (95% CI 24.3–28.9) No significant difference
Eskenazi et al., 2002	Residents of Seveso Zones A and B up to 30 years old in 1976; compared incidence of endometriosis across serum TCDD concentrations	Serum TCDD (ppt) 20.1–100 ppt (n = 8), OR = 1.2 (90% CI 0.3–4.5) > 100 ppt (n = 9), OR = 2.1 (90% CI 0.5–8.0)
Studies Reviewed in *Update 2002*		
Pauwels et al., 2001	Patients undergoing infertility treatment in Belgium; compared number of women with, without endometriosis who had serum dioxin levels up to 100 pg TEQ/g of serum lipid	Six exposed cases: OR = 4.6 (95% CI 0.5–43.6)
Mayani et al., 1997	Residents of Jerusalem being evaluated for infertility; compared number of women with high TCDD who had (n = 44), did not have (n = 35) diagnosis of endometriosis	Eight exposed cases: OR = 7.6 (95% CI 0.9–169.7)

ABBREVIATIONS: BMI, body mass index; CI, confidence interval; DLC, dioxin-like compound; OR, odds ratio; PCB, polychlorinated biphenyl; PCDD, polychlorinated dibenzodioxin; PCDF, polychlorinated dibenzofuran; TCDD, 2,3,7,8-tetrachlorodibenzo-*p*-dioxin; TEQ, toxicity equivalent quotient.
[a]TEQs calculated using the 1998 World Health Organization dioxin toxic equivalency factor (TEF) method (Van den Berg et al., 1998).

Environmental Studies

Three new studies concerning exposure to the compounds of interest and endometriosis have been conducted since the last update. The first two were conducted by the same research group that reported an increased risk of endometriosis with serum concentrations of dioxin-like compounds (DLCs) (Heilier et al., 2005). In the new studies, they sought to expand their findings by focusing on a possible biologic pathway (aromatase activity) and routes of exposure (such as diet and residential proximity to waste incinerators). However, neither study showed significant associations of endometriosis with the factors studied. The third new study (Tsuchiya et al., 2007), which looked at specific genes in addition to dioxin exposure, did not find an association between dioxin exposure and early stage-endometriosis regardless of genotype. In contrast with some earlier studies, it found dioxin exposure to be associated with a lower risk of advanced endometriosis. This lower risk was particularly strong in women who had a specific genotype.

In the study of Heilier et al. (2006), 47 women admitted to a university hospital in Belgium for the treatment of endometriosis agreed to participate in a study aimed at determining whether aromatase activity was associated with the concentration of DLCs in the endometriotic tissue. Aromatase is an enzyme important in the synthesis of estrogen, and drugs that block the synthesis of estrogen lead to a reduction in endometriotic tissue. The authors thought that DLCs might increase the aromatase, which would increase estrogen and lead to increased growth of endometrial tissue. Endometriotic tissue was surgically removed from the women, and DLCs and aromatase activity were measured in the laboratory. They found that the concentration of DLCs was not associated with higher aromatase activity in endometriotic tissue.

Heilier et al. (2007) studied a total of 264 women in the same gynecologic practice, divided equally into three groups matched on age; cases of pelvic endometriosis, cases of deep endometriotic nodules, and controls. Serum TEQ concentrations were available for 58 of these women who had participated in a previous study by the authors (Heilier et al., 2005), which found a risk of endometriosis associated with exposure to DLCs. Interviews conducted with patients and controls collected information on diet, occupation, and residential proximity to automobile traffic, waste incinerators, or other pollution sources. In the subset of women whose serum DLCs were measured, they found that those with higher concentrations were more likely to have consumed specific high-fat foods: pig meat, marine fish, and fresh cream. However, neither dietary fat consumption, body mass index (BMI), residential proximity to automobile traffic or waste incinerators, nor specific occupation was associated with pelvic endometriosis or with deep endometriotic nodules. The study used indirect measures of dioxin exposure that are expected to be less precise than measures of serum dioxin, so the results do not necessarily contradict those of their earlier study. The investigators were unable to identify any likely source of dioxin exposure that differed between cases and controls.

The third new study was conducted by Tsuchiya et al. (2007) in Japan to examine a possible association between genetic susceptibility to effects of exposure to DLCs and endometriosis. They studied a total of 138 women who sought treatment for infertility and had undergone laparoscopy. On the basis of laparoscopy, the women were classified as having early-stage endometriosis (stages I–II), advanced endometriosis (stages III–IV), or no evidence of endometriosis (controls). They measured serum dioxin and DLCs (TEQ per gram of lipids) and extracted DNA from serum to determine polymorphisms (different genetic versions) of two genes (cytochromes P450 [CYP] 1A1 and 1B1), which regulate the synthesis and metabolism of endogenous and exogenous estrogens. They hypothesized that differences in genetic makeup might confer differences in susceptibility to effects of

DLCs and might explain why studies of endometriosis and dioxins show inconsistent results. Overall, serum-dioxin concentrations did not differ significantly between cases with early or advanced endometriosis and controls (adjusted for age). Women who had advanced endometriosis were less likely to have high serum dioxins than controls (OR = 0.46, 95% CI 0.20–1.06), but the difference was of borderline statistical significance; the result was virtually unchanged by considering the total concentration of PCBs and dioxins. When genotype was considered, the authors found no significant interaction between genotype and serum dioxin in women who had early endometriosis. However, there was some evidence of interaction between CYP genes and dioxin exposure with respect to the risk of advanced endometriosis. There was a reduced risk of advanced endometriosis after high dioxin exposure in women who had the less common allele for CYP1A1, but the number of women in this group was very small. In summary, the study found some evidence of a gene–environment interaction related to the occurrence of endometriosis, but women who had higher concentrations of dioxin were found to be at *lower* risk for advanced endometriosis.

Biologic Plausibility

Laboratory studies that used animal models and examined gene-expression changes associated with human endometriosis and TCDD exposure provide evidence to support the biologic plausibility of a link between TCDD exposure and endometriosis. The first suggestion that TCDD exposure may be linked to endometriosis came as a secondary finding from a study that exposed female rhesus monkeys (*Macaca mulatta*) chronically to low concentrations of dietary TCDD for 4 years (Rier et al., 1993). Ten years after the exposure ended, the investigators documented an increased incidence of endometriosis in the monkeys that correlated with the dioxin exposure concentration. The small sample prevented a definitive conclusion that TCDD was a causal agent in the development of the endometriosis, but it led to numerous studies of the ability of TCDD to promote the growth of pre-existing endometriotic lesions.

When fragments of uterine tissue were implanted in the peritoneal cavity to mimic eutopic endometrial lesions, TCDD exposure was shown to promote the survival and growth of the lesions in monkeys and in rodents (Cummings et al., 1996; Johnson et al., 1997; Yang et al., 2000). In mice, direct treatment of endometrial tissue with TCDD before placement into the peritoneal cavity resulted in increased size and number of endometrial lesions (Bruner-Tran et al., 1999).

A number of proposed mechanisms by which TCDD may promote endometrial lesions provide additional biologic plausibility of the link between TCDD and endometriosis. Human endometrial tissue expresses the aryl hydrocarbon receptor (AHR) and its dimerization partner, the aryl hydrocarbon nuclear translocator (ARNT) (Khorram et al., 2002), and three AHR target genes: CYP1A1,

1A2, and 1B1 (Bulun et al., 2000). That suggests that endometrial tissue is responsive to TCDD. Furthermore, TCDD significantly decreases the ratio of progesterone receptor B to progesterone receptor A in normal human endometrial stromal cells and blocks the ability of progesterone to suppress matrix metalloproteinase (MMP) expression; these actions may promote endometrial-tissue invasion. Both the reduced ratio and the resistance to progesterone-mediated MMP suppression are observed in endometrial tissue from women who have endometriosis (Igarashi et al., 2005). Progesterone prevents endometrial breakdown before menstruation by down-regulating expression of endometrial matrix metalloproteins during the secretory phase of the menstrual cycle. Bruner-Tran et al. (2008) have proposed that environmental toxicants, such as TCDD, that disrupt progesterone action may predispose the endometrium to an inflammatory microenvironment that would promote a process of tissue loss at menstruation. Their hypothesis is supported by their evidence that TCDD inhibits expression of progesterone receptor and transforming growth factor $\beta2$ in the endometrium and possibly expression of other immune modulators regulated by progesterone.

TCDD induces changes in gene expression that mirror those observed in endometrial lesions. For example, TCDD can induce expression of histamine-releasing factor, which is increased in endometrial lesions and accelerates their growth (Oikawa et al., 2002, 2003). Similarly, TCDD stimulates expression of RANTES (regulated on activation, normal T cell–expressed, and secreted) in endometrial stromal cells, and RANTES concentration and bioactivity are increased in women who have endometriosis (Zhao et al., 2002). The two CC-motif chemokines (chemotactic cytokines), RANTES and macrophage-inflammatory protein (MIP)-1α, have been identified as potential contributors to the pathogenesis and progression of endometriosis. To probe the effect of dioxin exposure and estrogen on expression of those chemokines in endometriosis-associated cells and to explore the pathogenesis of endometriosis, endometrial stromal cells were exposed to a combination of 17β-estradiol and TCDD. The combined treatment increased the secretion of RANTES and MIP-1α, promoted the invasiveness of endometrial stromal cells, and increased the expression of matrix metalloproteins MMP-2 and MMP-9 in endometrial stromal cells, indicating that combined TCDD and estradiol may facilitate the onset of endometriosis and contribute to its development by increasing the invasion of endometrial stromal cells mediated by CC-motif chemokines (Yu et al., 2008). Those data are consistent with the evidence of an interaction between the AHR and the estrogen receptor that induces estrogen-mediated proliferative effects in the mouse uterus (Ohtake et al., 2008). Differences between the mouse uterus and the human endometrium prevent absolute extrapolation, but the data suggest that dioxins may induce changes in endometrial physiology. In summary, it may be expected that TCDD exposure would create an inflammatory endometrial microenvironment that could disrupt endometrial function and cause disease.

Although those studies do not establish the degree to which TCDD may cause or promote endometriosis, they do provide evidence that supports the biologic plausibility of a link between TCDD exposure and endometriosis.

Synthesis

The three new studies described above were designed to follow on previous studies showing an association between DLCs and endometriosis. Two of the studies (Heilier et al., 2006, 2007) were conducted by the same research group that had found a significant association between blood concentrations of DLCs and risk of endometriosis. They sought to shed light on possible biologic pathways and routes of exposure that might expand on the previous findings. However, neither the evaluation of an enzyme important in the synthesis of estrogen nor examination of routes of exposure to dioxin yielded evidence of association with endometriosis. The third new study (Tsuchiya et al., 2007) found a decreased risk of endometriosis in women with higher dioxin concentrations.

Overall, the studies linking dioxin exposure with endometriosis are few in number and inconsistent. The association in animal studies is biologically plausible, but it is possible that human exposures are too low to show an association consistently.

Conclusion

On the basis of the evidence reviewed here and in the previous VAO reports, the committee concludes that there is inadequate or insufficient evidence to support an association between exposure to the chemicals of interest and human endometriosis.

FERTILITY

Male reproductive function is under the control of several components whose proper coordination is important for normal fertility. Several of the components and some health outcomes related to male fertility, including reproductive hormones and sperm characteristics, can be studied as indicators of fertility. The reproductive neuroendocrine axis involves the central nervous system, the anterior pituitary gland, and the testis. The hypothalamus integrates neural inputs from the central and peripheral nervous systems and regulates the gonadotropins luteinizing hormone (LH) and follicle-stimulating hormone (FSH). Both are secreted into the circulation in episodic bursts by the anterior pituitary gland and are necessary for normal spermatogenesis. In the testis, LH interacts with receptors on Leydig cells, where it stimulates increased testosterone synthesis. FSH and the testosterone from the Leydig cells interact with the Sertoli cells in the seminiferous tubule epithelium to regulate spermatogenesis. More detailed reviews of the male reproductive hormones can be found elsewhere (Knobil et al., 1994; Yen and Jaffe, 1991). Several agents, such as lead and dibromochloropropane, affect the neuroendocrine system and spermatogenesis (for reviews, see Bonde and Giwercman, 1995; Tas et al., 1996).

Studies of the relationship between chemicals and fertility are less common in women than in men. Some chemicals may disrupt the female hormonal balance necessary for proper functioning. Normal menstrual-cycle functioning is also important in the risk of hormonally related diseases, such as osteopenia, breast cancer, and cardiovascular disease. Chemicals can have multiple effects on the female system, including modulation of hormone concentrations resulting in menstrual-cycle or ovarian-cycle irregularities, changes in menarche and menopause, and impairment of fertility (Bretveld et al., 2006a,b). In this section, we also discuss studies that have focused on menstrual-cycle characteristics and age at menarche or menopause. An affect on age at menarche would be of concern among the daughters of Vietnam veterans rather than among female veterans themselves, but the occurrence of this effect in other populations would demonstrate the ability of the chemicals in question to perturb functioning of the female reproductive system.

Conclusions from *VAO* and Updates

The committee responsible for the original *VAO* report (IOM, 1994) concluded that there was inadequate or insufficient evidence of an association between exposure to 2,4-D, 2,4,5-T, TCDD, picloram, or cacodylic acid and altered sperm characteristics or infertility. Overall, additional information available to the committees responsible for *Update 1996*, *Update 1998*, *Update 2000*, *Update 2002*, *Update 2004*, and *Update 2006* did not change that finding. Reviews of the relevant studies are presented in the earlier reports. Tables 7-2 and 7-3 summarize the studies related to male and female fertility, respectively.

Update of the Epidemiologic Literature

Male Fertility

Vietnam-Veteran Studies   One new Vietnam-veteran study has been published since *Update 2006*. Gupta et al. (2006) compared serum testosterone concentrations measured in 1987 with TCDD concentrations measured at the same time in veterans in the Air Force Health Study. A total of 971 Ranch Hand veterans and 1,266 comparison veterans with serum TCDD and serum testosterone measurements were included in the analyses. After adjustment for age and BMI in 1987 and for a percentage change in BMI from the end of their Southeast Asia tour to 1987, higher serum TCDD was significantly associated with lower testosterone concentrations in both Ranch Hands (slope for ln[TCDD] = −0.02, 95% CI

TABLE 7-2 Selected Epidemiologic Studies—Male Fertility (Altered Hormone Concentrations, Decreased Sperm Counts or Quality, Subfertility, or Infertility)

Reference	Study Population	Exposed Cases[a]	Measure of Risk (95% CI)[a]
VIETNAM VETERANS			
New Studies			
Gupta et al., 2006	AFHS (964 Ranch Hands, 1,259 comparison)		Coefficient (p-value) for ln(Testosterone) vs ln(TCDD) in 1987
	Comparison TCDD quartile I (mean, 2.14 ppt)	nr	0 (referent)
	Comparison TCDD quartile II (mean, 3.54 ppt)	nr	−0.063 (0.004)
	Ranch Hand TCDD quartile I (mean, 4.14 ppt)	nr	0.002 (0.94)
	Comparison TCDD quartile III (mean, 4.74 ppt)	nr	−0.048 (0.03)
	Comparison TCDD quartile IV (mean, 7.87 ppt)	nr	−0.079 (< 0.001)
	Ranch Hand TCDD quartile II (mean, 8.95 ppt)	nr	−0.052 (0.03)
	Ranch Hand TCDD quartile III (mean, 18.40 ppt)	nr	−0.029 (0.22)
	Ranch Hand TCDD quartile IV (mean, 76.16 ppt)	nr	−0.056 (0.02)
Studies Reviewed in *Update 1996*			
Henriksen et al., 1996	Effects on specific hormone concentrations or sperm count in Ranch Hands		
	Low testosterone		
	High dioxin (1992)	18	1.6 (0.9–2.7)
	High dioxin (1987)	3	0.7 (0.2–2.3)
	Low dioxin (1992)	10	0.9 (0.5–1.8)
	Low dioxin (1987)	10	2.3 (1.1–4.9)
	Background (1992)	9	0.5 (0.3–1.1)
	High FSH		
	High dioxin (1992)	8	1.0 (0.5–2.1)
	Low dioxin (1992)	12	1.6 (0.8–3.0)
	Background (1992)	16	1.3 (0.7–2.4)
	High LH		
	High dioxin (1992)	5	0.8 (0.3–1.9)
	Low dioxin (1992)	5	0.8 (0.5–3.3)
	Background (1992)	8	0.8 (0.4–1.8)
	Low sperm count		
	High dioxin	49	0.9 (0.7–1.2)
	Low dioxin	43	0.8 (0.6–1.0)
	Background	66	0.9 (0.7–1.2)
Studies Reviewed in *VAO*			
CDC, 1989	Vietnam Experience Study		
	Lower sperm concentration	42	2.3 (1.2–4.3)
	Proportion of abnormal sperm	51	1.6 (0.9–2.8)
	Reduced sperm motility	83	1.2 (0.8–1.8)
Stellman et al., 1988	American Legionnaires who served in SEA		
	Difficulty in having children	349[a]	1.3 (p < 0.01)

TABLE 7-2 Continued

Reference	Study Population	Exposed Cases[a]	Measure of Risk (95% CI)[a]
OCCUPATIONAL			
Newly considered study			
Egeland et al., 1994	Male chemical workers exposed to dioxin vs neighborhood controls in New Jersey, Missouri measured in 1987		Risk of extreme hormone concentration
	Testosterone (< 10.4 nmol/L)		
	Referents (TCDD < 20 ppt)	11	1.0
	Workers	25	2.1 (1.0–4.6)
	Quartile I (TCDD < 20 ppt)	2	0.9 (0.2–4.5)
	Quartile II (TCDD 20–75 ppt)	7	3.9 (1.3–11.3)
	Quartile III (TCDD 76–240 ppt)	6	2.7 (0.9–8.2)
	Quartile IV (TCDD 241–3,400 ppt)	10	2.1 (0.8–5.8)
	FSH (> 31 IU/L)	20	1.5 (0.7–3.3)
	LH (> 28 IU/L)	23	1.6 (0.8–3.3)
Studies Reviewed in *Update 2006*			
Oh et al., 2005	Male fertility, dioxin exposure with air monitoring	31	1.4 (nr)
Studies Reviewed in *Update 2000*			
Larsen et al., 1998	Danish farmers who used any potentially spermatotoxic pesticides, including 2,4-D		
	Farmers using pesticides vs organic farmers	523	1.0 (0.8–1.4)[b]
	Used three or more pesticides	nr	0.9 (0.7–1.2)[b]
	Used manual sprayer for pesticides	nr	0.8 (0.6–1.1)[b]
Studies Reviewed in *Update 1998*			
Heacock et al., 1998	Workers at sawmills using chlorophenates		
	Standardized fertility ratio	18,016 (births)	0.7 (0.7–0.8)[c]
	Mantel–Haenszel rate-ratio estimator	18,016 (births)	0.9 (0.8–0.9)[c]
	Cumulative exposure (hours)		
	120–1,999	7,139	0.8 (0.8–0.9)[c]
	2,000–3,999	4,582	0.9 (0.8–1.0)[c]
	4,000–9,999	4,145	1.0 (0.9–1.1)[c]
	≥ 10,000	1,300	1.1 (1.0–1.2)[c]
Lerda and Rizzi, 1991	Argentinean farmers exposed to 2,4-D	32	
	Sperm count (millions/mL)	exposed: 49.0 vs control: 101.6	
	Motility (%)	exposed: 24.8 vs control: 70.4	
	Sperm death (%)	exposed: 82.9 vs control: 37.1[d]	
	Anomalies (%)	exposed: 72.9 vs control: 33.4	
		(p < 0.01 overall)	
ENVIRONMENTAL			
New Studies			
Cok et al, 2008	Case–control study of infertile men in Ankara, Turkey; adipose-tissue samples assayed for dioxins, furans, dl PCBs	22 fertile 23 infertile	9.4 TEQ pg/g lipid 12.5 TEQ pg/g lipid (p = 0.065)
Mocarelli et al., 2008	Men exposed in Seveso, Zone A vs age-matched men residing outside the contamination zone, measured semen characteristics, estradiol, FSH, testosterone, LH, inhibin B		Authors' evaluation (data not shown)
	Age at 1976 exposure:		
	Infant/prepuberty (1–9 year), n = 71, 176		Sensitive

continued

TABLE 7-2 Continued

Reference	Study Population	Exposed Cases[a]	Measure of Risk (95% CI)[a]
	Puberty (10–17 year), n = 44, 136		Intermediate response
	Adult (18–26 year), n = 20, 60		No associations
Polsky et al., 2007	Case–control study of erectile dysfunction in urology patients patients in Ontario, Canada		Highest vs lowest PCB groups
	PCB-118 (TEF = 0.0001)		1.0 (0.5–2.1)
	PCB-156 (TEF = 0.0005)		0.9 (0.5–1.6)
	PCB-170		0.6 (0.3–1.2)
	PCB-180		0.7 (0.4–1.4)
Toft et al., 2007	Men in general population of Poland, Greenland, Ukraine, Sweden; AHR binding measured with CALUX assay		
	Measurements of semen quality (concentration, motility, percentage normal)		No consistent associations
Dhooge et al., 2006	Men in general population of Belgium; Association with 2-fold increase in		
	CALUX-TEQ		Change (p-value)
	Sperm concentration		25.2% (p = 0.07)
	Semen volume		–16.0% (p = 0.03)
	Total testosterone		–7.1% (p = 0.04)
	Free testosterone		–6.8% (p = 0.04)
Studies Reviewed in *Update 2006*			
Swan et al., 2003	Men in Missouri, US with or without low sperm quality		
	Increased urinary metabolite marker for 2,4-D	5	0.8 (0.2–3.0)
Studies Reviewed in *Update 2002*			
Staessen et al., 2001	Adolescents in communities close to industrial sources of heavy metals, PCBs, VOCs, and PAHs—delays in sexual maturity		
	In Hoboken, Belgium	8	4.0 (nr)
	In Wilrik, Belgium	15	1.7 (nr)

ABBREVIATIONS: 2,4-D, 2,4-dichlorophenoxyacetic acid; AFHS, Air Force Health Study; AHR, aryl hydrocarbon receptor; CALUX, assay for determination of dioxin-like activity; CI, confidence interval; dl, dioxin-like; FSH, follicle-stimulating hormone; IU, international unit; LH, luteinizing hormone; nr, not reported; PAH, polycyclic aromatic hydrocarbon; PCB, polychlorinated biphenyl; SEA, Southeast Asia; TCDD, 2,3,7,8-tetrachlorodibenzo-*p*-dioxin; TEF, toxicity equivalency factor; TEQ, toxicity equivalent quotient; VOC, volatile organic compounds.

[a]Given when available; results other than estimated risk explained individually.

[b]For this study, relative risk has been replaced with fecundability ratio, for which value less than 1.0 indicates adverse effect.

[c]For this study, relative risk has been replaced with standardized fertility ratio, for which value less than 1.0 indicates adverse effect.

[d]Table 1 in reference reverses these figures—control, 82.9%; exposed, 37.1%—but text ("The percentages of asthenospermia, mobility, necrosperma and teratospermia were greater in the exposed group than in controls. . .") suggests that this is a typographical error.

TABLE 7-3 Selected Epidemiologic Studies—Female Fertility (Altered Hormone Concentrations, Subfertility, or Infertility)

Reference	Study Population	Exposed Cases	Estimated Relative Risk (95% CI)[a]
OCCUPATIONAL			
Studies Reviewed in *Update 2006*			
Farr et al., 2006	Age of menopause women who self-reported pesticide exposure	8,038	0.9 (0.8–1.0)
Farr et al., 2004	Menstrual-cycle characteristics of premenopausal women in AHS 21–40 years old	1,754	
	Short menstrual cycle		0.8 (0.6–1.0)
	Long menstrual cycle		1.4 (0.9–2.1)
	Irregular		0.6 (0.4–0.8)
	Missed period		1.6 (1.3–2.0)
	Intermenstrual bleeding		1.1 (0.9–1.4)
ENVIRONMENTAL			
New Studies			
Chao et al., 2007	Pregnant women in Taiwan; measured placental dioxin TEQ, PCB TEQ		Regression adjusted for maternal age, BMI, parity
	Older of "regular menstrual cycle"		
	Dioxin TEQ		$p = 0.032$
	PCB TEQ		$p = 0.077$
	Longer "longest menstrual cycle"		
	Dioxin TEQ		$p = 0.269$
	PCB TEQ		$p = 0.006$
Eskenazi et al., 2007	Seveso Women's Health Study—fibroids among women from Zones A & B newborn to 40 yr in 1976		
	$\log_{10}$ TCDD (ppt)		Age-adjusted hazard ratio
	≤ 20.0		1.0
	20.1–75.0		0.6 (0.4–0.8)
	> 75.0		0.6 (0.4–0.9)
Warner et al., 2007	SWHS—ovarian function in women in Zones A and B, newborn to 40 years old in 1976		
	Ovarian follicles in follicular phase (age-adjusted OR)		1.0 (0.4–2.2)
	Ovulation (age-adjusted OR)		
	in luteal phase		1.0 (0.5–1.9)
	in midluteal phase		1.0 (0.4–2.7)
	Estradiol		slopes with $\log_{10}$ TCDD
	in luteal phase		−1.8 (−10.4 to 6.8)
	in midluteal phase		−3.1 (−14.1 to 7.8)
	Progesterone		
	in luteal phase		−0.7 (−2.4 to 1.0)
	in midluteal phase		−0.8 (−3.7 to 2.0)

continued

TABLE 7-3 Continued

Reference	Study Population	Exposed Cases	Estimated Relative Risk (95% CI)[a]
Studies Reviewed in *Update 2006*			
Eskanazi et al., 2005	Seveso cohort, serum-dioxin concentrations, stage of menopause	616	
	Premenopause	260	43.6 (0.2–0.9)
	Natural menopause	169	45.8 (0.3–1.0)
	Surgical menopause	83	43.4 (0.3–1.0)
	Impending menopause	13	43.8 (0.2–0.9)
	Perimenopause	33	36.5 (0.2–0.9)
	Other	58	39.6 (0.2–0.9)
Greenlee et al., 2003	Women in Wisconsin, US with or without infertility (maternal exposure)		
	Mixed or applied herbicides	21	2.3 (0.9–6.1)
	Used 2,4,5-T		9 cases (2.7%)
		9	11 controls (3.4%)
	Used 2,4-D		4 cases (1.2%)
		4	4 controls (1.2%)
Warner et al., 2004	SWHS—age at menarche	282	1.0 (0.8–1.1)

ABBREVIATIONS: 2,4-D, 2,4-dichlorophenoxyacetic acid; 2,4,5-T, 2,4,5-trichlorophenoxyacetic acid; AHS, Agricultural Health Study; BMI, body mass index; CI, confidence interval; OR, odds ratio; PCB, polychlorinated biphenyl; SWHS, Seveso Women's Health Study; TCDD, 2,3,7,8-tetrachlorodibenzo-*p*-dioxin; TEQ, toxicity equivalent quotient.
[a]Given when available; results other than estimated risk explained individually.

−0.04 to −0.002) and comparison veterans (slope for ln[TCDD] = −0.05, 95% CI −0.08 to −0.03). Because both TCDD and testosterone measurements were log transformed for analysis, it is difficult to convey the magnitude of the adjusted association; the comparison group had considerably lower TCDD than the Ranch Hands, but the inverse relationship with testosterone appeared at least as strong. The estimated slopes have overlapping confidence intervals, but given that testosterone levels appear more profoundly depressed in the comparison group, it would have been informative to determine the relationship with ln[TCDD] over the full range analyzing the data for both groups together. In the unadjusted quartile distributions, Ranch Hands with the highest exposure had average testosterone of 530 ng/dL, and the least exposed 583 ng/dL. Comparison veterans with the highest exposure had average testosterone of 491 ng/dL, and the least exposed, 606 ng/dL. The lead author (A Gupta, University of Texas Southwestern Medical Center, personal communication on March 29, 2009) confirmed that the single specification of a unit for testosterone concentration—in Table 2 as ng/mL—was an error. The adjusted mean testosterone measurements were significantly lower in the most exposed veterans in both groups, but they were still well within the normal range of 300–1,000 ng/dL for adult men (http://www.nlm. nih.gov/MEDLINEPLUS/ency/article/003707.htm).

Environmental Studies   To investigate TCDD's effect on reproductive hormones and sperm quality, Mocarelli et al. (2008) compared 135 men exposed to TCDD by the 1976 Seveso accident with 184 healthy men neither exposed to TCDD nor living in the Seveso contamination zones. Each group was divided into three categories that reflected age at the time of the Seveso accident: infancy–prepuberty (1–9 years), puberty (10–17 years), and adulthood (18–26 years). The study found that TCDD exposure in infancy–prepuberty was associated with lower sperm concentration and motility in adulthood, lower estradiol, and higher FSH. Exposure during puberty was associated with increased sperm concentration and motility but lower estradiol and higher FSH. The higher FSH triggered by low estradiol may be responsible for the increased sperm concentration. Exposure during adulthood was not associated with any differences in semen characteristics or hormone level concentrations but the data were not shown. The small number of men exposed in adulthood (20) limited the power to detect effects of exposure that took place in adulthood.

Dhooge et al. (2006) studied Belgian men several months after a 1999 contamination of the food chain with PCBs and dioxins. Men were randomly selected from population registries, and 30% agreed to participate. Semen samples and serum for determination of dioxin-like activity (CALUX assay) and reproductive-hormone concentrations were collected from 101 men. Information on age, BMI, abstinence time, and other demographic characteristics was collected and used to adjust for possible confounding. No association was found between serum dioxin-like activity and total sperm count, sperm morphology, or serum gonadotropins (FSH and LH). However, increasing serum-dioxin activity was associated with decreased semen volume (p = 0.02) and increased sperm concentration (p = 0.02). Increasing serum dioxin was also associated with decreasing testosterone. That association was of borderline statistical significance (p = 0.07) but became stronger (p = 0.04) when men with dioxin concentrations below 16 pg/L were excluded (n = 11). The cut point of 16 pg/L was near the assay's limit of detection, and readings in that range are subject to greater measurement error. The results were adjusted for age, BMI, and sampling date.

Polsky et al. (2007) conducted a case–control study of patients seen in urology practices in Ontario, Canada. Eligible participants were 50–80 years old, had normal prostate-specific antigen concentrations, were not taking hormonal medication, and had not received a diagnosis of prostate cancer. Of 335 eligible participants, 101 had a diagnosis of erectile dysfunction. The remaining 234 men served as controls. Controls had a variety of diagnoses of benign urologic conditions, including prostatic hyperplasia and urinary tract infections. Participants completed a questionnaire and had blood drawn for determination of concentrations of specific PCB congeners. Cases and controls did not differ in concentrations of total PCBs or of any of the 14 congeners examined (regardless of adjustment for lipids and potential confounders).

Toft et al. (2007) obtained semen and blood samples from 319 men in Poland, Ukraine, Greenland, and Sweden. Participants were recruited differently in different locations. Dioxin-like activity was measured with the CALUX assay. No consistent association was found between dioxin-like activity and semen characteristics. In Poland, dioxin-like activity was associated with increased sperm concentration but not sperm motility or sperm count.

Cok et al. (2008) collected adipose tissue samples from men who were undergoing abdominal surgical procedures (such as appendectomy) and compared the samples from infertile azoospermic men of normal karyotype with samples obtained from fertile men. They compared the concentrations of 29 congeners of dioxins, furans, and dioxin-like PCBs. The concentrations of two furans, 2,3,7,8-TCDF and 1,2,3,4,6,7,8,9-OCDF, were significantly higher in the infertile men than in the fertile men. However, the overall TEQ was significantly *lower* in the infertile men than in the fertile men (9.4 vs 12.5 pg/g); this difference remained statistically significant after controlling for age, BMI, smoking, and alcohol consumption.

Female Fertility

No new Vietnam-veteran or occupational studies addressing female fertility have been published since *Update 2006*.

Environmental Studies   Eskenazi et al. (2007) and Warner et al. (2007) studied women in the Seveso Women's Health Study. The study identified women who were up to 40 years old at the time of the dioxin explosion in 1976. Women who lived in the most contaminated zones (A and B) and had adequate stored serum were enrolled during 1996–1998. For the Eskanazi et al. study of fibroids, women who had a diagnosis of fibroids before 1976 were excluded; this left a total of 956 women for analyses. Fibroids were ascertained by self-report, medical records, and ultrasonographic examinations (634 women). The age-adjusted risk of fibroids was significantly *lower* in the high-exposure group (hazard ratio [HR] = 0.62, 95% CI 0.44–0.89) and in the middle-exposure group (HR = 0.58, 95% CI 0.41–0.81) than in the low-exposure group. The lower risk with higher exposure was not confounded by parity, family history of fibroids, age at menarche, current BMI, smoking, alcohol consumption, or education.

In a study of menstrual function (Warner et al., 2007), women who were 20–40 years old and not taking oral contraceptives were evaluated with ultrasonography (96 women), according to serum hormone concentrations (87), and according to the occurrence of ovulation (203). After adjustment for age and quality of the ultrasound, TCDD was not associated with the number or size of ovarian follicles, the occurrence of ovulation, or serum estradiol or progesterone.

Chao et al. (2007) determined the concentrations of dioxins, furans, and PCBs in the placentas of 119 Taiwanese women. Dioxin TEQ, but not PCB TEQ, was associated with greater age at attaining "regular menstrual cycle" whereas PCB TEQ, but not dioxin TEQ, was associated with greater "length of longest menstrual cycle." Those measures do not coincide exactly with the more common variables "age at first menstrual cycle" and "length of menstrual cycle," which were examined and found not to be associated with dioxin exposure. The analyses and data presentation in the publication were unclear.

Biologic Plausibility

There is little evidence that 2,4-D or 2,4,5-T has substantial effects on reproductive organs or fertility. In contrast, many diverse laboratory studies have provided evidence that TCDD can affect reproductive-organ function and reduce fertility in both males and females.

The administration of TCDD to male animals elicits reproductive toxicity by affecting testicular and seminal vesicle weight and function and by decreasing the rate of sperm production. The mechanisms of those effects are not known, but a primary hypothesis is that they are mediated through dysregulation of testicular steroidogenesis. Exposure to TCDD is associated with increased estradiol secretion and decreased testosterone secretion; both hormones regulate sperm production. Both the AHR and the ARNT are expressed in rat and human testes, and studies suggest that TCDD causes tissue damage by inducing oxidative stress. Prostate cells are also responsive to TCDD's inducting expression of various genes, including those involved in drug metabolism. Studies published since *Update 2006* have reinforced those findings. Single intraperitoneal injections of TCDD induced marked histological changes in the testis, impaired spermatogenesis, increased serum estradiol, and decreased testosterone in male rats (Choi JS et al., 2008; Park JS et al., 2008). The effects of TCDD on the reproductive system of the male rat are critically dependent on the developmental time of exposure; for example, when fetal male rats were exposed to a single dose on gestational day 15, no decrease in sperm counts was observed although other developmental effects were found (Bell et al., 2007b).

Many studies have examined the effects of TCDD on the female reproductive system. Two primary mechanisms that probably contribute to abnormal follicle development and decreased numbers of ova after TCDD exposure are cross-talk of the AHR with the estrogen receptor and dysregulation of the hypothalamic-pituitary-gonadal axis. Interaction of the activated AHR leads to inhibition of estradiol-induced gene expression and to enhancement of estrogen-receptor protein degradation; both activities may contribute to TCDD's antiestrogenic effects. TCDD also dysregulates the secretion pattern of preovulatory gonadotropin hormones, and this leads to abnormal and reduced follicle development. In addition, oocytes are directly responsive to TCDD. Thus, TCDD's effects on hormone concentrations, hormone-receptor signaling, and ovarian responsiveness to hormones all probably contribute to TCDD-induced female reproductive toxicity. Wang et al. (2006) showed that dioxins and dibenzofurans significantly correlate with dysregulation of estrogen metabolism in pregnant women.

The reproductive organs of female experimental animals are targets for the action of TCDD (IOM, 2007). The ovary expresses both the AHR and the ARNT and is responsive to TCDD-inducible CYP1A1 and 1B1 expression, which depends on the phase of the estrous cycle (IOM, 2005). TCDD alters ovarian steroidogenesis, reducing ovarian expression of LH and FSH receptors, reducing circulating progesterone and estradiol, and decreasing fertility. TCDD decreases uterine weight, alters endometrial structure, and blocks estrogen-mediated endometrial proliferation and hypertrophy via an AHR-dependent mechanism in rodents and increases the incidence of endometriosis in rhesus monkeys.

Since *Update 2006*, additional work addressing TCDD's effects on female reproduction in animal models has been published. The data of Heiden et al. (2008) on zebrafish suggest that TCDD inhibits follicle maturation via attenuated gonadotropin responsiveness or depression of estradiol biosynthesis and that interference of estrogen-regulated signal transduction may also contribute to TCDD's effects on follicular development, possibly by disrupting signaling pathways, such as glucose and lipid metabolism, and disrupting regulation of transcription.

Exposure of cultured luteinized human granulose cells to TCDD increased expression of inhibin A, which would be expected to produce a reduction in FSH-stimulatable estrogen secretion (Ho et al., 2006). The AHR has been found to be required for normal ovulation and gonadotropin responses in the mouse ovary, as shown in AHR-null mice, which have lower concentrations of LH-receptor and FSH-receptor expression than their wild-type counterparts. AHR-null mice produce fewer eggs than wild-type mice in response to human chorionic gonadotropin; this, suggests that their follicles have a lower capacity to ovulate than do follicles of wild-type mice because of reduced responsiveness to gonadotropins (Barnett et al., 2007a). Barnett et al. (2007b) had previously shown that the follicles of AHR-null mice grew more slowly than follicles of wild-type mice but that administration of estradiol restored the normal growth rate, perhaps because of the AHR affected follicular growth via mechanisms that involve estradiol regulation and responsiveness. Similarly, Ye and Leung (2008) showed that TCDD down-regulated expression of the CYP19 gene, which codes for the aromatase enzyme responsible for the conversion of androstenedione to estrone and of testosterone to estradiol, indicating that exposure to TCDD was directly antiestrogenic by decreasing estrogen. Ovarian endocrine disruption appears to be the predominant functional change induced by chronic exposure to the low doses of TCDD that are associated with premature reproductive senescence in female rats without depletion of ovarian follicular reserves (Shi et al., 2007).

TCDD exhibits antiestrogenic properties, including antiuterotrophic effects (such as inhibition of estrogen-induced uterine growth and proliferation), possibly by inhibiting estrogen-mediated gene expression through estrogen-receptor/ AHR cross-talk. The effects of TCDD on changes in the expression of uterine genes mediated by ethynyl estradiol (EE) were investigated by using cDNA microarrays and physiologic and histologic determinations. EE-TCDD cotreatment inhibited the increase in uterine wet weight and the reductions in stromal edema, hypertrophy, and hyperplasia induced by EE alone. The cotreatment also induced marked luminal epithelial-cell apoptosis. Of the 2,753 EE-mediated differentially expressed genes, only 133 were significantly modulated by TCDD cotreatment; the modulation might be because of a gene-specific inhibitory response. The EE-mediated induction of several genes, including trefoil factor 1 and keratin 14, was inhibited by more than 90% by TCDD. Comparison with public databases found that the genes whose expression was inhibited are known to have functions associated with cell proliferation, water and ion transport, and maintenance of cellular structure and integrity; this theoretical profile of functional impacts is consistent with the observed histological alterations and sheds light on possible mechanisms for TCDD's antiuterotrophic effects (Boverhof et al., 2008).

Although it would not constitute an adverse health outcome in an individual veteran, there is fairly strong evidence (see Table 7-4) that paternal exposure to dioxin may result in a lower sex ratio (that is, a smaller than expected proportion of male infants at birth). Pronounced reductions in sex ratio have been observed in the offspring of men exposed to dioxin after the Seveso accident, especially those under 19 years old at the time of the dioxin release (Mocarelli et al., 2000); this phenomenon was not observed in the offspring of young women exposed by the Seveso accident (Baccarelli et al., 2008). Similar results of a depression in the sex ratio concentrated among fathers who were under 20 years old at the time of the incident were following the Yucheng poisoning with oil contaminated with PCBs, PCDFs, and PCDDs (del Rio Gomez et al., 2002). Reductions in the expected number of male offspring have also been reported in several cohorts of men occupationally exposed to dioxin (Moshammer and Neuberger, 2000; Ryan et al., 2002), but other such cohorts did not manifest this relationship (Heacock et al., 1998; Savitz et al., 1997; Schnorr et al., 2001). In the single report relevant to this outcome in Vietnam veterans, however, the sex ratio was increased in the Ranch Hand group that had the highest serum dioxin concentrations (Michalek et al., 1998b).

There were three articles published after *Update 2006* that contributed information on whether TCDD exposure alters the sex ratio. Chao et al. (2007) mention that they did not find an association between sex ratio of the offspring and the TEQ concentrations of dioxins, furans, or PCBs in the placentas from 119 Taiwanese women. Crude sex ratios for all births in 1994–2005 to women who were less than 18 years old at the time of the Seveso accident are reported in Baccarelli et al. (2008), and the proportion of male births exceeds that of female births in Zones A and B. The only new evidence of an effect on sex ratio came from Hertz-Picciotto et al. (2008), who reported on serum concentrations of nine

TABLE 7-4 Selected Epidemiologic Studies—Sex Ratio[a]

Reference	Study Population	Sex Ratio of Offspring (boys/total)[b]	Comments
VIETNAM VETERANS			
Studies Reviewed in *Update 2002*			
Michalek et al., 1998b	Births from service through 1993 in AFHS		
	Comparison group	0.504	Not formally analyzed
	Dioxin level in Ranch Hand personnel		
	Background	0.502	
	Low	0.487	
	High	0.535	
OCCUPATIONAL			
Studies Reviewed in *Update 2004*			
Ryan et al., 2002	Russian workers manufacturing 2,4,5-trichlorophenol (1961–1988) or 2,4,5-T (1964–1967)	0.401 (91 boys: 136 girls)	$p < 0.001$, either parent exposed
		0.378 (71 boys: 117 girls)	$p < 0.001$, only father exposed
		0.513 (20 boys: 19 girls)	ns, only mother exposed
Studies Reviewed in *Update 2002*			
Schnorr et al., 2001	Workers producing trichlorophenol and derivatives, including 2,4,5-T		No difference on basis of age at first exposure
	Serum TCDD in fathers		
	Neighborhood controls (< 20 ppt)	0.544	Referent
	Worker fathers		
	< 20 ppt	0.507	None
	20–255 ppt	0.567	significantly
	255– < 1,120 ppt	0.568	decreased (or
	≥ 1,120 ppt	0.550	increased)
Moshammer and Neuberger, 2000	Austrian chloracne cohort		Fewer sons, especially if
	Children born after starting TCDD exposure in 1971	0.464 (26 boys: 30 girls)	father was under 20 years old
	Children born before 1971	0.613 (19 boys: 12 girls)	when exposed: SR = 0.20 (1 boy: 4 girls)
Savitz et al., 1997	OFFHS fathers' exposure during 3 mo before conception:		
	No chemical activity	0.503	Referent
	Crop herbicides (some phenoxy herbicides)	0.500	ns
	Protective equipment used not used	0.510	ns
	No protective equipment	0.450	ns
Studies Reviewed in *Update 1998*			
Heacock et al., 1998	Sawmill workers in British Columbia		
	Chlorophenate-exposed workers	0.515	
	Nonexposed workers	0.519	
	Province overall	0.512	

TABLE 7-4 Continued

Reference	Study Population	Sex Ratio of Offspring (boys/total)[b]	Comments
ENVIRONMENTAL			
New Studies			
Baccarelli et al., 2008	Births 1994–2005 in women 0–28 years old at time of Seveso accident		
	Zone A	0.571	
	Zone B	0.508	
	Zone R	0.495	
Hertz-Picciotto et al., 2008	San Francisco Bay area—serum concentrations in pregnant women during 1960s	OR for male birth (not SR)	SRs all < 0.5
	90th percentile vs 10th percentile		
	Total PCBs	0.4 (0.3–0.8)	p = 0.007
	dl PCBs		
	PCB 105	0.6 (0.4–0.9)	p = 0.02
	PCB 118	0.7 (0.5–1.2)	p = 0.17
	PCB 170	0.6 (0.4–0.9)	p = 0.02
	PCB 180	0.8 (0.5–1.2)	p = 0.32
Chao et al., 2007	Taiwan—placental TEQ concentrations of TCDDs, TCDFs, PCBs	nr	No association
del Rio Gomez et al., 2002	Births in individuals exposed to PCBs, PCDFs, PCDDs in 1979 Yucheng incident		vs unexposed with same demographics
	Father exposed (whether or not mother exposed)	0.490	p = 0.037
	Father under 20 years old in 1979	0.458	p = 0.020
	Father at least 20 years old in 1979	0.541	p = 0.60
	Mother exposed (whether or not father exposed)	0.504	p = 0.45
	Mother under 20 years old in 1979	0.501	p = 0.16
	Mother at least 20 years old in 1979	0.500	p = 0.40
Studies Reviewed in *Update 2002*			
Karmaus et al., 2002	Births after 1963 to Michigan fish-eaters with serum PCBs in both parents		
	Paternal PCBs > 8.1 µg/L	0.571	p < 0.05 (but for more sons)
	Maternal PCBs > 8.1 µg/L	0.494	ns
Yoshimura et al., 2001	Parents (one or both) exposed to PCBs, PCDFs in Yusho, Japan		
	All Japan in 1967	0.513	Referent
	Births 1967 (before poisoning incident)	0.516	ns
	Births 1968–1971 (after incident)	0.574	ns

continued

TABLE 7-4 Continued

Reference	Study Population	Sex Ratio of Offspring (boys/total)[b]	Comments
Revich et al., 2001	Residents near chemical plant in operation 1967–1987 in Chapaevsk, Russia		
	1983–1997	0.507	No clear pattern
	Minimum—in 1989	0.401	
	Maximums		
	in 1987	0.564	
	in 1995	0.559	
Studies Reviewed in *Update 2000*			
Mocarelli et al., 2000	Births 1977–1996 in people from Zones A, B, R, 3–45 years old at time of 1976		
	Seveso accident	0.514	Referent
	Neither parent exposed	0.608	ns
	Father exposed (whether or not mother exposed)	0.440	p = 0.03
	Father under 19 years old in 1976	0.382	p = 0.002
	Father at least 19 years old in 1976	0.469	ns
	Only mother exposed	0.545	ns
Studies Reviewed in *Update 1998*			
Mocarelli et al., 1996	Parent (either sex) from Seveso Zone A		
	Births 1977–1984	0.351 (26 boys: 48 girls)	p < 0.001, related to parental TCDD serum
	Births 1985–1994	0.484 (60 boys: 64 girls)	ns

ABBREVIATIONS: 2,4,5-T, 2,4,5-trichlorophenoxyacetic acid; AFHS, Air Force Health Study; dl, dioxin-like; ns, not significant; nr, not reported; OFFHS, Ontario Farm Family Health Study; OR, odds ratio; PCB, polychlorinated biphenyl; PCDD, polychlorinated dibenzodioxin; PCDF, polychlorinated dibenzofurans; SR, sex ratio; TCDD, 2,3,7,8-tetrachlorodibenzo-*p*-dioxin; TCDF, tetrachlorodibenzofuran; TEQ, toxicity equivalent quotient.

[a]*VAO* reports before *Update 1998* did not address association between perturbations in sex ratio of offspring and exposure to chemicals of interest.

[b]Given when available.

PCB congeners (four of which were dioxin-like: PCB 105, 118, 170, and 180) in blood gathered during the 1960s from 399 pregnant women in the San Francisco Bay area. The adjusted odds of a male birth were significantly decreased when the 90th percentile of the total concentration of all nine PCBs was compared with the 10th percentile (OR = 0.45, 95% CI 0.26–0.80). The proportion of male births was significantly reduced for two of the dioxin-like PCBs analyzed separately, and the decrease in the proportion of male babies was not significant for any of the five non–dioxin-like PCBs.

A population-level finding of a paternally mediated effect would be a strong indicator that dioxin exposure can interfere with the male reproductive process.

To date, however, the results for a reduced number of sons for exposed fathers are mixed. James (2006) has interpreted perturbation of sex ratios by dioxins and other agents as being an indicator of parental endocrine disruption. If James' hypothesis were demonstrated to hold, it would be concordant with observing a reduction in testosterone levels among exposed men. Another pathway to an altered sex ratio might involve male embryos experiencing more lethality with induction of mutations due to their unmatched X chromosome. A genotoxic mechanism has not been expected to apply to TCDD, but gender-specific adverse consequences of modified imprinting of gametes might be a possible mechanism leading to observation of altered sex ratios at birth.

There has been no work with experimental animals that specifically examines the effects of TCDD on sex ratios of offspring, nor have any alterations in sex ratio been reported in animal studies that examined developmental effects of TCDD on offspring.

Synthesis

Reproduction is sensitive to TCDD and DLCs in rodents. It is clear that the fetal rodent is more sensitive to adverse effects of TCDD than the adult rodent. The sensitivity in humans is less apparent. There is little evidence that exposure to dioxin is associated with a reduction in sperm quality or a reduction in fertility. However, the committee notes that the evidence that TCDD exposure reduces serum testosterone in men is consistent among several epidemiologic studies with appropriate consideration of confounders, including one of Vietnam veterans; shows a dose–response relationship; and is biologically plausible on the basis of concomitant increases observed in gonadotropins and biologic plausibility shown by animal studies. Human populations showing evidence of reduced testosterone with exposure to DLCs include a general population sample (Dhooge et al., 2006), occupationally exposed people (Egeland et al., 1994), and Vietnam veterans in the Air Force Health Study (Gupta et al., 2006). The evidence that DLCs may modify the sex ratio lends credence to the hypothesis that these chemicals affect male reproductive functioning.

Despite the general consistency of the findings of a reduction in testosterone concentration, the testosterone concentrations observed even in the most exposed groups studied are well within the normal range. The small reduction in testosterone is not expected to have adverse clinical consequences. There is evidence that compensatory physiologic mechanisms come into play. The occupational study of Egeland et al. (1994) found increased gonadotropins in addition to reduced testosterone. The gonadotropins stimulate the production of testosterone in men.

Conclusions

On the basis of the evidence reviewed here and in previous VAO reports, the committee concludes that there is inadequate or insufficient evidence of an association between exposure to the chemicals of interest and decreased sperm counts or sperm quality, subfertility, or infertility.

SPONTANEOUS ABORTION

Spontaneous abortion is the expulsion of a nonviable fetus, generally before 20 weeks of gestation, that is not induced by physical or pharmacologic means. The background risk of recognized spontaneous abortion is generally 7–15% (Hertz-Picciotto and Samuels, 1988), but it is established that many more pregnancies terminate before women become aware of them (Wilcox et al., 1988); such terminations are known as subclinical pregnancy losses and generally are not included in studies of spontaneous abortion. Estimates of the risk of recognized spontaneous abortion vary with the design and method of analysis. Studies have included cohorts of women asked retrospectively about pregnancy history, cohorts of pregnant women (usually those receiving prenatal care), and cohorts of women who are monitored for future pregnancies. The value of retrospective reports can be limited by memory loss, particularly of spontaneous abortions that took place long before. Studies that enroll women who appear for prenatal care require the use of life tables and specialized statistical techniques to account for differences in the times at which women seek medical care during pregnancy. Enrollment of women before pregnancy provides the theoretically most valid estimate of risk, but it can attract nonrepresentative study groups because protocols are demanding.

Conclusions from *VAO* and Updates

The committee responsible for the original *VAO* report concluded that there was inadequate or insufficient evidence of an association between exposure to 2,4-D, 2,4,5-T, TCDD, picloram, or cacodylic acid and spontaneous abortion. Additional information available to the committees responsible for *Update 1996*, *Update 1998*, and *Update 2000* did not change that conclusion.

The committee responsible for *Update 2002*, however, did conclude that there was enough evidence available concerning paternal exposure to TCDD specifically to conclude that there was suggestive evidence that paternal exposure to TCDD is *not* associated with the risk of spontaneous abortion. This conviction was based primarily on the National Institute for Occupational Safety and Health (NIOSH) study (Schnorr et al., 2001), which investigated a large number of pregnancies fathered by workers whose serum TCDD levels were extrapolated back to the time of conception; no association was observed up to the highest exposure group ($\geq 1,120$ ppt). Indications of positive association were seen in studies of Vietnam veterans (CDC, 1989; Field and Kerr, 1988; Stellman et al., 1988), but the committee for *Update 2002* asserted that they might be due to exposure to phenoxy herbicides rather than to TCDD and concluded that there was insufficient information to determine whether an association exists between maternal exposure to TCDD and the risk of spontaneous abortion or between maternal or paternal exposure to 2,4-D, 2,4,5-T, picloram, or cacodylic acid and the risk of spontaneous abortion.

The additional information (none of which concerned paternal exposures) reviewed by the committees responsible for *Update 2004* and *Update 2006* did not change that conclusion. The relevant studies are reviewed in the earlier reports. Table 7-5 summarizes their findings.

Update of the Epidemiologic Literature

No occupational or veterans studies on spontaneous abortion in relation to the chemicals of interest have been published since *Update 2006*.

Tsukimori et al. (2008) gathered the reproductive history back to 1958 of 214 women involved in the 1968 Yusho incident of ingestion of rice oil contaminated with PCBs and other dioxin-like compounds. Information was gathered on 512 pregnancies: 204 in 1958–1967 served as the referent group, 122 in the 10 years after the incident (1968–1977) were of primary interest, and 88 in 1978–1987 and 98 in 1988–2003 were used to show the degree to which adverse reproductive effects had abated. Blood samples were drawn from 97 of the women in 2001–2005; analyses focused on three DLCs: 2,3,4,7,8-pentachlorodibenzofuran (PeCDF), PCB 126 (total equivalency factor [TEF] = 0.1), and PCB 169 (TEF = 0.01). The risk of spontaneous abortion in all pregnancies (excluding induced abortions) in the 10 years after the incident was higher than the risk before it (OR = 2.09, 95% CI 0.84–5.18) but fell to more neutral values in 1978–1987 (OR = 1.00, 95% CI 0.32–3.09) and 1988–2003 (OR = 1.22, 95% CI 0.41–3.63). When the pregnancies of the women whose serum was reviewed for the DLCs were analyzed, an increased risk of spontaneous abortion were found for 10-fold increases in serum concentrations of all three: PeCDF (OR = 1.60, 95% CI 1.10–2.33), PCB 126 (OR = 2.52, 95% CI 0.92–6.87), and PCB 169 (OR = 2.28, 95% CI 1.09–4.75).

In studying pregnant Taiwanese women, Chao et al. (2007) mentioned that they did not find an association between placental dioxin, PCB TEQ, or indicator PCBs and spontaneous abortion, but the data were not presented.

Biologic Plausibility

Laboratory animal studies have demonstrate that TCDD exposure during pregnancy can alter concentrations of circulating steroid hormones and disrupt placental development and function and thus contribute to a reduction in survival of implanted embryos and to fetal death. However, the reproductive significance of those effects and the risk of recognized pregnancy loss before 20 weeks of gestation in humans are not clear. There is no evidence of a relationship between

TABLE 7-5 Selected Epidemiologic Studies—Spontaneous Abortion[a]

Reference	Study Population	Exposed Cases[b]	Estimated Relative Risk (95% CI)[b]
VIETNAM VETERANS			
Studies Reviewed in *Update 2002*			
Kang et al.,	Female Vietnam-era veterans (maternal exposure)		1.0 (0.82–1.21)
2000	Vietnam veterans (1,665 pregnancies)	278	nr
	Vietnam-era veterans who did not serve in		
	Vietnam (1,912 pregnancies)	317	nr
Studies Reviewed in *Update 2000*			
Schwartz,	Female Vietnam veterans (maternal exposure)		
1998	Women who served in Vietnam	113	nr
	Women who did not serve in the war zone	124	nr
	Civilian women	86	nr
Studies Reviewed in *Update 1996*			
Wolfe	Air Force Ranch Hand veterans	157	
et al., 1995	Background	57	1.1 (0.8–1.5)
	Low exposure	56	1.3 (1.0–1.7)
	High exposure	44	1.0 (0.7–1.3)
Studies Reviewed in *VAO*			
Aschengrau	Wives of Vietnam veterans presenting at Boston		
and	Hospital for Women		
Monson,	27 weeks of gestation	10	0.9 (0.4–1.9)
1989	13 weeks of gestation	nr	1.2 (0.6–2.8)
CDC, 1989	Vietnam Experience Study		
	Overall	1,566	1.3 (1.2–1.4)
	Self-reported low exposure	489	1.2 (1.0–1.4)
	Self-reported medium exposure	406	1.4 (1.2–1.6)
	Self-reported high exposure	113	1.7 (1.3–2.1)
Field and	Follow-up of Australian Vietnam veterans	199	1.6 (1.3–2.0)
Kerr, 1988			
Stellman	American Legionnaires with service 1961–1975		
et al., 1988	Vietnam veterans vs Vietnam-era veterans		
	All Vietnam veterans	231	1.4 (1.1–1.6)
	Low exposure	72	1.3 (1.0–1.7)
	Medium exposure	53	1.5 (1.1–2.1)
	High exposure	58	1.7 (1.2–2.4)
	Vietnam-era veterans vs herbicide handlers	9	1.6 (0.7–3.3)
	Vietnam veterans		
	Low exposure	72	1.0
	Medium exposure	53	1.2 (0.8–1.7)
	High exposure	58	1.4 (0.9–1.9)
OCCUPATIONAL			
Studies Reviewed in *Update 2002*			
Schnorr	Wives and partners of men in NIOSH cohort		
et al., 2001	Estimated paternal TCDD serum at time of		
	conception		
	< 20 ppt	29	0.8 (0.5–1.2)
	20 to < 255 ppt	11	0.8 (0.4–1.6)
	255 to < 1120	11	0.7 (0.3–1.6)
	≥ 1120 ppt	8	1.0 (0.4–2.2)

TABLE 7-5 Continued

Reference	Study Population	Exposed Cases[b]	Estimated Relative Risk (95% CI)[b]
Studies Reviewed in *Update 2000*			
Driscoll, 1998	Women employed by US Forest Service— miscarriages (maternal exposure)	141	2.0 (1.1–3.5)
Studies Reviewed in *VAO*			
Moses et al., 1984	Follow-up of 2,4,5-T production workers	14	0.9 (0.4–1.8)
Suskind and Hertzberg, 1984	Follow-up of 2,4,5-T production workers	69	0.9 (0.6–1.2)
Smith et al., 1982	Follow-up of 2,4,5-T sprayers vs nonsprayers	43	0.9 (0.6–1.3)[c]
Townsend et al., 1982	Wives of men employed involved in chlorophenol processing at Dow Chemical Co.	85	1.0 (0.8–1.4)
Carmelli et al., 1981	Wives of men occupationally exposed to 2,4-D		
	All reported work exposure to herbicides (high and medium)	63	0.8 (0.6–1.1)[c]
	Farm exposure	32	0.7 (0.4–1.5)[c]
	Forest and commercial exposure	31	0.9 (0.6–1.4)[c]
	Exposure during conception period		
	Farm exposure	15	1.0 (0.5–1.8)[c]
	Forest and commercial exposure	16	1.6 (0.9–1.8)[c]
	Fathers 18–25 years old		
	Farm exposure	1	0.7 (nr)
	Forest and commercial exposure	3	4.3 (nr)
	Fathers 26–30 years old		
	Farm exposure	4	0.4 (nr)
	Forest and commercial exposure	8	1.6 (nr)
	Fathers 31–35 years old		
	Farm exposure	10	2.9 (nr)
	Forest and commercial exposure	5	1.0 (nr)
ENVIRONMENTAL			
New Studies			
Chao et al., 2007	Pregnant Taiwanese women, placental TEQ of dioxins, PCBs (maternal exposure)		nr, but reported ns
Tsukimori et al., 2008	Spontaneous abortions among pregnancies (excluding induced abortions) of women in 1968 Yusho incident (maternal exposure)		
	10 years after vs 10 years before	nr	2.1 (0.8–5.2)
	10-fold increase in maternal blood concentration (drawn 2001–2005) of:		
	PeCDF	nr	1.6 (1.1–2.3)
	PCB–126 (TEF = 0.1)	nr	2.5 (0.9–6.9)
	PCB–169 (TEF = 0.01)	nr	2.3 (1.1–4.8)

continued

TABLE 7-5 Continued

Reference	Study Population	Exposed Cases[b]	Estimated Relative Risk (95% CI)[b]
Studies Reviewed in *Update 2006*			
Eskenazi et al., 2003	SWHS participants living in exposure Zones A, B in 1976 (maternal exposure)		
	Pregnancies 1976–1998	97	0.8 (0.6–1.2)
	Pregnancies 1976–1984	44	1.0 (0.6–1.6)
Studies Reviewed in *Update 2002*			
Arbuckle et al., 2001	Ontario farm families (maternal and paternal exposure)		
	Phenoxyacetic acid herbicide exposure in preconception period, spontaneous-abortion risk	48	1.5 (1.1–2.1)
Revich et al., 2001	Residents of Samara Region, Russia (maternal and paternal exposure)		
	Chapaevsk	nr	24.4% (20.0–29.5%)[d]
	Samara	nr	15.2% (14.3–16.1%)[d]
	Toliatti	nr	10.6% (9.8–11.5%)[d]
	Syzran	nr	15.6% (13.4–18.1%)[d]
	Novokuibyshevsk	nr	16.9% (14.0–20.3%)[d]
	Other small towns	nr	11.3% (9.4–13.8%)[d]
Tuyet and Johansson, 2001	Vietnamese women who were or whose husbands were exposed to herbicides sprayed during Vietnam War	nr	nr, anecdotal reports of miscarriage in pilot study

ABBREVIATIONS: 2,4-D, 2,4-dichlorophenoxyacetic acid; 2,4,5-T, 2,4,5-trichlorophenoxyacetic acid; CI, confidence interval; NIOSH, National Institute for Occupational Safety and Health; nr, not reported; ns, not significant (usually refers to p < 0.05); PCB, polychlorinated biphenyl; PeCDF, 2,3,4,7,8-pentachlorodibenzofuran; SWHS, Seveso Women's Health Study; TCDD, 2,3,7,8-tetrachlorodibenzo-*p*-dioxin; TEF, toxic equivalency factor; TEQ, toxicity equivalent quotient.
[a]Unless otherwise indicated, results are for paternal exposure.
[b]Given when available; results other than estimated risk explained individually.
[c]90% CI.
[d]Spontaneous abortion rate per 100 full-term pregnancies for 1991–1997.

paternal or maternal exposure to TCDD and spontaneous abortion. Exposure to 2,4-D or 2,4,5-T causes fetal toxicity and death after maternal exposure in experimental animals. However, that effect occurs only at high doses and in the presence of maternal toxicity. No fetal toxicity or death has been reported to occur after paternal exposure to 2,4-D.

Synthesis

The two new environmental studies with information on DLCs and spontaneous abortion had conflicting results and do not constitute motivation to change the assessment of the prior committees. Given the age of the Vietnam-veteran cohort, publication of additional information on this outcome in the target population of the VAO series is unlikely.

Conclusions

On the basis of the evidence reviewed here and in previous VAO reports, the committee concludes that paternal exposure to TCDD is *not* associated with risk of spontaneous abortion and that insufficient information is available to determine whether an association exists between the risk of spontaneous abortion and maternal exposure to TCDD or either maternal or paternal exposure to 2,4-D, 2,4,5-T, picloram, or cacodylic acid.

STILLBIRTH, NEONATAL DEATH, AND INFANT DEATH

Stillbirth or *late fetal death* typically refers to the delivery at or after 20 weeks of gestation of a fetus that shows no signs of life, including fetuses that weigh more than 500 g regardless of gestational age (Kline et al., 1989). *Neonatal death* refers to the death of a liveborn infant within 28 days of birth, and *infant death* includes deaths occurring before the first birthday.

Because the causes of stillbirth and early neonatal death overlap considerably, they are commonly analyzed together in a category referred to as perinatal mortality (Kallen, 1988). Stillbirths make up less than 1% of all births (CDC, 2000). The most common causes of perinatal mortality (Kallen, 1988) among low-birth-weight (500–2,500 g) liveborn and stillborn infants are placental and delivery complications—abruptio placenta, placenta previa, malpresentation, and umbilical-cord conditions. The most common causes of perinatal death of infants weighing more than 2,500 g at birth are complications of the cord, placenta, and membranes and congenital malformations (Kallen, 1988).

Conclusions from *VAO* and Updates

The committee responsible for *VAO* concluded that there was inadequate or insufficient evidence of an association between exposure to 2,4-D, 2,4,5-T, TCDD, picloram, or cacodylic acid and stillbirth, neonatal death, or infant death. Additional information available to the committees responsible for *Update 1996*, *Update 1998*, *Update 2000*, *Update 2002*, *Update 2004*, and *Update 2006* did not change that conclusion. Reviews of the relevant studies are presented in the earlier reports.

Update of the Epidemiologic Literature

No additional occupational or veterans studies on perinatal death in relation to the chemicals of interest have been published since *Update 2006*.

In the study of pregnancy results in women involved in the Yusho poisoning incident, Tsukimori et al. (2008) reported on the intensity of pregnancy loss, defined as the risk of stillbirth, neonatal death, or spontaneous abortion among all pregnancies after induced abortions had been excluded. The risk of pregnancy loss was higher in the 10 years after the incident than before the incident period (OR = 2.11, 95% CI 0.92–4.87) but fell to more neutral values in 1978–1987 (OR = 1.02, 95% CI 0.37–2.84) and in 1988–2003 (OR = 1.01, 95% CI 0.37–2.78). In women whose serum concentrations of the three DLCs had been measured, the risk of pregnancy loss increased with 10-fold increases in serum concentrations of each: PeCDF (OR = 1.70, 95% CI 1.18–2.46), PCB 126 (OR = 2.99, 95% CI 1.16–7.73), and PCB 169 (OR = 2.68, 95% CI 1.32–5.48). Inclusion of stillbirths and neonatal deaths made the risk higher than that of spontaneous abortions alone (see above), but spontaneous abortions appear to dominate the analyses.

Biologic Plausibility

Laboratory studies of maternal TCDD exposure during pregnancy have demonstrated the induction of fetal death; neonatal death, however, is only rarely observed and is usually the result of cleft palate, which leads to an inability to nurse. Studies addressing the potential for perinatal death as a result of paternal exposure to TCDD or herbicides are inadequate to support conclusions. One new study (Kransler et al., 2008) evaluated fetal and neonatal viability in rats exposed to various TCDD doses. Mortality in exposed rats was very high at gestation day 20 and postnatal day 7, but the causes of death were not determined in any of the cases.

Synthesis

The Yusho study reviewed for this update did find significant associations between maternal serum concentrations of three DLCs and rates of pregnancy loss, a variable that included stillbirth and neonatal death but was dominated by spontaneous abortion. The committee, however, considers studies of exposures to dioxin-like PCBs and furans as supportive studies of dioxin rather than presenting primary evidence. Given the age of the Vietnam-veteran cohort, publication of additional information on this outcome in the target population of the VAO series is highly unlikely.

Conclusions

On the basis of the evidence reviewed here and in previous VAO reports, the committee concludes that there is inadequate or insufficient evidence of an association between exposure to the chemicals of interest and stillbirth, neonatal death, or infant death.

BIRTH WEIGHT AND PRETERM DELIVERY

Birth weight and the length of the gestation period can have significant effects on neonatal morbidity and mortality. Defined by the World Health Organization as birth weights < 2,500 grams (Alberman, 1984), low birth weight is a health outcome resulting from one of two distinct causes. Intrauterine growth retardation (IUGR) occurs when fetal growth is diminished and a fetus or baby fails to attain a normal weight or is small for gestational age. The concept of IUGR represents birth weight adjusted for gestational age, resulting in a lower weight than average when compared to local or national fetal growth graphs (Romo et al., 2009). Low birth weight can also occur secondary to preterm delivery (PTD), which is delivery at less than 259 days, or 37 completed weeks, of gestation, calculated on the basis of the date of the first day of the last menstrual period (Bryce, 1991). Low birth weight resulting from either of these causes occurs in approximately 7% of live births. When no distinction is made between the causes of low birth weight (IUGR or PTD), the factors most strongly associated with it are maternal tobacco use during pregnancy, multiple births, and race or ethnicity. Other potential risk factors are low socioeconomic status (SES), malnutrition, maternal weight, birth order, maternal complications during pregnancy (such as severe pre-eclampsia or intrauterine infections) and obstetric history, job stress, and cocaine or caffeine use during pregnancy (Alexander and Slay, 2002; Alexander et al., 2003; Ergaz et al., 2005; Kallen, 1988; Peltier, 2003). Established risk factors for PTD include race (black), marital status (single), low SES, previous low birth weight or PTD, multiple gestations, tobacco use, and cervical, uterine, or placental abnormalities (Berkowitz and Papiernik, 1993).

Conclusions from *VAO* and Updates

The committee responsible for *VAO* concluded that there was inadequate or insufficient evidence of an association between exposure to the chemicals of interest and low birth weight or PTD. Additional information available to the committees responsible for *Update 1996*, *Update 1998*, *Update 2000*, *Update 2002*, *Update 2004*, and *Update 2006* did not change that conclusion. Reviews of the relevant studies are presented in the earlier reports.

Update of the Epidemiologic Literature

No new occupational or Vietnam-veteran studies concerning exposure to the chemicals of interest and low birth weight or PTD have been published since *Update 2006*.

In reporting on neonatal thyroid function among the births in 1994–2005 to women who had been less than 28 years old at the time of the Seveso accident, Baccarelli et al. (2008) noted that birth weight was similar among the three exposure zones. The data were not formally analyzed, but tabulated data indicated that the proportions of low-birth-weight infants (under 2,500 g) were not excessive: Zone A (1.8%, based on only 32 births), Zone B (5.2%), and Zone R (5.9%).

In the study of pregnancy results in women involved in the Yusho poisoning incident, Tsukimori et al. (2008) reported on the frequency of PTD. The risk of PTD in the 10 years after the incident was significantly higher than that before the incident (OR = 5.70, 95% CI 1.17–27.79) but was less pronounced in 1978–1987 (OR = 1.46, 95% CI 0.20–10.49) and in 1988–2003 (OR = 2.09, 95% CI 0.33–13.20). In the women whose serum concentrations of the three DLCs had been measured, the risk of PTD increased with 10-fold increases in serum concentrations of each: PeCDF (OR = 1.98, 95% CI 1.03–3.80), PCB 126 (OR = 4.90, 95% CI 0.93–25.75), and PCB 169 (OR = 4.12, 95% CI 1.19–14.30).

Sagiv et al. (2007) measured PCB congeners in the cord blood of 788 infants born in 1993–1998 to mothers at least 18 years old and residing around the PCB-contaminated harbor in New Bedford, Massachusetts. After adjustment for infant gestational age, sex, and year of birth and for maternal age, race, parity, BMI, smoking, and fish consumption, tests for trends in birth weight, crown-to-heel length, and head circumference with cord serum concentrations of dioxin-like PCB 118 (TEF = 0.0001) or with the sum of mono-ortho TEFs were all nonsignificant.

Similarly, Nishijo et al. (2008) studied 42 mother–infant pairs born at Toyama University Hospital, Japan, after at least 30 weeks of gestation. They did not find significant correlations between TEQ–total, TEQ–PCDD, or TEQ–PCDF in maternal breast milk and birth weight. There were also no patterns of correlation in these measures of dioxin-like activity and infant length, chest circumference, or head circumference at birth.

Biologic Plausibility

The available experimental evidence on animals indicates that TCDD exposure during pregnancy can reduce body weight at birth but only at high doses. Laboratory studies of the potential male-mediated developmental toxicity of TCDD and herbicides as a result of exposure of adult male animals are inadequate to permit conclusions. TCDD and herbicides are known to cross the placenta, and this leads to direct exposure of the fetus. Data from studies of experimental animals also suggest that the preimplantation embryo and developing fetus are sensitive to the toxic effects of 2,4-D and TCDD after maternal exposure. However, the significance of those animal effects for humans is not clear.

Synthesis

The four environmental studies reviewed here did not provide compelling evidence of an association between exposure to the chemicals of interest and the risk of low birth weight or prematurity. The increased risk of PTD in the 5 years after the Yusho incident and specifically in relation to measures of dioxin-like activity (Tsukimori et al., 2008) is of interest, but as the authors note, their sample included fewer than half the eligible women and the pregnancy information was gathered from the subjects long after the events. Otherwise, the results overall suggest a lack of an association with various measures of in utero development. Given the age of the Vietnam-veteran cohort, publication of additional information on this outcome in the target population of the VAO series is highly unlikely.

Conclusions

On the basis of the evidence reviewed here and in previous VAO reports, the committee concludes that there is inadequate or insufficient evidence of an association between exposure to the compounds of interest and low birth weight or preterm delivery.

BIRTH DEFECTS

The March of Dimes defines a birth defect as an abnormality of structure, function, or metabolism, whether genetically determined or as the result of an environmental influence during embryonic or fetal life (Bloom, 1981). Other terms, often used interchangeably, are *congenital anomaly* and *congenital malformation*. Major birth defects, which occur in 2–3% of live births, are abnormalities that are present at birth and are severe enough to interfere with viability or physical well-being. Birth defects are detected in another 5% of babies through the first year of life. The causes of most birth defects are unknown. Genetic factors, exposure to some medications, exposure to environmental contaminants, occupational exposures, and lifestyle factors have been implicated in the etiology of birth defects (Kalter and Warkany, 1983). Most etiologic research has focused on the effects of maternal and fetal exposures, but some work has addressed paternal exposures. Paternally mediated exposures might occur by several routes and exert effects in various ways. One way is through direct genetic damage to the male germ cell transmitted to the offspring and dominantly expressed as a birth defect. A hypothesized route is the transfer of toxic compounds through a man's body into his seminal fluid, resulting in intermittent fetal exposures throughout gestation (Chia and Shi, 2002). Another, even more indirect route of paternally mediated exposure could be contact of family members with contamination brought into the home from the workplace, but this would not be applicable to offspring of Vietnam veterans conceived after deployment.

Conclusions from *VAO* and Updates

The committee responsible for *VAO* determined that there was inadequate or insufficient evidence of an association between exposure to 2,4-D, 2,4,5-T or its contaminant TCDD, picloram, or cacodylic acid and birth defects in offspring. Additional information available to the committee responsible for *Update 1996* led it to conclude that there was limited or suggestive evidence of an association between at least one of the chemicals of interest and spina bifida in the children of veterans; there was no change in the conclusions regarding other birth defects. The committee for *Update 2002*, which reviewed the study of female Vietnam veterans (Kang et al., 2000) that reported significant increases in birth defects in their offspring, did not find those results adequate to modify prior conclusions. Later VAO committees have not encountered additional data to merit changing the conclusion that the evidence is inadequate to support an association between exposure to the chemicals of interest and birth defects (aside from spina bifida) in the offspring of either male or female veterans.

Summaries of the results of studies of birth defects and specifically neural-tube defects that were reviewed in the current report and in earlier VAO reports can be found in Tables 7-6 and 7-7, respectively.

Update of the Epidemiologic Literature

Vietnam-Veteran Studies

No Vietnam-veteran studies of exposure to the chemicals of interest and birth defects have been published since *Update 2006*.

Occupational Studies

One study published since *Update 2006* examined occupational exposures and birth defects. Weselak et al. (2008) reported results of the Ontario Farm Family Health Study. Spouses completed questionnaires that requested the history of pesticide use on the farm. Pregnancies resulting in birth defects were reported by the female study participants. All birth defects were combined for study analyses and exposure was examined by pesticide class, family, and active ingredient for two 3-month periods: before and after conception. After adjustment for infant sex, maternal age at conception, parity, and fever during pregnancy, no association was observed between phenoxy herbicide use and any birth defect during either period. Slightly increased ORs were observed for preconception use of 2,4-D (OR = 1.07, 95% CI 0.55–2.08) and dicamba (OR = 1.67, 95% CI 0.79–3.53). When the outcome was limited to birth defects in male offspring, the associations increased for both 2,4-D (OR = 1.25, 95% CI 0.56–2.81) and dicamba (OR = 2.42, 95% CI 1.06–5.53). No association with birth defects was observed in analyses that addressed direct use of phenoxy herbicides or 2,4-D specifically by fathers in the 3 months before conception.

Two additional articles describing the evaluation of occupational pesticide exposures and birth defects have been published since *Update 2006*. Lacasana

TABLE 7-6 Selected Epidemiologic Studies—Birth Defects in Offspring of Subjects[a]

Reference	Study Population	Exposed Cases[b]	Estimated Relative Risk (95% CI)[b]
VIETNAM VETERANS			
Studies Reviewed in *Update 2002*			
Kang et al., 2000	Female Vietnam-era veterans—deployed vs nondeployed (maternal exposure)		
	"Likely" birth defects	nr	1.7 (1.2–2.2)
	"Moderate-to-severe" birth defects	nr	1.5 (1.1–2.0)
Studies Reviewed in *Update 2000*			
AIHW, 1999	Australian Vietnam veterans—validation study		Cases expected (95% CI)
	Down syndrome	67	92 expected (73–111)
	Tracheo-esophageal fistula	10	23 expected (14–32)
	Anencephaly	13	16 expected (8–24)
	Cleft lip or palate	94	64 expected (48–80)
	Absent external body part	22	34 expected (23–45)
	Extra body part	74	74 expected (nr)
Michalek et al., 1998a	Air Force Ranch Hand veterans		
	Before service in SEA	nr	0.7 (nr)
	After service in SEA	nr	1.5 (nr)
Studies Reviewed in *Update 1996*			
Wolfe et al., 1995	High-exposure Ranch Hands relative to comparisons		
	All anomalies	57	1.0 (0.8–1.3)
	Nervous system	3	nr
	Eye	3	1.6 (0.4–6.0)
	Ear, face, neck	5	1.7 (0.6–4.7)
	Circulatory system, heart	4	0.9 (0.3–2.7)
	Respiratory system	2	nr
	Digestive system	5	0.8 (0.3–2.0)
	Genital system	6	1.2 (0.5–3.0)
	Urinary system	7	2.1 (0.8–5.4)
	Musculoskeletal	31	0.9 (0.6–1.2)
	Skin	3	0.5 (0.2–1.7)
	Chromosomal anomalies	1	nr
Studies Reviewed in *VAO*			
AFHS, 1992	Air Force Operation Ranch Hand veterans— birth defects in conceptions after service in SEA		
	Congenital anomalies	229	1.3 (1.1–1.6)
	Nervous system	5	1.9 (0.5–7.2)
	Respiratory system	5	2.6 (0.6–10.7)
	Circulatory system, heart	19	1.4 (0.7–2.6)

continued

TABLE 7-6 Continued

Reference	Study Population	Exposed Cases[b]	Estimated Relative Risk (95% CI)[b]
	Urinary system	21	2.5 (1.3–5.0)
	Chromosomal	6	1.8 (0.6–6.1)
	Other	5	2.6 (0.6–10.7)
Aschengrau and Monson, 1990	Vietnam veterans whose children were born at Boston Hospital for Women		
	All congenital anomalies (crude OR)		
	vs men without known military service	55	1.3 (0.9–1.9)
	vs non-Vietnam veterans	55	1.2 (0.8–1.9)
	One or more major malformations (crude OR)		
	vs men without known military service	18	1.8 (1.0–3.1)
	vs non-Vietnam veterans	18	1.3 (0.7–2.4)
CDC, 1989a	Vietnam Experience Study—interview data		
	Total anomalies	826	1.3 (1.2–1.4)
	Nervous system defects	33	2.3 (1.2–4.5)
	Ear, face, neck defects	37	1.6 (0.9–2.8)
	Integument	41	2.2 (1.2–4.0)
	Musculoskeletal defects	426	1.2 (1.1–1.5)
	Hydrocephalus	11	5.1 (1.1–23.1)
	Spina bifida	9	1.7 (0.6–5.0)
	Hypospadias	10	3.1 (0.9–11.3)
	Multiple defects	71	1.6 (1.1–2.5)
	Children of veterans reporting high exposure	46	1.7 (1.2–2.4)
CDC, 1989b	GBDS—hospital records		
	Birth defects	130	1.0 (0.8–1.3)
	Major birth defects	51	1.2 (0.8–1.9)
	Digestive system defects	18	2.0 (0.9–4.6)
	Birth defects—black Vietnam veterans only	21	3.4 (1.5–7.6)
Donovan et al., 1984	Australian Vietnam veterans		
	Vietnam veterans vs all other men	127	1.0 (0.8–1.3)
	National Service veterans—Vietnam service vs no Vietnam service	69	1.3 (0.9–2.0)
Erikson et al., 1984a	Vietnam veterans identified through CDC Metropolitan Atlanta Congenital Defects Program		
	Any major birth defects	428	1.0 (0.8–1.1)
	Multiple birth defects with reported exposure	25	1.1 (0.7–1.7)
	EOI-5: spina bifida	1	2.7 (1.2–6.2)
	EOI-5: cleft lip with or without cleft palate	5	2.2 (1.0–4.9)
OCCUPATIONAL			
New Studies			
Weselak et al., 2008	Pregnancies with one or more birth defects in OFFHS	108	
	Use on farm, during 3 months before conception, of:		
	Herbicides	24	0.7 (0.4–1.1)

TABLE 7-6 Continued

Reference	Study Population	Exposed Cases[b]	Estimated Relative Risk (95% CI)[b]
	Male offspring	19	0.9 (0.5–1.6)
	Direct paternal use	19	0.5 (0.3–1.0)
	Phenoxy herbicides	12	0.6 (0.3–1.1)
	Male offspring	9	0.8 (0.4–1.7)
	Direct paternal use	8	0.4 (0.2–0.9)
	2,4-D	10	1.1 (0.6–2.1)
	Male offspring	7	1.3 (0.6–2.8)
	Direct paternal use	6	0.6 (0.3–1.5)
	Dicamba	8	1.7 (0.8–3.5)
	Male offspring	7	2.4 (1.1–5.5)
	Use on farm, during 3 months after conception, of:		
	Herbicides	7	0.5 (0.2–1.2)
	Phenoxy herbicides	9	0.8 (0.4–1.5)
	2,4-D	7	1.0 (0.4–2.3)
Studies Reviewed in *Update 2006*			
Lawson et al., 2004	Wives of workers with measured serum TCDD in NIOSH cohort	14	nr
Studies Reviewed in *Update 1998*			
Kristensen et al., 1997	Norwegian farmers (maternal, paternal exposure)	4,189	1.0 (1.0–1.1)
Dimich-Ward et al., 1996	Sawmill workers with exposure in upper three quartiles for any job held up to 3 months before conception		
	Cataracts	11	5.7 (1.4–22.6)
	Genital organs	105	1.3 (0.9–1.5)
Garry et al., 1996	Private pesticide appliers		
	All births with anomalies	125	1.4 (1.2–1.7)
	Circulatory, respiratory	17	1.7 (1.0–2.8)
	Gastrointestinal	6	1.7 (0.8–3.8)
	Urogenital	20	1.7 (1.1–2.6)
	Musculoskeletal, integumental	30	
	Maternal age under 30 years	11	0.9 (0.5–1.7)
	Maternal age over 30 years	19	2.5 (1.6–4.0)
	Chromosomal	8	1.1 (0.5–2.1)
	Other	48	
	Maternal age under 35 years	36	1.1 (0.8–1.6)
	Maternal age over 35 years	12	3.0 (1.6–5.3)
Studies Reviewed in *VAO*			
Moses et al., 1984	Follow-up of 2,4,5-T male production workers	11	1.3 (0.5–3.4)
Suskind and Hertzberg, 1984	Follow-up of 2,4,5-T male production workers	18	1.1 (0.5–2.2)
Smith et al., 1982	Follow-up of 2,4,5-T sprayers—sprayers vs non-sprayers	13	90% CI 1.2 (0.6–2.5)

continued

TABLE 7-6 Continued

Reference	Study Population	Exposed Cases[b]	Estimated Relative Risk (95% CI)[b]
Townsend et al., 1982	Follow-up of Dow Chemical plant workers	30	0.9 (0.5–1.4)
ENVIRONMENTAL			
New Studies			
Meyer et al., 2006	Case–control study in eastern Arkansas of hypospadias as function of mother's residence within 500 m of agricultural pesticide use during gestation weeks 6–16		
	Dicamba (lb)		
	0	nr	1.0
	> 0– < 0.04	nr	0.5 (0.3–1.0)
	≥ 0.04	nr	0.9 (0.4–2.1)
Studies Reviewed in *Update 2006*			
Cordier et al., 2004	Residents of Rhône-Alpes region of France living near municipal solid-waste incinerators (maternal, paternal exposure)		
	Minor anomalies	518	0.9 (0.8–1.1)
	Chromosomal anomalies	204	1.0 (0.9–1.2)
	Monogenic anomalies	83	1.1 (0.8–1.4)
	Unknown or multifactorial etiology	964	1.1 (1.0–1.2)
Schreinemachers, 2003	Rural or farm residents of Minnesota, Montana, North Dakota, South Dakota (maternal, paternal exposure)		
	Any birth anomaly	213	1.1 (0.9–1.3)
	Central nervous system anomalies	12	0.8 (0.5–1.4)
	Circulatory, respiratory anomalies	39	1.7 (1.1–2.6)
	Digestive system anomalies	24	0.9 (0.6–1.5)
	Urogenital anomalies	44	1.0 (0.7–1.5)
	Musculoskeletal, integumental anomalies	70	1.5 (1.1–2.1)
	Chromosomal anomalies	17	0.9 (0.6–1.6)
Tango, 2004	Investigated multiple pregnancy outcomes in Japan-infant deaths from congenital defects	42	nr, but ns
Studies Reviewed in *Update 2002*			
Loffredo et al., 2001	Mothers in the BWIS exposed to herbicides during first trimester (maternal exposure)	8	2.8 (1.2–6.9)
Revich et al., 2001	Residents of Chapaevsk, Russia—congenital malformations	nr	nr, but ns
ten Tusscher et al., 2000	Infants born in Zeeburg, Amsterdam, clinics 1963–1965 with orofacial cleft (maternal exposure)		
	Births in 1963	5	nr, but said to be significant
	Births in 1964	7	nr, but said to be significant

TABLE 7-6 Continued

Reference	Study Population	Exposed Cases[b]	Estimated Relative Risk (95% CI)[b]
Studies Reviewed in *Update 2000*			
García et al., 1998	Residents of agricultural areas in Spain—at least median score on chlorophenoxy-herbicide exposure duration (months) index	14	3.1 (0.6–16.9)
Studies Reviewed in *VAO*			
Fitzgerald et al., 1989	Persons exposed to an electric-transformer fire—total birth defects (maternal, paternal exposure)	1	2.1 (0.05–11.85)
Mastroiacovo et al., 1988	Seveso residents (maternal, paternal, in utero exposure)		90% CI
	Zones A, B, R—total defects	137	1.0 (0.8–1.1)
	Zones A and B—total defects	27	1.2 (0.9–1.6)
	Zones A and B—mild defects	14	1.4 (0.9–2.2)
Stockbauer et al., 1988	Persons in Missouri with documented TCDD soil contamination near residence (maternal, paternal, in utero exposure)		
	Total birth defects	17	0.8 (0.4–1.5)
	Major defects	15	0.8 (0.4–1.7)
	Midline defects	4	0.7 (0.2–2.3)
Hanify et al., 1981	Residents of areas of northland New Zealand subject to aerial 2,4,5-T spraying		
	All birth malformations excluding dislocated or dislocatable hip	164	90% CI 1.7 (1.4–2.1)
	All heart malformations	20	3.9 (2.1–7.4)
	Hypospadias, epispadias	18	5.6 (2.7–11.7)
	Talipes	52	1.7 (1.2–2.3)
	Cleft lip	6	0.6 (0.3–1.3)
	Isolated cleft palate	7	1.4 (0.6–3.2)

ABBREVIATIONS: 2,4-D, 2,4-dichlorophenoxyacetic acid; 2,4,5-T, 2,4,5-trichlorophenoxyacetic acid; BWIS, Baltimore–Washington Infant Study; CI, confidence interval; EOI, exposure opportunity index; GBDS, General Birth Defects Study; NIOSH, National Institute for Occupational Safety and Health; nr, not reported; ns, not significant; OFFHS, Ontario Farm Family Health Study; OR, odds ratio; SEA, Southeast Asia; TCDD, 2,3,7,8-tetrachlorodibenzo-*p*-dioxin.
[a]Unless otherwise indicated, studies show paternal exposure.
[b]Given when available; results other than estimated risk explained individually.

et al. (2006) examined anencephaly and maternal and paternal agricultural work during pregnancy in a case–control study. However, exposure definition was limited to general job characteristics (such as agricultural work) rather than specific pesticides, so the study did not meet the level of exposure classification required for full review by the committee. Similarly, the work of Carbone et al. (2007) was limited by an exposure definition that considered the probability of exposure to

TABLE 7-7 Selected Epidemiologic Studies—Neural-Tube Defects in Offspring of Subjects[a]

Reference	Study Population	Exposed Cases[b]	Estimated Relative Risk (95% CI)[b]
VIETNAM VETERANS			
Studies Reviewed in *Update 2000*			
AIHW, 1999	Australian Vietnam veterans—validation study		Cases expected (95% CI)
	Spina bifida—maximums		33 expected
		50	(22–44)
	Anencephaly		16 expected
		13	(8–24)
Studies Reviewed in *Update 1996*			
Wolfe et al., 1995	Air Force Operation Ranch Hand personnel— neural-tube defects	4[c]	nr
Studies Reviewed in *VAO*			
CDC, 1989b	Vietnam Experience Study		
	Spina bifida		
	Vietnam veterans' children	9	1.7 (0.6–5.0)
	Non-Vietnam veterans' children	5	1.0
	Anencephaly		
	Vietnam Veterans' children	3	nr
	Non-Vietnam veterans' children	0	1.0
Erickson et al., 1984a,b	CDC birth defects case–control study Service in Vietnam		
	Spina bifida	19	1.1 (0.6–1.7)
	Anencephaly	12	0.9 (0.5–1.7)
	Military records indicate opportunity for exposure		
	Spina bifida	20	2.7 (1.2–6.2)
	Anencephaly	7	0.7 (0.2–2.8)
ADVA, 1983	Australian Vietnam veterans—neural-tube defects	16	0.9 (nr)
OCCUPATIONAL			
Studies Reviewed in *Update 1998*			
Blatter et al., 1997	Dutch farmers		
	Spina bifida—moderate, heavy exposure		
	Pesticide use	8	1.7 (0.7–4.0)
	Herbicide use	7	1.6 (0.6–4.0)[d]
Kristensen et al., 1997	Norwegian farmers—spina bifida (maternal, paternal exposure)		
	Tractor spraying equipment	28	1.6 (0.9–2.7)
	Tractor spraying equipment, orchards, greenhouses[e]	5	2.8 (1.1–7.1)

TABLE 7-7 Continued

Reference	Study Population	Exposed Cases[b]	Estimated Relative Risk (95% CI)[b]
Dimich-Ward et al., 1996	Sawmill workers with exposure in upper three quartiles for any job held up to 3 months before conception		
	Spina bifida, anencephaly	22	2.4 (1.1–5.3)
	Spina bifida only	18	1.8 (0.8–4.1)
Garry et al., 1996	Private pesticide appliers—central nervous system defects	6	1.1 (0.5–2.4)
ENVIRONMENTAL			
Studies Reviewed in *Update 2006*			
Cordier et al., 2004	Residents of Rhône-Alpes region of France (maternal, paternal exposure)	49	0.9 (0.6–1.2)
Studies Reviewed in *VAO*			
Stockbauer et al., 1988	Persons in Missouri with documented TCDD soil contamination—central nervous system defects (maternal, paternal, in utero exposure)	3	3.0 (0.3–35.9)
Hanify et al., 1981	Spraying of 2,4,5-T in New Zealand (all exposures)		90% CI
	Anencephaly	10	1.4 (0.7–2.9)
	Spina bifida	13	1.1 (0.6–2.1)

ABBREVIATIONS: 2,4,5-T, 2,4,5-trichlorophenoxyacetic acid; CDC, Centers for Disease Control and Prevention; CI, confidence interval; nr, not reported; TCDD, 2,3,7,8-tetrachlorodibenzo-*p*-dioxin.
[a]Unless otherwise indicated, studies show paternal exposure.
[b]Given when available; results other than estimated risk explained individually.
[c]Of four neural-tube defects reported in Ranch Hand offspring, two were spina bifida (high dioxin exposure), one spina bifida (low dioxin), one anencephaly (low dioxin); no neural-tube defects reported in comparison cohort; 454 postservice births studied in Ranch Hand veterans; 570 in comparison cohort.
[d]Calculated from data presented in the paper.
[e]Greenhouse workers would not have been exposed to chemicals of interest.

pesticides (all types combined) and was therefore unable to examine the associations related to the specific chemicals of interest for this review.

Environmental Studies

Meyer et al. (2006) examined maternal residential proximity to agricultural pesticide applications and hypospadias. This population-based study identified cases and controls born in eastern Arkansas in 1998–2002. A geographic-information-system approach was used as a surrogate for pesticide exposure, defined as applications within 500 m of each mother's residence during gestational weeks 6–16. Land-cover data, providing crop locations and type, and state-wide annual data on crop-specific pesticide use were used to classify maternal exposure during pregnancy. Of the 116 pesticides used during the study period, the authors focused on 38 pesticides with existing toxicologic evidence of reproductive, developmental, or endocrine-disrupting properties. Of the chemicals of interest in the VAO series, 2,4-D was considered as a possible endocrine disruptor that influenced LH and dicamba was tracked as a possible developmental toxicant. Dicamba, but not 2,4-D, was among the 16 pesticides used in proximity to maternal residences. No association with hypospadias was observed with all pesticides combined or with categories based on mode of action and target hormone. Dicamba was among four pesticides to which the cases had significantly lower average exposure than the controls ($p < 0.05$). Similarly, with the exception of diclofop-methyl (not a pesticide included as a chemical of interest for VAO committees), no dose–response relationships were found in analyses of specific pesticides adjusted for maternal age, race, smoking, and weight gain; timing of first prenatal visit; gestational age; and paternal education. 2,4-D was not examined separately.

Two additional articles published since *Update 2006* examined environmental exposure to pesticides and birth defects. Felix et al. (2008) defined exposure as herbicide and insecticide use combined, and Clementi et al. (2007) used an ecologic exposure definition (living in an area of high pesticide application). Those broad exposure definitions did not meet the level of exposure specificity required for full review by the committee.

Biologic Plausibility

Little information is available on the reproductive and developmental effects of exposure to the herbicides discussed in this report. Studies indicate that 2,4-D does not affect male or female fertility and does not produce fetal abnormalities. Offspring of pregnant rodents exposed to 4-(2,4-dichlorophenoxy) butyric acid exhibit a reduced growth rate and increased mortality (Charles et al., 1999) but only after very high doses. Exposure to 2,4-D also alters the concentration and function of reproductive hormones and prostaglandins. One study reported an increased incidence of malformed offspring of male mice exposed to a mixture of 2,4-D and picloram in drinking water; however, paternal toxicity was observed in the high-dose group, and there was no clear dose–response relationship (Blakley et al., 1989). Picloram alone produced fetal abnormalities in rabbits at doses that are also toxic to the pregnant animals (John-Greene et al., 1985), but that effect has not been seen in many studies. 2,4,5-T was toxic to fetuses when administered to pregnant rats, mice, and hamsters, but in early studies TCDD contamination confounded attribution of the observed toxicity specifically to the herbicide; its ability to interfere with calcium homeostasis in vitro has been documented and linked to its teratogenic effects on the early development of sea urchin eggs. Cacodylic acid is toxic to rat, mouse, and hamster fetuses at high doses that are also toxic to the pregnant mothers.

TCDD is a potent teratogen in all laboratory species that have been studied, but the pattern of induced birth defects is often species-specific. As demonstrated by continuing research, fish, mouse, and avian embryos exhibit substantial alterations in craniofacial development—shortened jaw in piscine species (Yamauchi et al., 2006), cleft palate in mice (Fujiwara et al., 2008; Jang et al., 2007, 2008; Keller et al., 2007b, 2008; Yamada et al., 2007), and beak malformations in birds (Blankenship et al., 2003). The developing cardiovascular system is also a common target for TCDD-induced teratogenicity (Lahvis et al., 2000; Mehta et al., 2008; Yamauchi et al., 2006). Effects on the fetal kidney (Choi et al., 2006; Keller et al., 2007a,b,c, 2008; Nishimura et al., 2008) and on dental or bone development (Bursian et al., 2006a,b; Gao et al., 2004, 2007; Ilvesaro et al., 2005; Lind et al., 1999, 2000a,b; Miettinen et al., 2005, 2006; Yasuda et al., 2005) have also been noted frequently after TCDD exposure.

The mechanisms by which TCDD induces various birth defects have not been exhaustively determined, but they appear to involve considerable species specificity and organ specificity. Studies have consistently demonstrated that TCDD-induced developmental toxicity required the AHR. That has been definitively established in mice that lack AHR expression. When pregnant AHR-null mice are exposed to TCDD, the fetuses fail to exhibit any of the typical developmental malformations associated with TCDD exposure. The activated AHR mediates changes in gene transcription, so the inappropriate and sustained activation of AHR by TCDD during development appears to be a key first step in mediating TCDD's developmental toxicity. Although structural differences in the AHR have been identified among species, it functions similarly in animals and humans. Therefore, a common mechanism mediated by the AHR in which tissue growth and differentiation processes are affected probably underlies the reproductive and developmental toxicity of TCDD in humans and animals.

It has been shown that cardiac myocytes and the endothelial lining of the heart and blood vessels are primary target sites of TCDD's effects on the developing cardiovascular system. CYP1A1 induction or alterations in pathways controlled by vascular endothelial growth factor might mediate the early lesions that result in TCDD-related vascular derangements. That antioxidant treatment provides protection against TCDD-induced embryotoxicity in some systems suggests that reactive oxygen species might be involved in the teratogenic effects of exposure to TCDD.

Studies in which effects of TCDD on the developing embryo or fetus were investigated after maternal exposure to TCDD; they include an array of animal models and a variety of experimental outcomes. Such laboratory studies have established that maternal exposure to TCDD during pregnancy is associated with a wide variety of birth defects, which depend on the timing of exposure and the species being studied. For instance, Hutt et al. (2008) identified the compaction stage of preimplantation rat embryogenesis as critically sensitive to the effects of TCDD, whereas survival to the blastocyst stage is not compromised.

Few laboratory studies of potential male-mediated developmental toxicity (and birth defects specifically) attributable to exposure to TCDD and herbicides have been conducted. Feeding of simulated Agent Orange mixtures to male mice produced no adverse effects in offspring; a statistically significant excess of fused sternebrae in the offspring of the two most highly exposed groups was attributed to an anomalously low rate of this defect in the controls (Lamb et al., 1981). It is notable, however, that both the AHR and the ARNT are expressed in the human testis and sperm (Khorram et al., 2004; Shultz et al., 2003), and studies in rodents have shown that TCDD exposure results in significant changes in gene expression in spermatocytes and Sertoli cells; hence, cells of the testis are responsive to TCDD exposure (Kuroda et al., 2005; Yamano et al., 2005). Thus, there is biologic potential for paternal exposure to contribute to TCDD-induced developmental toxicity.

Synthesis

Embryonic and fetal development is a sensitive toxic outcome of TCDD and DLCs in rodents. It is clear that the fetal rodent is more sensitive to adverse effects of TCDD than the adult rodent; human data are generally lacking, however, and the sensitivity of this outcome in humans is less apparent.

Overall, neither of the studies (Meyer et al., 2006; Weselak et al., 2008) considered by the committee provided evidence of an association between the chemicals of interest and birth defects. An association with dicamba exposure and birth defects in male offspring was observed in the study by Weselak et al. (2008), but the interpretation of this finding is limited by the inability to attribute the association with specific birth defects.

Given the age of the Vietnam-veteran cohort, publication of additional information on this outcome in the target population of the VAO series is highly unlikely.

Conclusions

There were no new relevant studies of the association between parental exposure to 2,4-D, 2,4,5-T, TCDD, cacodylic acid, or picloram and spina bifida in offspring. The committee concludes that the evidence of an association between exposure to the chemicals of interest and spina bifida is still limited or suggestive. The evidence of an association between exposure to the chemicals of interest and other birth defects is inadequate or insufficient.

CHILDHOOD CANCER

The American Cancer Society estimated that 10,730 children under 15 years old would have a diagnosis of cancer in the United States in 2008 (ACS, 2008). Treatment and supportive care of children with cancer have improved greatly, and mortality has declined by 49% over the last 30 years. Despite those advances, cancer remains the leading cause of death from disease in children under 15 years old, and 1,490 deaths were projected for 2008 (ACS, 2008).

Leukemia is the most common cancer in children. It accounts for about one-third of all childhood cancer cases; leukemia was expected to be diagnosed in nearly 3,540 children in 2008 (ACS, 2008). Of those, nearly 2,000 will have acute lymphocytic leukemia (ALL); most of the rest will have acute myelogenous leukemia. Acute myelogenous leukemia (ICD-9 205) is commonly referred to as acute myeloid leukemia and acute nonlymphocytic leukemia. For consistency, this report uses *acute myelogenous leukemia*, or simply *AML*, regardless of usage in the source materials. ALL is most common in early childhood, peaking at the ages of 2–3 years, and AML is most common during the first 2 years of life. ALL incidence is consistently higher in boys than in girls; AML incidence is similar in boys and girls (NCI, 2001). Through early adulthood, ALL rates are about twice as high in whites as in blacks; AML exhibits no consistent pattern in this respect. Chapter 6 contains additional information on leukemia as part of the discussion of adult cancer.

The second-most common group of cancers in children are those of the central nervous system—the brain and the spinal cord. Other cancers in children include lymphomas, bone cancers, soft-tissue sarcomas, renal cancers, eye cancers, and adrenal gland cancers. In contrast with adult cancers, relatively little is known about the etiology of most childhood cancers, especially about potential environmental risk factors and the effect of parental exposures.

Conclusions from *VAO* and Updates

The committee responsible for *VAO* concluded that there was inadequate or insufficient evidence of an association between exposure to 2,4-D, 2,4,5-T, TCDD, picloram, or cacodylic acid and childhood cancers. Additional information available to the committees responsible for *Update 1996* and *Update 1998* did not change that conclusion. The committee responsible for *Update 2000* reviewed the material in earlier VAO reports and newly available published literature and determined that there was limited or suggestive evidence of an association between exposure to at least one of the chemicals of interest and AML. After the release of *Update 2000*, investigators involved in one study discovered an error in their published data. The committee reconvened to evaluate the previously reviewed and new literature regarding AML, and *Acute Myelogenous Leukemia* (IOM, 2002) was produced. It reclassified AML from "limited/suggestive evidence of an association" to "inadequate evidence to determine whether an association exists." Table 7-8 summarizes the results of the relevant studies. The committees responsible for *Update 2000*, *Update 2002*, *Update 2004*, and *Update 2006* reviewed the material in earlier VAO reports and in newly available published literature and agreed that there remained inadequate or insufficient evidence of an association between exposure and childhood cancers.

TABLE 7-8 Selected Epidemiologic Studies—Childhood Cancers[a]

Reference	Study Population	Exposed Cases[b]	Estimated Relative Risk (95% CI)[b]
VIETNAM VETERANS			
Studies Reviewed in *Herbicide/Dioxin Exposure and AML in the Children of Veterans*			
AIHW, 2001	Australian Vietnam veterans' children—revised validation study—AML	12[c]	1.3 (0.8–4.0)
Studies Reviewed in *Update 2000*			
AIHW, 2000	*Australian Vietnam veterans' children—validation study—AML*		
	This study, which incorrectly calculated expected number of AML cases, is superseded by AIHW, 2001 above		
Wen et al., 2000	Case–control study of children's leukemia		
	AML, ALL		
	Father ever served in Vietnam, Cambodia	117	1.2 (0.9–1.6)
	< 1 year in Vietnam or Cambodia	61	1.4 (0.9–2.0)
	> 1 year in Vietnam or Cambodia	49	1.2 (0.8–1.7)
	AML only		
	Father ever served in Vietnam, Cambodia	40	1.7 (1.0–2.9)
	< 1 year in Vietnam, Cambodia	13	2.4 (1.1–5.4)
	> 1 year in Vietnam, Cambodia	16	1.5 (0.7–3.2)
Studies Reviewed in *VAO*			
CDC, 1989b	Vietnam Experience Study—outcomes in offspring of veterans		
	Cancer	25	1.5 (0.7–2.8)
	Leukemia	12	1.6 (0.6–4.0)
Field and Kerr, 1988	Cancer in children of Australian Vietnam veterans	4	nr
Erikson et al., 1984b	CDC Birth Defects Study—children of Vietnam veterans		
	"Other" neoplasms	87	1.8 (1.0–3.3)
OCCUPATIONAL			
New Studies			
Monge et al., 2007	Parental occupational exposure to pesticide, childhood leukemia in Costa Rica		
	Paternal exposure in year before conception to:		
	Herbicides	53	1.2 (0.8–1.7)
	Phenoxyacetic acids	28	1.0 (0.6–1.6)
	Picloram (all ALL)	11	1.6 (0.7–3.4)
	High vs low	8	6.3 (1.0–38.6)
	Maternal exposure to:		
	Herbicides		
	In year before conception	9	2.0 (0.8–5.0)
	In 1st trimester	8	5.3 (1.4–20.0)
	In 2nd trimester	8	5.3 (1.4–20.0)
	In 3rd trimester	7	2.3 (0.8–6.8)
	Phenoxyacetic acids in year before conception	4	1.3 (0.4–4.8)

TABLE 7-8 Continued

Reference	Study Population	Exposed Cases[b]	Estimated Relative Risk (95% CI)[b]
Studies Reviewed in *Update 2006*			
Chen et al., 2005	Parental occupational exposure to pesticide, childhood GCTs		
	Maternal	32	1.1 (0.7–1.6)
	Paternal	39	0.9 (0.6–1.3)
Reynolds et al., 2005b	Maternal exposure to agricultural pesticide in class of "probable human carcinogens" (including cacodylic acid) during 9 months before delivery		
	All sites	223	1.0 (0.9–1.2)
	Leukemias	179	1.2 (0.9–1.5)
	Central nervous system tumors	31	0.9 (0.5–1.4)
Studies Reviewed in *Update 2004*			
Flower et al., 2004	Offspring of male pesticide applicators in Iowa from AHS		
	Maternal exposure to chlorophenoxy herbicides	7	0.7 (0.3–1.5)
	Paternal exposure to chlorophenoxy herbicides	28	1.3 (0.6–2.6)
	Maternal exposure to 2,4-D	7	0.7 (0.3–1.6)
	Paternal exposure to 2,4-D	26	1.3 (0.7–2.4)
Studies Reviewed in *Update 2000*			
Heacock et al., 2000	Offspring of sawmill workers exposed to fungicides contaminated with PCDDs, PCDFs		
	Leukemia		
	All workers' offspring—incidence	11	1.0 (0.5–1.8)
	Chlorophenate exposure: high- vs low-exposure subjects	5	0.8 (0.2–3.6)
	Brain cancer		
	All workers' offspring—incidence	9	1.3 (0.6–2.5)
	Chlorophenate exposure: high- vs low-exposure subjects	5	1.5 (0.4–6.9)
Buckley et al., 1989	Children's Cancer Study Group—exposure to pesticides, weed killers—AML		
	Any paternal exposure	27	2.3 (p = 0.5)
	Paternal exposure over 1,000 days	17	2.7 (1.0–7.0)
	Maternal exposure over 1,000 days	7	undefined
ENVIRONMENTAL			
New Studies			
Cooney et al., 2007	Case–control study of Wilms' tumor in United States and Canada		
	Maternal report of household use of herbicides from month before conception through child's diagnosis	112	1.0 (0.7–1.4)
Rudant et al., 2007	Case–control study of childhood hematopoietic malignancies in France		
	Maternal household herbicide use during pregnancy		

continued

TABLE 7-8 Continued

Reference	Study Population	Exposed Cases[b]	Estimated Relative Risk (95% CI)[b]
	Acute leukemia	53	1.5 (1.0–2.2)
	Without paternal exposure	4	5.0 (1.3–19.0)
	All ALL	nr	1.7 (1.2–2.5)
	Common B-cell ALL	nr	1.9 (1.3–2.9)
	Mature B-cell ALL	nr	1.5 (0.3–6.4)
	T-cell ALL	nr	0.5 (0.1–2.0)
	AML	nr	1.2 (0.5–2.8)
	HD	9	1.1 (0.5–2.4)
	Without paternal exposure	0	nr
	Nodular sclerosis	nr	1.3 (0.5–3.1)
	Mixed cell	nr	0.8 (0.1–6.6)
	NHL	14	1.5 (0.8–2.7)
	Without paternal exposure	0	nr
	Burkitt's lymphoma	nr	1.7 (0.7–4.0)
	B-cell lymphoblastic	nr	0.7 (0.2–3.0)
	T-cell lymphoblastic	nr	2.6 (0.7–9.0)
	Anaplastic large cell	nr	1.4 (0.3–2.8)
Studies Reviewed in *Update 2006*			
Chen et al., 2006	Childhood GCTs residential exposure to herbicides 6 months before conception, during gestation, through breastfeeding period		
	Maternal exposure	47	1.3 (0.9–1.7)
	Daughters	36	1.4 (1.0–2.0)
	Sons	11	1.0 (0.5–1.8)
	Paternal exposure	90	1.0 (0.7–1.3)
	Daughters	32	1.2 (0.7–2.0)
	Sons	58	1.0 (0.7–1.4)
Studies Reviewed in *Update 2002*			
Daniels et al., 2001	Neuroblastoma risk in children (case–control study) (as reported by both parents)		
	Pesticides in home (used ever)	nr	1.6 (1.0–2.3)
	Herbicides in garden	nr	1.9 (1.1–3.2)
	Pesticides in garden	nr	2.2 (1.3–3.6)
Kerr et al., 2000	Neuroblastoma risk in children		
	Maternal occupational exposure to insecticides	40	2.3 (1.4–3.7)
	Paternal exposure to dioxin	7	6.9 (1.3–68.4)
Studies Reviewed in *Herbicide/Dioxin Exposure and AML in the Children of Veterans*			
Kristensen et al., 1996	Children of agricultural workers in Norway Children with AML whose parents purchased pesticides	12	1.4 (0.6–2.9)
Studies Reviewed in *Update 2000*			
Meinert et al., 2000	Childhood cancer—population-based case–control study		
	Leukemia		
	Paternal exposure year before pregnancy	62	1.5 (1.1–2.2)
	Paternal exposure during pregnancy	57	1.6 (1.1–2.3)

TABLE 7-8 Continued

Reference	Study Population	Exposed Cases[b]	Estimated Relative Risk (95% CI)[b]
	Maternal exposure year before pregnancy	19	2.1 (1.1–4.2)
	Maternal exposure during pregnancy	15	3.6 (1.5–8.8)
	Lymphomas		
	Paternal exposure year before pregnancy	11	1.5 (0.7–3.1)
	Paternal exposure during pregnancy	10	1.6 (0.7–3.6)
	Maternal exposure year before pregnancy	3	2.9 (0.7–13)
	Maternal exposure during pregnancy	4	11.8 (2.2–64)
Pearce and Parker, 2000	Renal cancer in subjects (1–15 years old) with paternal occupation in agriculture	21	0.9 (0.2–3.8)
Infante-Rivard et al., 1999	Childhood ALL in households using herbicides— population-based case–control study		
	Exposure during pregnancy	118	1.8 (1.3–2.6)
	Exposure during childhood	178	1.4 (1.1–1.9)
Studies Reviewed in *Update 1996*			
Pesatori et al., 1993	Seveso residents 0–19 years old—10-year follow-up, morbidity, all exposure zones		
	All cancers	17	1.2 (0.7–2.1)
	Ovary, uterine adnexa	2	nr (0 cases expected)
	Brain	3	1.1 (0.3–4.1)
	Thyroid	2	4.6 (0.6–32.7)
	HD	3	2.0 (0.5–7.6)
	Lymphatic leukemia	2	1.3 (0.3–6.2)
	Myeloid leukemia	3	2.7 (0.7–11.4)
Bertazzi et al., 1992	Seveso residents 0–19 years old—10-year follow-up, mortality, all exposure zones		
	All cancers	10	7.9 (3.8–13.6)
	Leukemias	5	3.9 (1.2–1.8)
	Lymphatic leukemia	2	1.6 (0.1–4.5)
	Myeloid leukemia	1	0.8 (0.0–3.1)
	Leukemia, others	2	1.6 (0.1–4.6)
	Central nervous system tumors	2	1.6 (0.1–4.6)

ABBREVIATIONS: 2,4-D, 2,4-dichlorophenoxyacetic acid; AHS, Agricultural Health Study; AIHW, Australian Institute for Health and Welfare; ALL, acute lymphocytic leukemia; AML, acute myeloid leukemia; CDC, Centers for Disease Control and Prevention; CI, confidence interval; GCT, germ-cell tumor; HD, Hodgkin's disease; NHL, non-Hodgkin's lymphoma; nr, not reported; PCDD, polychlorinated dibenzodioxin; PCDF, polychlorinated dibenzofuran.

[a]Unless otherwise indicated, studies show paternal exposure.

[b]Given when available; results other than estimated risk explained individually.

[c]Of the 12, nine were observed, three additional cases estimated to have occurred in portion of cohort whose data were not validated.

Update of Epidemiologic Literature

Vietnam-Veteran Studies

No Vietnam-veteran studies of exposure to the chemicals of interest and childhood cancer have been published since *Update 2006*.

Occupational Studies

One paper (Monge et al., 2007) addressed occupational exposure to pesticides and the risk of childhood leukemia in Costa Rica. All cases of leukemia in infants and children (up to 14 years old at diagnosis) in Costa Rica in 1995–2000 were identified at the Cancer Registry and at Children's Hospital of Costa Rica. Population-based controls were identified from the National Birth Registry by computerized randomization and were frequency-matched by year of birth. Data were collected via interviews with both parents of the 300 case and 579 control children. Parents who worked in agriculture or livestock production completed an additional interview. Pesticide use and agricultural tasks were ascertained from 12 months before conception until the diagnosis of cancer for the cases and the interview date for the controls. Exposures to any herbicides were assessed during all periods of interest to the researchers (the year before conception, the three trimesters of pregnancy, and the first year of life), but only paternal exposures before conception and maternal exposure before and during gestation could be of any possible relevance to the circumstances under which Vietnam veterans were exposed. Paternal exposure to herbicides during the year before conception was slightly associated with all types of leukemia (OR = 1.2, 95% CI 0.8–1.7). Picloram was one of only five pesticides to which the parents of more than three cases had recorded exposure, and all 11 cases of leukemia involving paternal exposure to picloram were specifically ALL; the association with any paternal exposure to picloram during the year before conception was increased (OR = 1.6, 95% CI 0.7–3.4). The association was greater, but of borderline significance, after high exposure than after low exposure (OR = 6.3, 95% CI 1.0–38.6). Paternal exposure to phenoxyacetic acids was not associated with total leukemia (OR = 1.0, 95% CI 0.6–1.6).

Overall, the ORs were higher, but less precise, for maternal exposure to all herbicides combined during the defined periods. The OR for maternal exposure to herbicides before conception and total leukemia was 2.0 (95% CI 0.8–5.0). An increased, but imprecise, risk was observed for maternal exposure to herbicides during the first two trimesters of pregnancy (OR = 5.3, 95% CI 1.4–20.0). Maternal exposure to phenoxyacetic acids, with four exposed cases, was weakly associated with total leukemia (OR = 1.3, 95% CI 0.4–4.8).

An additional study published since *Update 2006* examined paternal occupational exposure to "pesticides or herbicides" and childhood cancer (Pearce et al., 2006). However, the exposure definition for analysis was limited to job titles that were likely to include exposure to pesticides and therefore did not meet the level of exposure specificity required for full review by the committee.

Environmental Studies

Cooney et al. (2007) examined household pesticide use and Wilms' tumor in a population-based case–control study. Cases, all registered with the National Wilms' Tumor Study, were patients under 16 years old who had Wilms' tumor newly diagnosed in the United States or Canada in 1999–2002. After the exclusion of 512 cases lacking physician or hospital approval for participation, 653 eligible cases remained, and 523 case mothers completed interviews. Random-digit dialing (RDD) was used to identify 682 eligible controls, who were frequency-matched on age at diagnosis and geographic residence. Of the control mothers, 517 completed interviews. Structured computer-assisted telephone interviews were used to gather information from mothers of cases and controls, including information on use of household pesticides from the month before pregnancy to the date of the child's diagnosis (or referent date); only the month before conception is relevant for the exposures being evaluated in this report, but exposures would be dominated by the period of gestation and childhood. No association with that broader definition of herbicide exposure was observed in the study (OR = 1.0, 95% CI 0.7–1.4).

Rudant et al. (2007) also examined household pesticide use in relation to the risk of childhood hematopoietic cancers in the ESCALE study, a French national population-based case–control study designed to examine infectious, environmental, and genetic factors in childhood cancers (leukemia, lymphoma, neuroblastoma, and brain tumor). Cases less than 15 years old who received new diagnoses during the 2003–2004 study period were identified from each of the pediatric-oncology departments with support of the French National Registry of Childhood Blood Malignancies. The population-based controls were randomly selected and frequency-matched on age and sex. Subjects who were adopted or whose mother had died, had a psychiatric problem, or did not speak French were excluded. Structured telephone interviews were used to obtain data from the mothers of cases and controls and included questions about household pesticide use by the mothers during pregnancy. Pesticides were classified by functional groups (such as herbicides). Maternal exposure to herbicides (all types combined) during pregnancy was associated with acute leukemia (AL) (OR = 1.5, 95% CI 1.0–2.2) and non-Hodgkin's lymphoma (NHL) (OR = 1.5, 95% CI 0.8–2.7); no association was observed with Hodgkin's disease (HD) (OR = 1.1, 95% CI 0.5–2.4). The study's assessment of postconception paternal exposure, which was considerably more common than maternal exposure, is not relevant for the present review. However, the pattern of associations with paternal exposure was similar to the pattern of associations between maternal exposure and AL (OR = 1.2, 95% CI 1.0–1.4), NHL (OR = 1.5, 95% CI 1.0–2.2), and HD (OR = 1.3, 95% CI 0.8–2.2). When the definition of exposure was limited to maternal exposure, the number of exposed AL cases decreased to four, but the observed association with AL increased (OR = 5.0, 95% CI 1.3–19.0). No NHL or HD cases were considered to have had only maternal exposure. When malignancy subtypes were examined, maternal household use of herbicides was associated with all types of ALL (OR = 1.7, 95% CI 1.2–2.5) and with the common B-cell subtype of ALL (OR = 1.9, 95% CI 1.3–2.9).

The Centers for Disease Control and Prevention investigated environmental factors that might influence childhood leukemia in Churchill County, Nevada, where a higher than expected number of cases were diagnosed in 1997–2002 (Rubin et al., 2007). This cross-sectional case-comparison study enrolled 14 of the 15 eligible families of children who had leukemia. RDD was used to identify the 55 participating comparison families (child and caretaking adults living in the home), which were matched on case children's sex and years of birth. Biologic and environmental samples were collected from each of the families, and family members were interviewed. None of the 31 nonpersistent pesticides was associated with leukemia, although geometric mean urinary concentrations of 2,4-D and 2,4,5-T in the entire study sample were above the reference (National Health and Nutrition Examination Survey) geometric mean. No association between the 11 persistent pesticides measured in serum and cases status was observed.

Two additional studies—by Carozza et al. (2008) and Walker et al. (2007)—examined environmental exposure to pesticides and childhood cancer. They were limited by definition of exposure on the basis of residence in counties of greater agricultural activity and did not meet the level of exposure specificity required for full review by the committee.

Biologic Plausibility

Paternal or maternal exposure to xenobiotics potentially could increase the susceptibility of offspring to cancer through multiple mechanisms. Susceptibility could be increased by inheriting a genetic predisposition, which by itself could increase the development of cancer or the likelihood of developing cancer after future exposure to a carcinogen; the mother or father would transmit either an acquired genetic defect or an epigenetic alteration that predisposed the child to cancer. Alternatively, a maternally mediated increase in susceptibility to childhood cancer could result from direct exposure of a child in utero or via lactation to a xenobiotic that induces epigenetic alterations that increase cancer susceptibility or is itself carcinogic.

It has been shown that prenatal TCDD exposure of rats is associated with altered mammary gland differentiation and an increase in the number of mammary adenocarcinomas (Brown et al., 1998). A recent study's demonstration that early postnatal TCDD exposure does not increase mammary-cancer risk (Desaulniers et al., 2004) is consistent with the finding that TCDD-induced changes in utero mediate the increase in cancer susceptibility (Fenton et al., 2000, 2002). Developmental epigenetic alterations may be involved in those prenatal effects. TCDD has been shown to suppress the expression of two tumor-suppressor genes, $p16^{Ink4a}$ and p53, via an epigenetic mechanism that appears to involve DNA methylation (Ray and Swanson, 2004). Similarly, it was reported that prenatal TCDD exposure increases methylation of two growth-related imprinted genes, H19 and Igf2, in the developing fetus (Wu et al., 2004).

Although there is no direct evidence from animal models that TCDD increases the risk of childhood cancers, such as acute leukemia or germ-cell tumors, emerging research suggests that prenatal TCDD exposure can disrupt epigenetic imprinting patterns and alter organ differentiation, which could contribute to an increased susceptibility to cancer later in life. A recent study has shown that chromosomal rearrangements associated with childhood ALL are evident in the neonatal blood spots; this suggests that childhood leukemias begin before birth and that maternal and perinatal exposures to xenobiotics may contribute to genetic mutations (Smith et al., 2005).

Synthesis

Two of the four studies reviewed by the committee report increased ORs with respect to herbicide exposure and childhood cancer. Monge et al. (2007) found that paternal exposure to picloram was associated with ALL, but the finding was limited by the small number of exposed cases, which resulted in imprecise estimates of risk; no association between paternal exposure to phenoxyacetic acids and leukemia was observed. Maternal exposures in the same study showed an increased risk of total leukemia, but the maternal exposure definition was limited to all herbicides combined. Analyses by pesticide subtypes found no association with maternal exposure to phenoxyacetic acids. Similarly, Rudant et al. (2007) reported an increased OR for maternal exposure to herbicides during pregnancy and ALL. The interpretation of those findings for the purposes of this review is limited by the nonspecific nature of the definition of exposure to include all herbicides.

Conclusions

On the basis of the evidence reviewed here and in previous VAO reports, the committee concludes that there is inadequate or insufficient evidence of an association between exposure to the chemicals of interest and childhood cancers.

EFFECTS OCCURRING LATER IN OFFSPRING'S LIFE OR IN LATER GENERATIONS

In response to a special request from the Department of Veterans Affairs, continuing inquiries from the veterans themselves and their families, and somewhat more attention in research efforts, this update addresses whether it is now necessary and feasible to assess associations between exposure to the herbicides sprayed in Vietnam and health effects in the children and grandchildren of Vietnam veterans that have not been formally reviewed in the VAO series. The additional outcomes may include effects (other than cancer) in the children that become apparent after the first year of life and that may be related to maternal or paternal exposures (for example, cognitive and behavioral outcomes and effects on sexual development). In addition, the committee explored the possibility of transgenerational effects resulting from exposure-related epigenetic changes, either in the parents or fetuses, that would result in adverse health effects in later generations (such as grandchildren).

Problems Detected in Children After First Year of Life

There is growing evidence from laboratory animal and human studies that exposures during fetal development can lead to adverse effects later in life that are not immediately apparent as structural malformations or functional deficits. Several reports of studies in animals and exposed humans suggest that prenatal exposure to TCDD or to DLCs can impair brain development and induce neurobehavioral deficits. Outcomes can be subtle, ranging from altered learning and memory to modification of sex-related behavior. The mechanisms of those effects are unclear. Animal studies have shown that perinatal TCDD exposure can decrease neuron number (Hojo et al., 2006), modify gene expression in various parts of the brain (Chang SF et al., 2005; Fujita et al., 2006; Mitsui et al., 2006; Nayyar et al., 2003), and reduce or reverse sexual dimorphic brain development (Chang SF et al., 2005; Ikeda et al., 2005b). Such changes can be associated with altered behavior and learning in rodents (Ikeda et al., 2005b; Mitsui et al., 2006) and primates (Negishi et al., 2006).

Human studies have found correlations between maternal, placental, and breast-milk concentrations of dioxins and PCBs and children's behavior in several hundred Dutch mother–infant pairs since 1990 (Koopman-Essenboom et al., 1994; Vreugdenhil and Weisglas-Kuperus, 2000; Vreugdenhil et al., 2002). A study of human exposure to background concentrations of dioxins, furans, and PCBs during prenatal development (Nakajima et al., 2006) suggested a greater association between exposure and reduced motor development in 6-month-old infants than between exposure and mental development; however, few significant correlations among dozens of comparisons with specific congeners that have low relative potency (TEFs).

Animal studies have repeatedly shown adverse effects of prenatal TCDD exposure on various reproductive characteristics of the offspring. Studies in rodents have shown that a single maternal dose of TCDD produces malformations of the external genitalia and functional reproductive alterations in female progeny, including decreased fertility rate, reduced fecundity, cystic endometrial hyperplasia, and disrupted estrous cycles. Those effects depend on the timing of exposure. In agreement with earlier work (Dienhart et al., 2000; Gray et al.,

1997b), recent research (Kakeyama et al, 2008) found that prenatal exposure to a low dose of TCDD affected the onset of puberty in the female offspring of rats. Several reports (Gray et al., 1997a; Mably et al., 1992; Ohsako et al., 2002) have indicated that development of the male reproductive system is exceptionally sensitive to in utero and lactational TCDD exposure. Maternal exposure to TCDD impairs prostate growth and seminal vesicle weight and branching and decreases sperm production and caudal epididymal sperm number in offspring. Work on the differentiation of mammary tissue in rats (Brown et al., 1998; Fenton et al., 2000, 2002) has demonstrated that TCDD produces changes in utero that increase susceptibility to cancer in adulthood.

Similar effects on the reproductive characteristics of the offspring have been reported in humans. Reviewers (Damgaard et al., 2002; Landrigan et al., 2003; Teilmann et al., 2002; Wikiera et al., 2007) have hypothesized that the world-wide reports of precocious puberty, reduced semen quality, and other forms of reproductive dysfunction are related to exposure from before birth to endocrine disruptors, including dioxins, at environmental concentrations. Demonstration of precocious puberty in the daughters of women accidentally exposed to poly-brominated biphenyls (Blanck et al., 2000) suggested the plausibility of such activity of DLCs.

Human Effects in Later Generations

As the cohort of Vietnam veterans ages, the veterans'children are well into their reproductive years, and concerns have been expressed as to whether her-bicide exposures experienced in Vietnam might be having adverse effects on another generation. Growing awareness of the possibility of epigenetic changes (that is, heritable changes in genome function that occur without a change in primary DNA sequences) arising from exposure to the chemicals of interest now increases the plausibility of such transgenerational findings (Cordier, 2008), whereas in previous review cycles VAO committees had been confident that di-oxin (the primary suspect) would not directly produce heritable genetic damage. Epidemiologic investigation of this possibility will be even more challenging to conduct than research on adverse effects on the first generation, but recently recognized epigenetic mechanisms that are the focus of intensive research could consititute a mechanism by which such outcomes might occur.

Lasting gene expression changes responsible for the phenotypic changes associated with a disease state are the result of stable alterations of the genetic material by either genetic or epigenetic mechanisms. Several factors—such as chemotherapy, mutagenic agents, endocrine disruptors, and environmental tox-ins—alter DNA by one or the other mechanism (Anway et al., 2005; Barber et al., 2002). In mammalian development, long-lasting changes of gene expression result from alterations in DNA methylation patterns, the most common form of epigenetic change modification of the genome (Morgan et al., 2005). DNA methylation is associated with permanent changes in the genome (Baylin and Chen, 2005) and is thought to be a strong mechanism for modifying gene expression and to have an important role in normal development and in maintenance of genome stability (Jaenisch and Bird, 2003). Several diseases result from epigenetic imprinting malformations (Jiang YH et al., 2004), including some forms of cancer associated with DNA methylation aberrations (Roundtree et al., 2001). Current understanding is that epigenetic mechanisms are responsible for phenotypic changes induced by various chemicals and agents that act primarily through DNA damage, such as heavy metals, some base analogues, ionizing radiation, reactive oxygen species, and smoke components. Those and other stress-inducing factors, such as pesticides and some hormones (for example, estradiol), may alter DNA methylation states or histone acetylation states. A growing body of evidence suggests that epigenetic factors play a critical role in the development of cancer (Nagasaka et al., 2008).

The best-understood epigenetic alteration is DNA methylation that occurs in cytosine residues that form part of CpG islands, so called for their higher content of CpG dinucleotides. CpG dinucleotides occur in gene-promoter regions at frequencies greater than would be expected on the basis of random distribution. Addition of a methyl group to the 5′-carbon of the cytosine in a CpG dinucleotide, if it occurs at multiple cytosines in a particular CpG island, is often associated with silencing of the gene by recruitment of methyl-binding proteins that create a chromatin conformation that leads to gene repression. During cancer development, epigenetic silencing by promoter hypermethylation is one of the mechanisms that inactivate tumor-suppressor genes. Unlike promoters of tumor-suppressor genes, other DNA sequences of the genome are normally methylated, and their methylation is an important part of normal development, cellular differentiation, and X-chromosome inactivation; at an extreme, changes in their methylation status may lead to specific human disease states (Ehrlich, 2003). Methylation status is genetically determined, but recent work in animal model systems suggests that environmental exposures, particularly during fetal development and early life, also induce epigenetic changes in somatic tissues (Cutfield et al., 2007) that can be passed through multiple generations, although they do not cause DNA mutations (Anway and Skinner, 2008).

It is during embryonic development that the organism is most sensitive to injury by chemicals and environmental toxins (Yamazaki et al., 2003). That is when lineage-specific and germ-line–specific DNA-methylation patterns are established (Reik and Walter, 2001). The lineage-specific pattern establishes the DNA-methylation pattern for the various somatic cells after fertilization. The germ-line–specific pattern is established during gonadal sex determination (Reik et al., 2001) and is critical for gene imprinting (Lucifero et al., 2004). Unlike lineage-specific DNA-methylation programming, changes in germ-line–specific programming can alter heritable DNA-methylation profiles and result in a transgenerational phenotype. Alterations in lineage-specific DNA methylation potentially lead to developmental defects and, in the worst case, embryonic death (Reik et al., 2001).

Because of its status as a persistent environmental contaminant of great concern and its known estrogenic activity, dioxin is often mentioned as a chemical that might be expected to produce adverse effects via epigenetic mechanisms (Edwards and Myers, 2007). Research into dioxin's potential as an epigenetic agent is in its early stages, but there have been several reports that dioxin has such properties. For instance, Wu et al. (2004) have demonstrated that TCDD exposure of mouse embryos before implantation in unexposed females resulted in reduced fetal weight in association with reduced expression and increased methylation of imprinted genes. Another mode of epigenetic change is modification of the spatial arrangement of chromosomes, which correlates with gene expression and with how cells differentiate, and Oikawa et al. (2008) have found that TCDD, through the AHR, modifies the position of chromosomes in the interphase nuclei of human pre-adipocytes.

Failure to comprehend how something might happen is not a scientifically legitimate reason for not inquiring into whether it has occurred. Nonetheless, despite the profound concern of veterans and their families that herbicide exposures in Vietnam were having adverse effects on the health of their children and now grandchildren, the longstanding biologic conviction that there was no plausible mechanism by which non-genotoxic agents like the chemicals of concern in these VAO reports could produce paternally-mediated transgenerational effects could only discourage undertaking the arduous work of conducting epidemiologic studies on such health problems in older offspring and the second generation. The developing understanding of epigenetic mechanisms leads the committee to conclude that it is considerably more plausible than previously believed that exposure to the herbicides sprayed in Vietnam might have caused transgenerational effects. Such potential would most likely be attributable to the TCDD contaminant in Agent Orange. Consequently, this committee recommends that toxicologic research be conducted to address and characterize TCDD's potential for inducing epigenetic modifications and is more convinced that additional epidemiologic study would be a worthwhile investment of resources.

Efficient conduct of epidemiologic investigations into whether such effects are being manifested in the grandchildren of Vietnam veterans will probably require the development of some innovative techniques and protocols. The design of such studies poses additional challenges compared with the traditional case–cohort or cohort studies in that large numbers of subjects need to be tracked in multiple generations, exposures need to be reconstructed as specifically as possible for critical periods in each individual's life, and the effects to be appraised could be quite diverse. Although there could be problems of selection bias, starting with previously defined cohorts of deployed and nondeployed Vietnam-era veterans would probably be the most efficient way to address the question of whether the incidence of health problems is increased in the mature children and grandchildren of Vietnam veterans. Only a single temporal pattern of expo-sure—preconception exposure of fathers (almost exclusively)—would need to be contrasted with a cleanly defined absence of such preconception exposure, so the hypothesis could be tested more precisely than in instances in which paternal or maternal exposure could occur before conception, during gestation, and after birth. It can be expected that it is not going to be possible so many decades after potential exposure to herbicides in Vietnam to determine original exposures ac-curately, so it would be advantageous to continue work with study populations whose serum TCDD has been measured.

SUMMARY

Synthesis

The studies reviewed for this update did not find any significant associa-tions between the relevant exposures and reproductive outcomes. The scientific evidence supports the biologic plausibility of a connection between exposure to the chemicals of interest and reproductive effects, but the epidemiologic studies of occupational cohorts, exposed communities, and Vietnam veterans have not provided conclusive evidence of any additional associations between exposures and an array of reproductive outcomes and conditions in the offspring of exposed parents. The mechanisms by which the chemicals exert their biologic effects are still subjects of scientific investigation. With the aging of the Vietnam-veteran population, additional studies of fertility, spontaneous abortion, and sex ratio cannot be expected, although there may be additional studies of reproductive outcomes in other populations after exposure to the chemicals of interest. The possibility that structural or functional abnormalities will be manifested in the maturing offspring of exposed people will continue to be of interest. In addi-tion, the committee strongly recommends that careful consideration be given to systematically evaluating whether recently recognized mechanisms of epigenetic modification mean that there could be long-term consequences of herbicide expo-sure for the health of the progeny of Vietnam veterans into later generations.

Conclusions

There is inadequate or insufficient evidence of an association between ex-posure to 2,4-D, 2,4,5-T, TCDD, picloram, or cacodylic acid and endometriosis; semen quality; infertility; spontaneous abortion; late fetal, neonatal, or infant death; low birth weight or preterm delivery; birth defects other than spina bifida; and childhood cancers.

There is limited or suggestive evidence of an association between exposure to the chemicals of interest and spina bifida. There is some evidence of altered hormone concentrations, but the degree to which testosterone concentration may be modified is not great enough for clinical consequences to be expected.

There is limited or suggestive evidence that the specific combination of paternal exposure to TCDD is *not* associated with risk of spontaneous abortion.

REFERENCES[1]

ACS (American Cancer Society). 2008. *Cancer Facts and Figures 2008.* http://www.cancer.org/downloads/STT/2008CAFFfinalsecured.pdf (Accessed March 30).

ADVA (Australia Department of Veterans Affairs). 1983. *Case–Control Study of Congenital Anomalies and Vietnam Service.* Canberra, Australia.

AFHS (Air Force Health Study). 1992. *An Epidemiologic Investigation of Health Effects in Air Force Personnel Following Exposure to Herbicides. Reproductive Outcomes.* Brooks AFB, TX: USAF School of Aerospace Medicine. AL-TR-1992-0090. 602 pp.

AIHW (Australian Institute of Health and Welfare). 1999. *Morbidity of Vietnam Veterans: A Study of the Health of Australia's Vietnam Veteran Community: Volume 3: Validation Study.* Canberra, Australia.

AIHW. 2000. *Morbidity of Vietnam veterans. Adrenal gland cancer, leukaemia and non-Hodgkin's lymphoma: Supplementary report no. 2.* (AIHW cat. no. PHE 28). Canberra, Australia: AIHW.

AIHW. 2001. *Morbidity of Vietnam veterans. Adrenal gland cancer, leukaemia and non-Hodgkin's lymphoma: Supplementary report no. 2.* Revised edition (AIHW cat. No. PHE 34). Canberra, Australia: AIHW.

Alberman E. 1984. Low birth weight. In: Bracken MB, ed. *Perinatal Epidemiology.* New York: Oxford University Press. Pp. 86–98.

Alexander GR, Slay M. 2002. Prematurity at birth: Trends, racial disparities, and epidemiology. *Mental Retardation and Developmental Disabilities Research Reviews* 8(4):215–220.

Alexander GR, Kogan M, Bader D, Carlo W, Allen M, Mor J. 2003. US birth weight/gestational age-specific neonatal mortality: 1995–1997 rates for whites, Hispanics, and blacks. *Pediatrics* 111(1):e61–e66.

Anway MD, Skinner MK. 2008. Epigenetic programming of the germ line: Effects of endocrine disruptors on the development of transgenerational disease. *Reproductive and Biomedical Online* 16:23–25.

Anway MD, Cupp AS, Uzumcu M, Skinner MK. 2005. Epigenetic transgenerational actions of endocrine disruptors and male fertility. *Science* 308:1466–1469.

Arbuckle TE, Lin Z, Mery LS. 2001. An exploratory analysis of the effect of pesticide exposure on the risk of spontaneous abortion in an Ontario farm population. *Environmental Health Perspectives* 109(8):851–857.

Aschengrau A, Monson RR. 1989. Paternal military service in Vietnam and risk of spontaneous abortion. *Journal of Occupational Medicine* 31(7):618–623.

Aschengrau A, Monson RR. 1990. Paternal military service in Vietnam and the risk of late adverse pregnancy outcomes. *American Journal of Public Health* 80(10):1218–1224.

Axmon A, Rylander L, Strömberg U, Hagmar L. 2000. Miscarriages and stillbirths in women with a high intake of fish contaminated with persistent organochlorine compounds. *International Archives of Occupational and Environmental Health* 73(3):204–208.

Baccarelli A, Giacomini SM, Corbetta C, Landi MT, Bonzini M, Consonni D, Grillo P, Patterson Jr DG, Pesatori AC, Bertazzi PA. 2008. Neonatal thyroid function in Seveso 25 years after maternal exposure to dioxin. *PLoS Medicine* 5(7):1133–1142.

---

[1]Throughout the report the same alphabetic indicator following year of publication is used consistently for the same article when there were multiple citations by the same first author in a given year. The convention of assigning the alphabetic indicator in order of citation in a given chapter is not followed.

Barber R, Plumb MA, Boulton E, Roux I, Dubrova YE. 2002. Elevated mutation rates in the germ line of first- and second-generation offspring of irradiated male mice. *Proceeding of the National Academy of Sciences of the United States of America* 99:6877–6882.

Barnett KR, Tomic D, Gupta RK, Babus JK, Roby KF, Terranova PF, Flaws JA. 2007a. The aryl hydrocarbon receptor is required for normal gonadotropin responsiveness in the mouse ovary. *Toxicology and Applied Pharmacology* 223(1):66–72.

Barnett KR, Tomic D, Gupta RK, Miller KP, Meachum S, Paulose T, Flaws JA. 2007b. The aryl hydrocarbon receptor affects mouse ovarian follicle growth via mechanisms involving estradiol regulation and responsiveness. *Biology of Reproduction* 76(6):1062–1070.

Baylin SB, Chen WY. 2005. Aberrant gene silencing in tumor progression: Implications for control of cancer. *Cold Spring Harbor Symposia on Quantitative Biology* 70:427–433.

Bell DR, Clode S, Fan MQ, Fernandes A, Foster PM, Jiang T, Loizou G, MacNicoll A, Miller BG, Rose M, Tran L, White S. 2007b. Toxicity of 2,3,7,8-tetrachlorodibenzo-*p*-dioxin in the developing male Wistar(Han) rat. I: No decrease in epididymal sperm count after a single acute dose. *Toxicological Sciences* 99(1):214–223.

Berkowitz GS, Papiernik E. 1993. Epidemiology of preterm delivery. *Epidemiologic Reviews* 15: 414–443.

Bertazzi PA, Zocchetti C, Pesatori AC, Guercilena S, Consonni D, Tironi A, Landi MT. 1992. Mortality of a young population after accidental exposure to 2,3,7,8-tetrachlorodibenzodioxin. *International Journal of Epidemiology* 21(1):118–123.

Blakley PM, Kim JS, Firneisz GD. 1989. Effects of paternal subacute exposure to Tordon 202c on fetal growth and development in CD-1 mice. *Teratology* 39(3):237–241.

Blanck H, Marcus M, Tolbert PE, Rubin C, Henderson A, Hertzberg V, Zhang R, Cameron L. 2000. Age at menarche and tanner stage in girls exposed in utero and postnatally to polybrominated biphenyl. *Epidemiology* 11(6):642–647.

Blankenship AL, Hilscherova K, Nie M, Coady KK, Villalobos SA, Kannan K, Powell DC, Bursian SJ, Giesy JP. 2003. Mechanisms of TCDD-induced abnormalities and embryo lethality in white leghorn chickens. Comparative Biochemistry and Physiology. *Toxicology and Pharmacology* 136(1):47–62.

Blatter BM, Hermens R, Bakker M, Roeleveld N, Verbeek AL, Zielhuis GA. 1997. Paternal occupational exposure around conception and spina bifida in offspring. *American Journal of Industrial Medicine* 32(3):283–291.

Bloom AD, ed. 1981. *Guidelines for Studies of Human Populations Exposed to Mutagenic and Reproductive Hazards*. White Plains, NY: March of Dimes Foundation.

Bonde JP, Giwercman A. 1995. Occupational hazards to male fecundity. *Reproductive Medicine Review* 4:59–73.

Boverhof DR, Burgoon LD, Williams KJ, Zacharewski TR. 2008. Inhibition of estrogen-mediated uterine gene expression responses by dioxin. *Molecular Pharmacology* 73(1):82–93.

Bretveld RW, Thomas CMG, Scheepers PTJ, Zielhuis GA, Roeleveld N. 2006a. Pesticide exposure: The hormonal function of the female reproductive system disrupted? *Reproductive Biology and Endocrinology* 4:20.

Bretveld RW, Thomas CM, Scheepers PT, Zielhuis GA, Roeleveld N. 2006b. Pesticide exposure: The hormonal function of the female reproductive system disrupted? *Reproductive Biology and Endocrinology* 4:30.

Brown NM, Manzolillo PA, Zhang JX, Wang J, Lamartiniere CA. 1998. Prenatal TCDD and predisposition to mammary cancer in the rat. *Carcinogenesis* 19(9):1623–1629.

Bruner-Tran KL, Rier SE, Eisenberg E, Osteen KG. 1999. The potential role of environmental toxins in the pathophysiology of endometriosis. *Gynecologic and Obstetric Investigation* 48(1):45–52.

Bruner-Tran KL, Yeaman GR, Crispens MA, Igarashi TM, Osteen KG. 2008. Dioxin may promote inflammation-related development of endometriosis. *Fertility and Sterility* 89(Supplement 5): 1287–1298.

Bryce R. 1991. The epidemiology of preterm birth. In: Kiely M, ed. *Reproductive and Perinatal Epidemiology.* Boca Raton, FL: CRC Press. Pp. 437–444.

Buckley JD, Robison LL, Swotinsky R, Garabrant DH, LeBeau M, Manchester P, Nesbit ME, Odom L, Peters JM, Woods WG, Hammond GD. 1989. Occupational exposures of parents of children with acute nonlymphocytic leukemia: A report from the Childrens' Cancer Study Group. *Cancer Research* 49(14):4030–4037.

Bulun SE, Zeitoun KM, Kilic G. 2000. Expression of dioxin-related transactivating factors and target genes in human eutopic endometrial and endometriotic tissues. *American Journal of Obstetrics & Gynecology* 182(4):767–775.

Bursian SJ, Beckett KJ, Yamini B, Martin PA, Kannan K, Shields KL, Mohr FC. 2006a. Assessment of effects in mink caused by consumption of carp collected from the Saginaw River, Michigan, USA. *Archives of Environmental and Contaminated Toxicology* 50(4):614–623.

Bursian SJ, Sharma C, Aulerich RJ, Yamini B, Mitchell RR, Beckett KJ, Orazio CE, Moore D, Svirsky S, Tillitt DE. 2006b. Dietary exposure of mink (Mustela vison) to fish from the Housatonic River, Berkshire County, Massachusetts, USA: Effects on organ weights and histology and hepatic concentrations of polychlorinated biphenyls and 2,3,7,8-tetrachlorodibenzo-*p*-dioxin toxic equivalence. *Environmental Toxicology and Chemistry* 25(6):1541–1550.

Carbone P, Giordano F, Nori F, Mantovani A, Taruscio D, Lauria L, Figa-Talamanca I. 2007. The possible role of endocrine disrupting chemicals in the aetiology of cryptorchidism and hypospadias: A population-based case–control study in rural Sicily. *International Journal of Andrology* 30(1):3–13.

Carmelli D, Hofherr L, Tomsic J, Morgan RW. 1981. *A Case–Control Study of the Relationship Between Exposure to 2,4-D and Spontaneous Abortions in Humans.* SRI International. Prepared for the National Forest Products Association and the US Department of Agriculture, Forest Service.

Carozza SE, Li B, Elgethun K, Whitworth R. 2008. Risk of childhood cancers associated with residence in agriculturally intense areas in the United States. *Environmental Health Perspectives* 116(4):559–565.

CDC (Centers for Disease Control and Prevention). 1989a. *Health Status of Vietnam Veterans Vols I-V, Supplements A-C. Vietnam Experience Study.* Atlanta, GA: US Department of Health and Human Services.

CDC. 1989b. *Health Status of Vietnam Veterans. Vietnam Experience Study, Vol. V, Reproductive Outcomes and Child Health.* Atlanta, GA: US Department of Health and Human Services.

CDC. 2000. National Center for Health Statistics. National Vital Statistics System. *Vital Statistics of the United States, Vol. II, Mortality, Part A, for Data Years 1950–1993.* Washington, DC: US Government Printing Office. Data for 1994 to 1998, data are available on the NCHS Web site at http://www.cdc.gov/nchs/datawh/statab/unpubd/mortabs.htm.

Chang SF, Sun YY, Yang LY, Hu SY, Tsai SY, Lee WS, Lee YH. 2005. Bcl-2 gene family expression in the brain of rat offspring after gestational and lactational dioxin exposure. *Annals of the New York Academy of Sciences.* 1042:471–480.

Chao HR, Wang YF, Chen HT, Ko YC, Chang EE, Huang YJ, Tsai FY, Tsai CH, Wu CH, Tsou TC. 2007. Differential effect of arecoline on the endogenous dioxin-responsive cytochrome P450 1A1 and on a stably transfected dioxin-responsive element-driven reporter in human hepatoma cells. *Journal of Hazardous Materials* 149(1):234–237.

Charles JM, Henwood SM, Leeming NM. 1999. Developmental toxicity studies in rats and rabbits and two-generation reproduction study in rats on 4-(2,4-dichlorophenoxy) butyric acid. *International Journal of Toxicology* 18:177–189.

Chen Z, Stewart PA, Davies S, Giller R, Krailo M, Davis M, Robison L, Shu XO. 2005. Parental occupational exposure to pesticides and childhood germ-cell tumors. *American Journal of Epidemiology* 162(9):858–867.

Chen Z, Robison L, Giller R, Krailo M, Davis M, Davies S, Shu XO. 2006. Environmental exposure to residential pesticides, chemicals, dusts, fumes, and metals, and risk of childhood germ cell tumors. *International Journal of Hygiene and Environmental Health* 209(1):31–40.

Chia SE, Shi LM. 2002. Review of recent epidemiological studies on paternal occupations and birth defects. *Occupational and Environmental Medicine* 59(3):149–155.

Choi JS, Kim IW, Hwang SY, Shin BJ, Kim SK. 2008. Effect of 2,3,7,8-tetrachlorodibenzo-*p*-dioxin on testicular spermatogenesis-related panels and serum sex hormone levels in rats. *BJU International* 101(2):250–255.

Choi SS, Miller MA, Harper PA. 2006. In utero exposure to 2,3,7,8-tetrachlorodibenzo-*p*-dioxin induces amphiregulin gene expression in the developing mouse ureter. *Toxicological Sciences* 94(1):163–174.

Clementi M, Causin R, Marzocchi C, Mantovani A, Tenconi R. 2007. A study of the impact of agricultural pesticide use on the prevalence of birth defects in northeast Italy. *Reproductive Toxicology* 24(1):1–8.

Cok I, Donmez MK, Satiroglu MH, Aydinuraz B, Henkelmann B, Shen H, Kotalik J, Schramm KW. 2008. Concentrations of polychlorinated dibenzo-*p*-dioxins (PCDDs), polychlorinated dibenzofurans (PCDFs), and dioxin-like PCBs in adipose tissue of infertile men. *Archives of Environmental Contamination and Toxicology* 55(1):143–152.

Cooney MA, Daniels JL, Ross JA, Breslow NE, Pollock BH, Olshan AF. 2007. Household pesticides and the risk of Wilms tumor. *Environmental Health Perspectives* 115(1):134–137.

Cordier S, Chevrier C, Robert-Gnansia E, Lorente C, Brula P, Hours M. 2004. Risk of congenital anomalies in the vicinity of municipal solid waste incinerators. *Occupational and Environmental Medicine* 61(1):8–15.

Cummings AM, Metcalf JL, Birnbaum L. 1996. Promotion of endometriosis by 2,3,7,8-tetrachlorodibenzo-*p*-dioxin in rats and mice: Time-dose dependence and species comparison. *Toxicology and Applied Pharmacology* 138:131–139.

Cutfield WS, Hofman PL, Mitchell M, Morison IM. 2007. Could epigenetics play a role in the developmental origins of health and disease? *Pediatric Research* 61:68R–75R.

Damgaard IN, Main KM, Toppari J, Skakkebaek NE. 2002. Impact of exposure to endocrine disrupters in utero and in childhood on adult reproduction. *Best Practice and Research Clinical Endocrinology and Metabolism* 16(2):289–309.

Daniels JL, Olshan AF, Teschke K, Herz-Picciotto I, Savitz DA, Blatt J, Bondy ML, Neglia JP, Pollock BH, Cohn SL, Look AT, Seeger RC, Castleberry RP. 2001. Residential pesticide exposure and neuroblastoma. *Epidemiology* 12:20–27.

De Felip E, Porpora MG, di Domenico A, Ingelido AM, Cardelli M, Cosmi EV, Donnez J. 2004. Dioxin-like compounds and endometriosis: A study on Italian and Belgian women of reproductive age. *Toxicology Letters* 150(2):203–209.

del Rio Gomez I, Marshall T, Tsai P, Shao Y-S, Guo YL. 2002. Number of boys born to men exposed to polychlorinated byphenlys [sic]. *The Lancet* 360:143–144.

Desaulniers D, Leingartner K, Musicki B, Cole J, Li M, Charboneau M, Tsang BK. 2004. Lack of effects of postnatal exposure to a mixture of aryl hydrocarbon-receptor agonists on the development of methylnitrosourea-induced mammary tumors in Sprague-Dawley rats. *Journal of Toxicology and Environmental Health Part A* 67(18):1457–1475.

Dhooge W, van Larebeke N, Koppen G, Nelen V, Schoeters G, Vlietinck R, Kaufman JM, Comhaire F, Flemish E, Health Study G. 2006. Serum dioxin-like activity is associated with reproductive parameters in young men from the general Flemish population. *Environmental Health Perspectives* 114(11):1670–1676.

Dienhart MK, Sommer RJ, Peterson RE, Hirshfield AN, Silbergeld EK. 2000. Gestational exposure to 2,3,7,8-tetrachlorodibenzo-*p*-dioxin induces developmental defects in the rat vagina. *Toxicological Sciences* 56:141–149.

Dimich-Ward H, Hertzman C, Teschke K, Hershler R, Marion SA, Ostry A, Kelly S. 1996. Reproductive effects of paternal exposure to chlorophenate wood preservatives in the sawmill industry. *Scandinavian Journal of Work, Environment and Health* 22(4):267–273.

Donovan JW, MacLennan R, Adena M. 1984. Vietnam service and the risk of cogenital anomalies: A case–control study. *Medical Journal of Australia* 140(7):394–397.

Driscoll R, Donovan B, Esswein E, Mattorano D. 1998. Health hazard evaluation report. *US Department of Agriculture* 1–72.

Edwards TM, Myers JP. 2007. Environmental exposures and gene regulation in disease etiology. *Environmental Health Perspectives* 115(9):1264–1270.

Egeland GM, Sweeney MH, Fingerhut MA, Wille KK, Schnorr TM, Halperin WE. 1994. Total serum testosterone and gonadotropins in workers exposed to dioxin. *American Journal of Epidemiology* 139:272–281.

Ehrlich M. 2003. Expression of various genes is controlled by DNA methylation during mammalian development. *Journal of Cellular Biochemistry* 88:899–910.

Ergaz Z, Avgil M, Ornoy A. 2005. Intrauterine growth restriction—etiology and consequences: What do we know about the human situation and experimental animal models? *Reproductive Toxicology* 20(3):301–322.

Erickson J, Mulinare J, Mcclain P, Fitch T, James L, McClearn A, Adams M. 1984a. *Vietnam Veterans' Risks for Fathering Babies with Birth Defects*. Atlanta, GA: US Department of Health and Human Services, Centers for Disease Control.

Erickson JD, Mulinare J, McClain PW, Fitch TG, James LM, McClearn AB, Adams MJ. 1984b. Vietnam veterans' risks for fathering babies with birth defects. *Journal of the American Medical Association* 252(7):903–912.

Eskenazi B, Mocarelli P, Warner M, Samuels S, Vercellini P, Olive D, Needham LL, Patterson DG Jr, Brambilla P, Gavoni N, Casalini S, Panazza S, Turner W, Gerthoux PM. 2002. Serum dioxin concentrations and endometriosis: A cohort study in Seveso, Italy. *Environmental Health Perspectives* 110(7):629–634.

Eskenazi B, Mocarelli P, Warner M, Chee WY, Gerthoux PM, Samuels S, Needham LL, Patterson DG Jr. 2003. Maternal serum dioxin levels and birth outcomes in women of Seveso, Italy. *Environmental Health Perspectives* 111(7):947–953.

Eskenazi B, Warner M, Marks AR, Samuels S, Gerthoux PM, Vercellini P, Olive DL, Needham L, Patterson D Jr, Mocarelli P. 2005. Serum dioxin concentrations and age at menopause. *Environmental Health Perspectives* 113(7):858–862.

Eskenazi B, Warner M, Samuels S, Young J, Gerthoux PM, Needham L, Patterson D, Olive D, Gavoni N, Vercellini P, Mocarelli P. 2007. Serum dioxin concentrations and risk of uterine leiomyoma in the Seveso Women's Health Study. *American Journal of Epidemiology* 166(1):79–87.

Farr SL, Cooper GS, Cai J, Savitz DA, Sandler DP. 2004. Pesticide use and menstrual cycle characteristics among premenopausal women in the Agricultural Health Study. *American Journal of Epidemiology* 160(12):1194–1204.

Farr SL, Cai J, Savitz DA, Sandler DP, Hoppin JA, Cooper GS. 2006. Pesticide exposure and timing of menopause: The Agricultural Health Study. *American Journal of Epidemiology* 163(8): 731–742.

Felix JF, Van Dooren MF, Klaassens M, Hop WCJ, Torfs CP, Tibboel D. 2008. Environmental factors in the etiology of esophageal atresia and congenital diaphragmatic hernia: Results of a case–control study. *Birth Defects Research Part A—Clinical and Molecular Teratology* 82(2):98–105.

Fenton SE, Hamm JT, Birnbaum LS, Youngblood GL. 2000. Adverse effects of TCDD on mammary gland development in long evans rats: A two generational study. *Organohalogen Compounds* 48:157–160.

Fenton SE, Hamm JT, Birnbaum LS, Youngblood GL. 2002. Persistent abnormalities in the rat mammary gland following gestational and lactational exposure to 2,3,7,8-tetrachlorodibenzo-*p*-dioxin (TCDD). *Toxicological Sciences* 67(1):63–74.

Field B, Kerr C. 1988. Reproductive behaviour and consistent patterns of abnormality in offspring of Vietnam veterans. *Journal of Medical Genetics* 25:819–826.

Fierens S, Mairesse H, Heilier JF, de Burbure C, Focant JF, Eppe G, de Pauw E, Bernard A. 2003. Dioxin/polychlorinated biphenyl body burden, diabetes and endometriosis: Findings in a population-based study in Belgium. *Biomarkers* 8(6):529–534.

Fitzgerald EF, Weinstein AL, Youngblood LG, Standfast SJ, Melius JM. 1989. Health effects three years after potential exposure to the toxic contaminants of an electrical transformer fire. *Archives of Environmental Health* 44:214–221.

Flower KB, Hoppin JA, Lynch CF, Blair A, Knott C, Shore DL, Sandler DP. 2004. Cancer risk and parental pesticide application in children of Agricultural Health Study participants. *Environmental Health Perspectives* 112(5):631–635.

Fujita H, Samejima H, Kitagawa N, Mitsuhashi T, Washio T, Yonemoto J, Tomita M, Takahashi T, Kosaki K. 2006. Genome-wide screening of dioxin-responsive genes in fetal brain: Bioinformatic and experimental approaches. *Congenital Anomalies* 46(3):135–143.

Fujiwara K, Yamada T, Mishima K, Imura H, Sugahara T. 2008. Morphological and immunohistochemical studies on cleft palates induced by 2,3,7,8-tetrachlorodibenzo-*p*-dioxin in mice. *Congenital Anomalies* 48(2):68–73.

Gao Y, Sahlberg C, Kiukkonen A, Alaluusua S, Pohjanvirta R, Tuomisto J, Lukinmaa PL. 2004. Lactational exposure of Han/Wistar rats to 2,3,7,8-tetrachlorodibenzo-*p*-dioxin interferes with enamel maturation and retards dentin mineralization. *Journal of Dental Research* 83(2):139–144.

García AM, Benavides FG, Fletcher T, Orts E. 1998. Paternal exposure to pesticides and congenital malformations. *Scandinavian Journal of Work, Environment and Health* 24(6):473–480.

Garry VF, Schreinemachers D, Harkins ME, Griffith J. 1996. Pesticide appliers, biocides, and birth defects in rural Minnesota. *Environmental Health Perspectives* 104(4):394–399.

Gray L, Ostby J, Kelce WR. 1997a. A dose response analysis of reproductive effects of a single gestational dose of 2,3,7,8-tetrachlorodibenzo-*p*-dioxin in male Long Evans Hooded rat offspring. *Toxicology and Applied Pharmacology* 146:11–20.

Gray L, Wolf C, Mann P, Ostby J. 1997b. In utero exposure to low doses of 2,3,7,8-tetrachlorodibenzo-*p*-dioxin alters reproductive development of female Long Evans hooded rat offsprings. *Toxicology and Applied Pharmacology* 146:237–244.

Greenlee AR, Arbuckle TE, Chyou PH. 2003. Risk factors for female infertility in an agricultural region. *Epidemiology* 14(4):429–436.

Gupta VK, Ali I, Suhas, Saini VK. 2006. Adsorption of 2,4-D and carbofuran pesticides using fertilizer and steel industry wastes. *Journal of Colloid and Interface Science* 299(2):556–563.

Hanify JA, Metcalf P, Nobbs CL, Worsley KJ. 1981. Aerial spraying of 2,4,5-T and human birth malformations: An epidemiological investigation. *Science* 212:349–351.

Heacock H, Hogg R, Marion SA, Hershler R, Teschke K, Dimich-Ward H, Demers P, Kelly S, Ostry A, Hertzman C. 1998. Fertility among a cohort of male sawmill workers exposed to chlorophenate fungicides. *Epidemiology* 9(1):56–60.

Heacock H, Hertzman C, Demers PA, Gallagher R, Hogg RS, Teschke K, Hershler R, Bajdik CD, Dimich-Ward H, Marion SA, Ostry A, Kelly S. 2000. Childhood cancer in the offspring of male sawmill workers occupationally exposed to chlorophenate fungicides. *Environmental Health Perspectives* 108(6):499–503.

Heiden TCK, Struble CA, Rise ML, Hessner MJ, Hutz RJ, Carvan IMJ. 2008. Molecular targets of 2,3,7,8-tetrachlorodibenzo-*p*-dioxin (TCDD) within the zebrafish ovary: Insights into TCDD-induced endocrine disruption and reproductive toxicity. *Reproductive Toxicology* 25(1):47–57.

Heilier JF, Nackers F, Verougstraete V, Tonglet R, Lison D, Donnez J. 2005. Increased dioxin-like compounds in the serum of women with peritoneal endometriosis and deep endometriotic (adenomyotic) nodules. *Fertility and Sterility* 84(2):305–312.

Heilier JF, Donnez J, Defrere S, Van Kerckhove V, Donnez O, Lison D. 2006. Serum dioxin-like compounds and aromatase (CYP19) expression in endometriotic tissues. *Toxicology Letters* 167(3):238–244.

Heilier JF, Donnez J, Nackers F, Rousseau R, Verougstraete V, Rosenkranz K, Donnez O, Grandjean F, Lison D, Tonglet R. 2007. Environmental and host-associated risk factors in endometriosis and deep endometriotic nodules: A matched case–control study. *Environmental Research* 103(1):121–129.

Henriksen GL, Michalek JE, Swaby JA, Rahe AJ. 1996. Serum dioxin, testosterone, and gonadotropins in veterans of Operation Ranch Hand. *Epidemiology* 7(4):352–357.

Hertz-Picciotto I, Samuels SJ. 1988. Incidence of early loss of pregnancy. *New England Journal of Medicine* 319(22):483–484.

Hertz-Picciotto I, Jusko TA, Willman EJ, Baker RJ, Keller JA, Teplin SW, Charles MJ. 2008. A cohort study of in utero polychlorinated biphenyl (PCB) exposures in relation to secondary sex ratio. *Environmental Health: A Global Access Science Source* 7:37.

Ho HM, Ohshima K, Watanabe G, Taya K, Strawn EY, Hutz RJ. 2006. TCDD increases inhibin a production by human luteinized granulosa cells in vitro. *Journal of Reproduction and Development* 52(4):523–528.

Hojo R, Zareba G, Kai JW, Baggs RB, Weiss B. 2006. Sex-specific alterations of cerebral cortical cell size in rats exposed prenatally to dioxin. *Journal of Applied Toxicology* 26(1):25–34.

Hutt KJ, Shi Z, Albertini DF, Petroff BK. 2008. The environmental toxicant 2,3,7,8-tetrachlorodibenzo-*p*-dioxin disrupts morphogenesis of the rat pre-implantation embryo. *BMC Developmental Biology* 8(1).

Igarashi TM, Bruner-Tran KL, Yeaman GR, Lessey BA, Edwards DP, Eisenberg E, Osteen KG. 2005. Reduced expression of progesterone receptor-B in the endometrium of women with endometriosis and in cocultures of endometrial cells exposed to 2,3,7,8-tetrachlorodibenzo-*p*-dioxin. *Fertility and Sterility* 84(1):67–74.

Ikeda M, Tamura M, Yamashita J, Suzuki C, Tomita T. 2005b. Repeated in utero and lactational 2,3,7,8-tetrachlorodibenzo-*p*-dioxin exposure affects male gonads in offspring, leading to sex ratio changes in F2 progeny. *Toxicology and Applied Pharmacology* 206(3):351–355.

Ilvesaro J, Pohjanvirta R, Tuomisto J, Viluksela M, Tuukkanen J. 2005. Bone resorption by aryl hydrocarbon receptor-expressing osteoclasts is not disturbed by TCDD in short-term cultures. *Life Sciences* 77(12):1351–1366.

Infante-Rivard C, Labuda D, Krajinovic M, Sinnett D. 1999. Risk of childhood leukemia associated with exposure to pesticides and with gene polymorphisms. *Epidemiology* 10:481–487.

IOM (Institute of Medicine). 1994. *Veterans and Agent Orange: Health Effects of Herbicides Used in Vietnam.* Washington DC: National Academy Press.

IOM. 1996. *Veterans and Agent Orange: Update 1996.* Washington, DC: National Academy Press.

IOM. 1999. *Veterans and Agent Orange: Update 1998.* Washington, DC: National Academy Press.

IOM. 2001. *Veterans and Agent Orange: Update 2000.* Washington, DC: National Academy Press.

IOM. 2002. *Veterans and Agent Orange: Herbicide/Dioxin Exposure and Acute Myelogenous Leukemia in the Children of Vietnam Veterans.* Washington, DC: National Academy Press.

IOM. 2003. *Veterans and Agent Orange: Update 2002.* Washington, DC: The National Academies Press.

IOM. 2005. *Veterans and Agent Orange: Update 2004.* Washington, DC: The National Academies Press.

IOM. 2007. *Veterans and Agent Orange: Update 2006.* Washington, DC: The National Academies Press.

Jaenisch R, Bird A. 2003. Epigenetic regulation of gene expression: How the genome integrates intrinsic and environmental signals. *Nature Genetics* 33:245–354.

James WH. 2006. Offspring sex ratios at birth as markers of paternal endocrine disruption. *Environmental Research* 100:77–85.

Jang JY, Shin S, Choi BI, Park D, Jeon JH, Hwang SY, Kim JC, Kim YB, Nahm SS. 2007. Antiteratogenic effects of alpha-naphthoflavone on 2,3,7,8-tetrachlorodibenzo-*p*-dioxin (TCDD) exposed mice in utero. *Reproductive Toxicology* 24(3-4):303–309.

Jang JY, Park D, Shin S, Jeon JH, Choi Bi, Joo SS, Hwang SY, Nahm SS, Kim YB. 2008. Antiteratogenic effect of resveratrol in mice exposed in utero to 2,3,7,8-tetrachlorodibenzo-*p*-dioxin. *European Journal of Pharmacology* 591(1-3):280–283.

Jiang YH, Bressler J, Beaudet AL. 2004. Epigenetics and human disease. *Annual Review of Genomics and Human Genetics* 5:479–510.

John-Greene JA, Ouellette JH, Jeffries TK, Johnson KA, Rao KS. 1985. Teratological evaluation of picloram potassium salt in rabbits. *Food and Chemical Toxicology* 23(8):753–756.

Johnson KL, Cummings AM, Birnbaum LS. 1997. Promotion of endometriosis in mice by polychlorinated dibenzo-*p*-dioxins, dibenzofurans, and biphenyls. *Environmental Health Perspectives* 105(7):750–755.

Kallen B. 1988. *Epidemiology of Human Reproduction.* Boca Raton, FL: CRC Press.

Kalter H, Warkany J. 1983. Congenital malformations. Etiologic factors and their role in prevention (first of two parts). *New England Journal of Medicine* 308:424–431.

Kang HK, Mahan CM, Lee KY, Magee CA, Mather SH, Matanoski G. 2000. Pregnancy outcomes among US women Vietnam veterans. *American Journal of Industrial Medicine* 38(4): 447–454.

Karmaus W, Huang S, Cameron L. 2002 Parental concentration of dichlorodiphenyl dichloroethene and polychlorinated biphenyls in Michigan fish eaters and sex ratio in offspring. *Journal of Occupational and Environmental Medicine* 44(1):8–13.

Keller JM, Allen DE, Davis CR, Leamy LJ. 2007a. 2,3,7,8-Tetrachlorodibenzo-*p*-dioxin affects fluctuating asymmetry of molar shape in mice, and an epistatic interaction of two genes for molar size. *Heredity* 98(5):259–267.

Keller JM, Huang JC, Huet-Hudson Y, Leamy LJ. 2007b. The effects of 2,3,7,8-tetrachlorodibenzo-*p*-dioxin on molar and mandible traits in congenic mice: A test of the role of the Ahr locus. *Toxicology* 242(1-3):52–62.

Keller JM, Huet-Hudson YM, Leamy LJ. 2007c. Qualitative effects of dioxin on molars vary among inbred mouse strains. *Archives of Oral Biology* 52(5):450–454.

Keller JM, Huet-Hudson Y, Leamy LJ. 2008. Effects of 2,3,7,8-tetrachlorodibenzo-*p*-dioxin on molar development among non-resistant inbred strains of mice: A geometric morphometric analysis. *Growth, Development, and Aging* 71(1):3–16.

Kerr M, Nasca PC, Mundt KA, Michalek AM, Baptiste MS, Mahoney MC. 2000. Parental occupational exposures and risk of neuroblastoma: A case–control study (United States). *Cancer Causes and Control* 11:635–643.

Khorram O, Garthwaite M, Golos T. 2002. Uterine and ovarian aryl hydrocarbon receptor (ahr) and aryl hydrocarbon receptor nuclear translocator (arnt) mrna expression in benign and malignant gynaecological conditions. *Molecular Human Reproduction* 8(1):75–80.

Khorram O, Garthwaite M, Jones J, Golos T. 2004. Expression of aryl hydrocarbon receptor (AHR) and aryl hydrocarbon receptor nuclear translocator (ARNT) mRNA expression in human spermatozoa. *Medical Science Monitor* 10(5):BR135–BR138.

Kline J, Stein Z, Susser M. 1989. *Conception to Birth: Epidemiology of Prenatal Development.* New York: Oxford University Press.

Knobil E, Neill JD, Greenwald GS, Markert CL, Pfaff DW, eds. 1994. *The Physiology of Reproduction.* New York: Raven Press.

Koopman-Esseboom C, Huisman M, Weisglas-Kuperus N, Van der Paauw CG, Tuinstra L, Boersma ER, Sauer PJJ. 1994. PCB, dioxin levels in plasma and human milk of 418 Dutch women and their infants. Predictive value of PCB congener levels in maternal plasma for fetal and infant's exposure to PCBs and dioxins. *Chemosphere* 28:1721–1732.

Kransler KM, McGarrigle BP, Russell RJ, Olson JR. 2008. Effects of Helicobacter infection on developmental toxicity of 2,3,7,8-tetrachlorodibenzo-*p*-dioxin in Holtzman rats. *Lab Animal* 37(4):171–175.

Kristensen P, Andersen A, Irgens LM, Bye AS, Sundheim L. 1996. Cancer in offspring of parents engaged in agricultural activities in Norway: Incidence and risk factors in the farm environment. *International Journal of Cancer* 65(1):39–50.

Kristensen P, Irgens LM, Andersen A, Bye AS, Sundheim L. 1997. Birth defects among offspring of Norwegian farmers, 1967–1991. *Epidemiology* 8(5):537–544.

Kuroda M, Oikawa K, Ohbayashi T, Yoshida K, Yamada K, Mimura J, Matsuda Y, Fujii-Kuriyama Y, Mukai K. 2005. A dioxin sensitive gene, mammalian WAPL, is implicated in spermatogenesis. *FEBS Letters* 579(1):167–172.

Lacasana M, Vazquez-Grameix H, Borja-Aburto VH, Blanco-Munoz J, Romieu I, Aguilar-Garduno C, Garcia AM. 2006. Maternal and paternal occupational exposure to agricultural work and the risk of anencephaly. *Occupational and Environmental Medicine* 63(10):649–656.

Lahvis GP, Lindell SL, Thomas RS, McCuskey RS, Murphy C, Glover E, Bentz M, Southard J, Bradfield CA. 2000. Portosystemic shunting and persistent fetal vascular structures in aryl hydrocarbon receptor–deficient mice. *Proceedings of the National Academy of Sciences of the United States of America* 97(19):10442–10447.

Lamb JC 4th, Moore JA, Marks TA, Haseman JK. 1981. Development and viability of offspring of male mice treated with chlorinated phenoxy acids and 2,3,7,8-tetrachlorodibenzo-*p*-dioxin. *Journal of Toxicology and Environmental Health* 8(5-6):835–844.

Landrigan P, Garg A, Droller DBJ. 2003. Assessing the effects of endocrine disruptors in the National Children's Study. *Environmental Health Perspectives* 111(13):1678–1682.

Larsen SB, Joffe M, Bonde JP. 1998. Time to pregnancy and exposure to pesticides in Danish farmers. *Occupational and Environmental Medicine* 55(4):278–283.

Lawson CC, Schnorr TM, Whelan EA, Deddens JA, Dankovic DA, Piacitelli LA, Sweeney MH, Connally LB. 2004. Paternal occupational exposure to 2,3,7,8-tetrachlorodibenzo-*p*-dioxin and birth outcomes of offspring: Birth weight, preterm delivery, and birth defects. *Environmental Health Perspectives* 112(14):1403–1408.

Lerda D, Rizzi R. 1991. Study of reproductive function in persons occupationally exposed to 2,4-dichlorophenoxyacetic acid (2,4-D). *Mutation Research* 262(1):47–50.

Lind PM, Eriksen EF, Sahlin L, Edlund M, Örberg J. 1999. Effects of the antiestrogenic environmental pollutant 3,3′,4,4′,5-pentachlorobiphenyl (PCB 126) in rat bone and uterus: Diverging effects in ovariectomized and intact animals. *Toxicology and Applied Pharmacology* 154(3):236–244.

Lind PM, Larsson S, Oxlund H, Hakansson H, Nyberg K, Eklund T, Örberg J. 2000a. Change in bone tissue composition and impaired bone strength in rats exposed to 3,3′,4,4′,5-pentachlorobiphenyl (PCB 126). *Toxicology* 150:41–51.

Lind PM, Örberg J, Edlund U-B, Sjöblom L, Lind L. 2000b. Bone tissue composition, dimensions and strength in rats an increased dietary level of vitamin A or exposed to 3,3′,4,4′,5-pentachlorobiphenyl (PCB 126) alone or in combination with vitamin C. *Toxicology* 151:11–23.

Loffredo CA, Silbergeld EK, Ferencz C, Zhang J. 2001. Association of transposition of the great arteries in infants with maternal exposures to herbicides and rodenticides. *American Journal of Epidemiology* 153(6):529–536.

Lorber M, Phillips L. 2002. Infant exposure to dioxin-like compounds in breast milk. *Environmental Health Perspectives* 110(6):A325–A332.

Lucifero D, Mann MR, Bartolomei MS, Trasler JM. 2004. Gene-specific timing and epigenetic memory in oocyte imprinting. *Human Molecular Genetics* 13:839–849.

Mably TA, Moore RW, Goy RW, Peterson RE. 1992. In utero and lactational exposure of male rats to 2,3,7,8-tetrachlorodibenzo-*p*-dioxin. 2. Effects on sexual behavior and the regulation of luteinizing hormone secretion in adulthood. *Toxicology and Applied Pharmacology* 114:108–117.

Mastroiacovo P, Spagnolo A, Marni E, Meazza L, Betrollini R, Segni G, Brogna-Pignatti C. 1988. Birth deffects in Seveso area after TCDD contamination. *Journal of American Medical Association* 259:1668–1672 (published erratum appears in *JAMA* 1988, 260:792).

Mayani A, Barel S, Soback S, Almagor M. 1997. Dioxin concentrations in women with endometriosis. *Human Reproduction* 12(2):373–375.

Mehta V, Peterson RE, Heideman W. 2008. 2,3,7,8-Tetrachlorodibenzo-*p*-dioxin exposure prevents cardiac valve formation in developing zebrafish. *Toxicological Sciences* 104(2):303–311.

Meinert R, Schüz J, Kaletsch U, Kaatsch P, Michaelis J. 2000. Leukemia and non-Hodgkin's lymphoma in childhood and exposure to pesticides: Results of a register-based case–control study in Germany. *American Journal of Epidemiology* 151(7):639–646.

Meyer KJ, Reif JS, Veeramachaneni DN, Luben TJ, Mosley BS, Nuckols JR. 2006. Agricultural pesticide use and hypospadias in eastern Arkansas. *Environmental Health Perspectives* 114(10): 1589–1595.

Michalek JE, Albanese RA, Wolfe WH. 1998a. *Project Ranch Hand II: An Epidemiologic Investigation of Health Effects in Air Force Personnel Following Exposure to Herbicides—Reproductive Outcome Update.* US Department of Commerce, National Technical Information Service. Report number AFRL-HE-BR-TR-1998-0073.

Michalek JE, Rahe AJ, Boyle CA. 1998b. Paternal dioxin, preterm birth, intrauterine growth retardation, and infant death. *Epidemiology* 9(2):161–167.

Miettinen HM, Pulkkinen P, Jamsa T, Koistinen J, Simanainen U, Tuomisto J, Tuukkanen J, Viluksela M. 2005. Effects of in utero and lactational TCDD exposure on bone development in differentially sensitive rat lines. *Toxicological Sciences* 85(2):1003–1012.

Miettinen HM, Sorvari R, Alaluusua S, Murtomaa M, Tuukkanen J, Viluksela M. 2006. The effect of perinatal TCDD exposure on caries susceptibility in rats. *Toxicological Sciences* 91(2): 568–575.

Mitsui T, Sugiyama N, Maeda S, Tohyama C, Arita J. 2006. Perinatal exposure to 2,3,7,8-tetrachlorodibenzo-*p*-dioxin suppresses contextual fear conditioning-accompanied activation of cyclic AMP response element-binding protein in the hippocampal CA1 region of male rats. *Neuroscience Letters* 398(3):206–210.

Mocarelli P, Brambilla P, Gerthoux PM, Patterson DG Jr, Needham LL. 1996. Change in sex ratio with exposure to dioxin. *Lancet* 348(9024):409.

Mocarelli P, Gerthoux PM, Ferrari E, Patterson DG Jr, Kieszak SM, Brambilla P, Vincoli N, Signorini S, Tramacere P, Carreri V, Sampson EJ, Turner WE, Needham LL. 2000. Paternal concentrations of dioxin and sex ratio of offspring. *The Lancet* 355:1858–1863.

Mocarelli P, Gerthoux PM, Patterson DG Jr, Milani S, Limonta G, Bertona M, Signorini S, Tramacere P, Colombo L, Crespi C, Brambilla P, Sarto C, Carreri V, Sampson EJ, Turner WE, Needham LL. 2008. Dioxin exposure, from infancy through puberty, produces endocrine disruption and affects human semen quality. *Environmental Health Perspectives* 116(1):70–77.

Monge P, Wesseling C, Guardado J, Lundberg I, Ahlbom A, Cantor KP, Weiderpass E, Partanen T. 2007. Parental occupational exposure to pesticides and the risk of childhood leukemia in Costa Rica. *Scandinavian Journal of Work, Environment and Health* 33(4):293–303.

Morgan HD, Santos F, Green K, Dean W, Reik W. 2005. Epigenetic reprogramming in mammals. *Human Molecular Genetics* 14:R47–R58.

Moses M, Lilis R, Crow KD, Thornton J, Fischbein A, Anderson HA, Selikoff IJ. 1984. Health status of workers with past exposure to 2,3,7,8-tetrachlorodibenzo-*p*-dioxin in the manufacture of 2,4,5-trichlorophenoxyacetic acid: Comparison of findings with and without chloracne. *American Journal of Industrial Medicine* 5(3):161–182.

Moshammer H, Neuberger M. 2000. Sex ratio in the children of the Austrian chloracne cohort. *The Lancet* 356:1271.

Nagasaka T, Koi M, Kloor M, Gebert J, Vilkin A, Nishida N, Shin SK, Sasamoto H, Tanaka N, Matsubara N, Boland CR, Goel A. 2008. Mutations in both KRAS and BRAF may contribute to the methylator phenotype in colon cancer. *Gastroenterology* 134:1950–1960.

Nakajima S, Saijo Y, Kato S, Sasaki S, Uno A, Kanagami N, Hirakawa H, Hori T, Tobiishi K, Todaka T, Nakamura Y, Yanagiya S, Sengoku Y, Iida T, Sata F, Kishi R. 2006. Effects of prenatal exposure to polychlorinated biphenyls and dioxins on mental and motor development in Japanese children at 6 months of age. *Environmental Health Perspectives* 114(5):773–778.

Nayyar T, Wu J, Hood DB. 2003. Downregulation of hippocampal NMDA receptor expression by prenatal exposure to dioxin. *Cellular and Molecular Biology* 49(8):1357–1362.

NCI (National Cancer Institute). 2001. *Surveillance, Epidemiology, and End Results (SEER) database.* http://seer.cancer.gov/ScientificSystems/CanQues (Accessed March 19).

Negishi T, Shimomura H, Koyama T, Kawasaki K, Ishii Y, Kyuwa S, Yasuda M, Kuroda Y, Yoshikawa Y. 2006. Gestational and lactational exposure to 2,3,7,8-tetrachlorodibenzo-*p*-dioxin affects social behaviors between developing rhesus monkeys (Macaca mulatta). *Toxicology Letters* 160(3):233–244.

NICHD (National Institute of Child Health and Human Development). 2007. *Endometriosis.* National Institute of Health. http://www.nichd.nih.gov/health/topics/endometriosis.cfm (Accessed December 17, 2008).

Nishijo M, Tawara K, Nakagawa H, Honda R, Kido T, Nishijo H, Saito S. 2008. 2,3,7,8-Tetrachlorodibenzo-*p*-dioxin in maternal breast milk and newborn head circumference. *Journal of Exposure Science and Environmental Epidemiology* 18(3):246–251.

Nishimura N, Matsumura F, Vogel CFA, Nishimura H, Yonemoto J, Yoshioka W, Tohyama C. 2008. Critical role of cyclooxygenase-2 activation in pathogenesis of hydronephrosis caused by lactational exposure of mice to dioxin. *Toxicology and Applied Pharmacology* 231(3):374–383.

Oh E, Lee E, Im H, Kang HS, Jung WW, Won NH, Kim EM, Sul D. 2005. Evaluation of immuno- and reproductive toxicities and association between immunotoxicological and genotoxicological parameters in waste incineration workers. *Toxicology* 210(1):65–80.

Ohsako S, Miyabara Y, Sakaue M, Ishimura R, Kakeyama M, Izumi H, Yonemoto J, Tohyama C. 2002. Developmental stage–specific effects of perinatal 2,3,7,8-tetrachlorodibenzo-*p*-dioxin exposure on reproductive organs of male rat offspring. *Toxicological Sciences* 66(2):283–292.

Ohtake F, Baba A, Fujii-Kuriyama Y, Kato S. 2008. Intrinsic AhR function underlies cross-talk of dioxins with sex hormone signalings. *Biochemical and Biophysical Research Communications* 370(4):541–546.

Oikawa K, Ohbayashi T, Mimura J, Fujii-Kuriyama Y, Teshima S, Rokutan K, Mukai K, Kuroda M. 2002. Dioxin stimulates synthesis and secretion of IgE-dependent histamine-releasing factor. *Biochemical and Biophysical Research Communications* 290(3):984–987.

Oikawa K, Kosugi Y, Ohbayashi T, Kameta A, Isaka K, Takayama M, Kuroda M, Mukai K. 2003. Increased expression of IgE-dependent histamine-releasing factor in endometriotic implants. *Journal of Pathology* 199(3):318–323.

Oikawa K, Yoshida K, Takanashi M, Tanabe H, Kiyuna T, Ogura M, Saito A, Umezawa A, Kuroda M. 2008. Dioxin interferes in chromosomal positioning through the aryl hydrocarbon receptor. *Biochemical and Biophysical Research Communications* 374(2):361–364.

Park JS, Hwang SY, Hwang BY, Han K. 2008. The spermatogenic effect of 50% ethanol extracts of Yacon and its ameliorative effect against 2,3,7,8-tetrachlorodibenzo-*p*-dioxin induced testicular toxicity in the rat. *Natural Product Sciences* 14(2):73–80.

Pauwels A, Schepens PJC, Hooghe TD, Delbeke L, Dhont M, Brouwer A, Weyler J. 2001. The risk of endometriosis and exposure to dioxins and polychlorinated biphenyls: A case–control study of infertile women. *Human Reproduction* 16(10):2050–2055.

Pearce MS, Parker L. 2000. Paternal employment in agriculture and childhood kidney cancer. *Pediatric Hematology and Oncology* 17(3):223–230.

Pearce MS, Hammal DM, Dorak MT, McNally RJ, Parker L. 2006. Paternal occupational expo-sure to pesticides or herbicides as risk factors for cancer in children and young adults: A case–control study from the North of England. *Archives of Environmental and Occupational Health* 61(3):138–144.

Peltier MR. 2003. Immunology of term and preterm labor. *Reproductive Biology and Endocrinology* 1:122–132.

Pesatori AC, Consonni D, Tironi A, Zocchetti C, Fini A, Bertazzi PA. 1993. Cancer in a young popula-tion in a dioxin-contaminated area. *International Journal of Epidemiology* 22(6):1010–1013.

Petrelli G, Figa-Talamanca I, Tropeano R, Tangucci M, Cini C, Aquilini S, Gasperini L, Meli P. 2000. Reproductive male-mediated risk: Spontaneous abortion among wives of pesticide applicators. *European Journal of Epidemiology* 16(4):391–393.

Polsky JY, Aronson KJ, Heaton JP, Adams MA. 2007. Pesticides and polychlorinated biphenyls as potential risk factors for erectile dysfunction. *Journal of Andrology* 28(1):28–37.

Porpora MG, Ingelido AM, di Domenico A, Ferro A, Crobu M, Pallante D, Cardelli M, Cosmi EV, De Felip E. 2006. Increased levels of polychlorobiphenyls in Italian women with endometriosis. *Chemosphere* 63(8):1361–1367.

Ray SS, Swanson HI. 2004. Dioxin-induced immortalization of normal human keratinocytes and silencing of p53 and p16INK4a. *Journal of Biological Chemistry* 279(26):27187–27193.

Reik W, Walter J. 2001. Genomic imprinting: Parental influence on the genome. *Nature Review Genetics* 2:21–32.

Reik W, Dean W, Walter J. 2001. Epigenetic reprogramming in mammalian development. *Science* 293:1089–1093.

Revich B, Aksel E, Ushakova T, Ivanova I, Zuchenko N, Lyuev N, Brodsky B, Sotsov Y. 2001. Dioxin exposure and public health in Chapaevsk, Russia. *Chemosphere* 43(4-7):951–966.

Reynolds P, Von Behren J, Gunier RB, Goldberg DE, Harnly M, Hertz A. 2005b. Agricultural pesti-cide use and childhood cancer in California. *Epidemiology* 16(1):93–100.

Rier SE, Martin DC, Bowman RE, Dmowski WP, Becker JL. 1993. Endometriosis in rhesus monkeys (Macaca mulatta) following chronic exposure to 2,3,7,8-tetrachlorodibenzo-*p*-dioxin. *Funda-mental and Applied Toxicology* 21(4):433–441.

Romo A, Carceller R, Tobajas J. 2009. Intrauterine growth retardation (IUGR): Epidemiology and etiology. *Pediatric Endocrinology Reviews* 6(Supplement 3):332–336.

Roundtree MR, Bachman KE, Herman JG, Baylin SB. 2001. DNA methylation, chromatin inheri-tance, and cancer. *Oncogene* 20:3156–3165.

Rudant J, Menegaux F, Leverger G, Baruchel A, Nelken B, Bertrand Y, Patte C, Pacquement H, Verite C, Robert A, Michel G, Margueritte G, Gandemer V, Hemon D, Clavel J. 2007. Household exposure to pesticides and risk of childhood hematopoietic malignancies: The ESCALE study (SFCE). *Environmental Health Perspectives* 115(12):1787–1793.

Ryan JJ, Amirova Z, Carrier G. 2002. Sex ratios of children of Russian pesticide producers exposed to dioxin. *Environmental Health Perspectives* 110(11):A699–A701.

Sagiv SK, Tolbert PE, Altshul LM, Korrick SA. 2007. Organochlorine exposures during pregnancy and infant size at birth. *Epidemiology* 18(1):120–129.

Savitz DA, Arbuckle A, Kaczor D, Curtis KM. 1997. Male pesticide exposure and pregnancy out-come. *American Journal of Epidemiology* 146(12):1025–1036.

Schnorr TM, Lawson CC, Whelan EA, Dankovic DA, Deddens JA, Piacitelli LA, Reefhuis J, Sweeney MH, Connally LB, Fingerhut MA. 2001. Spontaneous abortion, sex ratio, and paternal occupational exposure to 2,3,7,8-tetrachlorodibenzo-*p*-dioxin. *Environmental Health Perspec-tives* 109(11):1127–1132.

Schreinemachers DM. 2003. Birth malformations and other adverse perinatal outcomes in four US wheat-producing states. *Environmental Health Perspectives* 111(9):1259–1264.

Schultz R, Suominen J, Varre T, Hakovirta H, Parvinen M, Toppari J, Pelto-Huikko M. 2003. Expression of aryl hydrocarbon receptor and aryl hydrocarbon receptor nuclear translocator messenger ribonucleic acids and proteins in rat and human testis. *Endocrinology* 144(3):767–776.

Schwartz LS. 1998. *Health Problems of Women Veterans of the Vietnam War*. Doctoral dissertation, Yale University.

Shi Z, Valdez KE, Ting AY, Franczak A, Gum SL, Petroff BK. 2007. Ovarian endocrine disruption underlies premature reproductive senescence following environmentally relevant chronic exposure to the aryl hydrocarbon receptor agonist 2,3,7,8-tetrachlorodibenzo-*p*-dioxin. *Biology of Reproduction* 76(2):198–202.

Smith AH, Fisher DO, Pearce N, Chapman CJ. 1982. Congenital defects and miscarriages among New Zealand 2,4,5-T sprayers. *Archives of Environmental Health* 37:197–200.

Staessen JA, Nawrot T, Hond ED, Thijs L, Fagard R, Hoppenbrouwers K, Koppen G, Nelen V, Schoeters G, Vanderschueren D, Van Hecke E, Verschaeve L, Vlietinck R, Roels HA. 2001. Renal function, cytogenetic measurements, and sexual development in adolescents in relation to environmental pollutants: A feasibility study of biomarkers. *Lancet* 357(9269):1660–1669. [Comment in *Lancet* 2001. 358(9295):1816–1817.]

Stellman SD, Stellman JM, Sommer JF Jr. 1988. Health and reproductive outcomes among American Legionnaires in relation to combat and herbicide exposure in Vietnam. *Environmental Research* 47:150–174.

Stockbauer JW, Hoffman RE, Schramm WF, Edmonds LD. 1988. Reproductive outcomes of mothers with potential exposure to 2,3,7,8-tetrachlorodibenzo-*p*-dioxin. *American Journal of Epidemiology* 128:410–419.

Suskind RR, Hertzberg VS. 1984. Human health effects of 2,4,5-T and its toxic contaminants. *Journal of the American Medical Association* 251:2372–2380.

Suzuki G, Nakano M, Nakano S. 2005. Distribution of PCDDs/PCDFs and Co-PCBs in human maternal blood, cord blood, placenta, milk, and adipose tissue: Dioxins showing high toxic equivalency factor accumulate in the placenta. *Bioscience, Biotechnology and Biochemistry* 69(10):1836–1847.

Swan SH, Kruse RL, Liu F, Barr DB, Drobnis EZ, Redmon JB, Wang C, Brazil C, Overstreet JW; Study for Future Families Research Group. 2003. Semen quality in relation to biomarkers of pesticide exposure. *Environmental Health Perspectives* 111(12):1478–1484.

Tango T, Fujita T, Tanihata T, Minowa M, Doi Y, Kato N, Kunikane S, Uchiyama I, Tanaka M, Uehata T. 2004. Risk of adverse reproductive outcomes associated with proximity to municipal solid waste incinerators with high dioxin emission levels in Japan. *Journal of Epidemiology* 14(3):83–93.

Tas S, Lauwerys R, Lison D. 1996. Occupational hazards for the male reproductive system. *Critical Reviews in Toxicology* 26(3):261–307.

Teilmann G, Juul A, Skakkebaek NE, Toppari J. 2002. Putative effects of endocrine disrupters on pubertal development in the human. *Best Practice and Research Clinical Endocrinology and Metabolism* 16(1):105–121.

ten Tusscher GW, Stam GA, Koppe JG. 2000. Open chemical combustions resulting in a local increased incidence of orofacial clefts. *Chemosphere* 40(9-11):1263–1270.

Toft G, Long M, Kruger T, Hjelmborg PS, Bonde JP, Rignell-Hydbom A, Tyrkiel E, Hagmar L, Giwercman A, Spano M, Bizzaro D, Pedersen HS, Lesovoy V, Ludwicki JK, Bonefeld-Jorgensen EC. 2007. Semen quality in relation to xenohormone and dioxin-like serum activity among Inuits and three European populations. *Environmental Health Perspectives* 115 (Supplement 1):15–20.

Townsend JC, Bodner KM, Van Peenen PFD, Olson RD, Cook RR. 1982. Survey of reproductive events of wives of employees exposed to chlorinated dioxins. *American Journal of Epidemiology* 115:695–713.

Tsuchiya M, Tsukino H, Iwasaki M, Sasaki H, Tanaka T, Katoh T, Patterson DG Jr, Turner W, Needham L, Tsugane S. 2007. Interaction between cytochrome P450 gene polymorphisms and serum organochlorine TEQ levels in the risk of endometriosis. *Molecular Human Reproduction* 13(6):399–404.

Tsukimori K, Tokunaga S, Shibata S, Uchi H, Nakayama D, Ishimaru T, Nakano H, Wake N, Yoshimura T, Furue M. 2008. Long-term effects of polychlorinated biphenyls and dioxins on pregnancy outcomes in women affected by the Yusho incident. *Environmental Health Perspectives* 116(5):626–630.

Tuyet LTN, Johansson A. 2001. Impact of chemical warfare with Agent Orange on women's reproductive lives in Vietnam: A pilot study. *Reproductive Health Matters* 9(18):156–164.

Van den Berg M, Birnbaum L, Bosveld AT, Brunstrom B, Cook P, Feeley M, Giesy JP, Hanberg A, Hasegawa R, Kennedy SW, et al. 1998. Toxic equivalency factors (TEFs) for PCBs, PCDDs, PCDFs for humans and wildlife. *Environmental Health Perspectives* 106:775–792.

Vreugdenhil H, Weisglas-Kuperus N. 2000. Effects of environmental exposure to polychlorinated biphenyls and dioxins on cognitive development in young children. *NeuroToxicology* 21(4):620.

Vreugdenhil HJI, Slijper FME, Mulder PGH, Weisglas-Duperus N. 2002. Effects of perinatal exposure to PCBs and dioxins on play behavior in Dutch children at school age. *Environmental Health Perspectives* 110(10):A593–A598.

Vreugdenhil HJ, Mulder PG, Emmen HH, Weisglas-Kuperus N. 2004. Effects of perinatal exposure to PCBs on neuropsychological functions in the Rotterdam cohort at 9 years of age. *Neuropsychology* 18(1):185–193.

Wang S-L, Chang Y-C, Chao H-R, Li C-M, Li L-A, Lin L-Y, Papke O. 2006. Body burdens of polychlorinated dibenzo-*p*-dioxins, dibenzofurans, and biphenyls and their relations to estrogen metabolism in pregnant women. *Environmental Health Perspectives* 114(5):740–745.

Warner M, Samuels S, Mocarelli P, Gerthoux PM, Needham L, Patterson DG Jr, Eskenazi B. 2004. Serum dioxin concentrations and age at menarche. *Environmental Health Perspectives* 112(13):1289–1292.

Warner M, Eskenazi B, Olive DL, Samuels S, Quick-Miles S, Vercellini P, Gerthoux PM, Needham L, Patterson DG Jr, Mocarelli P. 2007. Serum dioxin concentrations and quality of ovarian function in women of Seveso. *Environmental Health Perspectives* 115(3):336–340.

Wen WQ, Shu XO, Steinbuch M, Severson RK, Reaman GH, Buckley JD, Robison LL. 2000. Paternal military service and risk for childhood leukemia in offspring. *American Journal of Epidemiology* 151(3):231–240.

Weselak M, Arbuckle TE, Wigle DT, Walker MC, Krewski D. 2008. Pre-and post-conception pesticide exposure and the risk of birth defects in an Ontario farm population. *Reproductive Toxicology* 25(4):472–480.

Wikiera B, Basiak A, Barg E, Noczynska A. 2007. Precocious thelarche—Current opinions. *Advances in Clinical and Experimental Medicine* 16(2):329–334.

Wilcox AJ, Weinberg CR, O'Connor JF, Baird DD, Schlatterer JP, Canfield RE, Armstrong EG, Nisula BC. 1988. Incidence of early pregnancy loss. *New England Journal of Medicine* 319: 189–194.

Wolfe WH, Michalek JE, Miner JC, Rahe AJ, Moore CA, Needham LL, Patterson DG Jr. 1995. Paternal serum dioxin and reproductive outcomes among veterans of Operation Ranch Hand. *Epidemiology* 6:17–22.

Wu Q, Ohsako S, Ishimura R, Suzuki JS, Tohyama C. 2004. Exposure of mouse preimplantation embryos to 2,3,7,8-tetrachlorodibenzo-*p*-dioxin (TCDD) alters the methylation status of imprinted genes H19 and Igf2. *Biological Reproduction* 70(6):1790–1797.

Yamada T, Fujiwara K, Mishima K, Imura H, Sugahara T. 2007. Effects of 2,3,7,8-tetrachlorodibenzo-*p*-dioxin on the development of murine palate in organ culture. *Asian Journal of Oral and Maxillofacial Surgery* 19(4):185–189.

Yamano Y, Ohyama K, Ohta M, Sano T, Ritani A, Shimada J, Ashida N, Yoshida E, Ikehara K, Morishima I. 2005. A novel spermatogenesis related factor-2 (SRF-2) gene expression affected by TCDD treatment. *Endocrine Journal* 52(1):75–81.

Yamauchi M, Kim EY, Iwata H, Shima Y, Tanabe S. 2006. Toxic effects of 2,3,7,8-tetrachlorodibenzo-*p*-dioxin (TCDD) in developing red seabream (Pagrus major) embryo: An association of morphological deformities with AHR1, AHR2 and CYP1A expressions. *Aquatic Toxicology* 80(2): 166–179.

Yamazaki Y, Mann MR, Lee SS, Marh J, McCarrey JR, Yanagimachi R, Bartolomei MS. 2003. Reprogramming of primordial germ cells begins before migration into the genital ridge, making these cells inadequate donors for reproductive cloning. *Proceedings of the National Academy of Sciences of the United States of America* 100:12207–12212.

Yang JZ, Agarwal SK, Foster WG. 2000. Subchronic exposure to 2,3,7,8-tetrachlorodibenzo-*p*-dioxin modulates the pathophysiology of endometriosis in the cynomolgus monkey. *Toxicological Sciences* 56:374–381.

Yasuda I, Yasuda M, Sumida H, Tsusaki H, Arima A, Ihara T, Kubota S, Asaoka K, Tsuga K, Akagawa Y. 2005. In utero and lactational exposure to 2,3,7,8-tetrachlorodibenzo-*p*-dioxin (TCDD) affects tooth development in rhesus monkeys. *Reproductive Toxicology* 20(1):21–30.

Ye L, Leung LK. 2008. Effect of dioxin exposure on aromatase expression in ovariectomized rats. *Toxicology and Applied Pharmacology* 229(1):102–108.

Yen SC, Jaffe RB. 1991. *Reproductive Endocrinology*. Philadelphia: W.B. Saunders Company.

Yoshimura T, Kaneko S, Hayabuchi H. 2001. Sex ratio in offspring of those affected by dioxin and dioxin-like compounds: The Yusho, Seveso, and Yucheng incidents. *Occupational and Environmental Medicine* 58(8):540–541.

Yu J, Wang Y, Zhou W-H, Wang L, He Y-Y, Li D-J. 2008. Combination of estrogen and dioxin is involved in the pathogenesis of endometriosis by promoting chemokine secretion and invasion of endometrial stromal cells. *Human Reproduction* 23(7):1614–1626.

Zhao D, Lebovic DI, Taylor RN. 2002. Long-term progestin treatment inhibits RANTES (regulated on activation, normal T cell expressed and secreted) gene expression in human endometrial stromal cells. *Journal of Clinical Endocrinology and Metabolism* 87(6):2514–2519.

8

Neurologic Disorders

The nervous system is a complex organ system that allows human beings to interact with both the internal environment and the external environment. For convenience, we divide the nervous system into the central nervous system (CNS) and the peripheral nervous system (PNS). The CNS comprises the brain and spinal cord, and the PNS includes sensory and motor nerves that enter or leave the spinal cord and are responsible for our ability to sense the outside world and to move within it, and autonomic nerve fibers, which sense internal events such as changes in blood pressure or temperature, and which act to control these and other aspects of our internal environment. Neurologic disorders due to toxicant exposure may result in either immediate or delayed dysfunction of any component of the nervous system; immediate effects of toxicants may involve all aspects of the nervous system, whereas delayed effects are likely to produce more focal problems.

Diffuse damage to the CNS may cause alterations in thinking, consciousness, or attention, often combined with abnormalities in movement. Focal dysfunction can cause myriad syndromes, depending on which area is damaged. Although neurologic disorders can cause problems with thinking and emotional dysregulation, it is important to distinguish them from psychiatric conditions—such as posttraumatic stress disorder, depression, and anxiety—and from systemic conditions of uncertain cause, such as chronic fatigue syndrome. In this chapter, we will consider possible diffuse CNS effects of toxic exposure and specific clinical conditions that result from focal dysfunction. Examples of diseases that result from degeneration of specific brain areas are Parkinson's disease (PD), Alzheimer's disease (AD), spinocerebellar degeneration, and amyotrophic lateral sclerosis (ALS). All those diseases occur in the absence of any toxicant exposure; but all may be triggered by aspects of the environment, including toxicant exposure.

Disorders of the PNS are generally referred to as neuropathies. Neuropathies may be purely motor and affect only movement or purely sensory; most often, both motor and sensory fibers are affected. Neuropathies usually are symmetric and start with symptoms related to dysfunction of fibers that travel the greatest distance to their target organ. For that reason, symptoms of neuropathy generally start in the digits and travel toward the torso. Most neuropathies also affect autonomic fibers and thus can result in changes in blood pressure and heart rate and in symptoms related to the control of digestion.

Neurologic disorders related to toxicant exposure may be acute or delayed and may produce temporary or long-lasting problems. Timing is important in assessing the effects of chemical exposure on neurologic function and must be considered in the design and critique of epidemiologic studies. In the original *Veterans and Agent Orange* report, hereafter referred to as *VAO* (IOM, 1994), attention was deliberately focused on persistent neurobehavioral disorders. That focus was maintained in *Update 1996* (IOM, 1996), *Update 1998* (IOM, 1999), *Update 2000* (IOM, 2001), and *Update 2002* (IOM, 2003). A slight change in emphasis toward chronic neurodegenerative disorders was reflected in the change in the name of this chapter to "Neurologic Disorders" in *Update 2004* (IOM, 2005), which was carried forward in *Update 2006* (IOM, 2007). This present report reviews data pertinent to persistent neurologic disorders of all types.

Case identification in neurologic disorders is often difficult because there are few disorders for which there are specific diagnostic tests. Many disorders involve cellular or molecular biochemical effects, so even the most advanced imaging techniques can miss an abnormality. Because the nervous system is not readily accessible for biopsy, pathologic confirmation usually is not feasible. However, identifiable neurologic disorders always result in objective abnormalities that are reflected in anatomic or functional tests or discovered via clinical examination.

Many studies have addressed the possible contribution of various chemical exposures to neurologic disorders, but the committee's focus is on the health effects of a particular set of chemicals: four herbicides—2,4-dichlorophenoxyacetic acid (2,4-D), 2,4,5-trichlorophenoxyacetic acid (2,4,5-T), picloram (4-amino-3,5,6-trichloropicolinic acid), and cacodylic acid (dimethyl arsenic acid or [DMA])—and a contaminant of 2,4,5-T, 2,3,7,8-tetrachlorodibenzo-*p*-dioxin (TCDD). Thus, the specificity of exposure assessment is an important consideration in weighing evidence relevant to the committee's charge.

This chapter reviews the association between exposure to the chemicals of interest and neurobehavioral disorders, neurodegenerative disorders, and peripheral neuropathy. The scientific evidence supporting biologic plausibility is also reviewed here. More complete discussions of the categories of association and of this committee's approach to categorizing health outcomes are presented in

Chapters 1 and 2. For citations new to this update that revisit previously studied populations, design information can be found in Chapter 5.

NEUROBEHAVIORAL (COGNITIVE OR NEUROPSYCHIATRIC) DISORDERS

This section summarizes the findings of *VAO* and previous updates on neurobehavioral disorders and incorporates information published in the last 2 years into the evidence database.

Conclusions from *VAO* and Previous Updates

On the basis of the data available at the time, the committee responsible for *VAO*, *Update 1996*, *Update 1998*, *Update 2000*, *Update 2002*, *Update 2004*, and *Update 2006* concluded that there was inadequate or insufficient evidence to determine the existence of an association between exposure to the chemicals of interest and neurobehavioral disorders. Many of the data that informed that conclusion came from the Air Force Health Study (AFHS, 1991, 1995, 2000; Barrett et al., 2001, 2003). *VAO* and the updates offer more complete discussions of the results. The AFHS studies (AFHS, 1991, 1995) reviewed in *VAO* revealed no association between serum TCDD concentration and reported sleep disturbance or variables on the Symptom Checklist-90-Revised (SCL-90); in contrast, serum TCDD was significantly associated with responses on some scales of the Millon Clinical Multiaxial Inventory. Observations on 55 highly exposed Czech 2,4,5-T production workers (Pazderova-Vejlupkova et al., 1981) were found to suffer from methodologic problems.

Update 1996 reviewed two not particularly informative studies of Vietnam veterans (Decoufle et al., 1992; Visintainer et al., 1995) and a study of highly exposed German workers (Zober et al., 1994), which found a relationship between "mental disorders" and severity of chloracne, but not with blood TCDD concentrations. *Update 1998* considered a report on mental health problems in Australian Vietnam veterans, but not in the context of herbicide exposure (O'Toole et al., 1996).

In *Update 2000*, results from the AFHS (AFHS, 2000) indicated that although the frequency of several self-reported neuropsychiatric symptoms differed between exposure groups, the associations were not significant after adjustment for covariates. In addition, a repeat psychologic assessment with the SCL-90 in conjunction with self-reported psychologic disorders verified through medical-record review showed that among five diagnostic categories (psychosis, alcohol dependence, drug dependence, anxiety, and other neurosis), a dose–response pattern with serum TCDD concentration was found only for "other neuroses" in the enlisted ground crew. When the entire cohort was evaluated, there were no significant associations between serum TCDD and various psychologic diagnoses.

Update 2002 reviewed three studies. Neuropsychologic tests of cognitive functioning indicated significant group differences on some scales in the AFHS cohort during the 1982 examination, but the findings did not support a dose–response relationship with serum TCDD: poorer performance was seen in groups with background or low exposure, and the lower performance on only one memory test for one subgroup of subjects suggested a chance finding (Barrett et al., 2001). Gauthier et al. (2001) did not find a relationship between AD and exposure to herbicides and insecticides. The results of Pelclová et al. (2001) on a Czech 2,4,5-T-production cohort were not given much credence.

Update 2004 reviewed five new studies. Among them was a report on the AFHS cohort (Barrett et al., 2003) in which the authors concluded that there were "few consistent differences in psychological functioning" between groups categorized by serum-dioxin concentrations. Kim et al. (2003) described increased prevalence of posttraumatic stress disorder in Korean military who served in Vietnam, but there was no association with estimated exposure to Agent Orange. The remaining three studies (Baldi et al., 2003; Dahlgren et al., 2003; Pelclová et al., 2002) were found to be uninformative because of methodologic limitations.

Update 2006 considered two new studies of limited relevance. Park et al. (2005) analyzed cause of death as a function of subjects' "usual occupation" on 2.8 million death certificates, but the significantly increased odds ratio (OR) for presenile dementia and "pest control" was not sufficiently specific for the toxicants of interest. The increase in mortality from "mental disorders" reported in Australian Vietnam veterans (ADVA, 2005c) was based on such a broad diagnostic category that it was impossible to conclude whether subjects who were investigated had neurologic symptoms or signs.

Prior committees have maintained the conclusion that there has been inadequate or insufficient evidence of an association between exposure to the chemicals of interest and neurobehavioral disorders (cognitive or neuropsychiatric).

Update of the Epidemiologic Literature

No Vietnam-veteran or environmental studies concerning exposure to the chemicals of interest and neurobehavioral conditions have been published since *Update 2006*.

Occupational Studies

Since *Update 2006*, few studies relevant to the chemicals of interest and neurobehavioral disorders have been published. Kamel et al. (2007a) evaluated subjects participating in the Agricultural Health Study (AHS) and questionnaire responses from more than 18,000 subjects who listed a variety of neurologic symptoms, including memory and concentration. There was clear evidence of a dose-dependent relationship between pesticide use and neurologic symptoms but no increase in symptoms from herbicide exposure. Symptoms were considered as a group, so there was no evaluation of behavioral symptoms separated from the other neurologic complaints.

Solomon et al. (2007) received responses (43%) to a mailed questionnaire dealing with pesticide exposure and a variety of neurologic symptoms including neuropsychiatric ones from 9,844 men born in 1933–1977 identified in the 1991 census of three rural areas of England and Wales. There was an increased incidence of symptoms reported by those with the highest frequency of exposure to a variety of pesticides; neuropsychiatric symptoms clustered with other neurologic symptoms and correlated strongly with a tendency toward somatization as assessed with a separate instrument. The authors concluded that there was a relationship between pesticide use and symptoms but considered psychologic factors, as opposed to a toxic effect, to be a likely cause. Those who had reported herbicide use constituted 40% of the subjects in the "other pesticides" category and about 80% of those who had used sheep dip and those who had used insecticides; comparisons of these three groups did not show clear differences. In any case, there was no separate evaluation of herbicide use in general or specifically of the chemicals of interest in this volume.

In contrast with the large cohort studies described above, Urban et al. (2007) were able to gather follow-up information on 15 of the subjects who had became acutely ill after chronic exposure to TCDD in 1965–1968 at the Czech chemical plant, considered previously in methodologically limited studies (Pazderova-Vejlupkova et al., 1981; Pelclova et al., 2001, 2002). When examined in 2004, the mean plasma TCDD concentration was 128 ppt. The majority had abnormalities on neuropsychologic testing or single-photon emission computed tomography (SPECT) imaging. This study supports the idea that exposure to large amounts of TCDD over a period of years can produce neurologic abnormalities shortly after or during exposure that can continue for more than 30 years. However, it is not clear how the 15 subjects in this report were contacted or the extent to which this small sample was biased toward increased symptoms, and there was no comparison group. SPECT scans are nonspecific studies, and many other environmental or age-related factors could have affected the results.

Biologic Plausibility

Some animal studies have suggested possible involvement of the chemicals of interest in the occurrence of neurobehavioral effects For example, Mitsui et al. (2006) reported that hippocampus-dependent learning could be impaired in male rats exposed in utero to TCDD and the impairment could have affected fear conditioning. Lensu et al. (2006) examined areas in the hypothalamus for possible involvement in TCDD effects on food consumption, potentially related to wasting syndrome, and suggested that their results were not consistent with a primary role of the hypothalamus. Studies in rodents have also detected molecular effects in cerebellar granule cells or neuroblasts, which are involved in cognitive and motor processes (Kim and Yang, 2005; Williamson et al., 2005). Sturtz et al. (2008) found that 2,4-D affected rat maternal behavior. The specific relevance of those studies and studies cited in earlier updates to neurobehavioral effects is unclear. A general summary of the biologic plausibility of neurologic effects of exposure to the herbicides used in Vietnam is presented at the end of this chapter.

Synthesis

There is not consistent epidemiologic evidence of an association between Agent Orange exposure and neurobehavioral disorders (cognitive or neuropsychiatric).

Conclusion

On the basis of the evidence reviewed here and in previous VAO reports, the committee concludes that there is still inadequate or insufficient evidence to determine the existence of an association between exposure to the chemicals of interest and neurobehavioral disorders (cognitive or neuropsychiatric).

NEURODEGENERATIVE DISEASES

This section summarizes the findings of previous *VAO* reports on neurodegenerative diseases—specifically PD and ALS—and incorporates information published in the last two years into the evidence database.

Parkinson's Disease and Parkinsonism

PD is a progressive neurodegenerative disorder that affects millions of people worldwide. Its primary clinical manifestations are bradykinesia, resting tremor, cogwheel rigidity, and gait instability. Those signs were first described in 1817 as a single entity by James Parkinson. In recent years, many nonmotor manifestations of PD have been described, and in some cases they can be the presenting symptoms of the disease. These include cognitive dysfunction often progressing to frank dementia, sleep disturbances, hallucinations, psychosis, mood disorders, fatigue, and autonomic dysfunction (Langston, 2006).

In the nearly 2 centuries since the initial description, much has been learned regarding genetic predisposition and the pathophysiology of the disease. However, the etiology of PD in most patients is unknown, and specific environmental risk factors remain largely unproved. The diagnosis of PD is based primarily on clinical examination; in recent years, however, magnetic resonance imaging and functional brain imaging have been increasingly useful. PD must be distinguished from a variety of parkinsonian syndromes, including drug-induced parkinsonism and neurodegenerative diseases, such as multiple systems atrophy, which have parkinsonian features combined with other abnormalities. Ultimately, a diagnosis of PD can be confirmed with postmortem pathologic examination of brain tissue for the characteristic loss of neurons from the substantia nigra and telltale Lewy body intracellular inclusions. Pathologic findings in other causes of parkinsonism show different patterns of brain injury.

Estimates of population-based incidence of PD range from 2 to 22 per 100,000 person-years, and estimates of prevalence range from 18 to 182 per 100,000 person-years. It affects about 1% of all persons over 60 years old, and up to 5 million people worldwide. That makes PD the second-most common neurodegenerative disease (after AD). Age is a risk factor for PD, with peak incidence and prevalence consistently found in people 60–80 years old. A consensus statement from a 2007 meeting of PD experts (Bronstein et al., 2009) concluded that, in addition to firm evidence that the toxicant 1-methyl-4-phenyl-1,2,4,6-tetrahydropyridine (MPTP) can induce PD, there is substantial evidence that men are at greater risk and that smoking and coffee consumption are associated with reduced risk.

Heredity has long been suspected of being an important risk factor for PD; as many as 25% of all PD patients have at least one first-degree relative who has PD. At least 13 gene mutations have been identified in autosomal dominant PD, including mutations in parkin and α-synuclein (Klein and Lohmann-Hedrich, 2007). Mutations associated with an autosomal recessive inheritance pattern have also been described. Complex genetics may be found to account for an increasing number of PD cases in coming years, but environmental risk factors clearly are also important.

Conclusions from *VAO* and Previous Updates

On the basis of growing concerns about a possible link between PD and pesticide exposures, the original *VAO* committee suggested that attention be paid to the pattern of new cases in Vietnam veterans as they enter the decades when PD is most prevalent to determine whether there is evidence of an association between PD and exposure to the chemicals of interest. That recommendation has been echoed in each update; however, no study has systematically evaluated current or changing prevalence in the Vietnam-veteran population. Thus, all previous updates have reviewed epidemiologic studies from other populations potentially exposed to the chemicals of interest. Previously reviewed studies were found to be inconclusive because levels of exposure were not systematically evaluated and sufficiently specific exposures were not defined. Many studies have evaluated the risks posed by pesticides in general; although a relationship to risk of PD has often been found, dose dependence was either not investigated or not present if investigated.

For this update, we selectively re-reviewed all epidemiologic studies that specifically assessed herbicide exposures (none had evaluated exposures to the specific herbicides of interest in the VAO series) and reviewed in detail the studies published since *Update 2006*. The results are presented in Table 8-1. To gain a better insight into what specific exposures may underlie the many reports of association with pesticide exposure in general that have dominated the epidemiologic results for PD, estimated risks posed by other classes of pesticides are presented for comparison with those for herbicides. To provide perspective on the new results for phenoxy herbicides, findings on other specific herbicides are presented, particularly for paraquat, which has been a target of study because of its similarity in chemical structure to a drug contaminant found to induce a parkinsonian syndrome (see the discussion of MPTP below in the section "Biologic Plausibility").

Stern et al. (1991) performed a case–control study of 69 cases that developed symptoms before the age of 40 years (early onset) and 80 cases whose symptoms began after the age of 60 years (late onset). Herbicide exposure (classified as "any" or "none") was not more prevalent in either early-onset or late-onset cases. However, this study is limited in that the design specifically eliminated cases in the age ranges in which PD is most often diagnosed. In contrast, Semchuk et al. (1992) used a conditional logistic regression model to assess risk in 130 PD subjects in Canada; a statistically significant crude OR of 3.06 (95% confidence interval [CI], 1.34–7.00) was found for herbicide exposure; seven of the 17 cases reporting herbicide use were able to specify the particular product—one reported paraquat use, and the rest reported exclusive use of chlorophenoxy and thiocarbamate compounds. Butterfield et al. (1993), in another case–control study, also found a significant association between herbicide exposure and PD (OR = 3.22; p = 0.033). In a larger population-based case–control study, Gorell et al. (1998) found a significant association between PD and herbicide exposure, which increased after controlling for other confounding factors (OR = 4.10, p < 0.012). PD and control subjects were equally likely to report residential herbicide exposure, which presumably occurs at a lower level than occupational exposure, whereas risk of PD was increased in subjects who reported 10 years or more of occupational herbicide exposure (OR = 5.81, 95% CI 1.99–16.97). In contrast, Taylor et al. (1999) performed a case–control study of 140 cases at Boston City Hospital that showed no association between herbicide use and PD (OR = 1.1, 95% CI 0.7–1.7); this was probably a primarily urban sample, and there is no mention of how many cases or controls reported herbicide use. In addition, controls were identified by PD subjects and contacted by the subjects themselves—an unconventional way of accruing control subjects that may be subject to unknown bias.

Taken as a group, those studies suggest that there is a relationship between herbicide exposure and risk of PD. Evidence defined simply as herbicide exposure, however, lacks the level of exposure specificity the committee requires for contributing fully relevant evidence toward a finding of association. All the studies used case–control methods and thus depended on the rigor of matching between cases and controls. Most of the studies did not record specific herbicide

TABLE 8-1 Epidemiologic Studies of Herbicide[a] Exposure and Parkinson's Disease

Reference and Country	Cases in Study Group	Comparison Group	Exposure Assessment	Exposure(s)[a]	n	OR (95 % CI)	Diagnosis of Neurologic Dysfunction
Brighina et al., 2008; US (Mayo Clinic)	833 PD sequential cases from clinic; median age = 67.7 yr, 208 cases ≤ 59.8 yr	472 unaffected siblings and 361 unrelated controls	Self-report down to specific herbicides; 2,4-D said to most prevalent in cases, but published analysis not that detailed	For *youngest quartile* at diagnosis: Pesticides (ever): Herbicides (ever): Phenoxy herbicides Insecticides (ever): Fungicides (ever):	87	1.8 (1.1–2.9) 2.5 (1.3–4.5) 1.5 (1.0–2.2) 1.0 (0.6–1.7) 1.0 (0.3–3.2)	PD diagnosed by movement disorder specialist
Hancock et al., 2008; US (Duke)	319 cases	296 unaffected relatives and others	All comparisons referent to those who never applied any pesticide	Pesticide application: Insecticides: Botanical: Organophosphate: Herbicides: Chlorophenoxy: Phosphonoglycine: Triazine:	200 7 53 15 57 5	1.6 (1.1–2.3) 1.8 (1.2–2.8) 5.9 (0.6–56) 1.9 (1.1–3.6) 1.6 (1.0–2.5) 2.1 (0.7–6.2) 1.5 (0.9–2.5) 1.1 (0.3–3.6)	
Kamel et al., 2007b; US (Agricultural Health Study) [supersedes Kamel et al., 2005]	83 prevalent cases at enrollment; 78 incident cases during follow-up among private applicators and spouses	79,557 without PD at enrollment; 55,931 without PD followed up	Self-report of individual herbicides (2,4-D; 2,4,5-T; 2,4,5-TP) on detailed self-administered questionnaires at enrollment or telephone interview for follow-up	For incident cases: 2,4-D: 2,4,5-T: 2,4,5-TP: Dicamba: Paraquat: Trifuralin: Cyanazine: For prevalent cases: 2,4-D: 2,4,5-T: 2,4,5-TP:	49 24 7 32 11 32 26 47 16 4	1.0 (0.5–2.1) 1.8 (1.0–3.3) 0.9 (0.4–1.8) 1.5 (0.8–2.8) 1.0 (0.5–1.9) 1.7 (1.0–3.2) 1.0 (0.5–1.8) 0.9 (0.5–1.8) 0.9 (0.5–1.7) 0.8 (0.3–1.9)	Self-reported PD

Reference	Number	Method	Exposure	n	OR (95% CI)	Comments
			Dicamba:	26	0.9 (0.5–1.6)	Controlled for age, sex, smoking
			Paraquat:	14	1.8 (1.0–3.4)	
			Trifuralin:	31	0.9 (0.5–1.6)	
			Cyanazine:	30	2.6 (1.4–4.9)	
Firestone et al., 2005; Washington, USA	250 (156 men) newly diagnosed 1992–2002 at Group Health Cooperative	Interview determining occupational and home-based pesticide exposure characterized by chemical name or brand, duration, and frequency	Occupational, men only			
			Pesticides:	19	1.0 (0.5–1.9)	
			Insecticides:	15	0.9 (0.4–1.8)	
			Fungicides:	2	0.4 (0.1–3.9)	
			Herbicides:	9	1.4 (0.5–3.9)	
			Paraquat:	2	1.7 (0.2–12.8)	
			Home use, all subjects			
			Pesticides:	178	1.0 (0.7–1.4)	
			Insecticides:	141	0.8 (0.6–1.1)	
			Fungicides:	14	0.6 (0.3–1.1)	
			Herbicides:	116	1.1 (0.8–1.5)	
Behari et al., 2001; India	377 (301 men, 76 women)	377 matched for age (± 3 yr), but not sex	Structured interview			
			McNemar chi-square:			
			Herbicides:		$p = 0.010$	
			(**protective** effect—*not confirmed* by multivariate analysis)			
			Insecticide:		$p = 0.169$	
			Rodenticide:		$p = 0.662$	
Engel et al., 2001; US [cross-sectional, but otherwise fairly high-quality design]	238	72	Self-administered questionnaire for occupational exposure		[prevalence ratios]	Neurologic exam by trained nurse
			Any pesticide:		0.8 (0.5–1.2)	
			Herbicides:		0.8 (0.5–1.2)	
			Insecticides:		0.9 (0.6–1.5)	
			Fungicides:		0.8 (0.6–1.3)	

continued

TABLE 8-1 Continued

Reference and Country	Cases in Study Group	Comparison Group	Exposure Assessment	Exposure(s):[a]	n	OR (95 % CI)	Diagnosis of Neurologic Dysfunction

Kuopio et al., 1999; Finland	123 (onset of PD before 1984; 63 men, 60 women)	246 matched on sex, age (± 2 yr), and urban/rural	Interview—pesticides or herbicides regularly or occasionally used	Pesticide use:
				  Occasional use:
				  Regular use:
				Herbicide use:
				  Occasional use:
				  Regular use:
					39
					26
					13
					33
					20
					13
						1.0 (0.6–1.7)
						1.2 (0.7–2.0)
						0.7 (0.3–1.3)
						1.4 (0.8–2.5)
						1.7 (0.9–3.2)
						0.8 (0.4–1.7)
							Neurologic exam

Taylor et al., 1999; Boston Medical Center	140	147 controls referred by cases	Interview—exposure recorded as total days for lifetime	Logistic analysis adjusted for age, sex, family history, education, smoking, water source, head injury, depression. Pesticides: Herbicides:		1.0 (0.9–1.2) 1.1 (0.7–1.7)	Neurologic exam
Gorell et al., 1998; US	144 (age > 50 years)	464	Interview—herbicide and insecticide use while working on a farm or gardening	All occupations contributing exposure to: Herbicides: Insecticides: Fungicides:		4.1 (1.4–12.2) 3.6 (1.8–7.2) 1.6 (0.5–5.5)	Standard criteria of PD by history
Liou et al., 1997; Taiwan	120	240 hospital controls matched for age (± 2 yr) and sex	Interview—occupational exposures to herbicides or pesticides	Pesticides vs no pesticides: But no paraquat use: Paraquat use vs no paraquat:		2.9 (2.3–3.7) 2.2 (0.9–5.6) 4.7 (2.0–12) 3.2 (2.4–4.3)	Neurologic exam

Seidler et al., 1996; Germany	380 (age < 66 years with PD after 1987)	755 (379 neighborhood, 376 regional; Dick suggests neighborhood)	Interview—dose-years = years of application weighted by use	Pesticides:
				Herbicides—high dose:
				Dose trend
				  vs neighbor controls
				  vs regional controls
						2.1 (1.6–2.6)
						2.4 (1.0–6.0)
						
						p = 0.06
						p < 0.001
							Neurologic exam

Reference	Cases	Controls	Method	Exposure	Results	Diagnosis
Hertzman et al., 1994; Canada	127 (71 men and 56 women)	245 (121 with cardiac disease; 124 voters) controls over-matched)	Interview—occupation with probable pesticide exposure	Insecticides—high dose: Dose trend vs neighbor controls vs regional controls	2.1 (0.9–4.8) p = 0.12 p < 0.001	Neurologic exam
				vs voters—among men Pesticides: Herbicides: Chlorophenoxys: Paraquat: Insecticides: Fungicides:	2.3 (1.1–4.9) 1.2 (0.6–2.5) 1.2 (0.6–2.4) 1.3 (0.3–4.6) 0.3 (0.1–0.9) 0.5 (0.2–1.1)	
Butterfield et al., 1993; US	63 young onset cases (age < 50 years)	68	Questionnaire—pesticide or insecticide use 10 times in any year	Herbicides: Insecticides: Dwelling fumigated:	3.2 p = 0.033 5.8 p < 0.001 5.3 p = 0.45	Standard criteria of PD by history
Semchuk et al., 1992; Calgary, Alberta, Canada	130 living cases from register of Calgary residents (population-based)	260 community controls matched for age (± 2.5 yr) and sex, identified by RDD	Interview—self-report of exposure for each job held > 1 month	Pesticides: Herbicides: Exposed during age interval: 16–25 yr 26–35 yr 36–45 yr 46–55 yr Insecticides: Fungicides:	32 2.3 (1.3–4.0) 17 3.1 (1.3–7.0) 1.4 (0.5–4.3) 4.8 (1.5–15.0) 3.8 (1.2–13.0) 4.9 (1.3–19.0) 17 2.1 (1.0–4.1) 16 1.6 (0.8–3.3)	Neurologic exam confirming idiopathic PD without dementia (average 7.8 yr from diagnosis)

continued

TABLE 8-1 Continued

Reference and Country	Cases in Study Group	Comparison Group	Exposure Assessment	Exposure(s).[a]	n	OR (95 % CI)	Diagnosis of Neurologic Dysfunction
Stern et al., 1991; NJ & PA, US	69—all young onset cases identified (age < 40 years); 80—random selection of old onset cases (age > 59 years)	149 nominated by each case or picked from hospital; matched by age (± 6 yr), sex, and race	Interview—self-report of insecticide and pesticide use by self or others in home or garden	Insecticides: Onset < 40 years: Onset > 59 years: Herbicides: Onset < 40 years: Onset > 59 years: Adjusted for smoking, head injury, rural residence: Insecticides: Herbicides:		0.7 (0.3–1.4) 0.6 (0.2–1.7) 0.8 (0.3–2.1) 1.1 (0.7–1.7) 0.9 (0.5–1.7) 1.3 (0.7–2.4) 0.5 (0.2–1.1) 0.9 (0.6–1.5)	Review of medical records, responsive to PD medication (under treatment average of 8.2 yr), without
Hertzman et al., 1990; British Columbia, Canada	57 prevalent PD patients (age < 79 years) [50–54 had confirmed PD, not clear exactly how many]	122 aged 50–79 who responded from electoral rolls	Questionnaire—ever worked in an orchard	Work in orchards: Paraquat:	4/57	3.7 (1.3–10.3) (p = 0.01)	Neurologic exam confirmed diagnostic criteria in 55 of 69 cases identified by asking physicians in area

ABBREVIATIONS: CI, confidence interval; OR, odds ratio; PD, Parkinson's disease; RDD, random-digit dialing.

[a]For the objective of this Veterans and Agent Orange review series, only associations with herbicides are of possible relevance; only the phenoxy herbicides, cacodylic acid, and picloram are of specific interest.

use; there was some reporting of paraquat use, but for the chemicals of interest it is generally unclear how many subjects were exposed.

Update of the Epidemiologic Literature

Since *Update 2006*, several relevant studies have been reported. There are still no data on Vietnam veterans and PD, but in addition to the several population-based studies that suggest a relationship between herbicide exposure and PD, a number of studies have identified exposure to specific chemicals of interest as a potential risk factor.

Kamel et al. (2007b) studied the large cohort collected by the prospective AHS; this cohort was established from 1993 to 1997 and included 84,738 people of whom 57,259 were reached again 5 years later. During the enrollment telephone contact, in addition to extensive demographic information, a detailed pesticide-exposure history (including information about use of protective techniques) was collected. Subjects who reported a doctor's diagnosis of PD at enrollment were classified as prevalent cases, and those who reported a diagnosis of PD that occurred in the 5 years before the second contact were classified as incident cases. Among prevalent cases, there was not a positive relationship between reported use of any pesticide and PD (OR = 0.5, 95% CI 0.2–1.1). Among incident cases, there was a trend toward increased risk of PD in subjects exposed to pesticides (OR = 1.3, 95% CI 0.5–3.3); although the overall relationship did not reach statistical significance, there was a dose effect over the quartiles (p = 0.009), with subjects with the highest number of days of pesticide use showing the greatest risk (OR = 2.3, 95% CI 1.2–4.5). This study obtained information about specific compounds of exposure and reported on 47 individual pesticides. Although risks were not presented in association with overall use of the 18 reported herbicides, individual results were given for three phenoxy herbicides (2,4-D, 2,4,5-T, and 2,4,5-TP) and the structurally similar benzoic herbicide, dicamba. With the statistics for those four chemicals of interest, findings on paraquat and the only two other pesticides with significant findings, trifluralin and cyanazine (which are also herbicides), have been transcribed into Table 8-1 for comparison. For prevalent cases, the risk of PD was significantly increased after exposure to cyanazine and barely significantly increased after exposure to paraquat. For incident cases, a modest just-significant increase in risk was found after exposure to 2,4,5-T (OR = 1.8, 95% CI 1.0–3.3) and trifluralin (OR = 1.7, 95% CI 1.0–3.2) and a nonsignificant increase after exposure to dicamba (OR = 1.5, 95% CI 0.8–2.8).

That study is provocative but raises questions. The findings on prevalent and incident cases do not reinforce each other, but in this prospective design, prevalent cases were associated with considerably less reliable data than incident cases in several ways. Selection bias could have been operational in connection with the PD cases already diagnosed at the time of enrollment; those already having PD may have self-selected themselves out of agricultural occupations and hence disproportionately made themselves ineligible for enrollment in the AHS. Prevalent cases would also have been susceptible to recall bias when they provided their exposure profiles at enrollment; this would be consistent with the prevalent cases' having a higher risk after exposure to paraquat (whose structural relationship to a chemical known to cause PD had been discussed in the public media at the time of enrollment), whereas its risk estimate was neutral in the incident PD cases.

Another study (Brighina et al., 2008) investigated PD and pesticide exposure in light of new genetic insights. Mutations in the α-synuclein gene have been reported in families that have familial PD. That finding has led to the hypothesis that aggregation and formation of α-synuclein fibrils may lead to PD in sporadic disease. Brighina et al. (2008) tested the hypothesis that pesticide exposure might increase the aggregation and fibrillation of α-synuclein and thus lead to PD. A large case–control study was conducted, with 833 pairs; the REP1 genotype for α-synuclein was overrepresented in PD cases (OR = .18, 95% CI 1.02–1.37; p = 0.03). In this study, overall pesticide use was not associated with increased risk of PD (OR = 1.11, 95% CI 0.89–1.38; p = 0.37), but there was a trend toward increased risk in younger subjects. When herbicide, insecticide, and fungicide use was segregated, only herbicide use in younger subjects was associated with increased risk. Of the herbicides reported, those in the chlorophenoxy acid or esters chemical class was associated with the greatest risk (OR = 1.52, 95% CI 1.04–2.22; p = 0.004); 2,4-D was most commonly reported in this group. There was no clear interaction between specific haplotypes for α-synuclein and exposure in modifying the risk of PD.

Although the lack of interaction between specific haplotype and exposure may raise questions about the mechanism by which herbicides might increase the risk of PD, the relationship between chlorophenoxy-herbicide exposure and PD risk in younger subjects is an important finding. Environmental modifiers of neurodegenerative diseases often alter the onset of symptoms; the increased risk in younger subjects may be a clue in that regard.

Finally, Hancock et al. (2008) evaluated specific pesticide exposure and risk of PD by using a family-based case–control series of 319 PD patients and 296 controls. Overall pesticide use was significantly associated with PD (OR = 1.61, 95% CI 1.13–2.29). Organochlorine and organophosphorus compounds were associated with the greatest statistically significant risks. Exposure to chlorophenoxy acid or esters, including chemicals of interest in this review, were associated with increased ORs but the relationship was not statistically significant (OR = 2.07, 95% CI 0.69–6.23).

Biologic Plausibility

Several reviews of the literature have addressed the possible involvement of environmental chemicals in the etiology of PD. The very clear PD-like toxicity resulting from human MPTP exposure has indicated that select compounds can result in the same type of damage to dopaminergic neurons as PD does, and MPTP has become an important toxicant in studies that use animal and in vitro models. It is notable that MPTP's bioactive metabolite, MPP+, is similar in chemical structure to paraquat (a commonly used herbicide although not one used in Vietnam); but it is different from the chemicals of interest in this report. Pesticides that have been shown to produce PD-like toxicity in animal models include paraquat, rotenone, maneb, and dieldrin, and substantial research has gone into understanding the molecular mechanisms responsible for the toxicity, especially in connection with paraquat and rotenone, as reviewed recently by Drechsel and Patel (2008), Hatcher et al. (2008), and Nunomura et al. (2007) and by others in the past, including DiMonte et al. (2002) and Sherer et al. (2002a). The damage done to dopaminergic neurons in PD is probably from oxidative stress and probably also involves damage to mitochondria in the target cells (Liang et al., 2007; Sarnico et al., 2008). The chemicals of interest to this committee are known to be distributed to the CNS, but they have not been investigated in similar experimental systems, so there is no evidence that they could cause inflammation or oxidative stress similar to that caused by the compounds, such as paraquat, that have been investigated.

Research on the neurotoxicity of 2,4-D has been going on for a number of years, but most of it has focused on its effects on the developing rodent nervous system. The studies have often used high doses of 2,4-D that have resulted in adverse changes in the developing nervous system, both neurochemical (such as changes in D2 receptors, tyrosine hydroxylase and dopamine beta-hydroxylase) and behavioral (for example, Bortolozzi et al., 1999, 2002, 2003, 2004; Duffard et al., 1996; Evangelista de Duffard et al., 1990, 1995; Garcia et al., 2004, 2006; Rosso et al., 2000a,b). Injection of 2,4-D directly into the rat brain yielded toxicity in the basal ganglia (Bortolozzi et al., 2001), but this route of administration is highly artificial. Recent studies showed that postpartum dietary exposure of females to 2,4-D resulted in adverse alterations in maternal behavior and neurochemical changes including increases in dopamine and its metabolites 3,4-dihydroxyphenylacetic acid and homovanillic acid (Sturtz et al., 2008). Such an increase in dopamine is the reverse of what is seen in PD, in which degradation of the dopaminergic system occurs. In addition, a study of mice and 2,4-D yielded no evidence of neurochemical damage to the dopaminergic system (Thiffault et al., 2001). One study indicated that 2,4-D, among a variety of pesticides and metals, caused fibrillation of α-synuclein in vitro, but it used purified protein and did not report data on 2,4-D but only a generalized result (Uversky et al., 2002), so little confidence can be placed in it. Because the majority of the studies were on the developing nervous system, not the mature nervous system, and some studies yielded evidence of a lack of a role of 2,4-D in the development of PD, the existing studies are of little use in addressing the question of the etiology of PD.

A summary of biologic plausibility related to general mechanisms pertinent to neurologic effects, including PD, arising from exposure to the herbicides used in Vietnam is presented at the end of this chapter.

Synthesis

Many studies have found associations of PD with pesticides, but most of them have not determined what specific entities are responsible for generating these positive findings. Increasingly, an association between herbicide exposure and PD has been reported, and several studies since 2006 have suggested a specific relationship between exposure to the chemicals of interest and PD. However, the newer studies are not completely consistent with each other; Kamel et al. (2007b) found an increased risk in incident cases in farm workers exposed to 2,4,5-T but not 2,4-D, and Brighina et al. (2008) found that subjects exposed to phenoxyacetate esters most often reported exposure to 2,4-D. The study of Hancock et al. (2008) reported increased risks after exposure to multiple pesticides and herbicides, and the increased risk after exposure to chlorophenoxy acid or esters was not statistically significant.

Given the broad spectrum of environmental exposures that epidemiologic studies have found to be associated with PD, it has been hypothesized that interactions may play a prominent role in its etiology. That would be compatible with PD's arising from the interaction between herbicides and other substances to which people are exposed during service in Vietnam, such as insecticides. The charge of this committee, however, is limited to the herbicides sprayed in Vietnam; an extension to consideration and evaluation of the limitless universe of interactions is not feasible for a single health outcome, much less for the full array of adverse outcomes that the committee is responsible for examining.

Data strengthening the concept of inflammation, oxidative stress, and the involvement of mitochondria in the etiology of PD have been generated recently but not on the herbicides sprayed by the military in Vietnam. Research with 2,4-D in rats, although relatively extensive, has been either on the developing nervous system or on maternal behavior and neurochemistry, and the results do not support a definitive role of 2,4-D in the etiology of PD.

Studies reported before 2006 produced a preponderance of data suggesting that exposure to herbicides in general may be related to increased risk of PD. The studies reported since *Update 2006* support and extend those earlier observations. The lack of preclinical data on a specific mechanism by which herbicides in general or specific chemicals of interest may produce PD does not argue against such a relationship but should be a stimulus for further research. Similarly, the lack of data on Vietnam War veterans themselves does not suggest that the relationship does not exist but only that appropriate studies have not been performed.

The lack of data relating PD incidence to exposure in the Vietnam-veteran population is of concern to the committee, and we recommend strongly that studies to produce such data be performed. We are also concerned that a biologic mechanism by which the chemicals of interest may cause PD has not been demonstrated. Nevertheless, the preponderance of epidemiologic evidence now supports an association between herbicide exposure and PD and specifically implicates the chemicals of interest.

Conclusions

On the basis of the evidence reviewed here and in previous VAO reports, the committee concludes that there is limited or suggestive evidence of an association between exposure to the chemicals of interest and PD.

Amyotrophic Lateral Sclerosis

ALS is a progressive, adult-onset, motor neuron disease that presents with muscle atrophy, weakness, and fasciculations and with signs that implicate involvement of motor pathways in the CNS. The cause of most cases of ALS is unknown, but about 10% of cases report an autosomal dominant pattern of inheritance. One-fifth of familial-ALS patients have mutations in the gene that encodes superoxide dismutase-1 (Rosen et al., 1993). The incidence of sporadic ALS is 1–2 per 100,000 person-years, and the incidence of ALS peaks at the ages of 55–75 years (Brooks, 1996). The diagnosis of ALS is made through clinical examination and electrodiagnostic testing and has a high degree of accuracy when made by experienced neurologists (Rowland, 1998; Rowland and Shneider, 2001).

Summary of Previous Updates

ALS was first considered by the committee for *Update 2002*. Although multiple potential etiologic factors have been investigated (Breland and Currier, 1967; Deapen and Henderson, 1986; Gallagher and Sander, 1987; Hanisch et al., 1976; Kurtzke and Beebe, 1980; McGuire et al., 1997; Roelofs-Iverson et al., 1984; Savettieri et al., 1991), associations have not been consistently identified.

Pesticide or herbicide exposure has been associated with increased risk of ALS, including a doubling of the risk after long-term occupational exposure to pesticides (Deapen and Henderson, 1986) and a tripling of the risk after exposure to agricultural chemical products (Savettieri et al., 1991) and after exposure to herbicides (McGuire et al., 1997), although none of the risk estimates was statistically significant. A population-based case–control study demonstrated associations between exposure to agricultural chemical products and ALS in men, with an odds ratio of 2.4 and a trend with duration of exposure that were both statistically significant (McGuire et al., 1997). A mortality study of Dow Chemical Company employees exposed to 2,4-D included three deaths from ALS, with a significant positive association (relative risk, 3.45, 95% CI 1.10–11.11) (Burns et al., 2001).

In *Update 2006*, three additional studies were reviewed. Morahan and Pamphlett (2006) published a case–control study from Australia in which the cases were self-reported and the controls chosen in nonrandom fashion. The authors found an increased risk of ALS after exposure to pesticides or herbicides, but the lack of appropriate case and control ascertainment and the fact that specific chemicals of interest were not asked about make this study difficult to interpret. Weisskopf et al. (2005) followed vital status of subjects in the American Cancer Society's cohort for the Cancer Prevention Study II and demonstrated an increased risk of ALS in those who served in any of the armed services during times of conflict. They adjusted for a variety of confounding variables in their model, including exposure to herbicides, and found that none of them significantly altered their conclusions. Thus, in an indirect way, this large study suggests the lack of a strong effect of herbicide exposure on ALS. Finally, a case–control study of Australian Vietnam veterans reported an association between deployment in Vietnam and ALS (ADVA, 2005c) but did not specifically study exposure to pesticides or herbicides.

Table 8-2 summarizes the results of the relevant studies.

Update of the Epidemiologic Literature

No studies concerning exposure to the chemicals of interest and ALS have been published since *Update 2006*.

Biologic Plausibility

No studies concerning the chemicals of interest specifically relevant to ALS have been published since *Update 2006*. A summary of biologic plausibility of neurologic effects arising from exposure to the chemicals of interest is presented at the end of this chapter.

Synthesis

Epidemiologic studies of ALS have pursued a variety of occupational exposures as potential risk factors; pesticide and herbicide exposures are among those receiving the most attention. Although it has rarely been possible to isolate the effects of selected chemicals of interest, a study of a cohort of 2,4-D production workers did identify significantly increased risk (Burns et al., 2001); however, this result is considered unstable, given the low number of cases and the wide CI. Case–control studies of occupational exposures to pesticides and herbicides have identified significantly increased risks (McGuire et al., 1997; Morahan and Pamphlett, 2006), but they did not weigh heavily, because of imprecise exposure assessments and other design limitations. Although recent prospective (Weisskopf et al., 2005) and retrospective (ADVA, 2005b) studies have identified increased

TABLE 8-2 Epidemiologic Studies of Pesticide[a] Exposure and Amyotrophic Lateral Sclerosis

Reference; Country	Study Group	Comparison Group	Exposure Assessment	Significant Association with Pesticides[a]	Estimated Relative Risk (95% CI)	Neurologic Dysfunction
Morahan and Pamphlett, 2006; Australia	179	179	Questionnaire—exposure to environmental toxicants		Herbicide, pesticide exposure: 1.6 (1.0–2.4); industrial exposure: 5.6 (2.1–15.1)	Self-reported
ADVA, 2005c; Australia	nr	nr	Deployment to Vietnam		4.7 (1.0–22.8)	Self-reported military services, death certificates
Weisskopf et al., 2005; Australia	nr	nr	Self-administered questionnaire		1.5 (1.1–2.1); p = 0.007	
Burns et al., 2001; US	1,567	40,600	Industrial hygienist ranked jobs for exposure to 2,4-D to derive of years exposure and cumulative exposure	+	3.45 (1.1–11.1)	Death certificates
McGuire et al., 1997; US	174	348	Self-reported lifetime job history, workplace exposures reviewed by panel of four industrial hygienists	+	Herbicide exposure: 2.4 (1.2–4.8); significant trend analysis for dose–effect relationship with agricultural chemicals: p = 0.03	New diagnosis of ALS 1990–1994 in western Washington state
Chancellor et al., 1993; Scotland	103	103	Required regular occupational exposure to pesticides for 12 months or more		1.4 (0.6–3.1)	Scottish Motor Neuron Register
Savettieri et al., 1991; Italy	46	92	Continual exposure to agricultural chemicals		3.0 (0.4–20.3)	Cases reviewed by neurologists
Deapen and Henderson, 1986; US	518	518	Ever worked in presence of pesticides		2.0 (0.8–5.4)	ALS Society of America

ABBREVIATIONS: ALS, amyotrophic lateral sclerosis; CI, confidence interval; nr, not reported; OR, odds ratio.
[a]For the objective of the VAO review series, only associations with herbicides are of possible relevance; only phenoxy herbicides, cacodylic acid, and picloram are of specific interest.

risk in veterans who served in Vietnam, they tend to implicate military service itself rather than exposure to the specific chemicals of interest.

Conclusions

On the basis of the evidence reviewed here and in previous VAO reports, the committee concludes that the evidence of an association between exposure to the chemicals of interest and ALS remains inadequate or insufficient.

PERIPHERAL NEUROPATHY

Peripheral neuropathies comprise a spectrum of disorders caused by damage to nerve fibers (axonal neuropathies) or to the myelin sheath that surrounds many fibers (demyelinating neuropathies). Manifestations of neuropathy can include a combination of sensory changes, motor weakness, and autonomic instability. Clinically, various forms of peripheral neuropathy can be characterized by the distribution of nerve abnormalities and their patterns of progression.

Peripheral neuropathy resulting from toxic exposure usually affects nerve fibers in a symmetric pattern, beginning distally in the longest fibers (in the toes) and moving proximally (toward the spine). This kind of neuropathy is called symmetric axonal sensorimotor polyneuropathy. Sensory deficits begin at the toes, progress above the ankles, and affect the hands only later. Motor symptoms show the same general pattern. Physiologically, various forms of peripheral neuropathy can be characterized by results of electrodiagnostic testing to indicate which neural structures are affected. Most toxicant-induced neuropathies involve injury to the nerve-cell bodies (neurons) or nerve fibers (axons) that produces changes in the amplitude of a nerve's response to an electric stimulus.

The clinical appearances of most symmetric axonal neuropathies are quite similar except for variation in rates of progression and in whether pain is a prominent symptom. There is no specific signature that distinguishes a toxicant-related neuropathy from one induced by other causes. As many as 30% of neuropathies are "idiopathic"; that is, no etiology is determined despite exhaustive clinical evaluation.

The most common toxicant-induced neuropathy occurs as a result of chronic alcohol exposure. Peripheral neuropathy also occurs commonly as a complication of diabetes: its reported prevalence in people who have chronic diabetes is up to 50%. It is important to include assessment of alcohol use and diabetes as covariates in epidemiologic studies because the neuropathies that are related to these conditions are clinically and physiologically indistinguishable from other toxicant-induced neuropathies.

Clinically, in cases of toxicant-induced peripheral neuropathy, stabilization or improvement is the rule after exposure ends. Recovery may not be complete, however, and the degree of recovery can depend on the severity of the initial deficits and the particular exposure. Furthermore, there is a possibility of "subclinical" effects, and a person might be unaware of symptoms although evidence of nerve dysfunction can be found through detailed neurologic examination or electrodiagnostic testing.

In *VAO*, peripheral neuropathy was considered a single category of disease. Before revising the conclusion regarding neuropathies, the committee for *Update 1996* divided them into "acute and subacute" and "chronic" classifications (on the basis of when an outcome occurs relative to exposure). In this section of the present report, however, the terms *acute* (brief) and *chronic* (prolonged or protracted) describe the time course of toxicant exposure. *Early onset* and *delayed onset* are used to describe the time course of the neuropathy. The distinction between *transient* and *persistent* is not always clear, because recovery may be protracted and incomplete. The committee considers a neuropathy to be of early onset and transient if abnormalities appear and resolve within 2 years after cessation of external exposure.

Conclusions from *VAO* and Previous Updates

VAO and the previous updates noted that the literature on peripheral neuropathy had been difficult to integrate because it was characterized by variable methods that lacked uniform operational definitions. The techniques used to identify affected persons, to define comparison populations, and to assess exposures differ considerably among studies. Many of the studies are limited by nonrandom selection, which raises a concern about bias, and by the relatively small number of participants, which decreases confidence in risk estimates and limits the power to detect a true association. Results have been variable; some studies demonstrated abnormalities of peripheral nerve function, and others did not.

In the first update, the committee for *Update 1996* partitioned the new information and that which had been addressed in *VAO* between "chronic persistent peripheral neuropathy" and "acute and subacute transient peripheral neuropathy." With this information, that committee reached a conclusion of limited or suggestive evidence of association with exposure to the chemicals of interest and the "acute or subchronic" form. (To be more precise, the committee for *Update 2004* applied the designation "early-onset transient peripheral neuropathy" to this outcome, which will be used henceforth in this discussion.)

As reported in *VAO*, many occupational studies give an indication of early-onset transient peripheral neuropathy in conjunction with herbicide production. In a study of workers from Nitro, West Virginia, that did have a comparison group, Moses et al. (1984) demonstrated this among the workers with chloracne. This outcome was also established shortly after the Seveso accident (Boeri at al., 1978; Filippini et al., 1981; Gilioli et al., 1979), but the effect abated with time (Assennato et al., 1989; Barbieri et al., 1988). Findings were less clear among residents around contamination sites in Missouri (Hoffman et al., 1986; Stehr et al., 1986; Webb et al., 1987).

In addition, the committee responsible for *Update 1996* reviewed case reports that described peripheral neuropathy after exposures to the compounds of interest (Berkley and Magee, 1963; Goldstein et al., 1959; Todd, 1962). In each instance, the peripheral neuropathy improved gradually but had not resolved completely even after several months or years. The possibility cannot be entirely excluded that the five cases reported in those publications were unrelated to herbicide exposure and were examples of other disorders, such as idiopathic Guillain-Barré syndrome. The committee also considered several supportive animal models (Grahmann et al., 1993; Grehl et al., 1993; see "Biologic Plausibility" below). The committee concluded that there was limited or suggestive evidence of an association between exposure to the compounds of interest and early-onset transient peripheral neuropathy. In subsequent updates, there has not been substantively more information found on this type of peripheral neuropathy and the committees have maintained the conclusion of limited evidence of an association for this outcome. New cases of this condition would not be expected among veterans who received their exposure during the Vietnam era.

In addition to the short-term assessment done by Moses et al. (1984), the committee responsible for *VAO* reviewed results of three other occupational-cohort studies of workers who had been exposed to the chemicals of interest. Singer et al. (1982) reported decreased nerve conduction velocities (NCVs) in 2,4-D and 2,4,5-T production workers who were examined 2 months after exposures were reduced. In former 2,4,5-T production workers who had a history of chloracne (10 years after last exposure), Moses et al. (1984) found diminished pin-prick sensation, but Suskind and Hertzberg (1984) did not find differences in NCVs. Similarly, Sweeney et al. (1993) reported decreased pin-prick sensation but no differences in NCVs in former herbicide-production workers (evaluated 15 years or more after their last exposure).

VAO also reviewed epidemiologic studies of populations potentially exposed to TCDD in the environment. A series of studies in Italy evaluated peripheral neuropathy in the Seveso population after the industrial accident on July 10, 1976. Boeri et al. (1978) reported more frequent symptoms and signs of neuropathy in a cohort of residents living in the contaminated area than in a comparison group last examined 7–10 months after the explosion; there was no statistical difference in conduction velocity between groups. Gilioli et al. (1979) noted electrodiagnostic abnormalities in laboratory technicians potentially exposed to TCDD from analytic samples; however, the technicians were also exposed to solvents used in the analytic process. Filippini et al. (1981) reported an increased prevalence of peripheral neuropathy in Seveso residents with evidence of high exposure to TCDD (chloracne or liver enzyme abnormalities) who were last examined 21 months after the accident. Barbieri et al. (1988) reported a higher rate of abnormalities on neurologic examination and electrodiagnostic testing in subjects who had a history of chloracne and were examined 6 years after the accident, but there was no significant increase in peripheral neuropathy as defined by World Health Organization (WHO) criteria. Assennato et al. (1989) described electrodiagnostic evaluation of that group 9 years after the accident; no differences were observed in NCVs or neuropathy as defined by WHO criteria. Other environmental studies reviewed in *VAO* were of Missouri residents potentially exposed to TCDD in the early 1970s when waste oil was sprayed to control dust (Hoffman et al., 1986; Stehr et al., 1986; Webb et al., 1987). Although more frequent sensory abnormalities were reported in potentially exposed subjects, the differences were not statistically significant, and the semiecologic study design was not suited to causal inference. Some of the data from epidemiologic studies of environmental exposures have suggested an increased risk of peripheral nerve abnormalities, but evidence of an association between exposure to the chemicals of interest and peripheral neuropathy is inconsistent.

Studies of Vietnam veterans were also reviewed in *VAO* (AFHS, 1984, 1987, 1991; CDC, 1988). A study by the Centers for Disease Control (now the Centers for Disease Control and Prevention) (CDC, 1988) focused on service in Vietnam, not on exposure to the chemicals of interest, and therefore provided no evidence of the possible effects of specific exposures. There was no indication of increased risk of peripheral neuropathy in the first reports on Ranch Hand veterans (AFHS, 1984, 1987, 1991). Studies reviewed in *VAO* did not indicate an association between exposure and peripheral neuropathy in Vietnam veterans.

Update 1996 reviewed two new epidemiologic studies. Using an administrative database, Zober et al. (1994) found no evidence of increased use of medical services for diagnosis of peripheral neuropathy in workers previously exposed to TCDD at a BASF plant. Decoufle et al. (1992) reported no association between self-reported exposure to herbicides in Vietnam and peripheral neuropathy. The limitations of those studies were such that they did not confirm or refute a possible relationship between exposure and neuropathy.

Update 1998 reviewed no new studies. The context for the issue of peripheral neuropathy, its relationship with toxic exposures, and the occurrence of diabetes mellitus was discussed. In particular, it was noted that neuropathy is a common consequence of diabetes. That was particularly relevant in that the committee issued a special report a year later that concluded that there was limited or suggestive evidence of an association between exposure to Agent Orange and diabetes.

Update 2000 reviewed what was then the most recent report on Ranch Hand veterans (AFHS, 2000), which combined signs of peripheral neuropathy to produce increasingly specific, graded indexes of neuropathy—a common approach in epidemiologic studies. Ranch Hand veterans were significantly more likely than comparison subjects to have abnormalities in the indexes, and the prevalence of abnormalities increased with dioxin concentration. Although the clinical relevance of epidemiologic indexes of neuropathy is never certain, the strong associations described between the indexes and the conditions known to produce peripheral neuropathy, such as diabetes and alcohol use, supported their validity in this study. The AFHS investigators included those conditions as potential confounders in their statistical analysis. However, the effect of diabetes could not be eliminated in the most specific neuropathy index, because there were not enough nondiabetic subjects. It therefore was impossible, lacking any effect of diabetes, to estimate the association between dioxin exposure and neuropathy.

Update 2002 considered one peer-reviewed article that described the peripheral-neuropathy data on the AFHS cohort (Michalek et al., 2001). In a primary analysis, the investigators had included diabetes as a potential confounder in the statistical model. In a secondary analysis, subjects who had conditions that were known to be associated with neuropathy were excluded, and subjects who had diabetes were enumerated. In both analyses, there were strong and significant associations between dioxin concentrations and possible and probable neuropathy, and significant trends were found with increasing concentrations of dioxin. However, there were too few nondiabetic subjects to produce useful estimates of risk in the absence of the contribution of diabetes. Thus, questions remained about the specific association between exposure to the chemicals of interest and peripheral neuropathy in the absence of any effect of diabetes.

Update 2004 considered one peer-reviewed article (Kim et al., 2003), which reported an association between Korean veterans' service in Vietnam and peripheral neuropathy. Methodologic limitations, such as a concern about recall bias and residual confounding due to diabetes, and issues related to TCDD dose estimation prevented a strong inference.

Update 2006 (IOM, 2005) uncovered no reports dealing with peripheral neuropathy as a diagnosis. Kamel et al. (2005) queried the large AHS cohort about a battery of neurologic symptoms, some of which could arise from peripheral neuropathy. As mentioned in the section on PD, it is not clear how to interpret studies that rely on nonspecific clinical findings.

Update of the Scientific Literature

Since *Update 2006*, only a single study reported on outcomes related to peripheral neuropathy. Urban et al. (2007) evaluated the neurologic status of 15 subjects surviving since experiencing significant exposure to TCDD during 1965–1968. The subjects on the average still had grossly increased toxicant concentrations in blood and body fat, suggesting ongoing internal exposure since their occupational exposure. Clinical examination suggested neuropathy in nine subjects; however, nerve-conduction studies were abnormal in only three. Alcohol exposure was significant in the subjects, and the presence or absence of diabetes was not mentioned, so any etiologic relationship between neuropathy and TCDD exposure must be regarded as speculative.

Biologic Plausibility

No new studies directly pertinent to peripheral neuropathy were identified in the present update. However, it is worth reiterating findings from earlier updates.

Neuronal cell cultures treated with 2,4-D showed decreased neurite extension associated with intracellular changes, including a decrease in microtubules, inhibition of the polymerization of tubulin, disorganization of the Golgi apparatus, and inhibition of ganglioside synthesis (Rosso et al., 2000a,b). Those mechanisms are important for maintaining synaptic connections between nerve cells and supporting the mechanisms involved in axon regeneration during recovery from peripheral neuropathy. Grahmann et al. (1993) and Grehl et al. (1993) reported the observations of electrophysiologic and pathologic abnormalities, respectively, in the peripheral nerves of rats treated with TCDD. When the animals were sacrificed 8 months after exposure, there was pathologic evidence of persistent axonal nerve damage and histologic findings typical of toxicant-induced injury. Those results constitute evidence of the biologic plausibility of an association between exposure to the chemicals of interest and peripheral neuropathy. A summary of the biologic plausibility of neurologic effects arising from exposure to the chemicals of interest is presented at the end of this chapter.

Synthesis

Over the last 50 years, a body of literature has accumulated that suggests an association between the chemicals of interest and peripheral neuropathy. Past committees have concluded that there is evidence of an association between exposure to at least one chemical of interest and "acute and subacute transient" peripheral neuropathy (*Update 1996*). However, there remained questions about whether evidence supported an association with persistent neuropathy.

Human case reports have documented peripheral neuropathy, as shown by neurologic examination and electrodiagnostic testing, after acute exposure to large amounts of 2,4-D. Reports have indicated eventual symptom stabilization and improvement, but sensory and motor deficits have persisted in some people for months or years after exposure ended.

Several epidemiologic studies have reported increased risk of peripheral neuropathy in populations exposed to the chemicals of interest in a variety of occupational and environmental settings. However, the literature is inconsistent and suffers from methodologic limitations. The most dramatic exposures have involved industrial accidents that caused environmental contamination, such as the one in Seveso, Italy, in 1976. Studies of residents in that region have shown early-onset neuropathy, and subclinical abnormalities in some subjects have been demonstrated with electrodiagnostic testing.

Epidemiologic studies that used appropriate comparison groups and standard techniques for diagnosis and assessment of exposure have not demonstrated consistent associations between exposure to the chemicals of interest and peripheral neuropathy. Several reports have shown no significant association, and in the reports that did indicate an association, chance, bias, or confounding could not be ruled out with confidence. In particular, diabetes might confound the results, inasmuch as many of the subjects with neuropathy also had diabetes, which is a known cause of neuropathy. Controlling for the effects of diabetes is a technical challenge because there is evidence of an association between exposure to at least one of the chemicals of interest and diabetes (IOM, 2003); in many cases, diabetes could be in the causal pathway that links exposure and peripheral neuropathy.

Conclusions

On the basis of the evidence reviewed here and in previous VAO reports, the committee concludes that there is limited or suggestive evidence of an association between exposure to the chemicals of interest and early-onset transient peripheral neuropathy.

On the basis of the evidence reviewed here and previous VAO reports, the committee concludes that there is inadequate or insufficient evidence of an association between exposure to the chemicals of interest and delayed or persistent peripheral neuropathy.

SUMMARY

Biologic Plausibility

Experimental data continue to accrue regarding the biologic plausibility of a connection between exposure to the chemicals of interest and various neurologic disorders. This section summarizes in a general way some of the information reviewed in the current update and, to make the summary complete, includes information from prior updates.

Several studies have dealt with mechanisms of neurotoxicity that might be ascribed to the chemicals of concern, notably 2,4-D and TCDD. Molecular effects of the chemicals of concern are described in detail in Chapter 4. Some of the effects suggest possible pathways by which there could be effects on the neural systems. A number of the studies suggest that there are neurologic effects, both neurochemical and behavioral, of the chemicals of interest, primarily 2,4-D, in animal models if exposure occurs during development or in cultured nerve cells (Konjuh et al., 2008; Rosso et al., 2000a,b; Sturtz et al., 2008); older references described behavioral effects of developmental exposure of rodents to a 2,4-D–2,4,5-T mixture (Mohammad and St. Omer, 1986; St. Omer and Mohammad, 1987). TCDD has caused deficits in learning behavior in the rat after exposure during development (Hojo et al., 2008). However, caution against overinterpreting the significance of these studies is urged because the developing nervous system is different from the mature nervous system and may not be an appropriate model for the possible consequences of exposure of adults to the chemicals of interest.

Some studies further support suggestions that the level of reactive oxygen species could alter the functions of specific signaling cascades and may be involved in neurodegeneration (Drechsel and Patel, 2008). Such studies do not specifically concern the chemicals of interest but are potentially relevant to these chemicals inasmuch as TCDD and herbicides have been reported to elicit oxidative stress (Byers, 2006; Celik et al., 2006; Shen et al., 2005). In addition, TCDD has been shown to affect phosphokinase C biochemistry in nerve cells and therefore could affect the integrity and physiology of nerve cells (Kim et al., 2007; Lee HG et al., 2007). Cytochrome P450 1A1, the aryl hydrocarbon receptor (AHR), and the AHR nuclear transporter occur in the brain, so TCDD might be likely to exert effects in the brain (Huang et al., 2000). In addition, although they dealt with hepatocytes and not cells of the nervous system, earlier studies have indicated that 2,4-D affected aspects of mitochondrial energetics and mitochondrial calcium flux (Palmeira et al., 1994a,b, 1995a,b); if these effects can also occur with nervous system cell mitochondria, which is feasible, then the energy balance and pathways of cells in the nervous system could be affected, with later damage to nervous system function. Those mechanistic studies, although they did not produce convincing evidence of specific effects of the chemicals of interest in the neurologic outcomes of concern, suggest possible avenues to pursue to determine linkages between the chemicals of interest and the neurologic outcomes that could occur in adult humans.

Basic scientific studies have emphasized the importance of alterations in neurotransmitter systems as potential mechanisms that underlie TCDD-induced neurobehavioral disorders. Neuronal cultures treated with 2,4-D exhibited decreased neurite extension associated with intracellular changes, including a decrease in microtubules, inhibition of the polymerization of tubulin, disorganization of the Golgi apparatus, and inhibition of ganglioside synthesis. Those mechanisms are important for maintaining the connections between nerve cells that are necessary for neuronal function and that are involved in axon regeneration and recovery from peripheral neuropathy. Animal experiments have demonstrated that TCDD treatments affect the fundamental molecular events that underlie neurotransmission initiated by calcium uptake. Mechanistic studies have demonstrated that 2,4,5-T can alter cellular metabolism and the cholinergic transmission necessary for neuromuscular transmission.

TCDD treatment of rats at doses that do not cause general systemic illness or wasting disease produces electrodiagnostic changes in peripheral nerve function and pathologic findings that are characteristic of toxicant-induced axonal peripheral neuropathy.

As discussed in Chapter 4, extrapolation of observations of cells in culture or animal models to humans is complicated by differences in sensitivity and susceptibility among animals, strains, and species; by the lack of strong evidence of organ-specific effects among species; and by differences in route, dose, duration, and timing of chemical exposures. Thus, although the observations themselves cannot support a conclusion that the chemicals of interest produced neurotoxic effects in humans, they do suggest the biologic plausibility of an association and describe potential mechanisms that might have come into play.

Conclusions

On the basis of the evidence reviewed here and in previous VAO reports, the committee concludes that there is inadequate or insufficient evidence of an association between exposure to the chemicals of interest (2,4-D, 2,4,5-T, TCDD, picloram, and cacodylic acid) and neurobehavioral disorders (cognitive or neuropsychiatric) or ALS.

Previous VAO reports have concluded that there was inadequate or insufficient evidence of an association between exposure to the chemicals of interest and PD. In this report, we review both new data published after *Update 2006* and older studies investigating the relationship between herbicide exposure and PD risk. Although a compelling biologic mechanism has not been identified, the bulk of evidence suggests a risk posed by herbicide exposure in general with regard to PD. That impression is strengthened by recent studies that report a specific risk related to the chemicals of interest. The committee now concludes that there is limited or suggestive evidence of an association between exposure to the chemicals of interest and PD.

The committee responsible for *Update 1996* concluded that there was limited or suggestive evidence of an association between exposure to at least one of the chemicals of interest and "acute and subacute transient" peripheral neuropathy. The evidence was drawn from occupational and other studies in which subjects were exposed to a variety of herbicides and herbicide components. Information available to the committees responsible for *Update 1998*, *Update 2000*, and *Update 2002* supported that conclusion. The committee for *Update 2004* exhaustively reviewed the data on peripheral neuropathy and concluded that there was limited or suggestive evidence of an association between exposure and "early onset, transient" peripheral neuropathy but that the evidence was inadequate or insufficient to support an association between exposure to the chemicals of interest and "delayed or persistent" peripheral neuropathy. The committees responsible for *Update 2006* concurred and the current committee concurs with that conclusion.

In summary, the present committee, on the basis of its review of new data and a re-evaluation of older studies, has left the conclusions of previous committees concerning neurologic outcomes unchanged.

REFERENCES[1]

ADVA (Australian Department of Veterans' Affairs). 2005b. *The Third Australian Vietnam Veterans Mortality Study.* Canberra, Australia: Department of Veterans' Affairs.

---

[1]Throughout the report the same alphabetic indicator following year of publication is used consistently for the same article when there were multiple citations by the same first author in a given year. The convention of assigning the alphabetic indicator in order of citation in a given chapter is not followed.

ADVA. 2005c. *Australian National Service Vietnam Veterans Mortality and Cancer Incidence Study.* Canberra, Australia: Department of Veterans' Affairs.

AFHS (Air Force Health Study). 1984. *An Epidemiological Investigation of Health Effects in Air Force Personnel Following Exposure to Herbicides. Baseline Morbidity Study Results.* Brooks AFB, TX: USAF School of Aerospace Medicine. NTIS AD-A138 340.

AFHS. 1987. *An Epidemiological Investigation of Health Effects in Air Force Personnel Following Exposure to Herbicides. First Follow-up Examination Results.* Brooks AFB, TX: USAF School of Aerospace Medicine. USAFSAM-TR-87-27.

AFHS. 1991. *An Epidemiological Investigation of Health Effects in Air Force Personnel Following Exposure to Herbicides. Serum Dioxin Analysis of 1987 Examination Results.* Brooks AFB, TX: USAF School of Aerospace Medicine.

AFHS. 1995. *An Epidemiological Investigation of Health Effects in Air Force Personnel Following Exposure to Herbicides. 1992 Follow-up Examination Results.* Brooks AFB, TX: Epidemiological Research Division. Armstrong Laboratory.

AFHS. 2000. *An Epidemiological Investigation of Health Effects in Air Force Personnel Following Exposure to Herbicides. 1997 Follow-up examination and results.* Reston, VA: Science Application International Corporation. F41624-96-C1012.

Assennato G, Cervino D, Emmett E, Longo G, Merlo F. 1989. Follow-up of subjects who developed chloracne following TCDD exposure at Seveso. *American Journal of Industrial Medicine* 16:119–125.

Baldi I, Lebailly P, Mohammed-Brahim B, Letenneur L, Dartigues J-F, Brochard P. 2003. Neurodegenerative diseases and exposure to pesticides in the elderly. *American Journal of Epidemiology* 157(5):409–414.

Barbieri S, Pirovano C, Scarlato G, Tarchini P, Zappa A, Maranzana M. 1988. Long-term effects of 2,3,7,8-tetrachlorodibenzo-*p*-dioxin on the peripheral nervous system. Clinical and neurophysiological controlled study on subjects with chloracne from the Seveso area. *Neuroepidemiology* 7:29–37.

Barrett DH, Morriss RD, Akhtar FZ, Michalek JE. 2001. Serum dioxin and cognitive functioning among veterans of operation ranch hand. *NeuroToxicology* 22:491–502.

Barrett DH, Morris RD, Jackson WG Jr, Stat M, Michalek JE. 2003. Serum dioxin and psychological functioning in US Air Force veterans of the Vietnam War. *Military Medicine* 168:153–159.

Behari M, Srivastava AK, Das RR, Pandey RM. 2001. Risk factors of Parkinson's disease in Indian patients. *Journal of Neurological Sciences* 190(1-2):49–55.

Berkley MC, Magee KR. 1963. Neuropathy following exposure to a dimethylamine salt of 2,4-D. *Archives of Internal Medicine* 111:133–134.

Boeri R, Bordo B, Crenna P, Filippini G, Massetto M, Zecchini A. 1978. Preliminary results of a neurological investigation of the population exposed to TCDD in the Seveso region. *Rivista di Patologia Nervosa e Mentale* 99:111–128.

Bortolozzi AA, Duffard RO, Evangelista de Duffard AM. 1999. Behavioral alterations induced in rats by a pre- and postnatal exposure to 2,4-dichlorophenoxyacetic acid. *Neurotoxicol Teratol* 21(4):451–465.

Bortolozzi A, de Duffard AME, Dajas F, Duffard R, Silveira R. 2001. Intracerebral administration of 2,4-diclorophenoxyacetic acid induces behavioral and neurochemical alterations in the rat brain. *NeuroToxicology* 22(2):221–232.

Bortolozzi A, Duffard R, Antonelli M, Evangelista de Duffard AM. 2002. Increased sensitivity in dopamine D(2)-like brain receptors from 2,4-dichlorophenoxyacetic acid (2,4-D)-exposed and amphetamine-challenged rats. *Annals of the New York Academy of Sciences* 965:314–323.

Bortolozzi A, Duffard R, de Duffard AM. 2003. Asymmetrical development of the monoamine systems in 2,4-dichlorophenoxyacetic acid treated rats. *NeuroToxicology* 24(1):149–157.

Bortolozzi AA, Evangelista de Duffard AM, Duffard RO, Antonelli MC. 2004. Effects of 2,4-dichlorophenoxyacetic acid exposure on dopamine D2-like receptors in rat brain. *Neurotoxicology and Teratology* 26(4):599–605.

Breland AE, Currier RD. 1967. Multiple sclerosis and amyotrophic lateral sclerosis in Mississippi. *Neurology* 17:1011–1016.

Brighina L, Frigerio R, Schneider NK, Lesnick TG, de Andrade M, Cunningham JM, Farrer MJ, Lincoln SJ, Checkoway H, Rocca WA, Maraganore DM. 2008. Alpha-synuclein, pesticides, and Parkinson disease: A case–control study. *Neurology* 70(16 pt 2):1461–1469.

Bronstein J, Carvey P, Chen H, Cory-Slechta DA, DiMonte D, Duda J, English PB, Goldman S, Grate S, Hansen J, Hoppin J, Jewell S, Kamel F, Koroshetz W, Langston J, Logroscino G, Nelson L, Ravina B, Rocca WA, Ross G, Schettler T, Schwarzschild M, Scott B, Seegal R, Singleton A, Steenland, K, Tanner C, Eeden, S, Weisskopf M. 2009. Meeting report: Consensus statement—Parkinson's disease and the environment: Collaborative on Health and the Environment and Parkinson's Action Network (CHE PAN) conference 26-28 June 2007. *Environmental Health Perspectives* 117(1):117–121.

Brooks BR. 1996. Clinical epidemiology of amyotrophic lateral sclerosis. *Neurological Clinics* 14(2):399–420.

Burns CJ, Beard KK, Cartmill JB. 2001. Mortality in chemical workers potentially exposed to 2,4-dichlorophenoxyacetic acid (2,4-D) 1945–94: An update. *Occupational and Environmental Medicine* 58:24–30.

Butterfield PG, Valanis BG, Spencer PS, Lindeman CA, Nutt JG. 1993. Environmental antecedents of young-onset Parkinson's disease. *Neurology* 43:1150–1158.

Byers JP, Masters K, Sarver JG, Hassoun EA. 2006. Association between the levels of biogenic amines and superoxide anion production in brain regions of rats after subchronic exposure to TCDD. *Toxicology* 228(2-3):291–298.

CDC (Centers for Disease Control and Prevention). 1988. Health status of Vietnam veterans. II. Physical health. *Journal of the American Medical Association* 259:2708–2714.

Celik I, Tuluce Y, Isik I. 2006. Influence of subacute treatment of some plant growth regulators on serum marker enzymes and erythrocyte and tissue antioxidant defense and lipid peroxidation in rats. *Journal of Biochemical and Molecular Toxicology* 20(4):174–182.

Chancellor AM, Slattery JM, Fraser H. 1993. Risk factors for motor neuron disease: A case–control study based on patients from the Scottish motor neuron disease register. *Journal of Neurology, Neurosurgery, and Psychiatry* 56:1200–1206.

Dahlgren J, Warshaw R, Horsak RD, Parker FM 3rd, Takhar H. 2003. Exposure assessment of residents living near a wood treatment plant. *Environmental Research* 92(2):99–109.

Deapen DM, Henderson BE. 1986. A case–control study of amyotrophic lateral sclerosis. *American Journal of Epidemiology* 123:790–799.

Decoufle P, Holmgreen P, Boyle CA, Stroup NE. 1992. Self-reported health status of Vietnam veterans in relation to perceived exposed to herbicides and combat. *American Journal of Epidemiology* 135:312–323.

Di Monte D, Lavasani M, Manning-Bog A. 2002. Environmental factors in Parkinson's disease. *NeuroToxicology* 23(4-5):487–502.

Drechsel DA, Patel M. 2008. Role of reactive oxygen species in the neurotoxicity of environmental agents implicated in Parkinson's disease. *Free Radical Biology and Medicine* 44(11): 1873–1886.

Duffard R, Garcia G, Rosso S, Bortolozzi A, Madariaga M, Di Paolo O, Evangelista De Duffard A. 1996. Central nervous system myelin deficit in rats exposed to 2,4-dichlorophenoxyacetic acid throughout lactation. *Neurotoxicology and Teratology* 18(6):691–696.

Engel LS, Checkoway H, Keifer MC, Seixas NS, Longstreth WT, Scott KC, Hudnell K, Anger WK, Camicioli R. 2001. Parkinsonism and occupational exposure to pesticides. *Occupational and Environmental Medicine* 58:582–589.

Evangelista de Duffard AM, Orta C, Duffard RO. 1990. Behavioral changes in rats fed a diet containing 2,4-dichlorophenoxyacetic butyl ester. 1990. *Neurotoxicology* 11:563–572.

Evangelista de Duffard AM, Bortolozzi A, Duffard RO. 1995. Altered behavioral responses in 2,4-dichlorophenoxyacetic acid treated and amphetamine challenged rats. *Neurotoxicology* 16(3):479–488.

Filippini G, Bordo B, Crenna P, Massetto N, Musicco M, Boeri R. 1981. Relationship between clinical and electrophysiological findings and indicators of heavy exposure to 2,3,7,8-tetrachlorodibenzodioxin. *Scandinavian Journal of Work, Environment, and Health* 7:257–262.

Firestone JA, Smith-Weller T, Franklin G, Swanson P, Longstreth WT Jr, Checkoway H. 2005. Pesticides and risk of Parkinson disease: A population-based case–control study. *Archives of Neurology* 62(1):91–95.

Gallagher JP, Sander M. 1987. Trauma and amyotrophic lateral sclerosis: A report of 78 patients. *Acta Neurologica Scandinavia* 75:1041–1043.

Garcia C, Pascual JA, Mena E, Hernandez T. 2004. Influence of the stabilisation of organic materials on their biopesticide effect in soils. *Bioresource Technology* 95(2):215–221.

Garcia GB, Konjuh C, Duffard RO, De Duffard AME. 2006. Dopamine-beta-hydroxylase immunohistochemical study in the locus coeruleus of neonate rats exposed to 2,4-dichlorophenoxyacetic acid through mother's milk. *Drug and Chemical Toxicology* 29(4):435–442.

Gauthier E, Fortier I, Courchcesne F, Pepin P, Mortimer J, Gauvreau D. 2001. Environmental pesticide exposure as a risk factor for Alzheimer's disease: A case–control study. *Environmental Research* 86:37–45.

Gilioli R, Cotroneo L, Bulgheroni C, Genta PA, Rota E, Cannatelli P, Fereari E. 1979. Neurological monitoring of workers exposed to TCDD: Preliminary neurophysiological results. *Activitas Nervosa Superior* 21:288–290.

Goldstein NP, Jones PH, Brown JR. 1959. Peripheral neuropathy after exposure to an ester of dichlorophenoxyacetic acid. *Journal of the American Medical Association* 171:1306–1309.

Gorell JM, Johnson CC, Rybicki BA, Peterson EL, Richardson RJ. 1998. The risk of Parkinson's disease with exposure to pesticides, farming, well water, and rural living. *Neurology* 50:1346–1350.

Grahmann F, Claus D, Grehl H, Neundoerfer B. 1993. Electrophysiologic evidence for a toxic polyneuropathy in rats after exposure to 2,3,7,8-tetrachlorodibenzo-*p*-dioxin (TCDD). *Journal of Neurological Sciences* 115(1):71–75.

Grehl H, Grahmann F, Claus D, Neundorfer B. 1993. Histologic evidence for a toxic polyneuropathy due to exposure to 2,3,7,8-tetrachlorodibenzo-*p*-dioxin (TCDD) in rats. *Acta Neurologica Scandinavica* 88(5):354–357.

Hancock DB, Martin ER, Mayhew GM, Stajich JM, Jewett R, Stacy MA, Scott BL, Vance JM, Scott WK. 2008. Pesticide exposure and risk of Parkinson's disease: A family-based case–control study. *BMC Neurology* 8(6).

Hanisch R, Dworsky RL, Henderson BE. 1976. A search for clues to the cause of amyotrophic lateral sclerosis. *Archives of Neurology* 33:456–457.

Hatcher JM, Pennell KD, Miller GW. 2008. Parkinson's disease and pesticides: A toxicological perspective. *Trends in Pharmacological Sciences* 29(6):322–329.

Hertzman C, Wiens M, Snow B, Kelly S, Calne D. 1994. A case–control study of occupational of Parkinson's disease in a horticultural region of British Columbia. *Movement Disorders* 9:69–75.

Hoffman RE, Stehr-Green PA, Webb KB, Evans RG, Knutsen AP, Schramm WF, Staake JL, Gibson BB, Steinberg KK. 1986. Health effects of long-term exposure to 2,3,7,8-tetrachlorodibenzo-*p*-dioxin. *Journal of the American Medical Association* 255:2031–2038.

Hojo R, Kakeyama M, Kurokawa Y, Aoki Y, Yonemoto J, Tohyama C. 2008. Learning behavior in rat offspring after in utero and lactational exposure to either TCDD or PCB126. *Environmental Health and Preventive Medicine* 13(3):169–180.

Huang P, Rannug A, Ahlbom E, Haakansson H, Ceccatelli S. 2000. Effect of 2,3,7,8-tetrachlorodibenzo-*p*-dioxin on the expression of cytochrome P450 1A1, the aryl hydrocarbon receptor, and the aryl hydrocarbon receptor nuclear translocator in rat brain and pituitary. *Toxicology and Applied Pharmacology Academic Press* 169(2):159–167.

IOM (Institute of Medicine). 1994. *Veterans and Agent Orange: Health Effects of Herbicides Used in Vietnam.* Washington, DC: National Academy Press.

IOM. 1996. *Veterans and Agent Orange: Update 1996.* Washington, DC: National Academy Press.

IOM. 1999. *Veterans and Agent Orange: Update 1998.* Washington, DC: National Academy Press.

IOM. 2001. *Veterans and Agent Orange: Update 2000.* Washington, DC: National Academy Press.

IOM. 2003. *Veterans and Agent Orange: Update 2002.* Washington, DC: The National Academies Press.

IOM. 2005. *Veterans and Agent Orange: Update 2004.* Washington, DC: The National Academies Press.

IOM. 2007. *Veterans and Agent Orange: Update 2006.* Washington, DC: The National Academies Press.

Kamel F, Engel LS, Gladen BC, Hoppin JA, Alavanja MC, Sandler DP. 2005. Neurologic symptoms in licensed private pesticide applicators in the Agricultural Health Study. *Environmental Health Perspectives* 113(7):877–882.

Kamel F, Engel LS, Gladen BC, Hoppin JA, Alavanja MC, Sandler DP. 2007a. Neurologic symptoms in licensed pesticide applicators in the Agricultural Health Study. *Human and Experimental Toxicology* 26(3):243–250.

Kamel F, Tanner C, Umbach D, Hoppin J, Alavanja M, Blair A, Comyns K, Goldman S, Korell M, Langston J, Ross G, Sandler D. 2007b. Pesticide exposure and self-reported Parkinson's disease in the Agricultural Health Study. *American Journal of Epidemiology* 165(4):364–374.

Kim JS, Lim HS, Cho SI, Cheong HK, Lim MK. 2003. Impact of Agent Orange exposure among Korean Vietnam veterans. *Industrial Health* 41(3):149–157.

Kim SY, Yang JH. 2005. Neurotoxic effects of 2,3,7,8-tetrachlorodibenzo-*p*-dioxin in cerebellar granule cells. *Experimental and Molecular Medicine* 37:58–64.

Kim SY, Lee HG, Choi EJ, Park KY, Yang JH. 2007. TCDD alters PKC signaling pathways in developing neuronal cells in culture. *Chemosphere* 67(9):S421–S427.

Klein C, Lohmann-Hedrich K. 2007. Impact of recent genetic findings in Parkinson's disease. *Current Opinion in Neurology* 20(4):453–464.

Konjuh C, Garcia G, Lopez L, de Duffard AME, Brusco A, Duffard R. 2008. Neonatal hypomyelination by the herbicide 2,4-dichlorophenoxyacetic acid. Chemical and ultrastructural studies in rats. *Toxicological Sciences* 104(2):332–340.

Kuopio A, Marttila RJ, Helenius H, Rinne UK. 1999. Environmental risk factors in Parkinson's disease. *Movement Disorders* 14:928–939.

Kurtzke JF, Beebe GW. 1980. Epidemiology of amyotrophic lateral sclerosis: 1. A case–control comparison based on ALS deaths. *Neurology* 30:453–462.

Langston JW. 2006. The Parkinson's complex: Parkinsonism is just the tip of the iceberg. *Annals of Neurology* 59(4):591–596.

Lee HG, Kim SY, Choi EJ, Park KY, Yang JH. 2007. Translocation of PKC-betaII is mediated via RACK-1 in the neuronal cells following dioxin exposure. *NeuroToxicology* 28(2):408–414.

Lensu S, Miettinen R, Pohjanvirta R, Lindén J, Tuomisto J. 2006. Assessment by c-Fos immunostaining of changes in brain neural activity induced by 2,3,7,8-tetrachlorodibenzo-*p*-dioxin (TCDD) and leptin in rats. *Basic and Clinical Pharmacology and Toxicology.* 98:363–371.

Liang CL, Wang TT, Luby-Phelps K, German DC. 2007. Mitochondria mass is low in mouse substantia nigra dopamine neurons: implications for Parkinson's disease. *Experimental Neurology* 203(2):370–380.

Liou HH, Tsai MC, Chen CJ, Jeng JS, Chang YC, Chen SY, Chen RC. 1997. Environmental risk factors and Parkinson's disease: A case–control study in Taiwan. *Neurology* 48:1583–1588.

McGuire V, Longstreth WT, Nelson LM, Koepsell TD, Checkoway H, Morgan MS, van Belle G. 1997. Occupational exposure and amyotrophic lateral sclerosis: A population-based case–control study. *American Journal of Epidemiology* 145:1076–1088.

Michalek JE, Akhtar FZ, Arezzo JC, Garabrant DH, Albers JW. 2001. Serum dioxin and peripheral neuropathy in veterans of Operation Ranch Hand. *Neurotoxicology* 22:479–490.

Mitsui T, Sugiyama N, Maeda S, Tohyama C, Arita J. 2006. Perinatal exposure to 2,3,7,8-tetrachlorodibenzo-*p*-dioxin suppresses contextual fear conditioning-accompanied activation of cyclic AMP response element-binding protein in the hippocampal CA1 region of male rats. *Neuroscience Letters* 398(3):206–210.

Mohammad FK, St. Omer VE. 1985. Behavioral and developmental effects in rats following in utero exposure to 2,4-D/2,4,5-T mixture. *Neurobehavioral Toxicology and Teratology* 8:551–560.

Morahan JM, Pamphlett R. 2006. Amyotrophic lateral sclerosis and exposure to environmental toxins: An Australian case–control study. *Neuroepidemiology* 27(3):130–135.

Moses M, Lilis R, Crow KD, Thornton J, Fischbein A, Anderson HA, Selikoff IJ. 1984. Health status of workers with past exposure to 2,3,7,8-tetrachlorodibenzo-*p*-dioxin in the manufacture of 2,4,5-trichlorophenoxyacetic acid: Comparison of findings with and without chloracne. *American Journal of Industrial Medicine* 5:161–182.

Nunomura A, Moreira PI, Lee HG, Zhu X, Castellani RJ, Smith MA, Perry G. 2007. Neuronal death and survival under oxidative stress in Alzheimer and Parkinson diseases. *CNS and Neurological Disorders—Drug Targets* 6(6):411–423.

O'Toole BI, Marshall RP, Grayson DA, Schureck RJ, Dobson M, Ffrench M, Pulvertaft B, Meldrum L, Bolton J, Vennard J. 1996. The Australian Vietnam Veterans Health Study: III. Psychological health of Australian Vietnam veterans and its relationship to combat. *International Journal of Epidemiology* 25(2):331–340.

Palmeira CM, Moreno AJ, Madeira VM. 1994a. Interactions of herbicides 2,4-D and dinoseb with liver mitochondrial bioenergetics. *Toxicology and Applied Pharmacology* 127:50–57.

Palmeira CM, Moreno AJ, Madeira VMC. 1994b. Metabolic alterations in hepatocytes promoted by the herbicides paraquat, dinoseb and 2,4-D. *Archives of Toxicology* 68:24–31.

Palmeira CM, Moreno AJ, Madeira VM. 1995a. Effects of paraquat, dinoseb and 2,4-D on intracellular calcium and on vasopressin-induced calcium mobilization in isolated hepatocytes. *Archives of Toxicology* 69:460–466.

Palmeira CM, Moreno AJ, Madeira VM. 1995b. Thiols metabolism is altered by the herbicides paraquat, dinoseb and 2,4-D: A study in isolated hepatocytes. *Toxicology Letters* 81:115–123.

Park RM, Schulte PA, Bowman JD, Walker JT, Bondy SC, Yost MG, Touchstone JA, Dosemeci M. 2005. Potential occupational risks for neurodegenerative diseases. *American Journal of Industrial Medicine* 48(1):63–77.

Pazderova-Vejlupkova J, Lukas E, Nemcova M, Pickova J, Jirasek L. 1981. The development and prognosis of chronic intoxication by tetrachlorodibenzo-*p*-dioxin in men. *Archives of Environmental Health* 36:5–11.

Pelclová D, Fenclová Z, Dlasková Z, Urban P, Lukás E, Procházka B, Rappe C, Preiss J, Kocan A, Vejlupková J. 2001. Biochemical, neuropsychological, and neurological abnormalities following 2,3,7,8-tetrachlorodibenzo-*p*-dioxin (TCDD) exposure. *Archives of Environmental Health* 56(6):493–500.

Pelclová D, Fenclová Z, Preiss J, Prochazka B, Spacil J, Dubska Z, Okrouhlik B, Lukás E, Urban P. 2002. Lipid metabolism and neuropsychological follow-up study of workers exposed to 2,3,7,8-tetrachlordibenzo-*p*-dioxin. *International Archives of Occupational and Environmental Health* 75:S60–S66.

Roelofs-Iverson RA, Mulder DW, Elverback LR, Kurland LT, Craig AM. 1984. ALS and heavy metals: A pilot case–control study. *Neurology* 34:393–395.

Rosen DR, Siddique T, Patterson D, Figlewicz DA, Sapp P, Hentati A, Donaldson D, Goto J, O'Regan JP, Deng HX, Rahmani Z, Krizus A, McKenna-Yasek D, Cayabyab A, Gaston S, Tanzi R, Halperin JJ, Herzfeldt B, Van den Berg R, Hung WY, Bird T, Deng G, Mulder DW, Smith C, Laing NG, Soriano E, Pericak-Vance MA, Haines J, Rouleau GA, Gusella J, Horvitz HR, Brown RH. 1993. Mutations in Cu/Zn superoxide dismutase gene are associated with familial amyotrophic lateral sclerosis. *Nature* 362(6415):59–62.

Rosso SB, Caceres AO, Evangelista de Duffard AM, Duffard RO, Quiroga S. 2000a. 2,4-dichlorophenoxyacetic acid disrupts the cytoskeleton and disorganizes the Golgi apparatus of cultured neurons. *Toxicological Sciences* 56:133–140.

Rosso SB, Garcia GB, Madariaga MJ, De Duffard AME, Duffard RO. 2000b. 2,4-dichlorophenoxyacetic acid in developing rats alters behaviour, myelination and regions brain gangliosides pattern. *NeuroToxicology* 21(1-2):155–164.

Rowland LP. 1998. Diagnosis of amyotrophic lateral sclerosis. *Journal of the Neurological Sciences* 160 (Suppl 1):S6–S24.

Rowland LP, Shneider NA. 2001. Amyotrophic lateral sclerosis. *The New England Journal of Medicine* 344(22):1688–1700.

Sarnico I, Boroni F, Benarese M, Sigala S, Lanzillotta A, Battistin L, Spano P, Pizzi M. 2008. Activation of NF-kappaB p65/c-Rel dimer is associated with neuroprotection elicited by mGlu5 receptor agonists against MPP(+) toxicity in SK-N-SH cells. *Journal of Neural Transmission* 115(5):669–676.

Savettieri G, Salemi G, Arcara A, Cassata M, Castiglione MG, Fierro B. 1991. A case–control study of amyotrophic lateral sclerosis. *Neuroepidemiology* 10:242–245.

Seidler A, Hellenbrand W, Robra BP, Vieregge P, Nischan P, Joerg J, Oertel WH, Ulm G, Schneider E. 1996. Possible environmental, occupational, and other etiologic factors for Parkinson's disease: A case–control study in Germany. *Neurology* 46:1275–1284.

Semchuk KM, Love EJ, Lee RG. 1992. Parkinson's disease and exposure to agricultural work and pesticide chemicals. *Neurology* 42:1328–1335.

Shen D, Dalton TP, Nebert DW, Shertzer HG. 2005. Glutathione redox state regulates mitochondrial reactive oxygen production. *Journal of Biological Chemistry* 280(27):25305–25312.

Sherer T, Betarbet R, Stout A, Lund S, Baptista M, Panov A, Cookson M, Greenamyre J. 2002a. An in vitro model of Parkinson's disease: Linking mitochondrial impairment to altered alpha-synuclein metabolism and oxidative damage. *The Journal of Neuroscience: The Official Journal of the Society for Neuroscience* 22(16):7006–7015.

Singer R, Moses M, Valciukas J, Lilis R, Selikoff IJ. 1982. Nerve conduction velocity studies of workers employed in the manufacture of phenoxy herbicides. *Environmental Research* 29(2):297–311.

Solomon C, Poole J, Palmer KT, Peveler R, Coggon D. 2007. Neuropsychiatric symptoms in past users of sheep dip and other pesticides. *Occupational and Environmental Medicine* 64(4): 259–266.

St. Omer VEV, Mohammad FF. 1987. Ontogeny of swimming behavior and brain catecholamine turnover in rats prenatally exposed to a mixture of 2,4-dichlorophenoxyacetic and 2,4,5-trichlorophenoxyacetic acids. *Neuropharmacology* 9:1351–1358.

Stehr PA, Stein G, Webb K, Schramm W, Gedney WB, Donnell HD, Ayres S, Falk H, Sampson E, Smith SJ. 1986. A pilot epidemiologic study of possible health effects associated with 2,3,7,8-tetrachlorodibenzo-*p*-dioxin contaminations in Missouri. *Archives of Environmental Health* 41:16–22.

Stern M, Dulaney E, Gruber SB, Golbe L, Bergen M, Hurtig H, Gollomp S, Stolley P. 1991. The epidemiology of Parkinson's disease: A case–control study of young-onset and old-onset patients. *Archives of Neurology* 48:903–907.

Sturtz N, Deis RP, Jahn GA, Duffard R, Evangelista de Duffard AM. 2008. Effect of 2,4-dichlorophenoxyacetic acid on rat maternal behavior. *Toxicology* 247(2-3):73–79.

Suskind RR, Hertzberg VS. 1984. Human health effects of 2,4,5-T and its toxic contaminants. *Journal of the American Medical Association* 251(18):2372–2380.

Sweeney, MH, Fingerhut MA, Arezzo JC, Hornung RW, Connally LB. 1993. Peripheral neuropathy after occupational exposure to 2,3,7,8-tetrachlorodibenzo-*p*-dioxin (TCDD). *American Journal of Industrial Medicine* 23(6):845–858.

Taylor CA, Saint-Hilaire MH, Cupples LA, Thomas CA, Burchard AE, Feldman RG, Myers RH. 1999. Environmental, medical, and family history risk factors for Parkinson's disease: A New England-based case–control study. *American Journal of Medical Genetics (Neuropsychiatric Genetics)* 88:742–749.

Todd RL. 1962. A case of 2,4-D intoxication. *Journal of the Iowa Medical Society* 52:663–664.

Thiffault C, Langston WJ, Di Monte DA. 2001. Acute exposure to organochlorine pesticides does not affect striatal dopamine in mice. *Neurotoxicity Research* 3(6):537–543.

Urban P, Pelclova D, Lukas E, Kupka K, Preiss J, Fenclova Z, Smerhovsky Z. 2007. Neurological and neurophysiological examinations on workers with chronic poisoning by 2,3,7,8-TCDD: Follow-up 35 years after exposure. *European Journal of Neurology* 14(2):213–218.

Uversky V, Kiowa Bower JL, Fink AL. 2002. Synergistic effects of pesticides and metals on the fibrillation of α-synuclein: Implications for Parkinson's disease. *NeuroToxicology* 23:527–536.

Visintainer PF, Barone M, McGee H, Peterson EL. 1995. Proportionate mortality study of Vietnam-era veterans of Michigan. *Journal of Occupational and Environmental Medicine* 37:423–428.

Webb KB, Evans RG, Stehr P, Ayres SM. 1987. Pilot study on health effects of environmental 2,3,7,8-TCDD in Missouri. *American Journal of Industrial Medicine* 11:685–691.

Weisskopf MG, O'Reilly EJ, McCullough ML, Calle EE, Thun MJ, Cudkowicz M, Ascherio A. 2005. Prospective study of military service and mortality from ALS. *Neurology* 64(1):32–37.

Williamson MA, Gasiewicz TA, Opanashuk LA. 2005. Aryl hydrocarbon receptor expression and activity in cerebellar granule neuroblasts: Implications for development and dioxin neurotoxicity. *Toxicological Sciences* 83:340–348.

Zober A, Ott MG, Messerer P. 1994. Morbidity follow-up study of BASF employees exposed to 2,3,7,8-tetrachlorodibenzo-*p*-dioxin (TCDD) after a 1953 chemical reactor incident. *Occupational and Environmental Medicine* 51:479–486.

9

Other Health Effects

This chapter discusses data on the possible association between exposure to the herbicides used in Vietnam—2,4-dichlorophenoxyacetic acid (2,4-D), 2,4,5-trichlorophenoxyacetic acid (2,4,5-T), picloram, and cacodylic acid—and 2,3,7,8-tetrachlorodibenzo-*p*-dioxin (TCDD), a contaminant of 2,4,5-T, and several noncancer health outcomes: chloracne, porphyria cutanea tarda (PCT), respiratory disorders, immune-system disorders, diabetes, lipid and lipoprotein disorders, gastrointestinal and digestive disease (including liver toxicity), circulatory disorders, and adverse effects on thyroid homeostasis.

For each type of health outcome, background information is followed by a brief summary of the findings described in earlier reports by the Institute of Medicine (IOM) Committee to Review the Health Effects in Vietnam Veterans of Exposure to Herbicides. In the discussion of the most recent scientific literature, studies are grouped by exposure type (Vietnam veteran, occupational, or environmental). For articles that report on only a single health outcome and that are not revisiting a previously studied population, design information is summarized with the results; design information on other studies can be found in Chapter 5. A synopsis of toxicologic and clinical information related to the biologic plausibility that the chemicals of interest can influence the occurrence of a health outcome is presented next and followed by a synthesis of all the material reviewed. Each health-outcome section ends with the present committee's conclusions regarding the strength of the evidence that supports an association with the chemicals of interest. The categories of association and the committee's approach to categorizing the health outcomes are discussed in Chapters 1 and 2.

CHLORACNE

Chloracne is a skin disease that is characteristic of exposure to TCDD and other diaromatic organochlorine chemicals. It shares some pathologic processes (such as the occlusion of the orifice of the sebaceous follicle) with more common forms of acne (such as acne vulgaris), but it can be differentiated by the presence of epidermoid inclusion cysts, which are caused by proliferation and hyperkeratinization (horn-like cornification) of the epidermis and sebaceous gland epithelium. Although chloracne is typically distributed over the eyes, ears, and neck, it can also occur on the trunk, genitalia, and buttocks of chemical-industry workers exposed to TCDD (Neuberger et al., 1998).

Chloracne has been exploited as a marker of exposure in epidemiologic studies of populations exposed to TCDD and related chemicals. It is one of the few findings in humans that are consistently associated with such exposure, and it is a well-validated indicator of high-dose exposure to TCDD and related chemicals (Sweeney et al., 1997/1998). If chloracne occurs, it appears shortly after the chemical exposure, not after a long latent period; therefore, new cases of chloracne among Vietnam veterans would not be the result of exposure during the Vietnam War. Although it is resistant to acne treatments, it usually regresses. It should be noted that absence of chloracne does not necessarily indicate absence of substantial exposure to TCDD, as is apparent from studies of people with documented exposure to TCDD after the Seveso incident (Baccarelli et al., 2005a), nor is there necessarily a correlation between serum TCDD concentration and the occurrence or severity of chloracne.

Conclusions from *VAO* and Previous Updates

The committee responsible for *Veterans and Agent Orange: Health Effects of Herbicides Used in Vietnam*, hereafter referred to as *VAO* (IOM, 1994), determined that there was sufficient evidence of an association between exposure to at least one chemical of interest (TCDD) and chloracne. Additional information available to the committees responsible for *Veterans and Agent Orange: Update 1996* (IOM, 1996), *Update 1998* (IOM, 1999), *Update 2000* (IOM, 2001), *Update 2002* (IOM, 2003), *Update 2004* (IOM, 2005), and *Update 2006* (IOM, 2007) has not modified that conclusion.

Even in the absence of full understanding of the cellular and molecular mechanisms that lead to the disease, several notable reviews (Panteleyev and Bickers, 2006; Sweeney and Mocarelli, 2000) have deemed the clinical and epidemiologic evidence of dioxin-induced chloracne to be strong. The occupational epidemiologic literature has many examples of chloracne in workers after reported industrial exposures (Beck et al., 1989; Bond et al., 1987, 1989a,b; Cook et al., 1980; Goldman, 1972; May, 1973, 1982; Oliver, 1975; Pazderova-Vejlupkova et al., 1981; Poland et al., 1971; Suskind and Hertzberg, 1984; Suskind et al.,

1953; Zober et al., 1990). With relative risk (RR) estimates as high as 5.5 in exposed workers compared with referent nonexposed workers, Bond et al. (1989a) identified a dose–response relationship between probable exposure to TCDD and chloracne. Not everyone exposed to relatively high doses develop chloracne, and some with lower exposure may demonstrate the condition (Beck et al., 1989).

Almost 200 cases of chloracne were recorded among those residing in the vicinity of the accidental industrial release of dioxin in Seveso, Italy; most cases were in children, were in people who lived in the highest-exposure zone, and had resolved within 7 years (Assennato et al., 1989a,b; Caramaschi et al., 1981; Mocarelli et al., 1991). No cases of chloracne were identified in conjunction with the nonextreme environmental dioxin contamination at Times Beach, Missouri (Webb et al., 1987).

Exposures of Vietnam veterans were substantially lower than those observed in occupational studies and in environmental disasters, such as in Seveso. The long period since the putative exposure has imposed methodologic limitations on studies of Vietnam cohorts for chloracne. Nonetheless, the Vietnam Experience Study (VES; CDC, 1988) found that chloracne was self-reported more often by Vietnam veterans than by Vietnam-era veterans (odds ratio [OR] = 3.9). Excess risk was also found in Vietnam vs era veterans among subjects who were physically examined (OR = 7.3). In comparison with a nonexposed group, Air Force Ranch Hand personnel potentially exposed to Agent Orange reported significant excess of acne (OR = 1.6) (Wolfe et al., 1990), but no cases of chloracne or postinflammatory scars were found on physical examination 20 years after the potential herbicide exposure (AFHS, 1991b).

Biologic Plausibility

Previous updates have reported that chloracne-like skin lesions have been observed in several animal species in response to exposure to TCDD but not to purified phenoxy herbicides. Data accruing over the last several decades demonstrated that TCDD alters differentiation of human keratinocytes, and more recent studies have illuminated how. Geusau et al. (2005) found that TCDD accelerates the events associated with early differentiation but also obstructs completion of differentiation. Panteleyev and Bickers (2006) proposed that the major mechanism of TCDD induction of chloracne is activation of the stem cells in the basal layer of the skin to differentiate and inhibition of their ability to commit fully to a differentiated status. Recent work with a constitutively activated form of the aryl hydrocarbon receptor (AHR) implicated additional inflammation-related mechanisms by which TCDD exposure may lead to chloracne (Tauchi et al., 2005). The data provide a biologically plausible mechanism for the induction of chloracne by TCDD.

Synthesis

No epidemiologic data in the last decade have refuted the conclusion of prior VAO committees that the evidence of an association between exposure to dioxin and chloracne is sufficient. The formation of chloracne lesions after administration of TCDD has been observed in some species of laboratory animals.

Conclusion

On the basis of numerous epidemiologic studies of occupationally and environmentally exposed populations and supportive toxicologic information, previous VAO committees have consistently concluded that there is sufficient evidence of an association between exposure to at least one chemical of interest and chloracne. Because TCDD-associated chloracne becomes evident shortly after exposure, there is no risk of new cases long after service in Vietnam. Given the established relationship of an association between TCDD and chloracne and the long period that has elapsed since service in Vietnam, the present committee concludes that the emergence of additional biologic or epidemiologic evidence that would merit review and deliberation by later VAO committees is unlikely.

PORPHYRIA CUTANEA TARDA

Porphyrias are uncommon disorders caused by deficiencies of enzymes involved in the pathway of biosynthesis of heme, the iron-containing nonprotein portion of the hemoglobin molecule. PCT is a heterogeneous group of disorders caused by a deficiency of a specific enzyme, uroporphyrinogen decarboxylase. PCT, the most common of this group of disorders, can be inherited but usually is acquired. Type I PCT, which accounts for 80–90% of all cases, is an acquired disease that typically becomes evident in adulthood. It can occur spontaneously but usually occurs in conjunction with environmental factors, such as alcohol consumption, exposure to estrogens, or use of some medications.

The most important clinical finding in PCT is cutaneous photosensitivity. Sensitivity to sunlight is thought to result from the excitation of excess porphyrins in the skin by long-wave ultraviolet radiation, which leads to cell damage. Fluid-filled vesicles and bullae develop on sun-exposed areas of the face and on the dorsa surfaces of the hands, feet, forearms, and legs. Other features include hypertrichosis (excess hair) and hyperpigmentation (increased pigment), especially on the face. People with PCT have increased porphyrins in the liver, plasma, urine, and stools. Iron, estrogens, alcohol, viral hepatitis, and chlorinated hydrocarbons can aggravate the disorder. Iron overload is almost always present in people who have PCT.

Conclusions from *VAO* and Previous Updates

On the basis of strong animal studies and case reports demonstrating TCDD-induced PCT and resolution after cessation of exposure, the committee responsible for *VAO* determined that there was sufficient evidence of an association between exposure to TCDD and PCT in genetically susceptible people.

Epidemiologic studies of occupational populations have indicated inconsistent association between the chemicals of interest and increased urinary uroporphyrin. Bleiberg et al. (1964) reported the increased urinary uroporphyrin in 11 of 29 workers in a factory that manufactured 2,4-D and 2,4,5-T and the manifestation of some clinical evidence of PCT in three of them. In a follow-up study of the same facility 6 years later, no abnormalities in urinary porphyrin were observed (Poland et al., 1971). Calvert et al. (1992) reported no difference in porphyrinuria or the occurrence of PCT between 281 workers in the National Institute for Occupational Safety and Health (NIOSH) cohort who were involved in the production of trichlorophenol and were exposed to TCDD and 260 nonexposed workers. Serum TCDD concentration was not associated with uroporphyrin or coproporphyrin concentrations.

Among people who were exposed to TCDD as a result of the 1976 chemical-plant explosion in Seveso, Italy, clinical PCT was observed only in a brother and a sister who had a mutant enzyme that confers susceptibility in the heterozygous state. In 1977, 60 Seveso residents were tested for increased porphyrins, and 13 had secondary coproporphyrinuria; increased concentrations persisted in only three cases that were thought to be due to liver damage and alcohol consumption (Doss et al., 1984). In the Quail Run mobile-home park in Missouri, residents exposed to dioxin as a result of the spraying of waste oil contaminated with TCDD were found to have higher urinary uroporphyrins than compared to controls, but no cases of clinical PCT were diagnosed (Hoffman et al., 1986; Stehr-Green et al., 1987).

The baseline study of the US Air Force Ranch Hands (AFHS, 1984) showed no difference in uroporphyrin or coproporphyrin concentrations in urine between Ranch Hands and controls. There were no indications of the clinical appearance of PCT in Ranch Hands. Follow-up studies of the Ranch Hand cohort revealed that mean uroporphyrin was greater in the comparison group than in the Ranch Hands, whereas mean coproporphyrin was higher in Ranch Hands. The clinical significance of the small differences between the Ranch Hands and the comparison groups was uncertain.

The committee responsible for *Update 1996* considered three additional nonpositive citations of populations that had substantial exposure to TCDD. Jung et al. (1994) presented porphyrin data on former workers in a German pesticide plant that had manufactured 2,4-D and 2,4,5-T. Of 170 men tested, 27 had present or past chloracne. The study found no difference in porphyrin concentrations between subjects with and without chloracne. There was also no relationship between abnormal results of liver-function tests and porphyrin concentrations and the presence of chloracne and no relationship between porphyrin concentrations in urine, red blood cells or plasma, and TCDD concentrations in adipose tissue. Three cases of chronic hepatic porphyria (none with overt PCT and none with chloracne) were identified—a number that did not exceed the expected prevalence in this population. Von Benner et al. (1994) found no indication of clinical porphyria in self-referred workers at six other German chemical plants. Another report on the NIOSH cohort (Calvert et al., 1994) was negative. On the basis of the cumulative findings, the committee responsible for *Update 1996* concluded that there was only limited or suggestive evidence of an association. *Update 1998*, *Update 2000*, *Update 2002*, *Update 2004*, and *Update 2006* did not change the revised conclusion.

Because PCT is manifested shortly after exposure to TCDD, new cases of PCT attributable to exposure during the Vietnam War are not expected to occur.

Biologic Plausibility

PCT has not been replicated in animal studies of effects of TCDD, although other porphyrin abnormalities have been reported. However, administration of TCDD to mice results in an accumulation of uroporphyrin that occurs in a manner that requires the AHR, Cytochrome P450 1A1 (CYP1A1), and CYP1A2 (Robinson et al., 2002; Smith et al., 2001; Uno et al., 2004).

Synthesis

No epidemiologic data have emerged in the last decade that refute the conclusion of previous VAO committees that there is limited or suggestive evidence of an association between the chemicals of interest and PCT.

Conclusion

On the basis of the evidence reviewed here and in previous VAO reports, the committee concludes that there is limited or suggestive evidence of an association between exposure to at least one chemical of interest and PCT. The occurrence of PCT is rare and may be influenced by genetic predisposition in people who have low concentrations of protoporphyrinogen decarboxylase. Because TCDD-associated changes in porphyrin excretion become evident shortly after exposure, there is no risk that new cases will occur long after service in Vietnam. Given the recognized association between TCDD and porphyrin excretion and the long period that has elapsed since service in Vietnam, the committee concludes that additional biologic and epidemiologic evidence meriting review and deliberation by this or by later VAO committees is unlikely to occur.

RESPIRATORY DISORDERS

For the purposes of this report, nonmalignant respiratory disorders comprise acute and chronic lung diseases other than cancer. Acute nonmalignant respiratory disorders include pneumonia and other respiratory infections; they can increase in frequency and severity when the normal defense mechanisms of the lower respiratory tract are compromised. Chronic nonmalignant respiratory disorders generally take two forms: airways disease and parenchymal disease. Airways disease encompasses disorders, among them asthma and chronic obstructive pulmonary disease (COPD), characterized by obstruction of the flow of air out of the lungs. COPD is also known as chronic obstructive airways disease and includes emphysema and chronic bronchitis. Parenchymal disease, or interstitial disease, generally includes disorders that cause inflammation and scarring of the deep lung tissue, including the air sacs and supporting structures; parenchymal disease is less common than airways disease and is characterized by reductions in lung capacity, although it can include a component of airway obstruction. Some severe chronic lung disorders, such as cystic fibrosis, are hereditary. Because Vietnam veterans received health screenings before entering military service, few severe hereditary chronic lung disorders are expected in that population.

The most important risk factor for many nonmalignant respiratory disorders is inhalation of cigarette smoke. Although exposure to cigarette smoke is not associated with all diseases of the lungs, it is the major cause of many airways disorders, especially COPD; it contributes to some interstitial disease; and it compromises host defenses in such a way that people who smoke are generally more susceptible to some types of pneumonia. Cigarette-smoking also makes almost every respiratory disorder more severe and symptomatic than it would otherwise be. The frequency of habitual cigarette-smoking varies with occupation, socioeconomic status, and generation. For those reasons, cigarette-smoking can be a major confounding factor in interpreting the literature on risk factors for respiratory disease. Vietnam veterans are reported to smoke more heavily than are non-Vietnam veterans (McKinney et al., 1997).

It is well known that causes of death from respiratory diseases, especially chronic diseases, are frequently misclassified on death certificates. Grouping various respiratory diseases for analysis, unless they all are associated with a given exposure, will lead to attenuation of the estimates of RR and to a diminution of statistical power. Moreover, deaths from respiratory and cardiovascular diseases (CVDs) are often confused. In particular, when persons have both conditions concurrently and both contributed to death, there may be some uncertainty about which cause should be selected as the primary underlying cause. In other instances, errors may arise in selecting one underlying cause in a complex chain of health events (for example, if COPD leads to congestive heart failure and then to respiratory failure). Many study populations were small, so investigators grouped deaths from all nonmalignant respiratory diseases into one category that combined pneumonia, influenza, and other diseases with COPD and asthma.

Conclusions from *VAO* and Previous Updates

The committee responsible for *VAO* concluded that there was inadequate or insufficient information to determine whether there is an association between exposure to the chemicals of interest and the respiratory disorders specified above. Additional information available to the committees responsible for *Update 1996* and *Update 1998* did not change that finding.

Update 2000 drew attention to findings on the Seveso cohort that suggested a higher mortality from nonmalignant respiratory disorders in study subjects, particularly males, who were more heavily exposed to TCDD. Those findings were not replicated in several other relevant studies, although one showed an increase that did not attain statistical significance. The committee responsible for *Update 2000* concluded that although new evidence suggested an increased risk of nonmalignant respiratory disorders, particularly COPD, in people exposed to TCDD, the observation was tentative and the information insufficient to determine whether there is an association between exposures to the chemicals of interest and respiratory disorders. Additional information available to the committee responsible for *Update 2002* did not change that finding.

Update 2004 included a new cross-sectional study of residents near a wood-treatment plant (Dahlgren et al., 2003). Soil and sediment samples from a ditch in the neighborhood contained dioxins and furans. Although exposed residents reported a greater frequency of chronic bronchitis by history (17.8% vs 5.7%; $p < 0.0001$) and asthma by history (40.5% vs 11.0%; $p < 0.0001$) than a "non-exposed" control group, the committee concluded that selection bias and recall bias limited the utility of the results and that there was a possibility of confounding in that history of tobacco use was not accounted for adequately.

Update 2006 reviewed a number of studies of veterans of the Vietnam War. Mortality from respiratory diseases was not found to be higher than expected in the Centers for Disease Control and Prevention VES (Boehmer et al., 2004), in the Air Force Health Study (Ketchum and Michalek, 2005), and in two Australian studies of Vietnam veterans (ADVA, 2005b,c). In contrast, in the US Army Chemical Corps cohort of Vietnam veterans, Kang et al. (2006) found that the prevalence of self-reported nonmalignant respiratory problems diagnosed by a doctor was significantly increased by about 40–60%, although no differences in the prevalence of respiratory problems was found in the subset of veterans whose serum TCDD was above 2.5 ppt.

In addition, *Update 2006* addressed new studies of potentially exposed occupational cohorts. No associations with respiratory mortality were found in a small subcohort of New Zealand phenoxy-herbicide sprayers included in the International Agency for Research on Cancer (IARC) cohort ('t Mannetje et al., 2005). In the Agricultural Health Study (AHS), no associations between the herbicide and mortality from COPD were found in private applicators or their spouses (Blair et al., 2005). A cross-sectional analysis of the AHS with data collected at enrollment among commercial pesticide applicators showed an association between "current" exposure to 2,4-D and the prevalence of wheeze. The committee was concerned about interpreting this finding because self-reported health conditions may not be reported accurately and there may be overreporting if people believe that their exposures were hazardous. As a result, the committee responsible for *Update 2006* did not change the original conclusion.

Table 9-1 summarizes the results of the relevant studies.

Update of the Epidemiologic Literature

Vietnam-Veteran Studies

Since *Update 2006*, there have been no publications concerning nonmalignant respiratory outcomes in Vietnam veterans.

Occupational Studies

The continuing AHS has generated several new publications concerning respiratory health problems. A common method was used: at time of enrollment, questionnaires regarding use of pesticides and health outcomes were administered, and subjects who returned both of them (about 40%) were included in the analyses. Subjects were then classified as having different health outcomes: wheeze, chronic bronchitis, farmer's lung, and asthma. Wheeze was defined as a positive response to the question "How many episodes of wheezing or whistling in your chest have you had in the past 12 months?" Farmer's lung and chronic bronchitis were defined if the subject reported having a doctor's diagnosis. Exposures to 40 specific chemicals used in the year before enrollment were assessed from the questionnaires. The analyses were cross-sectional studies of disease prevalence at the time of enrollment that compared the frequency of reported exposures in those who had the health outcome of interest versus the remainder of the cohort or a subset of the cohort; such an analysis is not equivalent to a case–control study.

There are now two reports of wheeze from the AHS: one that was reported in *Update 2006* and a new one. Wheeze is a cardinal sign of asthma. In the previous report (Hoppin et al., 2006a), the authors reported an OR of 1.3 (95% confidence interval [CI] 1.0–1.7) in commercial applicators for exposure to 2,4-D in the preceding year, adjusted for age, smoking status, asthma or atopy status, and body-mass index (BMI). In the later report (Hoppin et al., 2006b), the association with 2,4-D was attenuated (OR = 1.0, 95% CI 0.7–1.3), but the covariables included in the model were different (age, smoking status, asthma or atopy status, BMI, previous use of pesticides, and exposure to the herbicide chlorimuron-ethyl); the authors noted that adjustment for use of chlorimuron-ethyl attenuated the risk of wheeze reported to be significant in commercial applicators for seven pesticides in the earlier report. No associations with 2,4-D or dicamba were found in the private applicators.

TABLE 9-1 Selected Epidemiologic Studies—Nonmalignant Respiratory Disease

Reference	Study Population	Exposed Cases[a]	Estimated Relative Risk (95% CI)[a]
VIETNAM VETERANS			
Studies Reviewed in *Update 2006*			
Boehmer et al., 2004	Vietnam Experience Cohort Nonmalignant respiratory mortality (ICD-9 460–519)	20	0.8 (0.5–1.5)
Ketchum and Michalek, 2005	AFHS Nonmalignant respiratory mortality (ICD-9 460–519)	8	1.2 (0.6–2.5)
Kang et al., 2006	US Army Chemical Corps personnel Self-reported nonmalignant respiratory problems diagnosed by doctor		
	Deployed vs nondeployed	267	1.4 (1.1–1.8)
	Sprayed herbicides in Vietnam vs never	140	1.6 (1.3–2.1)
ADVA, 2005b	Third Australian Vietnam Veterans Mortality Study Deployed veterans vs Australian population		
	All branches		
	Respiratory system diseases	239	0.8 (0.7–0.9)
	COPD	128	0.8 (0.7–1.0)
	Navy		
	Respiratory system diseases	50	0.8 (0.6–1.0)
	COPD	28	0.9 (0.6–1.3)
	Army		
	Respiratory system diseases	162	0.8 (0.7–0.9)
	COPD	81	0.8 (0.7–1.0)
	Air Force		
	Respiratory system diseases	28	0.6 (0.4–0.9)
	COPD	18	0.8 (0.4–1.2)
ADVA, 2005c	Australian National Service Vietnam Veterans: Mortality and Cancer Incidence Study		
	National Serviceman (SMR)		
	Respiratory diseases	38	0.5 (0.3–0.6)
	COPD	18	0.9 (0.5–1.4)
	National Serviceman, deployed (SMR)		
	Respiratory diseases	18	0.5 (0.3–0.8)
	COPD	8	0.9 (0.4–1.8)
	National Serviceman, nondeployed (SMR)		
	Respiratory diseases	20	0.4 (0.2–0.6)
	COPD	10	0.9 (0.4–1.7)
Boehmer et al., 2004	Vietnam Experience Cohort Nonmalignant respiratory mortality (ICD-9 460–519)	20	0.8 (0.5–1.5)

continued

TABLE 9-1 Continued

Reference	Study Population	Exposed Cases[a]	Estimated Relative Risk (95% CI)[a]
Studies Reviewed in *Update 1998*			
Bullman and Kang, 1996	Male Vietnam veterans who were wounded in combat vs US population Nonmalignant respiratory mortality (ICD 9 460–519)	43	0.9 (0.7–1.2)
O'Toole et al., 1996	Australian Army Vietnam veterans self-reported health status (1989–1990) vs Australian population—prevalence		
	Acute conditions that required recent medical intervention		
	Asthma	nr	1.4 (0.6–2.1)
	Bronchitis, emphysema	nr	2.1 (0.2–4.0)
	Other	nr	2.1 (1.6–2.8)
	Chronic conditions		
	Asthma	nr	0.9 (0.5–1.4)
	Bronchitis, emphysema	nr	4.1 (2.8–5.5)
	Other	nr	4.0 (2.2–5.9)
Watanabe et al., 1996;	Mortality of US Vietnam veterans who died during 1965–1988, PMR analysis of nonmalignant respiratory mortality (ICD 8 460–519)		
	Army	648	0.8 (p < 0.05)
	Marine Corps	111	0.7 (p < 0.05)
Crane et al., 1997a	Mortality of male Australian Vietnam veterans vs Australian population		
	Non-malignant respiratory mortality (ICD-9 460–519)		
	1964–1979	3	0.1 (0.0–0.3)
	1980–1994	92	0.9 (0.7–1.1)
	Chronic obstructive airways disease (ICD-9 490–496)		
	1980–1994	47	0.9 (0.7–1.2)
Crane et al., 1997b	Mortality of deployed Australian National Servicemen vs those who did not serve in Vietnam		
	1965–1982	2	2.6 (0.2–30.0)
	1982–1994	6	0.9 (0.3–2.7)
AFHS, 1996	Cause-specific mortality in Rand Hand personnel vs Air Force veterans	2	0.5 (0.1–1.6)
Studies Reviewed in *VAO*			
Anderson et al., 1986	White males with Wisconsin death certificate (1968–1978), mortality from nonmalignant respiratory disease (ICD-8 460–519)		
	Vietnam veterans vs expected deaths calculated from proportions for:		
	Nonveterans	10	0.5 (0.3–0.8)
	All veterans		0.8 (0.4–1.5)
	Vietnam-era veteran		1.0 (0.5–1.8)

TABLE 9-1 Continued

Reference	Study Population	Exposed Cases[a]	Estimated Relative Risk (95% CI)[a]
CDC, 1988	Cross-sectional study, with medical examinations, of US Army Vietnam veterans vs nondeployed US Army veterans		
	Odds ratios from pulmonary-function tests (case definition: ≤ 80% predicted value)		
	FEV$_1$	254	0.9 (0.7–1.1)
	FVC	177	1.0 (0.8–1.3)
	FEV$_1$/FVC	152	1.0 (0.8–1.3)
Eisen et al., 1991	Incidence in deployed vs nondeployed monozygotic twins who served in US military during Vietnam era		
	Respiratory conditions		
	Present at time of survey	nr	1.4 (0.8–2.4)
	At any time since service	nr	1.4 (0.9–2.0)
	Required hospitalization	nr	1.8 (0.7–4.2)

OCCUPATIONAL
New Studies

Reference	Study Population	Exposed Cases[a]	Estimated Relative Risk (95% CI)[a]
Hoppin et al., 2008	US AHS—prevalence at enrollment among farm women of:		
	Atopic asthma having exposure to:		
	2,4-D	52	1.5 (1.1–2.1)
	Dicamba	11	1.1 (0.6–2.1)
	Nonatopic asthma having exposure to:		
	2,4-D	66	1.1 (0.8–1.4)
	Dicamba	13	0.7 (0.4–1.3)
Hoppin et al., 2007a	US AHS—prevalence at enrollment of self-reported farmer's lung (hypersensitivity pneumonitis)		
	Private applicators exposed to phenoxy herbicides	392	1.2 (0.8–1.7)
	Spouses exposed to phenoxy herbicides	16	1.4 (0.7–2.7)
Hoppin et al., 2007b	US AHS—prevalence at enrollment of chronic bronchitis in private applicators exposed to:		
	2,4-D	78	1.1 (0.9–1.4)
	2,4,5-T (lifetime days)	28	1.5 (1.3–1.8)
	None	74	1.0
	1–14	16	1.4 (1.1–1.8)
	15–55	6	1.3 (0.9–1.8)
	> 55	4	1.0 (0.6–1.5)
	2,4,5-TP (lifetime days)	9	1.7 (1.3–1.3)
	None	92	1.0
	1–14	3	1.1 (0.7–1.8)
	15–55	3	1.6 (1.0–2.8)
	> 55	2	1.4 (0.8–2.5)
	Dicamba	48	1.0 (0.8–1.2)

continued

TABLE 9-1 Continued

Reference	Study Population	Exposed Cases[a]	Estimated Relative Risk (95% CI)[a]
Valcin et al., 2007	US AHS—prevalence at enrollment of chronic bronchitis in nonsmoking farm women exposed to:		0.9 (0.7–1.1)
	2,4-D	16	1.2 (0.9–1.6)
	2,4,5-T	1	1.0 (0.4–2.5)
	Dicamba	5	1.1 (0.6–2.0)
Hoppin et al., 2006b	US AHS—prevalence at enrollment of wheeze (added adjustment for exposure to herbicide chlorimuron-ethyl)		
	Private applicators with current use of:		
	2,4-D	nr	1.0 (0.9–1.1)
	Dicamba	nr	1.1 (0.9–1.2)
[supercedes Hoppin et al., 2006a]	Commercial applicators with current use of:		
	2,4-D	nr	1.0 (0.7–1.3)
	Dicamba	nr	0.8 (0.6–1.1)
Studies Reviewed in ***Update 2006***			
Hoppin et al., 2006a	US AHS—cross-sectional study of wheeze in commercial applicators with current use of:		
	2,4-D	225	1.3 (1.0–1.7)
	Dicamba	167	1.1 (0.9–1.4)
't Mannetje et al., 2005	New Zealand phenoxy herbicide workers, nonmalignant respiratory mortality (ICD-9 480–519)		
	Producers	9	0.9 (0.4–1.8)
	Sprayers	6	0.7 (0.2–1.2)
Blair et al., 2005	US AHS—COPD mortality		
	Private applicators	50	0.2 (0.2–0.3)
	Spouses	15	0.3 (0.2–0.7)
Studies Reviewed in ***Update 2002***			
Burns et al., 2001	Males employees of Dow Chemical Company— manufacture exposed to 2,4-D in 1945–1994, nonmalignant respiratory mortality (ICD-8 460–519)		
	All nonmalignant respiratory	8	0.4 (0.2–0.7)
	Pneumonia	4	0.6 (0.2–1.4)
Studies Reviewed in ***Update 2000***			
Steenland et al., 1999	NIOSH mortality study of chemical workers at 12 plants in US exposed to TCDD, nonmalignant respiratory mortality (ICD-9 460–519)	86	0.9 (0.7–1.1)
Sweeney et al., 1997/98 *[supersedes Calvert et al., 1991]*	NIOSH follow-up study of workers in production of sodium trichlorophenol, 2,4,5-T ester contaminated with TCDD, chronic bronchitis and COPD	2	nr

TABLE 9-1 Continued

Reference	Study Population	Exposed Cases[a]	Estimated Relative Risk (95% CI)[a]
Studies Reviewed in *Update 1998*			
Becher et al., 1996	Four German facilites for production of phenoxy herbicides, chlorophenols, nonmalignant respiratory mortality (ICD-9 460–519)		
	Boehringer Ingelheim	10	0.5 (0.3–1.0)
	Bayer Uerdingen	2	0.9 (0.1–3.1)
	Bayer Dormagen	0	0.0
	BASF Ludwigshafen	4	0.6 (0.2–1.6)
Svensson et al., 1995	Swedish fishermen exposed to TCDD, mortality from bronchitis or emphysema (ICD-7 490–493)		
	East coast	4	0.5 (0.2–1.2)
	West coast	43	0.8 (0.6–1.1)
Ott and Zober, 1996 *[supersedes Zober et al., 1994]*	German workers exposed to trichlorophenol contaminated with TCDD from accident at BASF plant, 1953–1993, nonmalignant respiratory mortality	1	0.1 (0.0–0.8)
Ramlow et al., 1996	Mortality of workers at Dow Chemical plant, Michigan, producing PCP contaminated with PCDDs, 1940–1989		
	Nonmalignant respiratory mortality (ICD-8 460–519)		
	Cumulative PCP exposure	14	0.9 (0.5–1.5)
	< 1 unit	3	0.6 (0.2–1.9)
	≥ 1 unit	11	1.4 (0.8–2.5)
	Pneumonia (ICD-8 480–486)	6	1.1 (0.4–2.4)
	Emphysema (ICD-8 492)	4	1.3 (0.4–3.3)
Kogevinas et al., 1997	Mortality in international workers producing or applying phenoxy herbicides, nonmalignant respiratory mortality (ICD-9 460–519), 1939–1992		
	Men	252	0.8 (0.7–0.9)
	Women	7	1.1 (0.4–2.2)
Studies Reviewed in *Update 1996*			
Senthilselvan et al., 1992	Cross-sectional study of self-reported prevalence of asthma in male farmers in Saskatchewan (1982–1983)		
	Chlorinated hydrocarbons	31	0.8 (0.5–1.3)
Zober et al., 1994	German workers exposed to trichlorophenol contaminated with TCDD from an accident at BASF plant, 1953–1989; exposed vs unexposed workers—prevalence		Illness episodes per 100 person-years (cohort/reference)
	All nonmalignant respiratory diseases (ICD-9 460–51)	nr	33.7/31.0 (p = 0.22)
	Upper respiratory tract infections (ICD-9 460–478)	nr	12.0/9.0 (p = 0.00)

continued

TABLE 9-1 Continued

Reference	Study Population	Exposed Cases[a]	Estimated Relative Risk (95% CI)[a]
	Pneumonia or influenza (ICD-9 480–487)	nr	17.4/18.8 (p = 0.08)
	COPD (ICD-9 490–496)	nr	8.0/7.5 (p = 0.31)
Studies Reviewed in *VAO*			
Coggon et al., 1991	Production of phenoxy herbicides, chlorophenols in four British plants, mortality from nonmalignant respiratory diseases, 1963–1985	8	0.7 (0.3–1.3)
Coggon et al., 1986	British plant manufacturing MCPA, mortality from nonmalignant respiratory diseases (ICD-9 460–519), 1947–1983	93	0.6 (0.5–0.8)
Alavanja et al., 1989	PMR study of USDA soil, forest conservationists, mortality 1970–1979 from nonmalignant respiratory diseases (ICD-9 460–519)	80	0.8 (0.6–1.0)
Calvert et al., 1991	NIOSH cross-sectional study of workers in production of sodium trichlorophenol, 2,4,5-T ester contaminated with TCDD comparing exposed with nonexposed workers; odds ratios for increase in 1 ppt of serum TCDD		
	Chronic bronchitis	nr	0.5 (0.1–2.6)
	COPD	nr	1.2 (0.5–2.8)
Suskind and Hertzberg, 1984	Cross-sectional study of Nitro, West Virginia, plant that manufactured 2,4,5-T, comparing exposed with nonexposed workers, 1979; odds ratios comparing exposed with nonexposed for "abnormal" outcome on pulmonary-functions tests:		
	FEV$_1$ (< 80% predicted)	32	2.82 (p = 0.02)
	FVC (< 80% predicted)	35	2.25 (p = 0.32)
	FEV$_1$/FVC (< 70%)	32	2.97 (p = 0.01)
	FEF$_{25-75}$ (< 80% predicted)	47	1.86 (p = 0.05)
Blair et al., 1983	Licensed pesticide applicators, Florida, nonmalignant respiratory diseases, (ICD-8 460–519)		
	Analyses by length of licensure	20	0.9 (nr)
	≤ 10 years	8	0.6 (nr)
	10–19 years	8	1.5 (nr)
	≥ 20 years	4	1.7 (nr)
ENVIRONMENTAL			
New Studies			
Consonni et al., 2008	25-year follow-up of Seveso residents—mortality from respiratory disease (ICD-9 460–519)		
	Zone A	9	1.4 (0.7–2.7)
	Zone B	48	1.0 (0.8–1.4)
	Zone R	341	1.0 (0.9–1.1)

TABLE 9-1 Continued

Reference	Study Population	Exposed Cases[a]	Estimated Relative Risk (95% CI)[a]
	Mortality from COPD (ICD-9 490–493)		
	Zone A	7	2.5 (1.2–5.3)
	Zone B	26	1.3 (0.9–1.9)
	Zone R	175	1.2 (1.0–1.4)
Studies Reviewed in *Update 2004*			
Dahlgren et al., 2003	Cross-sectional study of residents near wood-treatment plant (creosote, PCP) in Mississippi, who were plaintiffs in lawsuit against plant vs subjects in comparable area with no known chemical exposures		Adjusted scores of exposed vs nonexposed; (< 0 means exposed subjects had more symptoms)
	Shortness of breath		
	Adults	nr	−2.5 (p < 0.05)
	Children	nr	−3.8 (p < 0.05)
Studies Reviewed in *Update 2000*			
Bertazzi et al., 2001	20-year follow-up of Seveso residents—mortality from respiratory disease (ICD-9 460–519)	44	1.0 (0.8–1.4)
	Zone A	9	1.9 (1.0–3.6)
	Zone B	35	1.3 (0.9–2.0)
	COPD (ICD-9 490–493)	29	1.5 (1.1–2.2)
	Zone A	7	3.3 (1.6–6.9)
	Zone B	22	1.3 (0.9–2.0)
Bertazzi et al., 1998; Pesatori et al., 1998 (results from Bertazzi)	15-year follow-up of Seveso residents—mortality from respiratory disease (ICD-9 460–519)		
	Zone A		
	Men	5	2.4 (1.0–5.7)
	Women	2	1.3 (0.3–5.3)
	Zone B		
	Men	13	0.7 (0.4–1.2)
	Women	10	1.0 (0.5–1.9)
	Zone R		
	Men	133	1.1 (0.9–1.3)
	Women	84	1.0 (0.8–1.2)
	COPD (ICD-9 490–493)		
	Zone A		
	Men	4	3.7 (1.4–9.8)
	Women	1	2.1 (0.3–14.9)
	Zone B		
	Men	9	1.0 (0.5–1.9)
	Women	8	2.5 (1.2–5.0)
	Zone R		
	Men	74	1.2 (0.9–1.5)
	Women	37	1.3 (0.9–1.9)

continued

TABLE 9-1 Continued

Reference	Study Population	Exposed Cases[a]	Estimated Relative Risk (95% CI)[a]
Studies Reviewed in *VAO*			
Bertazzi	10-year follow-up on Seveso residents—mortality		
et al., 1989a;	from respiratory disease (ICD-9 460–519)		
Bertazzi	Men	55	1.0 (0.7–1.3)
et al., 1989b	Women	24	1.0 (0.7–1.6)
(results from	Pneumonia (ICD-9 480–486)		
Bertazzi	Men	14	0.9 (0.5–1.5)
et al.,	Women	9	0.8 (0.4–1.6)
1989a)	COPD (ICD-9 490–493)		
	Men	31	1.1 (0.8–1.7)
	Women	8	1.0 (0.5–2.2)

ABBREVIATIONS: 2,4-D, 2,4-dichlorophenoxyacetic acid; 2,4,5-T, 2,4,5-trichlorophenoxyacetic acid; 2,4,5-TP, 2-(2,4,5-trichlorophenoxy) propionic acid; AFHS, Air Force Health Study; AHS, Agricultural Health Study; CI, confidence interval; COPD, chronic obstructive pulmonary disease; FEF_{25-75}, forced midexpiratory flow; FEV_1, forced expiratory volume in 1 second; FVC, forced vital capacity; ICD-8, *International Classification of Diseases, 8th revision*; ICD-9, *International Classification of Diseases, 9th revision*; MCPA, 2-methyl-4-chlorophenoxyacetic acid; NIOSH, National Institute for Occupational Safety and Health; nr, not reported; PCDD, polychlorinated dibenzo-*p*-dioxin; PCP, pentachlorophenol; PMR, proportionate mortality ratio; SMR, standardized mortality ratio; TCDD, 2,3,7,8-tetrachlorodibenzo-*p*-dioxin; USDA, US Department of Agriculture.
[a]Given when available; results other than estimated risk explained individually.
Studies in italics have been superseded by newer studies of same cohort.

In another publication from the AHS, Hoppin et al. (2008) conducted an analysis of the 702 women among the 25,814 farm women who reported at enrollment that they had had a diagnosis of asthma after the age of 19 years. Of the 702, 282 had atopic asthma (asthma with eczema or hay fever), and 420 had nonatopic asthma. A significantly increased risk of atopic asthma was observed in association with exposure to 2,4-D (OR = 1.4, 95% CI 1.1–1.8) but not with exposure to dicamba (OR = 1.1, 95% CI 0.9–1.3). For nonatopic asthma, the risk associated with exposure to 2,4-D was increased slightly (OR = 1.1, 95% CI 0.9–1.3), and no association was found with exposure to dicamba.

In a study of the prevalence of farmer's lung (hypersensitivity pneumonitis) at enrollment in the AHS population, Hoppin et al. (2007a) did not find significantly increased risks among private pesticide applicators (OR = 1.2, 95% CI 0.8–1.7) or their spouses (OR = 1.4, 95% CI 0.7–2.7) who had ever been exposed to phenoxy herbicides. Adjustment was made for age, state, smoking, and all other exposures.

Chronic bronchitis was the outcome of interest in two publications from the AHS. Among the 20,908 private pesticide applicators (who were mostly male farmers), Hoppin et al. (2007b) found significant increases in the prevalence of self-reported chronic bronchitis that was diagnosed by a physician in people more than 19 years old who had been exposed to 2,4,5-T (OR = 1.5, 95% CI 1.3–1.8) or to 2-(2,4,5-trichlorophenoxy) propionic acid (2,4,5-TP) (OR = 1.7, 95% CI 1.3–2.3). Statistically significant associations with exposures to 2,4-D and dicamba were not observed. Analyses according to the number of days on which 2,4,5-T or 2,4,5-TP was sprayed did not reveal monotonic increases in the odds of prevalence, but there were few exposed cases in each category of use, so the statistical power to detect monotonic trends was low. Similar analyses of 21,541 nonsmoking women in the AHS by Valcin et al. (2007) did not find increased risks of chronic bronchitis in those exposed to 2,4-D, to 2,4,5-T, or to dicamba.

Environmental Studies

In the 25-year follow-up of the mortality of the Seveso population through 2001, Consonni et al. (2008) estimated associations by using Poisson regression for three exposure zones (A, B, and R) and comparing rates among residents of nonexposed areas in 11 surrounding municipalities. They found that mortality from all types of respiratory disease (*International Classification of Diseases, 9th revision* [ICD-9] 460–493) was not increased, although there was an increase in the most highly exposed but relatively small group from Zone A (RR = 1.4, 95% CI 0.7–2.7). For the more specific diagnosis of COPD (ICD-9 490–493), however, there was a marked increase in Zone A (RR = 2.5, 95% CI 1.2–5.3), and increased rates were found in the intermediate-exposure Zone B (RR = 1.3, 95% CI 0.9–1.9) and the least exposed Zone R (RR = 1.2, 95% CI 1.0–1.4).

Biologic Plausibility

Acute nonmalignant respiratory disorders, including pneumonia and other respiratory infections, can be increased in frequency and severity when the normal defense mechanisms of the lower respiratory tract are compromised. Thus exposure to chemicals that affect those mechanisms could exacerbate respiratory disorders. There is no evidence that the herbicides used in Vietnam alter such defense mechanisms. However, inasmuch as TCDD has been shown to suppress immune function in a variety of animal models, exposure to TCDD could be expected to increase the incidence or severity of respiratory infections. Several laboratory studies have shown that treatment of mice with TCDD increased their mortality after infection with influenza virus (Burleson et al., 1996; Lawrence et al., 2003). Treatment with TCDD also suppressed the animals' ability to generate an immune response to the virus (Mitchell and Lawrence, 2003). The mechanism underlying increased influenza mortality was not related to the suppression of the immune response to influenza by TCDD but appeared to involve an increase in the inflammatory response associated with an increased flow of neutrophils into the lung (Mitchell and Lawrence, 2003). Neutrophils produce several toxic products (which kill pathogens), so it is possible that excess numbers of neutrophils in the lung produce excess collateral damage and pathologic changes that increase mortality. Later studies to test that hypothesis showed that prevention of the neutrophilia (increase in the number of neutrophils) with an antineutrophil antibody provided partial protection of TCDD-treated mice from influenza-induced mortality (Teske et al., 2005). Furthermore, the increased mortality and increased neutrophilia were AHR-dependent and not observed in TCDD-treated AHR-knockout mice (Teske et al., 2005). However, TCDD exposure did not alter the concentrations of common lung neutrophil chemoattractants, the expression of adhesion molecules, or the normal neutrophil apoptotic process. Likewise, concentrations of reactive oxygen species and myeloperoxidase activity were normal in neutrophils from TCDD-treated mice (Teske et al., 2005).

In the absence of evidence of TCDD effects at the level of neutrophil recruitment or function, several indicators of lung damage were assessed (Bohn et al., 2005). TCDD exposure did not alter the concentration of lactate dehydrogenase (a marker of lung-cell damage) or increase edema (measured by protein in bronchioalveolar lavage fluid and wet-weight to dry-weight ratios).

Although AHR expression was shown to be required for TCDD to increase neutrophils in the lungs, the cells expressing AHR were not the neutrophils themselves or other immune cells, and this suggests that lung parenchyma was being directly affected by TCDD (Teske et al., 2008). However, the concentration of Clara cell secretory protein, an inflammatory mediator produced by lung-associated Clara cells, was not altered by TCDD. Thus, the mechanisms underlying the increase in mortality after influenza infection remain to be determined. Despite the lack of functional changes in the lung, TCDD induced cytochrome P450 1A1 (CYP1A1) expression in the Clara cells of the lung, in lung endothelial cells, and in type II pneumocytes—indications of the ability of TCDD to affect the lung directly via AHR activation (Bohn et al., 2005). CYP1A1 and CYP1B1 were also induced in the lungs of rats given a single dose (5 µg/kg of body weight) of TCDD 4 hours before termination (Harrigan et al., 2006). On the basis of those findings, it is biologically plausible that exposure to TCDD results in exacerbation of acute lung disease that is associated with reduced immune responses or of chronic lung diseases including COPD, that is associated with increased inflammatory responses. It is also plausible that the induction of CYP1A1 and CYP1B1 enzymes in the lung by TCDD result in the metabolism of several chemicals found in tobacco smoke to more toxic intermediates. Exposure to TCDD would thus increase the toxic effects of tobacco smoke and increase respiratory disease.

Synthesis

Results of the studies of mortality from nonmalignant respiratory diseases reported in *Update 2006* and earlier VAO reports (ADVA, 2005b,c; Anderson et al., 1986; Becher et al., 1996; Blair et al., 1983, 2005; Bullman and Kang,

1996; Burns et al., 2001; Coggon et al., 1986, 1991; Crane et al., 1997a; Ketchum and Michalek, 2005; Kogevinas et al., 1997; Ott and Zober, 1996; Ramlow et al., 1996; Steenland et al., 1999; Svensson et al., 1995; 't Mannetje et al., 2005; Zober et al., 1994) do not support the hypothesis that herbicides are associated with respiratory mortality. The recent studies of the Seveso incident showed a positive association (Consonni et al., 2008) based on nine deaths in the high-exposure area (Zone A); this finding could have been due to chance or to misclassification of causes of death. More important, as the committee recognizes that mortality studies are limited by small numbers of events and misclassification of causes of death (especially respiratory conditions), it does not believe that scientific conclusions can be based on health outcomes that are defined vaguely, for example, by combining a wide array of disparate respiratory health outcomes into one large category.

In *Update 2006*, when Kang et al. (2006) compared deployed to nondeployed Vietnam-era veterans in a study of US Army Chemical Corps personnel, they found an association between exposure and the prevalence of self-reported physician-confirmed respiratory problems (OR = 1.41, 95% CI 1.13–1.76). The association was also significant when those who reported spraying herbicides in Vietnam were compared to those who did not (OR = 1.62, 95% CI 1.26–2.05). In the subset of subjects for whom serum TCDD concentrations had been determined, individuals with respiratory problems were evenly distributed above and below the median, which argues against the association arising from herbicide exposure. As in the case of the mortality studies cited in the preceding paragraph, the issue of nonspecificity is key to interpreting this study. The nonspecificity of the types of respiratory conditions reported in Kang et al. (2006) makes it exceedingly difficult to draw any conclusions regarding specific respiratory conditions.

The present committee found an additional five papers on the prevalence of various respiratory conditions, all from the AHS. Those respiratory outcomes now include wheeze, asthma, COPD, and farmer's lung. The following summarizes the evidence on those outcomes.

- **COPD.** The findings from the Seveso incident showed increased risks of death from COPD (Consonni et al., 2008), with higher RRs found in the zone (A) closest to the accident and slightly lower RRs for the outlying zones. No associations with mortality from COPD were found in the recent Australian studies (ADVA, 2005b,c; Crane et al., 1997a). A 4-fold excess prevalence in chronic bronchitis and emphysema was found in a health-status study of Australian army Vietnam veterans (O'Toole et al., 1996). In the AHS, Hoppin et al. (2007b) found associations between exposure to 2,4,5-T and 2,4,5-TP and the prevalence of physician-diagnosed COPD in private applicators, and Valcin et al. (2007) found that the prevalence of physician-diagnosed COPD in nonsmoking farm women was 20% higher in those persons exposed to 2,4-D. Other cross-sectional prevalence studies considered in previous updates that bear on this matter include the study of an accident at a BASF plant (Zober et al., 1994) that showed no association of exposure with episodes of COPD and the NIOSH cross-sectional study of production workers exposed to 2,4,5-T ester contaminated with TCDD (Calvert et al., 1991) that also did not show an increase in COPD associated with serum TCDD concentration. In addition, the study of residents exposed environmentally to emissions from a plant that produced creosote and pentachlorophenol (Dahlgren et al., 2003) showed positive associations with chronic bronchitis, but the study was judged in *Update 2004* to have been biased.

- **Wheeze and asthma.** These related health outcomes were the subject of two reports from the AHS (Hoppin et al., 2006a,b). The study new to the present update (Hoppin et al., 2006b) stated that the first study's associations between "current" exposure to 2,4-D and several other pesticides and the prevalence of self-reported wheeze (adjusted OR = 1.3) did not persist (OR = 1.0) after adjustment for exposure to chlorimuron-ethyl. Previous updates noted that a cross-sectional study in Saskatchewan (Senthilselvan et al., 1992) showed no association between exposure to chlorinated hydrocarbons and the prevalence of self-reported asthma. The study by Hoppin et al. (2006b) is unclear about what wheeze represents: the definition of *wheeze* was very broad and included any episode in the year before administration of the questionnaire, and the authors reported that only 28% of subjects with wheeze reported having asthma or atopic conditions.
- **Farmer's lung.** There was only one study on this outcome (Hoppin et al., 2007a), and no conclusions can be drawn.

Conclusion

On the basis of the evidence reviewed here and in previous VAO reports, the committee concludes that there is inadequate or insufficient evidence of an association between exposure to the chemicals of interest and mortality from all nonmalignant respiratory diseases or the prevalence of wheeze or asthma, COPD, and farmer's lung.

IMMUNE-SYSTEM DISORDERS

The immune system defends the body against infection by pathogens—viruses, bacteria, and other disease-producing microorganisms. It also plays a role in cancer surveillance, destroying mutated cells that might otherwise develop into tumors. To recognize the wide array of pathogens in the environment, the immune system relies on many cell types that operate together to generate immune responses. Those cells arise from stem cells in the bone marrow, they are found throughout the body's lymphoid tissues, and they circulate in the blood as white blood cells (WBCs). The main types of WBCs are granulocytes, monocytes, and lymphocytes.

Immune Suppression

Suppression of immune responses can reduce resistance to infectious disease and increase the risk of cancer. Infection with the human immunodeficiency virus (HIV) is a well-recognized example of an acquired immune deficiency in which a specific type of lymphocyte (CD4+ T cells) is the target of the virus. The decline in the number of CD4+ T cells after HIV infection correlates with an increased incidence of infectious diseases, including fatal opportunistic infections, and with an increased incidence of several types of cancer. Treatment of cancer patients with toxic chemotherapeutic drugs suppresses the immune system by inhibiting the generation of new WBCs from the bone marrow and by blocking proliferation of lymphocytes during an immune response. Immune suppression can result from exposure to chemicals in the workplace or in the environment, including dioxin (see Chapter 4). However, unless the immune suppression is severe, it is often difficult to obtain clinical evidence that directly links chemical-induced changes in immune function to increased infectious disease or cancer, because many confounding factors can influence a person's ability to combat infection. Such confounders include age, vaccination status, the virulence of the pathogen, the presence of other diseases (such as diabetes), stress, smoking, and the use of drugs or alcohol.

Allergy

The immune system sometimes responds to a foreign substance that is not pathogenic. Such immunogenic substances are called allergens. The response to some allergens, such as pollen and bee venom, results in the production of immunoglobulin E (IgE) antibodies. Once produced, IgE antibodies bind to specialized cells—mast cells—that occur in tissues throughout the body, including lung airways, the intestinal wall, and blood-vessel walls. When a person is exposed again to the allergen, the allergen binds to the antibodies on the mast cells, causing them to release histamine and leukotrienes, which produce the symptoms associated with an allergic response. Other allergens, such as poison ivy and nickel, activate allergen-specific lymphocytes at the site of contact (usually the skin) that release substances that cause inflammation and tissue damage. Although inflammation is advantageous in fighting infectious diseases, tissue damage can result when it is inappropriately increased or prolonged. Inflammation is known to contribute to coronary arterial disease and appears to play a role in promoting the growth of cancer.

Autoimmune Disease

Autoimmune disease is another example of the immune system's causing rather than preventing disease. The immune system attacks the body's own cells and tissues as though they are foreign, and this leads to the generation of inflammatory substances that cause damage to the tissues. For example, the autoimmune reaction in multiple sclerosis is directed against the myelin sheath of the nervous system; in Crohn's disease, the intestine is the target of attack; in type 1 diabetes mellitus, the insulin-producing cells of the pancreas are destroyed by the immune response. Rheumatoid arthritis (RA) is an autoimmune disease that arises from immune attack on the joints. Genetic predisposition and such environmental factors as infectious diseases and stress are thought to facilitate the development of autoimmune diseases.

Systemic lupus erythematosus (SLE) is an autoimmune disease that has no specific target organ of immune attack. Instead, patients have a variety of symptoms that often occur in other diseases, and this makes diagnosis difficult. A characteristic rash across the cheeks and nose and sensitivity to sunlight are common symptoms; oral ulcers, arthritis, pleurisy, proteinuria, and neurologic disorders may be present. Almost all people who have SLE test positive for antinuclear antibodies in the absence of drugs known to induce them. The causes of SLE are unknown, but environmental and genetic factors have been implicated. Some of the environmental factors that may trigger it are infections, antibiotics (especially those in the sulfa and penicillin groups) and some other drugs, ultraviolet radiation, extreme stress, and hormones. Occupational exposures to such chemicals as crystalline silica, solvents, and pesticides have also been associated with SLE (Cooper and Parks, 2004; Parks and Cooper, 2005).

Conclusions from *VAO* and Previous Updates

The committees responsible for *VAO*, *Update 1996*, *Update 1998*, *Update 2000*, *Update 2002*, *Update 2004*, and *Update 2006* concluded that there was inadequate or insufficient information to determine whether there is an association between exposure to the chemicals of interest and immune-system disorders. Reviews of the studies that underlay that conclusion are presented in the previous reports (IOM, 1994, 1996, 1999, 2001, 2003, 2005, 2007). The committee responsible for *Update 2006* reviewed a report by Boehmer et al. (2004) that found no excess in postservice mortality in male US Army Vietnam veterans related to endocrine, nutritional, and metabolic diseases or to immune disorders and concurred with the conclusion of the previous review committees.

Update of the Epidemiologic Literature

No Vietnam-veteran or occupational studies addressing exposure to the chemicals of interest and the immune system have been published since *Update 2006*.

Environmental Studies

One study of potential effects on the immune system of adults has been published since *Update 2006*. In addition, two studies of perinatal and childhood exposures have been described.

Lee DH et al. (2007a) investigated the concentrations of persistent organic pollutants in adipose tissue of 1,721 adults in the 1999–2002 National Health and Nutrition Examination Survey (NHANES), their effect on the immune system, and the possibility of an association with self-reported arthritis, either RA or osteoarthritis. The study focused on pollutants that were found in at least 60% of study subjects, which included three polychlorinated dibenzo-*p*-dioxins (PCDDs) and four dioxin-like polychlorinated biphenyls (PCBs, PCB-74, -118, -126, and -169). Women had higher serum concentrations of all classes of those organic pollutants, including the PCDDs and their dioxin-like congeners, than man. PCDDs were not associated with arthritis in either sex. However, women who had higher concentrations of dioxin-like PCBs had a higher prevalence of arthritis. After adjustment for possible confounders, ORs for all types of arthritis were 1.0, 2.1, 3.5, and 2.9 across quartiles of dioxin-like PCBs (quartiles 2–4 each significantly higher than quartile 1; p for trend = 0.02). The adjusted ORs for RA specifically were 1.0, 7.6, 6.1, and 8.5 for dioxin-like PCBs (quartiles 2–4 each significantly higher than quartile 1; p for trend = 0.05). For the nondioxin-like PCBs, however, the individual quartile risks of RA were not as high, but the pattern was monotonic: 1.0, 2.2, 4.4, and 5.4 (not significantly higher in quartile 2; p for trend < 0.01). No associations of dioxin-like PCBs or other substances with RA were observed in men.

Smith AG et al. (2008) reported on the consequences of exposure of 13 members of two Spanish families poisoned by cooking oil greatly contaminated with highly chlorinated dioxins (PCDD). Originally, all the people had chloracne as an early symptom. Analyses of the pattern of lymphocyte subpopulations were performed on whole blood. In family members with the highest body burdens of hexachlorinated to octachlorinated PCDDs, no changes in immunologic markers in comparison with a reference population were noted. Four of the children had significantly higher numbers of total blood lymphocytes.

Biologic Plausibility

Exposure of laboratory animals to phenoxy herbicides or cacodylic acid has not been associated with immunotoxicity. In contrast, the immune system has been recognized as a sensitive target for the toxicity of TCDD in laboratory animals for many years. Many cell types make up the immune system, and most of the cells have been shown to express the AHR, which is required for initiating the toxicity of TCDD (see Chapter 4). Identifying the specific cells of the immune system that are altered by TCDD and how they contribute to TCDD-induced alterations in immune function is of great interest to the research community.

Understanding how TCDD affects the immune system in rodents increases the ability to extrapolate experimental results to assessment of human risks.

TCDD is a potent immunosuppressive chemical in laboratory animals, and exposure to it has been shown to increase the incidence and severity of various infectious diseases and to increase the development of cancer. Consistent with its immunosuppressive effects, TCDD exposure suppresses the allergic immune response of rodents, and this in turn results in decreased allergen-associated pathologic lung conditions and has recently been shown to suppress the development of experimental autoimmune disease (Quintana et al., 2008). Thus, depending on the particular disease, TCDD exposure could result in exacerbation or amelioration of symptoms. The demonstration in recent studies that AHR activation by TCDD leads to the development of regulatory T cells helps to explain the diversity of effects seen after exposure to TCDD (Funatake et al., 2008; Marshall et al., 2008; Quintana et al., 2008).

In contrast, under some conditions, exposure of laboratory animals to TCDD has been associated with increased inflammatory responses and increased production of inflammatory mediators. That could potentially increase the severity of autoimmune disease and promote the growth of cancer cells. The AHR appears to regulate the expression of several genes associated with inflammation that could explain the influence of TCDD on inflammatory diseases.

Taken together, results of experimental laboratory studies indicate that TCDD exposure can have diverse effects on the immune response—some that are detrimental to health and others that appear to be beneficial, depending on the disease in question.

Synthesis

TCDD is a well-known immunosuppressive agent in laboratory animals. Therefore, one would expect exposure of humans to substantial doses of TCDD to result in immune suppression. However, several studies of various measures of human immune function failed to reveal consistent correlations with TCDD exposure, probably because the exposures were inadequate to produce immune suppression. No detectable pattern of an increase in infectious disease has been documented in veterans exposed to TCDD or the herbicides used in Vietnam. Suppression of the immune response by TCDD might increase the risk of some kinds of cancer in Vietnam veterans, but there is no evidence to support that connection.

Epidemiologic studies have been inconsistent with regard to TCDD's influence on IgE production in humans. No animal or human studies have specifically addressed the influence of TCDD on autoimmune disease. In studying postservice mortality, Boehmer et al. (2004) found no increase in deaths of Vietnam veterans that could be attributed to immune-system disorders. The present review included a study that found a significant association between concentrations of dioxin-like

PCBs and the prevalence of arthritis (thought to be an autoimmune disorder) in women but not in men (Lee DH et al., 2007a). There is no experimental evidence to support that finding, and future studies are needed to determine a potential mechanism of TCDD-induced RA.

Few effects of phenoxy herbicide or cacodylic acid exposure on the immune system have been reported in animals or humans, and no clear association between such exposure and autoimmune or allergic disease has been found.

Conclusion

On the basis of the evidence reviewed here and in previous VAO reports, the committee concludes that there is inadequate or insufficient evidence to determine whether there is an association between exposure to the chemicals of interest and immune suppression, allergy, or autoimmune disease.

TYPE 2 DIABETES

Diabetes mellitus is a group of heterogeneous metabolic disorders characterized by hyperglycemia and quantitative or qualitative deficiency of insulin action (Orchard et al., 1992). Although all forms share hyperglycemia, the pathogenic processes involved in its development differ. Most cases of diabetes mellitus are in one of two categories: type 1 diabetes is characterized by a lack of insulin caused by the destruction of insulin-producing cells in the pancreas (β cells), and type 2 diabetes is characterized by a combination of resistance to the actions of insulin and inadequate secretion of insulin (called relative insulin deficiency). In old classification systems, type 1 diabetes was called insulin-dependent diabetes mellitus or juvenile-onset diabetes mellitus, and type 2 was called non–insulin-dependent diabetes mellitus or adult-onset diabetes mellitus. The modern classification system recognizes that type 2 diabetes can occur in children and can require insulin treatments. Long-term complications of both types can include CVDs, nephropathy, retinopathy, neuropathy, and increased vulnerability to infections. Keeping blood sugar concentrations within the normal range is crucial for preventing complications.

About 90% of all cases of diabetes mellitus are of type 2. Onset can occur before the age of 30 years, and incidence increases steadily with age. The main risk factors are age, obesity, central fat deposition, a history of gestational diabetes (in women), physical inactivity, ethnicity (prevalence is greater in blacks and Hispanics than in whites), and—perhaps most important—family history. The relative contributions of those features are not known. Prevalence and mortality statistics in the US population for 2006 are presented in Table 9-2.

The etiology of type 2 diabetes is unknown, but three major components have been identified: peripheral insulin resistance (thought by many to be primary) in target tissues (muscle, adipose tissue, and liver), a defect in β-cell se-

TABLE 9-2 Prevalence and Mortality in United States for 2006 from Diabetes, Lipid Disorders, and Circulatory Disorders

ICD-9 Range	Diseases of Circulatory System	Prevalence (% of Americans 20 years old and older)		Mortality (no. deaths, all ages)	
		Men	Women	Men	Women
250	Diabetes	nr	nr	36,500	38,600
	Physician-diagnosed	7.4[a]	8.0[a]	nr	nr
	Undiagnosed	3.8[a]	2.1[a]	nr	nr
	Prediabetes	31.7[a]	19.9[a]	nr	nr
	Lipid disorders				
	Total cholesterol ≥ 200 mg/dL	42.6	47.1.	nr	nr
	Total cholesterol ≥ 240 mg/dL	13.8	17.3	nr	nr
	LDL cholesterol ≥ 130 mg/dL	33.8	31.7	nr	nr
	HDL cholesterol < 40 mg/dL	24.9	6.7	nr	nr
390–459	All circulatory disorders	37.6	34.9	409,900	454,600
390–398	Rheumatic fever and rheumatic heart disease	nr	nr	1,022	2,226
401–404[b]	Hypertensive disease			24,000	33,300
401	Essential hypertension	nr	nr	nr	nr
402	Hypertensive heart disease	nr	nr	nr	nr
403	Hypertensive renal disease	nr	nr	nr	nr
404	Hypertensive heart and renal disease	nr	nr	nr	nr
410–414, 429.2	Ischemic, coronary heart disease	8.6	6.8	232,100	213,600
410, 412	Acute, old myocardial infarction	4.7	2.7	80,100	70,900
411	Other acute, subacute forms of ischemic heart disease	nr	nr	nr	nr
413	Angina pectoris	4.3	4.5	nr	nr
414	Other forms of chronic ischemic heart disease	nr	nr	nr	nr
429.2	Cardiovascular disease, unspecified	8.6	6.8	232,100	213,600
415–417[b]	Diseases of pulmonary circulation	nr	nr	nr	nr
420–429	Other forms of heart disease (such as pericarditis, endocarditis, myocarditis, cardiomyopathy)	nr	nr	nr	nr
426–427	Arrhythmias	nr	nr	nr	nr
428	Heart failure	3.2	2.0	126,200	166,100
430–438[b]	Cerebrovascular disease (such as hemorrhage, occlusion, transient cerebral ischemia; includes mention of hypertension in ICD-401)	2.6	3.2	56,600	87,000
440–448[b]	Diseases of arteries, arterioles, capillaries	nr	nr	nr	nr
451–459	Diseases of veins, lymphatics, other diseases of circulatory system	nr	nr	nr	nr

ABBREVIATIONS: HDL, high-density lipoprotein; ICD, International Classification of Diseases; LDL, low-density lipoprotein; nr, not reported.
[a]For ages 18 years and above.
[b]Gap in ICD-9 sequence follows.
SOURCE: AHA, 2009 (pp. e175–e176).

cretion of insulin, and overproduction of glucose by the liver. In states of insulin resistance, insulin secretion is initially higher for each concentration of glucose than in people without diabetes. That hyperinsulinemic state is a compensation for peripheral resistance and in many cases maintains normal glucose concentrations for years. Eventually, β-cell compensation becomes inadequate, and there is progression to overt diabetes with concomitant hyperglycemia. Why the β cells cease to produce sufficient insulin is not known.

Type 1 diabetes occurs as a result of immunologically mediated destruction of β cells in the pancreas, which often occurs during childhood but can occur at any age. As in many autoimmune diseases, genetic and environmental factors influence pathogenesis. Some viral infections are believed to be important environmental factors that can trigger the autoimmunity associated with type 1 diabetes.

Pathogenetic diversity and diagnostic uncertainty are among the important problems associated with epidemiologic study of diabetes mellitus. Given the multiple likely pathogenetic mechanisms that lead to diabetes mellitus—which include diverse genetic susceptibilities (as varied as autoimmunity and obesity) and all sorts of potential environmental and behavioral factors (such as viruses, nutrition, and activity)—many agents or behaviors can contribute to risk, especially in genetically susceptible people. The multiple mechanisms also can lead to heterogeneous responses to various exposures. Because up to half the cases of diabetes are undiagnosed, the potential for ascertainment bias in population-based surveys is high (more intensively followed groups or those with more frequent health-care contact are more likely to get the diagnosis); this emphasizes the need for formal standardized testing (to detect undiagnosed cases) in epidemiologic studies.

Conclusions from *VAO* and Previous Updates

The committee responsible for *VAO* concluded that there was inadequate or insufficient information to determine whether an association between exposure to the chemicals of interest and diabetes mellitus exists. Additional information available to the committees responsible for *Update 1996* and *Update 1998* did not change that conclusion.

In 1999, in response to a request from the Department of Veterans Affairs, IOM called together a committee to conduct an interim review of the scientific evidence regarding type 2 diabetes. That review focused on information published after the deliberations of the *Update 1998* committee and resulted in the report *Veterans and Agent Orange: Herbicide/Dioxin Exposure and Type 2 Diabetes*, hereafter referred to as *Type 2 Diabetes* (IOM, 2000). The committee responsible for that report determined that there was limited or suggestive evidence of an association between exposure to at least one chemical of interest and type 2 diabetes. The committees responsible for *Update 2000*, *Update 2002*, *Update*

2004, and *Update 2006* upheld that finding. Reviews of the pertinent studies are found in the earlier reports; Table 9-3 presents a summary.

Update of the Epidemiologic Literature

Vietnam-Veteran Studies

Michalek and Pavuk (2008) published an updated analysis of the Air Force Health Study (AFHS) that related participation in Operation Ranch Hand to the onset of diabetes, incorporated additional follow-up time (through December 31, 2004), and refined the stratification of exposure categories compared with those used in the previous report (Henriksen et al., 1997). The study population included military personnel who were part of Operation Ranch Hand, did not have a diagnosis of diabetes before the end of their service in Vietnam, and participated in at least one of five in-person examinations conducted in 1982–1997. Data on a comparison cohort of other Air Force veterans who served in Southeast Asia (SEA) in 1962–1971 and were not involved in spraying herbicides were included. TCDD exposure was estimated by extrapolating TCDD concentrations measured in 1987 to the time of the end of the tour of duty, assuming a half-life of 7.6 years. Relative exposure effects were also assessed by date of service (through 1969 or after 1969) and number of days of spraying that occurred while participants were stationed in Vietnam (fewer than 90 days and 90 days or more). The authors hypothesized that Agent Orange was more heavily contaminated earlier in the war, but their choice of differing cutpoints for analogous analyses in their paper suggests that they were selected in a fashion that influenced the results. (In contrast with what was done for diabetes, for cancer, 1968 or before was the cutpoint for the date-of-service variable, days of spraying were counted through 1967 and the distribution was partitioned at 30 days.) Measured TCDD was significantly lower ($p < 0.001$) in AFHS participants who served after 1969 or were exposed to fewer than 90 days of spraying.

Overall, the RR of diabetes was 21% higher in AFHS participants than in the SEA comparison cohort (RR = 1.21, $p = 0.16$) after adjustment for BMI at follow-up and during the qualifying tour in Vietnam or SEA, family history of diabetes, smoking history in 1982, year of birth, last year of service in the Ranch Hand Unit or in SEA, ratio of the number of days spent in Vietnam to the number spent in SEA, and military occupation. Among those who served before 1970, AFHS participants had a 65% higher risk of diabetes than the SEA comparison group (RR = 1.65, $p = 0.005$). No association with diabetes was seen in those serving after 1970 (RR = 0.85, $p = 0.45$). Similarly, AFHS participants who had at least 90 days of spraying had a 32% higher risk of diabetes (RR = 1.32, $p = 0.04$). A proportional-hazards model of time-to-diabetes applied to the individual log(TCDD) values of all the Ranch Hand and SEA subjects generated a significant slope for diabetes incidence with serum dioxin (hazard ratio [HR] = 1.29,

TABLE 9-3 Selected Epidemiologic Studies—Diabetes and Related Health Outcomes

Reference	Study Population	Exposed Cases[a]	Estimated Relative Risk (95% CI)[a]
VIETNAM VETERANS			
New Studies			
Michalek and Pavuk, 2008	AFHS—follow-up through 2004 Ranch Hand veterans vs SEA comparison group		
	Calendar period in Vietnam		
	During or before 1969	130	1.7 (p = 0.005)
	Background (serum TCDD ≤ 10 ppt)	39	1.3 (0.8–2.0)
	Low (10–91 ppt)	40	1.9 (1.2–2.9)
	High (> 91 ppt)	51	2.0 (1.3–3.1)
	After 1969	50	0.9 (p = 0.45)
	Spraying during tour		
	≥ 90 days	170	1.3 (p = 0.04)
	Background (serum TCDD ≤ 10 ppt)	42	1.0 (0.7–1.4)
	Low (10–91 ppt)	60	1.5 (1.0–2.0)
	High (> 91 ppt)	68	1.6 (1.1–2.2)
	< 90 days	10	0.6 (p = 0.12)
Studies Reviewed in *Update 2006*			
Kang et al., 2006	US Army Chemical Corps personnel		
	Deployed vs nondeployed	226	1.2 (0.9–1.5)
	Sprayed herbicides in Vietnam vs never	123	1.5 (1.1–2.0)
AFHS, 2005	AFHS—2002 examination cycle Ranch Hand veterans—relative risk with 2-fold increase in 1987 TCDD		1.3 (1.1–1.5)
ADVA, 2005b	Australian Vietnam veterans vs Australian population—mortality	55	0.5 (0.4–0.7)
	Navy	12	0.5 (0.3–0.9)
	Army	37	0.5 (0.4–0.7)
	Air Force	6	0.5 (0.2–1.0)
ADVA, 2005c	Australian men conscripted into Army National Service—deployed vs nondeployed—mortality	6	0.3 (0.1–0.7)
Boehmer et al., 2004	Follow-up of CDC Vietnam Experience Cohort		
Kern et al., 2004	AFHS—Ranch Hand–comparison subject pairs—within-pair differences: lower Ranch Hand insulin sensitivity with greater TCDD levels		
	1997 examination (29 pairs)		(p = 0.01)
	2002 examination (71 pairs)		(p = 0.02)

continued

TABLE 9-3 Continued

Reference	Study Population	Exposed Cases[a]	Estimated Relative Risk (95% CI)[a]
CDC, 1988	VES—deployed vs nondeployed		
	Interviewed—self-reported diabetes	155	1.2 (p > 0.05)
	Subset with physical examinations		
	Self-reported diabetes	42	1.1 (p > 0.05) geometric means (mg/dL)
	Fasting serum glucose		93.4 vs 92.4 (p < 0.05)
Studies Reviewed in *Update 2004*			
Kim JS et al., 2003	Korean veterans of Vietnam—Vietnam veterans	154	2.7 (1.1–6.7)
Michalek et al., 2003	Air Force Ranch Hand veterans (n = 343)	92	ns
Studies Reviewed in *Update 2000*			
AFHS, 2000[b]	AFHS—1997 exam cycle Ranch Hand veterans and comparisons	(Numerous analyses discussed in the text of *Type 2 Diabetes*)	
Longnecker and Michalek, 2000[b]	AFHS—comparison veterans only, OR by quartiles of serum dioxin concentration		
	Quartile 1: < 2.8 ng/kg	26	1.0
	Quartile 2: 2.8– < 4.0 ng/kg	25	0.9 (0.5–1.7)
	Quartile 3: 4.0– < 5.2 ng/kg	57	1.8 (1.0–3.0)
	Quartile 4: ≥ 5.2 ng/kg	61	1.6 (0.9–2.7)
CDVA, 1998a[b]	Australian Vietnam veterans—male		Cases expected (95% CI)
	Self-report of doctor's diagnosis	2,391	1,780
	(proportion of respondents)	(6%)	(1,558–2,003)
CDVA, 1998b[b]	Australian Vietnam veterans—female		Cases expected (95% CI)
	Self-report of doctor's diagnosis	5	10
	(proportion of respondents)	(2%)	(9–11)
Studies Reviewed in *Update 1998*			
Henriksen et al., 1997[b]	AFHS—through 1992 examination cycle Ranch Hand veterans—high-exposure group		
	Glucose abnormalities	60	1.4 (1.1–1.8)
	Diabetes prevalence	57	1.5 (1.2–2.0)
	Use of oral medications for diabetes	19	2.3 (1.3–3.9)
	Serum insulin abnormalities	18	3.4 (1.9–6.1)
O'Toole et al., 1996	Australian Vietnam veterans		
	Self-report of doctor's diagnosis	12	1.6 (0.4–2.7)
Studies Reviewed in *VAO*			
AFHS, 1991	AFHS—1987 examination cycle—elevation in blood glucose with serum TCDD		Significance of slope
	Ranch Hand veterans and comparisons	85	p = 0.001, p = 0.028

TABLE 9-3 Continued

Reference	Study Population	Exposed Cases[a]	Estimated Relative Risk (95% CI)[a]
AFHS, 1984	AFHS—1982 examination cycle—elevation in blood glucose with serum TCDD		
	Ranch Hand veterans and comparisons	158	p = 0.234
OCCUPATIONAL			
New Studies			
Montgomery et al., 2008	US AHS—self-reported incident diabetes (1999–2003) in licensed applicators		
	2,4-D	73	0.9 (0.8–1.1)
	2,4,5-T	28	1.0 (0.9–1.2)
Saldana et al., 2007	US AHS—self-reported gestational diabetes in wives of licensed applicators		
	Documented exposure during 1st trimester		ORs read from graph
	2,4-D	10	~1.0 (ns)
	2,4,5-T	3	~5 (p < 0.05)
	2,4,5-TP	2	~7 (p < 0.05)
	Dicamba	7	~3 (p ~ 0.06)
Studies Reviewed in *Update 2006*			
Blair et al., 2005	US Agriculture Health Study—mortality		
	Private applicators (male and female)	26	0.3 (0.2–0.5)
	Spouses of private applicators (> 99% female)	18	0.6 (0.4–1.0)
Studies Reviewed in *Update 2002*			
Steenland et al., 2001	Ranch Hand veterans, workers exposed to TCDD-contaminated products compared with nonexposed comparison cohorts		
	Ranch Hands	147	1.2 (0.9–1.5)
	Workers	28	1.2 (0.7–2.3)
Kitamura et al., 2000	Workers exposed to PCDD at municipal waste incinerator	8	nr, but ns
Studies Reviewed in *Update 2000*			
Calvert et al., 1999[b]	Workers exposed to 2,4,5-T, derivatives	26	1.5 (0.8–2.9)
	Serum TCDD pg/g of lipid		
	< 20	7	2.1 (0.8–5.8)
	20–75	6	1.5 (0.5–4.3)
	75–238	3	0.7 (0.2–2.6)
	238–3,400	10	2.0 (0.8–4.9)
Steenland et al., 1999[b]	Highly exposed industrial cohorts (n = 5,132)		
	Diabetes as underlying cause	26	1.2 (0.8–1.7)
	Diabetes among multiple causes	89	1.1 (0.9–1.3)
	Chloracne subcohort (n = 608)	4	1.1 (0.3–2.7)
Vena et al., 1998[b]	IARC cohort of production workers and sprayers in 12 countries—mortality[c]	33	2.3 (0.5–9.5)

continued

TABLE 9-3 Continued

Reference	Study Population	Exposed Cases[a]	Estimated Relative Risk (95% CI)[a]
Steenland et al., 1992[b]	NIOSH cohort of dioxin-exposed workers—mortality[c]		
	Diabetes as underlying cause	16	1.1 (0.6–1.8)
	Diabetes among multiple causes	58	1.1 (0.8–1.4)
Studies Reviewed in *Update 1998*			
Sweeney et al., 1997/1998	Dioxin-exposed workers in two chemical plants		1.1, p < 0.003
Ramlow et al., 1996	PCP production workers—mortality	4	1.2 (0.3–3.0)
Studies Reviewed in *Update 1996*			
Ott et al., 1994	TCP production workers		p = 0.06
Von Benner et al., 1994	West German chemical production workers	nr	nr
Zober et al., 1994	BASF production workers	10	0.5 (0.2–1.0)
Studies Reviewed in *VAO*			
Sweeney et al., 1992	NIOSH production workers	26	1.6 (0.9–3.0)
Henneberger et al., 1989	Paper and pulp workers	9	1.4 (0.7–2.7)
Cook et al., 1987	Production workers—mortality	4	0.7 (0.2–1.9)
Moses et al., 1984	2,4,5-T, TCP production workers with chloracne	22	2.3 (1.1–4.8)
May, 1982	TCP production workers	2	nr
Pazderova-Vejlupkova et al., 1981	2,4,5-T, TCP production workers	11	nr
ENVIRONMENTAL			
New Studies			
Consonni et al., 2008	Seveso residents (men and women)— 25-year mortality follow-up		
	Zone A	3	1.0 (0.3–3.1)
	Zone B	26	1.3 (0.9–1.9)
	Zone R	192	1.3 (1.1–1.5)
Everett et al., 2007	NHANES 1999–2002 participants Total diabetes (self-report or HbA1c > 6.1%)		
	HxCDD (TEF = 0.1)		
	> 42.0–99.1 pg/g		1.8 (1.1–2.8)
	> 99.1 pg/g		2.0 (0.9–4.4)
	PCB 126 (TEF = 0.1)		
	> 31.3–83.8 pg/g		1.7 (1.0.–2.7)
	> 83.8 pg/g		3.7 (2.1–6.5)

TABLE 9-3 Continued

Reference	Study Population	Exposed Cases[a]	Estimated Relative Risk (95% CI)[a]
Uemura et al., 2008a	Survey of Japanese adults		
	Total dioxins (pg TEQ/g lipid)		
	≥ 20.00–31.00	17	2.1 (0.9–5.4)
	≥ 31.00	39	3.8 (1.6–10.1)
Lee DH et al., 2006	NHANES 1999–2002 participants		
	HpCDD > 90th percentile vs nondetectable	46	2.7 (1.3–5.5)
	OCDD > 90th percentile vs nondetectable	31	2.1 (0.9–5.2)
Studies Reviewed in *Update 2006*			
Chen HL et al., 2006	Residents around 12 municipal waste incinerators in Taiwan—prevalence of physician-diagnosed diabetes with TEQs for serum TCDD/Fs in logistic model adjusted for age, sex, smoking, BMI	29	2.4 (0.2–31.9)
Baccarelli et al., 2005b	Children residing in Seveso at time of incident—development of diabetes		
	101 with chloracne	1	nr
	211 without chloracne	2	nr
Studies Reviewed in *Update 2004*			
Fierens et al., 2003	Belgium residents (142 women, 115 men) exposed to dioxins, PCBs		
	Subjects in top decile for dioxins		5.1 (1.2–21.7)
Studies Reviewed in *Update 2002*			
Masley et al., 2000	Population-based survey in Saskatchewan	28	nr
Studies Reviewed in *Update 2000*			
Bertazzi et al., 2001	Seveso residents—20-year follow-up		
	Zones A, B—males	6	0.8 (0.3–1.7)
	—females	20	1.7 (0.1–2.7)
Cranmer et al., 2000[b]	Vertac/Hercules Superfund site residents (n = 62)—OR for high insulin in nondiabetic subjects at various times, levels for TCDD > 15 ppt compared with persons with TCDD < 15 ppt		
	Fasting (insulin > 4.5 μIU/mL)	3	8.5 (1.5–49.4)
	30-min (insulin > 177 μIU/mL)	3	7.0 (1.3–39.0)
	60-min (insulin > 228 μIU/mL)	4	12 (2.2–70.1)
	120-min (insulin > 97.7 μIU/mL)	6	56 (5.7–556)
Bertazzi et al., 1998[b]	Seveso residents—15-year follow-up		
	Zone A—females	2	1.8 (0.4–7.0)
	Zone B—males	6	1.2 (0.5–2.7)
	—females	13	1.8 (1.0–3.0)

continued

TABLE 9-3 Continued

Reference	Study Population	Exposed Cases[a]	Estimated Relative Risk (95% CI)[a]
Pesatori	Zone R—males	37	1.1 (0.8–1.6)
et al., 1998[b]	—females	74	1.2 (1.0–1.6)

ABBREVIATIONS: 2,4-D, 2,4-dichlorophenoxyacetic acid; 2,4,5-T, 2,4,5-trichlorophenoxyacetic acid; 2,4,5-TP, 2-(2,4,5-trichlorophenoxy) preopionic acid; AFHS, Air Force Health Study; AHS, Agricultural Health Study; BMI, body mass index; CDC, Centers for Disease Control and Prevention; CI, confidence interval; HbA1c, hemoglobin A1c; HDL, high-density lipoprotein; HpCDD, 1,2,3,4,6,7,8-heptachlorodibenzo-*p*-dioxin; HxCDD, 1,2,3,6,7,9-hexachlorodibenzo-*p*-dioxin; IU, international unit; NHANES, National Health and Nutrition Examination Survey; NIOSH, National Institute for Occupation Safety and Health; nr, not reported; ns, not significant; OCDD, 1,2,3,4,6,7,8,9-octachlorodibenzo-*p*-dioxin; OR, odds ratio; PCB, polychlorinated biphenyl; PCDD, polychlorinated dibenzo-*p*-dioxin; PCP, pentachlorophenol; SEA, Southeast Asia; TCDD, 2,3,7,8-tetrachlorodibenzo-*p*-dioxin; TCDD/Fs, dioxins and furans combined; TCDF, tetrachlorodibenzofuran; TCP, trichlorophenol; TEF, toxicity equivalency factor; TEQ, total equivalent quotient; VES, Vietnam Experience Study.
[a]Given when available; results other than estimated risk explained individually.
[b]Study is discussed in greater detail in *Veterans and Agent Orange: Herbicide/Dioxin Exposure and Type 2 Diabetes* (IOM, 2000).
[c]Includes some subjects covered in other references cited in the category occupational cohorts.
Studies in italics have been superseded by newer studies of same cohort.

$p < 0.001$). The results were very similar in the strata expected to have a greater potential for high exposure and strongest when limited to subjects in the "high" group for both calendar time and number of spraying days (HR = 1.39, 95% CI 1.21–1.58).

Occupational Studies

Saldana and colleagues reported (2007) on the cross-sectional relationship between pesticide and herbicide exposure and a history of gestational diabetes in the AHS, a study of licensed pesticide applicators and their spouses who lived in Iowa and North Carolina. Women (n = 11,273) were asked about their health during their pregnancies closest to enrollment, and 506 (4.5%) reported gestational diabetes. Exposure to 2,4,5-T and 2,4-D was assessed by questionnaire. Data on women exposed to 2,4-D and 2,4,5-T were shown only for 337 women with documented exposure during the first trimester of pregnancy and then only in graphic form. The figure provided indicates that self-reported 2,4-D exposure was not associated with gestational diabetes but that 2,4,5-T exposure was associated after adjustment for BMI, mother's age, parity, race, state and commonly used pesticides.

Also in the AHS, Montgomery et al. (2008) reported on the relationship between pesticide and herbicide exposure and self-reported incident diabetes in 31,787 licensed pesticide applicators and their spouses. Physician-diagnosed incident diabetes (n = 1,176) was assessed during a follow-up by questionnaire. With adjustment for age, BMI, and state, neither the use of 2,4,5-T nor the use of 2,4-D was associated with the 5-year risk of diabetes (OR = 1.02, 95% CI 0.88–1.19; and OR = 0.92, 95% CI 0.79–1.06, respectively).

Environmental Studies

Consonni and colleagues (2008) reported on the 25-year mortality follow-up of persons exposed to dioxin accidentally in Seveso, Italy. Mortality experience was assessed relative to residence and intensity of exposure. Over the 25 years of follow-up, only three residents of the highest-exposed location died of diabetes mellitus (ICD-9 250). In comparison with nonexposed residents of surrounding localities, the estimated risk of diabetes mortality adjusted for sex, age, and period (5-year intervals for time of death) was significantly increased only in the most populated but least exposed zone (RR = 1.01, 95% CI 0.33–3.14; RR = 1.32, 95% CI 0.89–1.94; and RR = 1.26, 95% CI 1.08–1.47 for the highest-exposed, middle-exposed, and lowest-exposed zones, respectively).

Several surveys of diabetes and diabetes-related metabolic changes in relation to exposure to PCBs with dioxin-like activity have been published in the 2 years since *Update 2006*. Four studies analyzed NHANES data from 1999–2002. The NHANES data are based on a series of probability samples of the noninstitutionalized US population. In the 1999–2002 survey, dioxins, furans, and coplanar PCBs were measured in a random one-third sample of people at least 20 years old (n = 2,016).

Lee DH et al. (2006) studied the association between blood concentrations of six persistent organic pollutants including two dioxin congeners (1,2,3,4,6,7,8-heptacholorodibenzo-*p*-dioxin [HpCDD] and 1,2,3,4,6,7,8,9-octachlorodibenzo-*p*-dioxin [OCDD]), selected from 49 assessed. The six chemicals were selected because at least 80% of the study subjects had concentrations more than the limit of detection of the analytic method. A history of diabetes was reported by 217 of the 2,016 subjects analysed in this study. The authors reported that there was no association between diabetes and TCDD, but no statistics were presented because TCDD concentrations were above the limit of detection for only 7% of the population studied. The prevalence of diabetes was high in those who had HpCDD at or above the 90th percentile (26%) compared with those who did not have detectable HpCDD (4.6%). The adjusted prevalence OR was 2.7 (95% CI 1.3–5.5) and the test of trend for a dose–response relationship was significant (p = 0.007). A similar finding was reported for OCDD although the test for trend was not statistically significant (p = 0.094). However, association with diabetes was not specific to dioxin-like compounds inasmuch as the four non–dioxin-like organic pollutants assessed (PCB-153, oxychlorodane, *p,p'*-dichlorodiphenyltri-chloroethane [DDT], and *trans*-nonachlor) were all more strongly related to the prevalence of diabetes than either OCDD or HpCDD.

Everett et al. (2007) reported on the association between hexachlorodibenzo-*p*-dioxin, PCB-126, and *p,p'*-dichlorodiphenyltrichloroethane (DDT). PCB-126 has dioxin-like activity, but DDT does not. Serum concentrations were related to diagnosed and undiagnosed diabetes (based on a reading of hemoglobin A1c [HbA1c] over 6.1%). Lipid-adjusted concentrations of all three chemicals were associated with diagnosed diabetes, and PCB-126 and DDT were associated with undiagnosed diabetes. In a multivariate analysis in which all three substances were included to predict total diabetes, PCB-126 and DDT remained significantly associated.

Uemura et al. (2008a) assessed the association between exposure to persistent organic pollutants and the prevalence of diabetes in a survey of 1,274 Japanese adults 15–73 years old. Participants were required to have lived in their area for at least 10 years and not to have a known occupational exposure to dioxins. Participants were volunteers recruited through a mass-media campaign in the sample areas. The authors used the measurements of 29 pollutants with dioxin-like activity to calculate a dioxin TEQ that weights the concentration of a substance by the relative strength of its dioxin-like activity. There was a strong association between total dioxin TEQs and the prevalence of diabetes (OR = 3.81, 95% CI 1.56–10.1) after adjustment for age, sex, the log of BMI, region, residential area, and survey year. The association was stronger for dioxin-like PCBs (OR = 6.82, 95% CI 2.59–20.1) than for PCDDs and PCDFs (OR = 2.21, 95% CI 1.02–5.04) although the population was exposed to a higher dioxin TEQ from PCDDs and PCDFs than from PCBs. Total dioxin TEQs was also correlated with HbA1c (r = 0.103; p < 0.001).

Other Reviewed Studies

Rather than investigating the occurrence of diabetes itself, several additional studies addressed association of serum concentrations of persistent environmental pollutants to two indicators of increased diabetes risk: insulin resistance (Chen JW et al., 2008; Lee DH et al., 2007b) and the metabolic syndrome (Lee DH et al., 2007c). The reporting with respect to dioxin-like chemicals in several other studies of diabetes (Codru et al., 2007; Karouna-Renier et al., 2007; Wang et al., 2008) did not meet the threshold for the committee's evidentiary database. The results of these studies were not entered in the results table for diabetes (Table 9-3), but the committee did considered them as supportive information.

Insulin resistance was assessed in 749 nondiabetic participants by using a homeostasis-model assessment of insulin resistance (HOMA-IR) that is based on fasting glucose and insulin measurements (Lee DH et al., 2007b). The pollutant analysis was restricted to 19 substances that were above the assay limit of detection in at least 60% of the samples. Individual pollutants were combined on the basis of chemical class: three polychlorinated dibenzo-*p*-dioxins (PCDDs), three polychlorinated dibenzofurans (PCDFs), four dioxin-like PCBs, five non–dioxin-like PCBs, and four organochlorine (OC) pesticides. After adjustment for age, sex, race, and economic status, there was an association between HOMA-IR and PCDDs (p = 0.05) and OC pesticides (p < 0.01) but not the other three classes of compounds. Adjustment for body composition, smoking, exercise, and alcohol consumption reduced the association between HOMA-IR and PCDDs substantially (p = 0.25). Further analysis in which HOMA-IR was dichotomized into high and low showed that very high exposures to all the chemical classes except for OC pesticides were associated with a very high HOMA-IR; none of the associations was statistically significant.

The metabolic syndrome is a collection of metabolic changes, including increased waist circumference, blood pressure, serum triglyceride, and fasting glucose and reduced serum high-density lipoprotein cholesterol. People who have three or more of those abnormalities are said to have the metabolic syndrome, which is associated with the risk of diabetes and CVD. Lee DH et al. (2007c) found that dioxin-like PCBs, non–dioxin-like PCBs, and OC pesticides were associated with the metabolic syndrome, but PCDDs and PCDFs were not.

Chen JW et al. (2008) assessed the relationship between concentrations of 29 PCDDs, PCDFs, and PCBs and insulin sensitivity in 40 pregnant women from a contaminated part of Tainan City, Taiwan. In their small sample, neither PCDD TEQs nor PCDF TEQs correlated with measures of insulin sensitivity. PCB TEQs correlated inversely with insulin sensitivity (r = −0.42; p = 0.009). Of the 12 PCBs examined, only the dioxin-like PCBs-123, -126, and -169 were associated with both measures of insulin sensitivity—HOMA-IR and the quantitative insulin sensitivity check index.

Dioxins and furans were among the soil contaminants at a Superfund site in Pensacola, Florida, resulting from operations at a wood-treating company that was in operation from 1942 to 1982. In 2000, Karouna-Renier et al. (2007) gathered health and exposure histories and measured serum concentrations of 17 PCDD and PCDF congeners in 47 potentially exposed people. The study sample was selected in a nonsystematic fashion from among former workers, their families, and residents. Logistic analysis of the prevalence of several health problems in terms of toxicity equivalents (TEQs) with adjustment for age, race, sex, BMI, tobacco and alcohol use, and worker status permitted investigation of dose–response relationships. No significant association was found between exposure to the chemicals in question and the occurrence of diabetes (statistics not provided), defined by self-report, use of prescribed mediation, or serum glucose greater than 126 mg/dL.

Codru et al. (2007) report on the association between hexachlorobenzene,

PCB-153, PCB-74, and DDE and diabetes in a cross-sectional sample of 352 adult Americans Indians. The serum concentrations of all four chemicals were associated with the prevalence of diabetes, although none has dioxin-like activity.

Wang et al. (2008) reported on the 24-year follow-up of the Yucheng cohort in Taiwan. The cohort was exposed to high concentrations of PCBs and PCDFs (some congeners of both have dioxin-like activity) through contaminated rice oil. Cohort members were matched to a nonexposed referent population matched on age, sex, and neighborhood. In men, there was no association between being in the Yucheng cohort and diabetes risk. Women in the Yucheng cohort had over twice the odds of developing diabetes. The study also contrasted the lifetime prevalence of several medical conditions on the basis of whether the Yucheng cohort members had a history of chloracne. The risk of diabetes was higher in men (OR = 1.7, 95% CI 0.7–4.6) and in women (OR = 5.5, 95% CI 2.3–13.4) who had chloracne than in cohort members who had not had chloracne; the risks in those with chloracne compared with the referent population would be more extreme. The results of the study were not reported in terms of dioxin-like activity, so they do not directly contribute to the evidence considered for Vietnam veterans; however, in light of the well-known association between chloracne and AHR activation and dioxin-like activity, they are consistent with an association between exposure to the chemicals of interest and diabetes.

Biologic Plausibility

The toxicity of TCDD in laboratory animals has been historically linked with body-weight loss through inhibition of gluconeogenesis and increased lipid metabolism. Despite alterations in those key metabolic processes, diabetes has not been reported in TCDD-exposed rodents.

Several biologic mechanisms that have been studied in cell culture and animal models may explain the potential diabetogenic effects of TCDD in humans. TCDD is known to alter glucose and lipid metabolism in animal models (Dalton et al., 2001), to modify expression of genes related to insulin transport and signaling pathways in human adipose tissue (Fujiyoshi et al., 2006), and to produce oxidative stress at high concentrations (Kern et al., 2002; Matsumura, 2003). The present committee's literature review included several new studies that had increased mechanistic biologic plausibility. Sato et al. (2008) found that exposure of mice to dioxin resulted in significant changes in genes that are expressed in the liver and code for cholesterol biosynthesis, lipogenesis, and glucose metabolism. Dabir et al. (2008) found that glucose stimulates AHR signaling pathways associated with the expression of thrombospondon-1, which is associated with atherosclerosis. Arsenescu et al. (2008) found that the dioxin-like PCB-77 increased body weight in C57BL/6 ApoE mice, altered serum lipid profiles, and increased atherosclerosis. Those investigators found that PCB-77 in vitro stimulated the release of inflammatory cytokines and adipokines and increased the maturation of

3T3-L1 adipocytes. Thus, numerous mechanisms associated with insulin signaling, glucose, and lipid metabolism may be under the influence of the AHR and can be modulated by TCDD. Many of them are also risk factors for hypertension and ischemic heart disease.

Synthesis

A large number of relevant studies have been published since *Update 2006.* Michalek and Pavuk (2008) updated a series of reports on the AFHS. Their work is important because of its direct relevance to Vietnam veterans, its longitudinal design, and the dose–response analyses included. The primary dose–response analysis is related to categories of putative exposure based on serum TCDD measured in 1987. In this analysis, Ranch Hand veterans with higher circulating concentrations clearly are at higher risk. About 19% of potentially eligible Ranch Hand veterans were not included in the study, including some 10% who were excluded because of nonparticipation in the follow-up examinations. Hypothetically, if Ranch Hand veterans who had diabetes and high exposure were more likely to participate in the follow-up examinations than those in the SEA veteran comparison group, the association between Agent Orange exposure and TCDD would be overestimated. Such a bias could also generate spurious evidence on a dose–response relationship. The concern is mitigated by the inclusion of alternative analyses of the diabetes risk of Ranch Hand veterans based on calendar year of service and days of spraying. Differential-selection effects would be less likely in such an internal comparison. From the publication, it can be calculated that the risk of diabetes was 19.8% (130 of 657 in Ranch Hand veterans who served in 1969 or before) compared with 13.8% (50 of 363) in those who served after 1969. Similarly, the risk of diabetes was 18.7% (170 of 909) in those exposed to 90 days or more of spraying compared with 9.0% (10 of 111) in those exposed less than 90 days. The authors did not calculate adjusted RRs, but both unadjusted RRs are statistically significant (1.4 and 2.1, respectively; $p < 0.05$).

Consonni et al. (2008) updated previous analyses of findings from Seveso, Italy. The data provide some evidence of an excess of diabetes deaths in Seveso residents, but the residents in the most intensely exposed zone did not have higher mortality than the reference population; however, diabetes is a relatively unusual cause of death, and few such deaths were reported in the small population of the high-exposure zone.

An analysis of gestational diabetes in the wives of pesticide applicators in the AHS cohort (Saldana et al., 2007) found evidence of significantly increased risks among women who were exposed to 2,4,5-T or to 2,4,5-T during the first trimester of pregnancy, but these finding were based on only three and two exposed cases, respectively. With ten exposed cases, exposure to 2,4-D during this period had a neutral risk of gestational diabetes, whereas the risk associated with exposure to the related herbicide, dicamba, approached significance (seven exposed cases). (The estimated risks and confidence intervals in this paper were only presented graphically, so precise statistics cannot be presented.)

Neither 2,4,5-T nor 2,4-D was associated with incident diabetes in a 5-year follow-up of the entire AHS cohort (Montgomery et al., 2008). The confidence intervals are narrow; this indicates good precision for ruling out all but the most modest increases in risk. However, exposure estimates are based on questionnaire results, so exposure misclassification could lead to estimates biased toward no effect.

There were a number of surveys of blood concentrations of various persistent organic pollutants that have dioxin-like activity and the prevalence of diabetes or related metabolic derangements (such as insulin resistance and the metabolic syndrome). The series of papers from NHANES (Everett et al., 2007; Lee DH et al., 2006, 2007b,c) show that prevalent diabetes is associated with at least some substances that have dioxin-like activity. However, the effect is nonspecific in that several pollutants with and without dioxin-like activity are associated with diabetes. That suggests that there is something about the diabetic phenotype that is associated with either greater accumulation or slower elimination of fat-soluble organic pollutants. BMI, a measure of adiposity, is associated with a longer PCDD elimination half-life and is also a strong risk factor for diabetes. Because those studies are cross-sectional, the temporal relationship between pollutant concentrations and diabetes cannot be determined. However, TCDD was not related to either insulin resistance or the metabolic syndrome as would be expected if dioxin caused diabetes (Lee DH et al., 2007b,c). The statistical analyses of the NHANES data did not weight exposures according to the extent of their dioxin-like activity (TEQ). If that had been done, and if the associations with diabetes had been stronger, this would have helped to address the specificity issue.

The Japanese survey (Ueruma et al., 2008a,b) used TEQs to analyze data and found a strong overall association with diabetes prevalence. The data are not entirely consistent with the hypothesis that dioxin increases diabetes risk, inasmuch as the association was seen strongly for TEQs from PCBs, but not TEQs from PCDDs even though the population was exposed to more TEQs from PCDDs. The strong and preferential cross-sectional association between PCBs with dioxin-like activity and diabetes or insulin resistance was seen in several other studies (Chen et al., 2008; Everett et al., 2007; Lee DH et al., 2007b), and thus suggests a basis for the association other than a dioxin-mediated mechanism.

In the aggregate, the newly added studies do not counter previous findings with respect to the association between exposure and diabetes risk. The new data suggest that the herbicides 2,4,5-T and 2,4-D are not important contributors to diabetes risk. The new data are broadly consistent with the view that PCDDs may increase diabetes risk. The new longitudinal data reviewed represent updates of previously considered studies and therefore cannot be considered to be completely new. Thus, the new studies are not sufficient to merit a stronger conclusion with respect to the association.

Conclusion

On the basis of the evidence reviewed here and in previous VAO reports, the committee concludes that there is limited or suggestive evidence of an association between exposure to at least one chemical of interest and diabetes.

LIPID AND LIPOPROTEIN DISORDERS

Concentrations of plasma lipid—notably cholesterol—have been shown to predict CVD and are considered fundamental to the underlying atherosclerotic process (Roberts, 2000). Cholesterol and triglycerides, the two major types of lipids, are carried in the blood attached to proteins to form lipoproteins, which are classified by density. Very-low-density lipoprotein (VLDL, the major triglyceride particle) is produced in the liver and is progressively catabolized (hydrolyzed), mainly by an insulin-stimulated enzyme (lipoprotein lipase), to form intermediate-density lipoprotein (IDL), or VLDL remnants. Most of the VLDL remnants are rapidly cleared by low-density lipoprotein (LDL) receptors (types B and E) in the liver, and the rest form LDL, the major "bad cholesterol." LDL is cleared by LDL receptors in the liver and other tissues. High-density lipoprotein (HDL), the "good cholesterol," is produced in the small intestine and liver. It also results from the catabolism of VLDL. LDL is involved in the delivery of cholesterol to the tissues, and HDL is involved in "reverse" transport and facilitates the return of cholesterol to the liver for biliary excretion (Vergès, 2005).

Disorders of lipoprotein metabolism usually result from overproduction or decreased clearance of lipoproteins or both. Common examples are hypercholesterolemia, which can be familial (because of an LDL-receptor genetic defect) or polygenic (because of multiple minor genetic susceptibilities); familial hypertriglyceridemia (sometimes linked to susceptibility to diabetes); and mixed hyperlipidemias, in which both cholesterol and triglycerides are high. The mixed hyperlipidemias include familial combined hyperlipidemia, which could result from hepatic overproduction of VLDL and apoprotein B, and type III dyslipidemia, which involves defective clearance of IDL and VLDL remnants and a buildup of these atherogenic particles. Although the bulk of blood lipid concentration is genetically determined, diet, activity, and other factors (such as concurrent illness, use of drugs, age, sex, and hormones) have major effects. In particular, the saturated-fat content of the diet might raise LDL concentrations through decreased LDL-receptor activity; obesity and a high-carbohydrate diet can increase VLDL and possibly are linked to insulin resistance and reduced lipoprotein lipase activity. Diabetes mellitus and the metabolic syndrome are associated with increased triglycerides and decreased HDL. Other diseases (thyroid and renal disorders) often result in hypercholesterolemia. It is evident that multiple host and environmental factors influence lipid and lipoprotein concentrations and must be considered before the effect of a new factor can be assessed

(Verges, 2005). Any analysis should control for obesity as a primary determinant of triglyceride and TCDD concentrations. Finally, the ability of chronic diseases to raise triglycerides, glucose, and LDL or to lower HDL must be recognized.

Table 9-2 presents statistics on the 2006 US prevalence of readings in the ranges that define various lipid disorders.

Conclusions from *VAO* and Previous Updates

The committee responsible for *VAO* concluded that there was inadequate or insufficient information to determine whether there is an association between exposure to the chemicals of concern and lipid and lipoprotein disorders. Additional information available to the committees responsible for *Update 1996*, *Update 1998*, *Update 2000*, *Update 2002*, *Update 2004*, and *Update 2006* did not change that conclusion. Table 9-4 provides a summary of relevant studies that have been reviewed.

Update of the Epidemiologic Literature

No Vietnam-veteran or occupational studies concerning exposure to the chemicals of interest and lipid and lipoprotein disorders have been published since *Update 2006*.

Environmental Studies

Two environmental studies relevant to lipid and lipoprotein disorders have been published since *Update 2006*.

Uemura et al. (2008b) examined metabolic and dietary correlates of serum concentrations of persistent organic pollutants in a survey of 1,274 Japanese adults 15–73 years old. The authors used the measurements of 29 pollutants with dioxin-like activity to calculate a dioxin TEQ weighs the concentration of a substance by the relative strength of its dioxin-like activity. After adjustment for BMI alanine aminotransferase, creatinine, meat and egg consumption, fish and shellfish consumption, green-yellow vegetable consumption, and cigarette-smoking—and parity and breastfeeding status for women—there was a weak association between dioxin TEQs and log-triglyceride concentrations in men and a moderately strong association with total cholesterol concentrations in women.

Using data from the NHANES, Lee DH et al. (2007c) studied the association between blood concentrations of 19 persistent organic pollutants (of 49 assessed by the survey) and components of the metabolic syndrome, including increased triglyceride concentrations and low HDL-cholesterol concentrations. The 19 analytes were selected because at least 60% of the study subjects had concentrations of them that were greater than the limits of detection of the analytic method. After adjustment for age, sex, race, income, cigarette-smoking, serum cotinine, alcohol

TABLE 9-4 Selected Epidemiologic Studies—Lipid and Lipoprotein Disorders

Reference	Study Population	Exposed Cases[a]	Estimated Relative Risk (95% CI)[a]
VIETNAM VETERANS			
Studies Reviewed in *Update 2006*			
AFHS, 2005	Air Force Ranch Hand veterans (2002 exam data)	762	
	Model 3: low + high TCDD exposure vs comparisons		
	Cholesterol		reduced, p = 0.039
	Model 1: Ranch Hand vs comparisons		
	Triglycerides		increased in enlisted groundcrew, p = 0.034
	Model 3: low + high TCDD exposure vs comparisons		
	Triglycerides		increased, p = 0.001
	Model 4: Ranch Hand subjects' 1987 serum TCDD concentrations		
	Triglycerides		increased, p = 0.02
Studies Reviewed in *Update 2000*			
AFHS, 2000	Air Force Ranch Hand veterans (1997 exam data)	858	
	Cholesterol		ns
	Triglycerides		ns
Studies Reviewed in *Update 1998*			
AFHS, 1996	Air Force Ranch Hand veterans (1992 exam data)— change over time, Ranch Hand vs comparison group	884	
	Cholesterol (cholesterol:LDL ratio)		ns
	Triglycerides		ns
	HDL cholesterol (cholesterol:HDL ratio)		ns
O'Toole et al., 1996	Australian Vietnam veterans compared with Australian population	20	
	Cholesterol		3.0 (1.3–4.7)
Studies Reviewed in *VAO*			
AFHS, 1991	Air Force Ranch Hand veterans (1987 exam data)— Ranch Hands subjects with "high" lipid values	283–304	
	Serum-dioxin levels over lipid groups		
	Cholesterol		p = 0.175
	Triglycerides		p < 0.001
	HDL cholesterol		p < 0.001
AFHS, 1990	Air Force Ranch Hand veterans (1987 exam data)		
	Model 1: Ranch Hand vs comparisons		
	Cholesterol		1.2 (0.9–1.5)
	Triglycerides		1.3 (0.9–1.8)
	HDL cholesterol		1.0 (0.4–2.4)

continued

TABLE 9-4 Continued

Reference	Study Population	Exposed Cases[a]	Estimated Relative Risk (95% CI)[a]
AFHS, 1984; Wolfe et al., 1990	Air Force Ranch Hand veterans (1982 exam data)		
	Model 1: Ranch Hand vs comparisons	1,027	
	Cholesterol		ns
	Triglycerides		ns
	HDL cholesterol		ns
OCCUPATIONAL			
Studies Reviewed in *Update 2004*			
Hu et al., 2003	Workers exposed to PCDD/Fs in Taipei City— above median vs below median	133	
	Total cholesterol		2.8 (1.0–7.9)
	Triglycerides		1.5 (0.5–4.3)
Pelclová et al., 2002	Workers exposed to TCDD in Spolana, Czech Republic	12	
	Maximum value (1968–2001) vs 1966 serum TCDD level		Correlation coefficient
	Cholesterol		r = 0.78, p = 0.01
	Triglycerides		r = 0.66, p = 0.02
Studies Reviewed in *Update 2002*			
Kitamura et al., 2000	Workers exposed to PCDDs—hyperlipidemia	8	6.1, p = 0.02
Studies Reviewed in *Update 1998*			
Calvert et al., 1996	Workers exposed to 2,4,5-T derivatives vs matched referents OR		
	Abnormal total cholesterol		
	Overall	95	1.1 (0.8–1.6)
	High TCDD	18	1.0 (0.5–1.7)
	Abnormal HDL cholesterol		
	Overall	46	1.2 (0.7–2.1)
	High TCDD	16	2.2 (1.1–4.7)
	Abnormal mean total; HDL cholesterol ratio		
	Overall	131	1.1 (0.8–1.6)
	High TCDD	36	1.5 (0.8–2.7)
	Abnormal mean triglyceride		
	Overall	20	1.0 (0.5–2.0)
	High TCDD	7	1.7 (0.6–4.6)
Ott and Zober, 1996	Production workers exposed to TCDD	42	
	Cholesterol		ns[b]
	Triglycerides		ns[b]
	HDL cholesterol		Increased; p = 0.05
Studies Reviewed in *VAO*			
Martin, 1984	Production workers exposed to TCDD vs controls		
	No chloracne	53	
	Cholesterol		Increased; p < 0.005
	Triglycerides		Increased; p < 0.005

TABLE 9-4 Continued

Reference	Study Population	Exposed Cases[a]	Estimated Relative Risk (95% CI)[a]
	HDL cholesterol		ns
	With chloracne	39	
	Cholesterol		Increased; p < 0.05
	Triglycerides		Increased; p < 0.01
	HDL cholesterol		ns
Moses et al., 1984	TCP and 2,4,5-T production workers—those who developed chloracne vs those who did not	118	
	Cholesterol		ns
	Triglycerides		ns
Suskind and Hertzberg, 1984	TCP production workers		
	Cholesterol	204	ns
	Triglycerides		ns
	HDL cholesterol		ns
May, 1982	TCP production workers	94	
	Cholesterol		ns
	Triglycerides		ns
Pazderova-Vejlupkova et al., 1981	TCP, 2,4,5-T production workers	55	
	Cholesterol		ns
	Triglycerides		Increased VLDL; p = 0.01

ENVIRONMENTAL
New Studies

Reference	Study Population	Exposed Cases[a]	Estimated Relative Risk (95% CI)[a]
Uemura et al., 2008b	Survey of Japanese Adults—regression of log measured lipid with log of total dioxins (pg TEQ)		regression coefficients
	Men		
	Cholesterol		0.08 (p = 0.47)
	HDL cholesterol		0.04 (p = 0.68)
	Triglycerides		0.09 (p = 0.04)
	Women		
	Cholesterol		0.39 (p < 0.01)
	HDL cholesterol		−0.13 (p = 0.18)
	Triglycerides		−0.05 (p = 0.32)
Lee DH et al., 2007c	NHANES cross-sectional survey of persistent organic pollutants (≥ 75th percentile vs < 25th percentile)		
	HDL (< 1.1 mmol/L in men or < 1.4 mmol/L in women)		
	PCDDs		0.8 (0.5–1.5)
	PCDFs		0.9 (0.5–1.5)
	Dioxin-like PCBs		1.1 (0.6–2.1)
	Triglycerides (≥ 1.7 mmol/L)		
	PCDDs		1.0 (0.6–1.8)
	PCDFs		0.7 (0.4–1.2)
	Dioxin-like PCBs		2.0 (1.1–3.9)

continued

TABLE 9-4 Continued

Reference	Study Population	Exposed Cases[a]	Estimated Relative Risk (95% CI)[a]
Studies Reviewed in *VAO*			
Assennato	Seveso Zone A adult subjects, chloracne	193	
et al., 1989a	Cholesterol		ns
	Triglycerides		ns
Mocarelli	Children exposed near Seveso	63	
et al., 1986	Cholesterol		ns
	Triglycerides		ns

ABBREVIATIONS: 2,4,5-T, 2,4,5-trichlorophenoxyacetic acid; CI, confidence interval; HDL, high-density lipoprotein; LDL, low-density lipoprotein; NHANES, National Health and Nutrition Examination Survey; ns, not significant; OR, odds ratio; PCB, polychlorinated biphenyl; PCDD, polychlorinated dibenzo-*p*-dioxin; PCDD/F, dioxins and furans combined; PCDF, polychlorinated dibenzofuran; TCDD, 2,3,7,8-tetrachlorodibenzo-*p*-dioxin; TCP, trichlorophenol; TEQ, toxicity equivalent quotient; VLDL, very-low-density lipoprotein.
[a]Given when available; results other than estimated risk explained individually.

use, and exercise, HDL levels were not found to be associated with dioxin-like PCBs, PCDDs, or PCDFs; triglyceride concentrations were found to increase only with the levels of dioxin-like PCBs, but not PCDDs or PCDFs.

Biologic Plausibility

The induction of lipid mobilization and alterations in lipid metabolism are well-known effects of high-dose exposure to TCDD in laboratory animals that result in hyperlipidemia and loss of body fat. For example, Boverhof et al. (2005) found that exposure of mice to a single high dose of TCDD (30 μg/kg of body weight) increased serum triglycerides 1–7 days after exposure, and the increase was associated with changes in hepatic gene expression that were consistent with mobilization of peripheral fat. Similarly, Dalton et al. (2001) found that exposure of mice to a cumulative TCDD dose of 15 μg/kg over 3 days increased serum triglycerides and LDL that were measured 4 weeks after exposure. Increases in serum triglycerides have also been seen in TCDD-exposed rhesus monkeys (Rier et al., 2001). The mechanism underlying altered lipid metabolism has not been elucidated, but the high-dose studies in animal models provide some evidence of biologic plausibility that TCDD exposure can directly alter serum lipid and lipoprotein concentrations.

Synthesis

Previously reviewed literature showed inconsistent changes in serum lipids or lipoproteins after exposure to the chemicals of interest, and in most cases the sample sizes were insufficient to support any conclusions. The recently reviewed relevant literature does not clarify the situation with respect to the effect of Agent Orange on lipid and lipoprotein levels.

Conclusion

On the basis of the evidence reviewed here and in previous VAO reports, the committee concludes that there is insufficient or inadequate evidence to determine whether there is an association between exposure to the chemicals of interest and lipid or lipoprotein disorders.

GASTROINTESTINAL AND DIGESTIVE DISEASE, INCLUDING LIVER TOXICITY

This section discusses a variety of conditions encompassed by ICD-9 520–579: diseases of the esophagus, stomach, intestines, rectum, liver, and pancreas. Details on peptic ulcer and liver disease, the two conditions most often discussed in the literature reviewed, are provided below. The symptoms and signs of gastrointestinal disease and liver toxicity are highly varied and often vague.

The essential functions of the gastrointestinal tract are to absorb nutrients and eliminate waste. Those complex tasks involve numerous chemical and molecular interactions on the mucosal surface and complex local and distant neural and endocrine activity. One common condition of the gastrointestinal tract is motility disorder, which might be present in 15% of adults. The most convenient way to categorize diseases that affect the gastrointestinal system is according to the affected anatomic segment. Esophageal disorders predominantly affect swallowing; gastric disorders are related to acid secretion; and conditions that affect the small and large intestines are reflected in alterations in nutrition, mucosal integrity, and motility. Some systemic disorders (inflammatory, vascular, infectious, and neoplastic conditions) also affect the gastrointestinal system.

Peptic-Ulcer Disease

Peptic-ulcer disease refers to ulcerative disorders of the gastrointestinal tract that are caused by the action of acid and pepsin on the stomach or duodenal mucosa. Peptic-ulcer disease is characterized as gastric or duodenal ulcer, depending on the site of origin. Peptic-ulcer disease occurs when the corrosive action of gastric acid and pepsin overcomes the normal mucosal defense mechanisms that protect against ulceration. About 10% of the population have clinical evidence of duodenal ulcer at some period in life; a similar percentage are affected by gastric ulcer. The incidence of duodenal ulcer peaks in the 5th decade, and the incidence of gastric ulcer about 10 years later.

Evidence increasingly indicates that the bacterium *Helicobacter pylori* is linked to peptic-ulcer disease (both duodenal and gastric). *H. pylori* colonizes the gastric mucosa in 95–100% of patients with duodenal ulcer and in 75–80%

of patients with gastric ulcer. Healthy subjects in the United States under 30 years old have gastric colonization rates of about 10%. Over the age of 60 years, colonization rates exceed 60%. Colonization alone, however, is not sufficient for the development of ulcer disease; only 15–20% of subjects with *H. pylori* colonization will develop ulcers in their lifetimes. Other risk factors include genetic predisposition (such as some blood and HLA [human leukocyte antigen] types), cigarette-smoking, and psychologic factors (chronic anxiety and stress).

Liver Disease

Blood tests that reflect liver function are the mainstay of diagnosis of liver disease. Increases in serum bilirubin and in the serum concentrations of some hepatic enzymes—aspartate aminotransferase, alanine aminotransferase, alkaline phosphatase, and γ-glutamyltransferase (GGT)—are commonly noted in liver disorders. The relative sensitivity and specificity of those enzymes for diagnosing liver disease vary, and diagnosis can require several tests. The only regularly reported abnormality in liver function associated with TCDD exposure in humans is an increase in GGT. Estimated serum activity of that enzyme is a sensitive indicator of a variety of conditions, including alcohol and drug hepatotoxicity, infiltrative lesions of the liver, parenchymal liver disease, and biliary tract obstruction. Increases are noted after many chemical and drug exposures that are not followed by evidence of liver injury. The confounding effects of alcohol use (often associated with increased GGT) make interpretation of changes in GGT in exposed people difficult (Calvert et al., 1992). An increase in GGT can be considered a normal biologic adaptation to chemical, drug, or hormone exposure.

Cirrhosis is the most commonly reported liver disease in epidemiologic studies of herbicide or TCDD exposure. Cirrhosis is irreversible chronic injury of the liver with extensive scarring and resulting loss of liver function. Clinical symptoms and signs include jaundice, edema, abnormalities in blood clotting, and metabolic disturbances. Cirrhosis can lead to portal hypertension with associated gastroesophageal varices, enlarged spleen, abdominal swelling attributable to ascites, and ultimately hepatic encephalopathy that can progress to coma. It generally is impossible to distinguish the various causes of cirrhosis by using clinical signs and symptoms or pathologic characteristics. The most common cause of cirrhosis in North America and many parts of western Europe and South America is excessive alcohol consumption. Other causes are chronic viral infection (hepatitis B or hepatitis C), the poorly understood condition primary biliary cirrhosis, chronic right-sided heart failure, and a variety of less common metabolic and drug-related conditions.

Conclusions from *VAO* and Previous Updates

Studies that have been reviewed by previous committees have consisted of those focusing on liver enzymes and others that have reported specific liver diseases. Evaluation of the effect of herbicide and TCDD exposure on noncancer gastrointestinal ailments is challenging in that clinical experience suggests that medical history and physical examination are undependable diagnostic tools for some ailments, so incidence data are sometimes problematic. The strong interdependence among the characteristics of a given person (such as weight and laboratory indexes of hepatic function and health) and TCDD body burden complicates the already difficult task of assessing association.

Most of the analyses of occupational or environmental cohorts have had insufficient numbers of cases to support confident conclusions. The International Agency for Research on Cancer cohort of phenoxy herbicide and chlorophenol production workers and sprayers (Vena et al., 1998), the only study with a relatively large number of observations, found less digestive system disease and cirrhosis mortality in exposed workers than in nonexposed controls. A study comparing Australian veterans to the general population (O'Toole et al., 1996) suggested a higher incidence of stomach and duodenal ulcers in both men and women, but the information was self-reported and the analyses were not controlled for confounding influences.

A report from the AFHS (2000) found a significantly higher percentage of other liver disorders in the Ranch Hand veterans in the high-dioxin category than in the SEA comparison subjects. The excesses were primarily of transaminase and other nonspecific liver abnormalities. Data were consistent with an interpretation of a dose–response relationship, but other explanations were also plausible. Studies continue to report some abnormalities in liver enzymes in the Ranch Hand cohort (AFHS, 2005) including decreasing C4 complement as dioxin increased. Abnormal triglyceride concentrations increased as the 1987 dioxin concentration increased.

A study of Vietnam veterans reported in *Update 2006* found an increased rate of hepatitis associated with Vietnam service but not with a history of spraying herbicide (Kang et al., 2006). Likewise, the Australian Vietnam-veterans study (ADVA, 2005b) did not find an increase in liver disease in military personnel who served in Vietnam compared with the general population of Australia. Mortality studies of the Ranch Hand cohort have not found increased mortality related to gastrointestinal or liver disease (Ketchum and Michalek, 2005).

The reports to date have been inconsistent, and interpretation of individual studies is difficult because of a lack of information on alcohol consumption and other risk factors. In the studies that showed the strongest association between potential exposure and gastrointestinal disease (specifically cirrhosis), there was strong evidence that excess alcohol consumption was the cause of the cirrhosis.

The committee responsible for *VAO* concluded that there was inadequate or insufficient information to determine whether there is an association between exposure to the chemicals of interest and gastrointestinal and digestive disease, including liver toxicity. Additional information available to the committees responsible for *Update 1996*, *Update 1998*, *Update 2000*, *Update 2002*, *Update 2004*, and *Update 2006* did not change that conclusion.

Update of the Epidemiologic Literature

No Vietnam-veteran or occupational studies addressing gastrointestinal disorders have been published since *Update 2006*.

Environmental Studies

Consonni et al. (2008) reported on mortality in the cohort exposed to high environmental TCDD contamination in Seveso, Italy, starting in 1976 and followed up through 2001. The study cohort of 273,108 subjects who were resident at the time of the incident or immigrated or were born in the 10 years thereafter were analyzed according to three zones with increasing soil TCDD. In the overall sample, no statistically significant increases in deaths related to digestive diseases (ICD-9 520–579) were observed. In Zone A (highest TCDD contamination), five deaths from digestive disease were observed (RR = 0.72, 95% CI 0.30–1.74); the middle-contamination zone had 45 deaths from digestive disease (RR = 0.99, 95% CI 0.74–1.33); and the lowest-contamination zone had 366 deaths from digestive disease (RR = 1.11, 95% CI 1.00–1.24). The analysis of the subset of deaths related to cirrhosis did not find any statistically significant associations.

Karouna-Renier et al. (2007) gathered health and exposure histories from 47 potentially exposed people at a dioxin- and furan-contaminated Superfund site in Pensacola, Florida. Serum concentrations of 17 PCDD and PCDF congeners were measured. Analysis of covariance was used to assess the relationship between TEQ and several measures of liver function (alanine amino transferase, aspartate amino transferase, and GGT) with adjustment for age, sex, BMI, and alcohol use. No significant associations were found (statistics were not provided).

Biologic Plausibility

The liver is a primary target for the toxicity of many chemicals. It is the first organ that encounters chemicals absorbed from the gastrointestinal tract and is responsible for metabolizing them to water-soluble chemicals that can be excreted in the urine. Because the liver has many detoxifying enzymes that efficiently metabolize many chemicals, liver toxicity is usually associated only with high-dose acute exposure or chronic exposure to lower doses. The liver can be damaged if metabolism of a chemical results in the production of a reactive intermediate that is more toxic than the parent chemical. Changes in serum concentrations of liver enzymes are biomarkers for liver toxicity, and their magnitude correlates with the degree of liver damage. Exposure of laboratory animals to high doses of 2,4-D, 2,4,5-T, and TCDD is known to cause liver damage. The mechanisms by which the phenoxy herbicides damage the liver is based on inhibition of mitochondrial function by blocking of oxidative phosphorylation; this leads to loss of generation of adenosine triphosphate, and death of cells, and hepatic necrosis and fibrosis.

TCDD-induced hepatotoxicity is mediated by activation of the AHR, which leads to changes in gene transcription and associated changes in cell function. Changes in gene expression are associated with several physiologic processes, oxidative stress, and apoptosis (Boverhof et al., 2005, 2006). Histopathology of the liver after high doses of TCDD shows the development of a fatty liver associated with mobilization of peripheral fat and increased uptake of fatty acids in the liver. Exposure of rats to lower doses of TCDD over a 2-year period (NTP, 2004) also produced several changes in the liver, including hepatocyte hypertrophy, multinucleated hepatocytes, inflammation, pigmentation, diffuse fatty change, necrosis, bile duct hyperplasia, bile duct cyst, nodular hyperplasia, portal fibrosis, and cholangiofibrosis.

Few health-relevant effects of phenoxy herbicides or TCDD on the gastrointestinal tract, even after high levels of exposure, have been reported. Thus, the animal data do not support a plausible link between herbicide exposure and gastrointestinal toxicity in Vietnam veterans.

Synthesis

There is no evidence that Vietnam veterans are at greatly increased risk for serious liver disease, and reports of increased risk of abnormal liver-function tests have been mixed. Although increased rates of gastrointestinal disease have not been reported, the possibility of a relationship between dioxin exposure and subtle alterations in the liver and in lipid metabolism cannot be ruled out.

Conclusion

On the basis of the evidence reviewed here and in previous VAO reports, the committee concludes that there is inadequate or insufficient evidence to determine whether there is an association between exposure to the chemicals of interest and gastrointestinal and digestive diseases.

CIRCULATORY DISORDERS

This section covers a variety of conditions encompassed by ICD-9 390–459, such as acute and chronic rheumatic fever (ICD-9 390–398), hypertension (ICD-9 401–404), ischemic heart disease (ICD-9 410–414), heart failure (ICD-9 428), cerebrovascular disease (ICD-9 430–438), and peripheral vascular disease (ICD-9 443). *Coronary heart disease* is a specific term related to atherosclerosis; *ischemic heart disease* is a broader term and typically includes atherosclerosis and its symptoms. The American Heart Association reports mortality related to coronary heart disease, not to its symptoms, which include angina and myocardial infarction. Table 9-2 contains estimates of prevalence of and mortality from individual disorders of the circulatory system in the US population in 2006.

The methods used in morbidity studies can involve the direct assessment of the circulatory system, including analysis of symptoms or history, physical examination of the heart and peripheral arteries, Doppler measurements of peripheral pulses, electrocardiography (ECG), and chest radiography. Doppler measurements and physical examination of pulses in the arms and legs are used to detect decreases in pulse strength, which can be caused by thickening and hardening of the arteries. ECG can be used to detect heart conditions and abnormalities, such as arrhythmias (abnormal heart rhythms), heart enlargement, and heart attacks. Chest radiography can be used to assess the consequences of ischemic heart disease and hypertension, such as the enlargement of the heart seen with heart failure. However, clinical testing is often nonspecific; various medical conditions can yield similar test results. It is also sometimes difficult to determine the time of onset of clinical findings, so the temporal relationship between exposure and disease occurrence may be uncertain. Cardiovascular-disease epidemiologists prefer to observe cohorts over time for the incidence of discrete clinical events, such as an acute myocardial infarction (ideally verified on the basis of changes in ECG readings and enzyme concentrations) and death due to heart disease. The onset of new angina symptoms or the performance of a revascularization procedure in a person without a history of disease is also used as evidence of incident disease. In many occupational studies, only mortality information is available. The attribution of death to a vascular cause is often based on a death certificate, whose accuracy can be uncertain.

Conclusions from *VAO* and Previous Updates

The committee responsible for *VAO* concluded that there was inadequate or insufficient information to determine whether there is an association between exposure to the chemicals of interest and circulatory disorders. Additional information available to the committees responsible for *Update 1996*, *Update 1998*, *Update 2000*, *Update 2002*, and *Update 2004* did not change that conclusion. The committee responsible for *Update 2006* reviewed both new studies and intensively revisited all the studies related to ischemic heart disease and hypertension that had been discussed in previous updates and concluded that there is limited or suggestive evidence to support an association between exposure to the herbicides used in Vietnam and hypertension. That committee was unable to reach a consensus as to whether that was also the case for ischemic heart disease, however, so that outcome remained in the category of inadequate evidence. The previous studies and studies published since *Update 2006* are all summarized in Table 9-5.

TABLE 9-5 Selected Epidemiologic Studies—Circulatory Disorders

Reference[a]	Study Population[b]	Exposed Cases[c]	Estimated Relative Risk (95% CI)[c]	Comments
Studies of Vietnam Veterans				
	Studies of US Vietnam veterans			
Kang et al., 2006 and supplemental data	**Army Chemical Corps—morbidity**			Diagnoses not confirmed by medical record review.
	Vietnam veterans vs nonVietnam veterans			Adjusted for age, race, rank, BMI, and smoking.
	Hypertension requiring medication	496	1.06 (0.89–1.27)	
	Heart disease diagnosed by physician	243	1.09 (0.87–1.38)	Serum TCDD levels were measured in a subset of
	Sprayers vs nonsprayers			subjects, and those self-reported to have been sprayers
	All (diabetics, nondiabetics)			did have significantly higher
	Hypertension requiring medication	247	1.26 (1.00–1.58)	concentrations than others.
	Heart disease diagnosed by physician	129	1.41 (1.06–1.89)	Therefore, the sprayer
	All veterans, contribution of spraying to logistic regression model			category is regarded as a valid surrogate for elevated exposure.
	All (diabetics, nondiabetics)			
	Hypertension requiring medication		1.32 (1.08–1.61)	
	Heart disease diagnosed by physician		1.52 (1.18–1.94)	
	Non-diabetics only			
	Hypertension requiring medication		1.23 (0.99–1.52)	
	Heart disease diagnosed by physician		1.52 (1.14–2.01)	
	Controlling for diabetic status			
	Hypertension requiring medication		1.27 (1.04–1.55)	
	Heart disease diagnosed by physician		1.45 (1.13–1.86)	

continued

TABLE 9-5 Continued

Reference[a]	Study Population[b]	Exposed Cases[c]	Estimated Relative Risk (95% CI)[c]	Comments
Thomas and Kang, 1990	**Army Chemical Corps vs US male population—mortality**			Not adjusted for known risk factors.
	Circulatory diseases (ICD 390–458)	6	0.55	
AFHS, 2005 [*Largely supersedes* AFHS, 1984, 1987, 1990, 1992, 1995, 2000]	**Air Force Health Study, 2002 exam cycle** (1,951 participants)—**morbidity** [results largely supersede those of 1982, 1985, 1987, 1997, and 1997 exams cycles]			All analyses adjusted for age, race, rank, smoking, alcohol history, HDL, cholesterol, cholesterol HDL ratio, uric acid, diabetes, BMI or percent body fat, waist-hip ratio, family history of heart disease.
Number in analysis	Model 1: RH subjects vs SEA comparisons (also available separately for officer, enlisted flyer, enlisted groundcrew)			
1,885	Essential hypertension	412 of 759	0.92 (0.53–1.13)	
1,902	Heart disease (except essential hypertension)	644 of 767	1.20 (0.94–1.54)	
308	Enlisted flyer	120 of 131	2.46 (1.19–5.11)	
1,902	Myocardial infarction	77 of 767	0.81 (0.59–1.12)	
1,902	Stroke or transient ischemic attack	29 of 767	1.39 (0.82–2.34)	
	Model 2: RH subjects with extrapolated initial serum TCDD (> 10 ppt in 1987)		Relative risk for 2-fold increase in serum TCDD	
406	Essential hypertension	244	1.12 (0.91–1.37)	
411	Heart disease (except essential hypertension)	344	1.08 (0.85–1.38)	
411	Myocardial infarction	42	1.31 (0.97–1.77)	
411	Stroke or transient ischemic attack	17	1.26 (0.78–2.03)	

continued

Model 3: All subjects with serum TCDD readings (RH group vs comparisons)

			Relative risk
Essential hypertension	1,344		
Comparison		644	1.0
RH background	(< 10 ppt, 1987)	168	0.88 (0.67–1.16)
RH low	(10–118 ppt, initial)	109	0.74 (0.53–1.04)
RH high	(> 118 ppt, initial)	135	1.32 (0.94–1.87)
Heart disease (except essential hypertension)	1,355		
Comparison		937	1.0
RH background	(< 10 ppt, 1987)	299	1.33 (0.94–1.89)
RH low	(10–118 ppt, initial)	171	1.03 (0.68–1.54)
RH high	(> 118 ppt, initial)	173	1.21 (0.81–1.82)
Myocardial infarction	1,355		
Comparison		132	1.0
RH background	(< 10 ppt, 1987)	34	0.81 (0.53–1.25)
RH low	(10–118 ppt, initial)	18	0.60 (0.34–1.04)
RH high	(> 118 ppt, initial)	24	1.04 (0.63–1.74)
Stroke or transient ischemic attack	1,355		
Comparison		36	1.0
RH background	(< 10 ppt, 1987)	12	1.21 (0.59–2.45)
RH low	(10–118 ppt, initial)	7	1.10 (0.47–2.57)
RH high	(> 118 ppt, initial)	10	2.16 (0.98–4.77)

Model 4: RH subjects with 1987 serum TCDD readings

		Relative risk for 2-fold increase in serum TCDD
Essential hypertension	748	1.11 (0.98–1.25)
Heart disease (except essential hypertension)	755	0.90 (0.78–1.06)
Myocardial infarction	755	1.03 (0.85–1.24)
Stroke or transient ischemic attack	755	1.04 (0.76–1.44)

TABLE 9-5 Continued

Reference[a]	Study Population[b]	Exposed Cases[c]	Estimated Relative Risk (95% CI)[c]	Comments
Ketchum and Michalek, 2005 [*Supersedes Michalek et al., 1990, 1998*]	**Air Force Health Study—circulatory disease—mortality**			
	Ranch Hand subjects vs all SEA veterans	66	1.3 (1.0–1.6)	Not adjusted for known risk factors.
	Pilots and navigators	18	1.1 (0.7–1.8)	
	Administrative officers	2	1.8 (0.4–7.8)	
	Enlisted flight engineers	6	0.5 (0.2–1.1)	
	Ground crew	40	1.7 (1.2–2.4)	
	Atherosclerosis	28	1.7 (1.1–2.5)	
	Hypertensive disease	2	2.5 (0.6–10.8)	
	Stroke	5	2.3 (0.9–6.0)	
	Subjects with serum TCDD measures			Adjusted for smoking and family history of heart disease.
	SEA comparison group	31	1.0	
	Background (0.6–10.0 ppt)	8	0.8 (0.4–1.8)	
	Low (10.0–29.2 ppt)	12	1.8 (0.9–3.5)	
	High (18.0–617.8 ppt)	9	1.5 (0.7–3.3)	
Cypel and Kang, 2008—new study [*Supersedes Thomas et al., 1991; Dalager et al., 1995*]	**Female US Vietnam-era veterans—mortality** (through 2004)			
	Circulatory system diseases			Adjusted for duration of service, year of birth, race.
	Vietnam vs non-SEA veterans	129	0.8 (0.6–1.0)	
	Nurses only	102	0.8 (0.6–1.0)	
Watanabe and Kang, 1996	**US Army and Marine Corps Vietnam-era veterans—mortality** (PMR, 1965–1988)			
	Served in Vietnam vs never-deployed to SEA			Not adjusted for known risk factors.
	Circulatory diseases (ICD-8 390–458)			
	Army	5,756	0.97 (p > 0.05)	
	Marine Corps	1,048	0.92 (p < 0.05)	

continued

		N		Comments
Bullman and Kang, 1996	**US wounded Vietnam veterans vs US men—mortality** (through 1981, focus on suicide)			
	Circulatory disease	246	0.72 (0.55–0.91)	
Boehmer et al., 2004	**CDC** Vietnam Experience Study—**mortality**			
	<u>Deployed vs nondeployed</u>			
	Circulatory disease	185	1.01 (0.82–1.24)	Adjusted for age, race, military occupation.
	Year of death			
	1970–1984	nr	0.56 (0.28–1.15)	
	1985–2000 (partition at 1970 arbitrary)	nr	1.06 (0.85–1.32)	
	Discharged before 1970	nr	0.83 (0.62–1.12)	
	Discharged after 1970	125	1.43 (1.02–1.99)	
	Ischemic heart diseases	8		
	0–15 years since discharge	117	0.77 (0.31–1.55)	
	>15 years since discharge		1.14 (0.87–1.50)	
CDC, 1988	**CDC** Vietnam Experience Study—**morbidity**			
	<u>Deployed vs nondeployed</u>			
	Hypertension after discharge			
	Interviewed	2,013	1.3 ($p < 0.05$)	Not adjusted for known risk factors.
	Examined	623	1.2 ($p < 0.05$)	
Stellman et al., 1988	**American Legionnaires serving during Vietnam era—morbidity**			
	<u>Service in SEA vs not, with medically diagnosed</u>			
	High blood pressure	592	1.12 ($p > 0.05$)	Not age adjusted.
	Heart disease	97	1.45 ($p < 0.05$)	Age adjusted.

TABLE 9-5 Continued

Reference[a]	Study Population[b]	Exposed Cases[c]	Estimated Relative Risk (95% CI)[c]	Comments
Anderson et al., 1986	**Wisconsin Vietnam veterans—all diseases of circulatory system—mortality**			
	White male Vietnam veterans vs	100		
	National population		0.69 (p < 0.05)	
	State population		0.62 (p < 0.05)	
	Nonveterans		0.58 (p < 0.05)	
	All veterans		0.86 (p > 0.05)	
	Vietnam-era veterans		0.99 (0.80–1.20)	
Kogan and Clapp, 1985	**Massachusetts Vietnam-era veterans (1958–1973)—mortality (1972–1983)**			
	Deployed vs nondeployed			
	Deaths 1972–1983			
	Circulatory system (except cerebrovascular)	139	PMR = 0.88 (p > 0.05)	Not adjusted for age; Vietnam veterans thought to be younger.
	Cerebrovascular	28	PMR = 1.11 (p > 0.05)	
	Deaths 1978–1983			
	Circulatory system (except cerebrovascular)	85	PMR = 0.80 (p < 0.05)	Expected less "diluted" effect for later time.
	Cerebrovascular	19	PMR = 1.64 (p < 0.05)	
ADVA, 2005b	**Studies of Australian Vietnam veterans**			
	Australian Vietnam veterans vs general male population—mortality			
	Circulatory disease	1,767	0.88 (0.84–0.92)	Pattern of increasing risks with time could perhaps indicate dissipation of healthy warrior effect.
	1963–1979	186	0.69 (0.59–0.79)	
	1980–1990	546	0.88 (0.80–0.95)	
	1991–2001	1,035	0.93 (0.87–0.99)	

continued

Reference	Outcome	N	Ratio (95% CI)	Comments
	Ischemic heart disease	1,297	0.94 (0.89–0.99)	
	1963–1979	124	0.70 (0.58–0.82)	
	1980–1990	421	0.95 (0.86–1.04)	
	1991–2001	753	0.99 (0.92–1.06)	
	Stroke	223	0.80 (0.70–0.91)	
	1963–1979	35	0.81 (0.54–1.07)	
	1980–1990	59	0.73 (0.54–0.92)	
	1991–2001	129	0.83 (0.69–0.97)	
ADVA, 2005c	**Australian National Service veterans—deployed vs nondeployed—mortality**			
	Circulatory disease	208	1.05 (0.87–1.27)	
	Ischemic heart disease	159	1.18 (0.94–1.47)	
	Stroke	15	0.61 (0.30–1.15)	Not adjusted for known risk factors.
Crane et al., 1997a [largely superseded by ADVA, 2005b]	**Australian Vietnam veterans—mortality** (1980–1994)			
	Circulatory disease		0.96 (0.88–1.05)	
	Ischemic heart disease		1.04 (0.94–1.14)	
	Cerebral hemorrhage		0.80 (0.53–1.22)	
Crane et al., 1997b [largely superseded by ADVA, 2005c]	**Australian National Service Vietnam-era veterans—mortality** (1982–1994)			Not adjusted for known risk factors.
	Deployed vs nondeployed			
	Circulatory disease	77	0.95 (0.70–1.28)	
	Ischemic heart disease	57	0.97 (0.68–1.39)	
	Cerebral hemorrhage	3	0.96 (0.14–5.66)	
	Other	17	0.88 (0.44–1.69)	

TABLE 9-5 Continued

Reference[a]	Study Population[b]	Exposed Cases[c]	Estimated Relative Risk (95% CI)[c]	Comments
O'Toole et al., 1996	**Australian male Army Vietnam veterans** (random sample)—**morbidity**			Adjusted for non-response, but not adjusted for known risk factors.
	Self-report in telephone interview		99% CIs	
	Hypertension	nr	2.17 (1.71–2.62)	
	Heart disease	nr	1.98 (0.91–3.05)	
	Other circulatory diseases (excluding above and hemorrhoids)	nr	2.39 (1.61–3.17)	
Kim JS et al., 2003	**Korean veterans of Vietnam—morbidity**			Concerns of selection bias, quality of diagnosis, low participation. Gross pooling of blood samples made TCDD concentrations useless.
	Deployed *vs* nondeployed (unadjusted)			
	Valvular heart disease	8	p = 0.0019	
	Congestive heart failure	5	p = 0.5018	
	Ischemic heart disease	34	p = 0.0045	
	Hypertension	383	p = 0.0143	
	Adjusted for age, smoking, alcohol, BMI, education, and marital status		2.29 (1.33–3.95)	
Occupational Studies				
Pelclová et al., 2007—new study	**2,4,5-T production workers at Spolana plant in Czech Republic 1965–1968**—vascular function measured by microvascular reactivity in response to flow-mediated or thermal hyperemia	15	Reactivity lower in workers compared to controls (p < 0.05)	Concerns about selection bias and the role of comorbidity.
McLean et al., 2006	**IARC cohort of pulp and paper workers—** circulatory disease—**mortality**			Not adjusted for known risk factors.
	Never exposed to nonvolatile organochlorines	2,727	0.92 (0.89–0.96)	
	Ever exposed to nonvolatile organochlorines	2,157	0.99 (0.95–1.04)	

Reference	Study	N	Risk estimate	Comments
Blair et al., 2005	**US Agricultural Health Study—mortality**			Adjusted for age, race, state, sex, and calendar year of death.
	Private applicators (farmers), spouses			
	Circulatory disease (1994–2000)	619	0.5 (0.5–0.6)	
't Mannetje et al., 2005 [IARC subcohort]	**New Zealand phenoxy herbicide workers—mortality**			Not adjusted for known risk factors.
	Producers (1969–2000)			
	Circulatory disease	51	1.0 (0.7–1.3)	
	Hypertensive disease	0	0.0 (0.0–3.5)	
	Ischemic heart disease	38	1.0 (0.7–1.4)	All-causes SMR = 1.0 (0.8–1.2).
	Sprayers (1973–2000)			
	Circulatory disease	33	0.5 (0.4–0.7)	
	Hypertensive disease	1	0.8 (0.0–4.5)	
	Ischemic heart disease	22	0.5 (0.3–0.8)	All-causes SMR = 0.6 (0.5–0.8).
Vena et al., 1998 [same dataset as Kogevinas et al., 1997 (emphasis on cancer) reviewed in *Update 1998*]	**IARC cohort of phenoxy herbicide workers—mortality** (1939–1992)			Not adjusted for known risk factors.
	All male phenoxy herbicide workers			
	All circulatory disease (ICD 390–459)	1,738	0.91 (0.87–0.95)	
	Ischemic heart disease (ICD 410–414)	1,179	0.92 (0.87–0.98)	
	Cerebrovascular disease (ICD 430–438)	254	0.86 (0.76–0.97)	
	Other diseases of heart (ICD 415–429)	166	1.11 (0.95–1.29)	
	All female phenoxy herbicide workers			
	All circulatory disease (ICD 390–459)	48	1.00 (0.73–1.32)	
	Ischemic heart disease (ICD 410–414)	24	1.07 (0.68–1.59)	
	Cerebrovascular disease (ICD 430–438)	9	0.73 (0.33–1.38)	
	Other diseases of heart (ICD 415–429)	6	0.92 (0.34–2.00)	
	Workers with phenoxy herbicide exposure only			
	All circulatory disease (ICD 390–459)	588	0.86 (0.79–0.93)	
	Ischemic heart disease (ICD 410–414)	394	0.85 (0.77–0.94)	

continued

TABLE 9-5 Continued

Reference[a]	Study Population[b]	Exposed Cases[c]	Estimated Relative Risk (95% CI)[c]	Comments
	Cerebrovascular disease (ICD 430–438)	96	0.86 (0.70–1.05)	
	Other diseases of heart (ICD 415–429)	32	0.80 (0.55–1.13)	
	TCDD-exposed workers			
	All circulatory disease (ICD 390–459)	1,170	0.94 (0.88–0.99)	
	Ischemic heart disease (ICD 410–414)	789	0.97 (0.90–1.04)	
	Cerebrovascular disease (ICD 430–438)	162	0.84 (0.71–0.98)	
	Other diseases of heart (ICD 415–429)	138	1.20 (1.01–1.42)	
	Contribution of TCDD exposure to Poisson regression analysis			
	All circulatory disease	1,151	1.51 (1.17–1.96)	Adjusted for age, timing of exposure.
	Ischemic heart disease	775	1.67 (1.23–2.26)	
	Cerebrovascular disease	161	1.54 (0.83–2.88)	
Hooiveld et al., 1998	**Dutch herbicide factory workers (IARC subcohort)—mortality (1955–1991)**			
	<u>549 exposed vs 482 nonexposed male workers</u>			
	All circulatory diseases (ICD 390–459)	45	1.4 (0.8–2.5)	Adjusted for age, timing of exposure.
	TCDD > 124 ng/kg	nr	1.5 (0.8–2.9)	
	Ischemic heart diseases (ICD 410–414)	33	1.8 (0.9–3.6)	
	TCDD > 124 ng/kg	nr	2.3 (1.0–5.0)	
	Cerebrovascular diseases (ICD 430–438)	9	1.4 (0.4–5.1)	
	TCDD > 124 ng/kg	nr	0.8 (0.2–4.1)	
	Other heart disease (ICD 415–429)	3	0.7 (0.1–4.3)	
	TCDD > 124 ng/kg	nr	0.4 (0.0–4.9)	

Flesch-Janys et al.,
1995

Hamburg, Germany herbicide production workers (*IARC subcohort*) *vs gas workers—mortality* (1952–1992; estimated blood PCDD, PCDF, TCDD from work history, measures on 190 of 1,189 men, divided into four lowest quintiles, top two deciles)

Gas workers provide a more appropriate comparison group for the data on production workers than the national population data used in the analysis in Flesch-Janys, 1997/1998; Flesch-Janys et al., 1998.

Not adjusted for known risk factors.

Potential for exposure misclassification.

Estimated final PCDD, PCDF TEQs (ng/kg)

Circulatory disease (ICD 390–459)   156

1.0–12.2	0.93 (0.57–1.50)
12.3–39.5	0.92 (0.59–1.46)
39.6–98.9	1.48 (1.01–2.17)
99.0–278.5	1.55 (1.07–2.24)
278.6–545.0	1.63 (1.01–2.64)
545.1–4361.9	2.06 (1.23–3.45)
	p-trend < 0.01

Ischemic heart disease (ICD 410–414)   76

1.0–12.2	1.02 (0.54–1.95)
12.3–39.5	0.96 (0.51–1.82)
39.6–98.9	0.97 (0.52–1.81)
99.0–278.5	1.13 (0.64–2.00)
278.6–545.0	1.73 (0.92–3.27)
545.1–4361.9	2.72 (1.49–4.98)
	p-trend < 0.01

continued

TABLE 9-5 Continued

Reference[a]	Study Population[b]	Exposed Cases[c]	Estimated Relative Risk (95% CI)[c]	Comments
	Estimated final TCDD (ng/kg)			
	Circulatory disease (ICD 390–459)	156		
	0–2.8		1.22 (0.81–1.83)	
	2.81–14.4		0.88 (0.54–1.44)	
	14.5–49.2		1.35 (0.91–2.01)	
	49.3–156.7		1.64 (1.12–2.39)	
	156.8–344.6		1.53 (0.95–2.44)	
	344.7–3890.2		1.96 (1.15–3.34)	
			p-trend = 0.01	
	Ischemic heart disease (ICD 410–414)	76		
	0–2.8		1.43 (0.83–2.44)	
	2.81–14.4		0.81 (0.41–1.61)	
	14.5–49.2		1.18 (0.65–2.16)	
	49.3–156.7		0.90 (0.47–1.75)	
	156.8–344.6		1.61 (0.85–3.04)	
	344.7–3890.2		2.48 (1.32–4.66)	
			p-trend < 0.01	
Becher et al., 1996 [mortality through 1992 for Hamburg plant reported above by Flesch-Janys]	**Phenoxy herbicide workers at four German plants** (four IARC subcohorts, including Hamburg)—**mortality** (through 1989)			
	Circulatory diseases (ICD 390–458)			
	Bayer Uerdingen	12	0.74 (0.38–1.30)	
	Bayer Dormagen	3	0.34 (0.07–0.99)	
	BASF Ludwigshafen	32	0.78 (0.53–1.10)	

continued

Reference	Disease/cohort	No.	Risk (95% CI)	Comments
Coggon et al., 1991	**British Chemical Manufacturers at four plants** (four IARC subcohorts)—**mortality**			
	Circulatory disease	74	1.16 (0.91–1.46)	
	Plant A (1975–1987)	34	1.67 (adjusted = 1.39, p ≈ 0.05)	
	Plant B (1969–1987)	5	0.95	
	Plant C (1963–1987)	12	0.84	
	Plant D (1969–1987)	23	0.97	
Coggon et al., 1986	**British MCPA manufacturers** (5th of seven UK IARC cohorts)—**mortality**			
	Hypertensive, ischemic heart disease (ICD 401–414, 428–429)	337		
	vs national rates		0.81 (0.73–0.90)	
	with rural adjustment		0.86 (0.77–0.96)	
	US cohorts in NIOSH cohort (also in IARC cohort)			
Burns et al., 2001 [part of IARC & NIOSH cohorts]	**Dow 2,4-D production workers—mortality** (1945–1994)			Not adjusted for known risk factors.
	Circulatory disease			
	0 years latency	158	0.95 (0.80–1.11)	
	≥ 20 years latency	130	1.05 (0.87–1.24)	
Ramlow et al., 1996	**Dow PCP workers (1930–1980)** (subcohort)—**mortality** (1940–1989)			
	Circulatory diseases (ICD 390–458)	115	0.95 (0.79–1.14)	
	Arteriosclerotic heart disease (ICD 410–414)	86	1.02 (0.82–1.26)	
	Cerebrovascular disease (ICD 430–438)	15	1.02 (0.57–1.68)	

TABLE 9-5 Continued

Reference[a]	Study Population[b]	Exposed Cases[c]	Estimated Relative Risk (95% CI)[c]	Comments
Steenland et al., 1999	**NIOSH cohort (subcohorts of IARC cohort at 12 US plants)—mortality** (through 1993)			
	Total cohort (5,132) vs US population			
	Cerebrovascular disease (ICD 430–438)	69	0.96 (0.74–1.21)	Not adjusted for known risk factors.
	Ischemic heart disease (ICD 410–414)	456	1.09 (1.00–1.20)	
	Chloracne subcohort (608) vs US population	92	1.17 (0.94–1.44)	
	Exposure subcohort (3,538)			
	< 19 cumulative TCDD	nr	1.0	Adjusted for age.
	19–139	nr	1.23 (0.75–2.00)	No units given for exposure derived from job–exposure matrix.
	139–580	nr	1.34 (0.83–2.18)	
	581–1,649	nr	1.30 (0.79–2.13)	
	1,650–5,739	nr	1.39 (0.86–2.24)	
	5,740–20,199	nr	1.57 (0.96–2.56)	
	≥ 20,200	nr	1.75 (1.07–2.87)	
			p-trend cumulative exposure = 0.05	
			p-trend log[cumulative exposure] < 0.001	
Calvert et al., 1998	**Two US chemical plants (part of NIOSH, IARC cohorts)—morbidity**			
	Verified conditions			
	TCDD-exposed (281) vs nonexposed (260)			
	Myocardial infarction	17	1.33 (0.62–2.84)	Not adjusted for known risk factors.
	Current systolic hypertension	64	1.05 (0.70–1.58)	
	Current diastolic hypertension	77	1.23 (0.83–1.82)	

TCDD effect vs nonexposed in logistic model
Self-reported and verified conditions combined

Myocardial infarction		
Serum TCDD < 238 pg/g of lipid	nr	1.14 (0.29–4.49)
Serum TCDD ≥ 238 pg/g of lipid	nr	1.09 (0.23–5.06)
Hypertension		
Serum TCDD < 238 pg/g of lipid	nr	1.34 (0.89–2.02)
Serum TCDD ≥ 238 pg/g of lipid	nr	1.05 (0.58–1.89)
Verified conditions		
Current systolic hypertension		
Serum TCDD < 238 pg/g of lipid	nr	1.09 (0.65–1.83)
Serum TCDD ≥ 238 pg/g of lipid	nr	1.20 (0.61–2.34)
Current diastolic hypertension		
Serum TCDD < 238 pg/g of lipid	nr	1.35 (0.88–2.09)
Serum TCDD ≥ 238 pg/g of lipid	nr	0.97 (0.51–1.87)

Adjusted for age, sex, BMI, smoking, drinking, diabetes, triglycerides, total cholesterol, HDL, family history of heart disease, and chemical plant.

Suskind and Hertzberg, 1984

Monsanto workers at Nitro, West Virginia—morbidity

Workers exposed to 2,4,5-T production (204) vs nonexposed (163) (self-report)

Hypertension	70	(p > 0.05)
Coronary artery disease	22	(p > 0.05)

Adjusted for age.

Zack and Gaffey, 1983

Monsanto workers at Nitro, West Virginia (884)—mortality (1955–1977)

Circulatory diseases (ICD 390–458)	92	1.11 (p > 0.05)
Atherosclerosis and CHD (ICD 410–413)	79	1.33 (p < 0.05)
All other	13	0.56 (p < 0.05)

Not adjusted for known risk factors.

continued

TABLE 9-5 Continued

Reference[a]	Study Population[b]	Exposed Cases[c]	Estimated Relative Risk (95% CI)[c]	Comments
Zack and Suskind, 1980	**Monsanto workers at Nitro, West Virginia—mortality (1955–1978)**			Not adjusted for known risk factors.
	Workers with chloracne (121)			
	Circulatory diseases (ICD 390–458)	17	0.68 (p > 0.05)	
	Atherosclerosis and CHD (ICD 410–413)	13	0.73 (p > 0.05)	
Swaen et al., 2004 [*Supersedes Swaen et al., 1992*]	**Dutch licensed herbicide applicators—mortality (1980–2000)**			
	Circulatory disease	70	0.68 (0.53–0.86)	
Ott and Zober, 1996	**Cleanup workers at German TCP reactor (BASF)—mortality (1953–1992)**			Reliability of estimated body burden is questionable.
[*Supersedes Zober et al., 1994 and Von Benner et al., 1994 (translation from German)*]	Circulatory diseases	37	0.8 (0.6–1.2)	
	< 0.1 estimated TCDD µg/kg bw	13	0.8 (0.4–1.4)	
	0.1–0.99	11	1.0 (0.5–1.7)	
	≥ 1.0	13	0.8 (0.4–1.3)	
	Ischemic heart disease	16	0.7 (0.4–1.1)	
	< 0.1 estimated TCDD µg/kg bw	7	0.9 (0.3–1.8)	
	0.1–0.99	4	0.7 (0.2–1.7)	
	≥ 1.0	5	0.6 (0.2–1.3)	
	Other Occupational Studies			
Kitamura K et al., 2000	**Municipal waste-incinerator workers—morbidity**			Adjusted for age, BMI, and smoking.
	Hypertension by PCDD, PCDF	14 of 94	No increases observed	

Gambini et al., 1997	**Italian rice growers—mortality** (1957–1992) (Phenoxy herbicide use common 1960–1980)			
	Myocardial infarction	67	0.72 (0.56–0.92)	
	Other ischemic heart diseases	72	0.41 (0.32–0.52)	
	Stroke	155	0.96 (0.81–1.12)	
Alavanja et al., 1989	**US forest and soil conservationists—mortality**		PMRs	
	Ischemic heart disease (ICD 410–414)	543	1.0 (0.9–1.1)	Not adjusted for known risk factors.
	Cerebrovascular disease (ICD 430–438)	99	0.9 (0.8–1.1)	
Blair et al., 1983	**Florida, US licensed pesticide applicators—mortality**			
	Circulatory diseases (ICD 390–458)	159	0.88 (p > 0.05)	Not adjusted for known risk factors.
Environmental Studies				
Consonni et al., 2008—new study [*Supersedes Betazzi et al., 1989a,b, 1998, 2001; Pesatori et al., 1998*]	**Seveso, Italy—mortality—25 years** (1976–2001) **Zone A, sexes combined**			
	All circulatory diseases (ICD 390–459)	45	1.1 (0.8–1.4)	Adjusted for gender, age, period.
	Chronic rheumatic heart diseases (ICD 393–398)	3	5.7 (1.8–18.0)	
	Hypertension (ICD 400–405)	5	2.2 (0.9–5.3)	
	Ischemic heart diseases (ICD 410–414)	13	0.8 (0.5–1.4)	
	Acute myocardial infarction (ICD 410)	6	0.6 (0.3–1.4)	
	Chronic ischemic heart diseases (ICD 412, 414)	7	1.1 (0.5–2.3)	
	Cerebrovascular diseases (ICD 430–438)	11	0.9 (0.5–1.6)	

continued

TABLE 9-5 Continued

Reference[a]	Study Population[b]	Exposed Cases[c]	Estimated Relative Risk (95% CI)[c]	Comments
	Zone B, sexes combined			
	All circulatory diseases (ICD 390–459)	289	1.0 (0.9–1.1)	
	Chronic rheumatic heart diseases (ICD 393–398)	1	0.3 (0.0–2.2)	
	Hypertension (ICD 400–405)	11	0.7 (0.4–1.3)	
	Ischemic heart diseases (ICD 410–414)	102	1.0 (0.8–1.2)	
	Acute myocardial infarction (ICD 410)	54	0.9 (0.7–1.1)	
	Chronic ischemic heart diseases (ICD 412, 414)	47	1.1 (0.8–1.4)	
	Cerebrovascular diseases (ICD 430–438)	101	1.2 (1.0–1.5)	
	Zone R, sexes combined			
	All circulatory diseases (ICD 390–459)	2,357	1.1 (1.0–1.1)	
	Chronic rheumatic heart diseases (ICD 393–398)	24	1.0 (0.6–1.5)	
	Hypertension (ICD 400–405)	144	1.1 (1.0–1.4)	
	Ischemic heart diseases (ICD 410–414)	842	1.1 (1.0–1.1)	
	Acute myocardial infarction (ICD 410)	447	1.0 (0.9–1.1)	
	Chronic ischemic heart diseases (ICD 412, 414)	390	1.2 (1.0–1.3)	
	Cerebrovascular diseases (ICD 430–438)	695	1.1 (1.0–1.2)	
Lee DH et al., 2007c—new study	NHANES, 1999–2002—721 nondiabetics ≥ 20 years old with fasting blood samples and measured POPs **high blood pressure** (≥ 130/85 mmHg)	nr	≥ 75th percentile vs those with nondetectable levels	Adjusted for age, race, sex, income, cigarette-smoking, serum cotinine, alcohol consumption, exercise.
	PCDDs		1.7 (1.0–3.1)	
	HxCDD		1.2 (0.7–2.2)	
	HpCDD		2.6 (1.3–5.0)	
	OCDD		1.1 (0.6–2.0)	

continued

PCDFs		1.9 (1.2–3.3)
	PtCDF	1.3 (0.7–2.4)
	HxCDF	2.3 (1.3–4.0)
	HpCDF	1.4 (0.8–2.3)
Dioxin-like PCBs		1.4 (0.8–2.7)
	PCB-74	1.2 (0.6–2.4)
	PCB-118	1.8 (1.0–3.5)
	PCB-126	2.1 (1.2–3.7)
	PCB-169	0.6 (0.3–1.1)
Everett et al., 2008b—new study [*supercedes Everett et al., 2008a*]	**NHANES, 1999–2004—prevalent hypertension** (self-report that told by doctor, ≥ 140/90 mmHg, or antihypertensive medications)—3,398–3,712 individuals depending on congener	See text for determination of cutpoints
	PCB-118 (ng/g of lipid) (TEF = 0.0001)	
	≤ 12.5	1.0
	> 12.5–27.5	1.4 (1.1–1.8)
	> 27.5	2.0 (1.3–3.0)
	PCB-126 (pg/g of lipid) (TEF = 0.1)	
	≤ 26.1	1.0
	26.1–59.1	1.1 (0.9–1.4)
	> 59.1	1.8 (1.2–2.6)
	PCB-156 (ng/g of lipid) (TEF = 0.0005)	
	≤ 12.5	1.0
	12.5–15.4	1.3 (0.9–1.9)
	> 15.4	1.2 (0.8–1.9)
	PCB-169 (pg/g of lipid) (TEF = 0.01)	
	≤ 27.0	1.0
	27.0–46.4	1.1 (0.9–1.5)
	> 46.4	1.3 (0.9–1.9)

Adjusted for age, sex, race, smoking status, BMI, exercise, total cholesterol, family history of myocardial infarction.

TABLE 9-5 Continued

Reference[a]	Study Population[b]	Exposed Cases[c]	Estimated Relative Risk (95% CI)[c]	Comments
Ha et al., 2007— new study	NHANES, 1999–2002—self-reported cardiovascular disease (excluding hypertension)— 889 nondiabetics ≥ 40 years old		≥ 75th percentile vs < 25th percentile	Adjusted for age, race, income, BMI, cigarette-smoking, serum cotinine, alcohol, exercise HDL, total cholesterol, triglycerides hypertension, C-reactive protein.
	Men			
	HxCDD	18	2.5 (0.8–7.7)	
	HpCDD	18	2.4 (0.5–10.3)	
	OCDD	16	2.1 (0.6–7.7)	
	PCDDs	23	2.2 (0.8–6.1)	
	PCDFs	19	0.7 (0.3–1.7)	
	Dioxin-like PCBs	22	1.7 (0.6–5.5)	
	Women			
	HxCDD	21	2.8 (0.9–8.6)	
	HpCDD	14	1.9 (0.3–10.8)	
	OCDD	17	0.7 (0.2–2.8)	
	PCDDs	19	2.0 (0.7–6.4)	
	PCDFs	15	1.0 (0.3–2.8)	
	Dioxin-like PCBs	23	5.0 (1.2–20.4)	
Karouna-Renier et al., 2007—new study	**Superfund site caused by wood-treatment facility in Pensacola, Florida—47 workers, residents—prevalence**			
	Hypertension defined by self-report, medication use, or two readings of systolic blood pressure greater than 140 mmHg or diastolic blood pressure greater than 90 mmHg		1.1 (1.1–1.2) [error likely; published OR and lower confidence limit identical to three decimal places]	Adjusted for age, race, sex, BMI, tobacco and alcohol use, worker status.
	Serum PCDD/F (TEQs in logistic model)			

Chen HL et al., 2006	**Residents around 12 municipal waste incinerators in Taiwan—prevalence**			
	Hypertension diagnosed by a physician	118	5.6 (1.6–19.6)	Adjusted for age, sex, smoking, BMI.
	Serum PCDD/F (TEQs in logistic model)		0.9 (0.2–3.7)	

ABBREVIATIONS: BMI, body mass index; CDC, Centers for Disease Control and Prevention; CHD, coronary heart disease; HDL, high-density lipoprotein; HpCDD, 1,2,3,4,6,7,8-heptachlorodibenzo-*p*-dioxin; HpCDF, 1,2,3,4,6,7,8-heptachlorodibenzofuran; HxCDD, 1,2,3,6,7,8-hexachlorodibenzo-*p*-dixion; HxCDF, 1,2,3,4,7,8-hexachlorodibenzofuran; IARC, International Agency for Research on Cancer; ICD, International Classification of Diseases; MCPA, 2-methyl-4,chlorophenoxyacetic acid; NHANES, National Health and Nutrition Examination Survey; NIOSH, National Institute for Occupational Safety and Health; nr, not reported; OCDD, 1,2,3,4,6,7,8,9-octachlorodibenzo-*p*-dioxin; OR, odds ratio; PCB, polychlorinated biphenyl; PCDD, polychlorinated dibenzo-*p*-dioxin; PCDD/F, dioxins and furans combined; PCDF, polychlorinated dibenzofuran; PCP, pentachlorophenol; PMR, proportional mortality ratio; POP, persistent organic pollutant; PrCDF, 2,3,4,7,8-pentachlorodibenzofuran; RH, Ranch Hand; SEA, Southeast Asia; SMR, standardized mortality ratio; TCDD, 2,3,7,8-tetrachlorod-ibenzo-*p*-dixion; TCP, trichlorophenol; TEF, toxicity equivalency factor for individual congener; TEQ, toxicity equivalent quotient.

*a*New citations labeled as such and bolded; section shaded for citations with dose-response information on TCDD..

*b*Subjects male unless otherwise noted.

*c*Given when available; results other than estimated risk explained individually.

Update of the Epidemiologic Literature

The practice of evaluating the evidence on hypertension separately from that on other circulatory diseases, established in *Update 2006*, is continued in this update.

Hypertension

No Vietnam-veteran or occupational studies addressing hypertension have been published since *Update 2006*.

Environmental Studies   Consonni and colleagues (2008) reported the 25-year mortality follow-up of people exposed to dioxin accidentally in Seveso, Italy. The area surrounding the point of release has been divided into Zones A, B, and R in descending order of soil contamination. For analysis, deaths were allocated to people's zones of residence at the time of the incident. The aggregate experience of the residents was compared with that of residents of surrounding localities. The RRs for mortality from hypertension were 2.2 (95% CI 0.9–5.2), 0.7 (95% CI 0.4–1.3), and 1.2 (95% CI 1.0–1.4) for the zones ranked from highest to lowest exposure and adjusted for sex, age, and period (5-year intervals for time of death).

Several papers reported on association between blood concentrations of organic pollutants and the prevalence of hypertension in the ongoing NHANES. The NHANES data are collected from probability samples of the noninstitutionalized US population.

Lee DH et al. (2007c) studied the association between blood concentrations of dioxins, furans, and coplanar PCBs and components of the metabolic syndrome in a random one-third sample of people at least 20 years old from the 1999–2002 NHANES. The five defining components of the metabolic syndrome included high blood pressure (blood pressure above 135/85 mmHg or use of antihypertensive medication). Of the 49 persistent organic pollutants measured in the survey, the 19 analytes studied in detail were selected because at least 60% of the study subjects had concentrations of them greater than the limit of detection of the analytic method: three PCDDs, four dioxin-like PCBs, five non–dioxin-like PCBs, three PCDFs, and four organochlorine pesticides. Those who had combined concentrations of the three PCDDs at or above the 75th percentile had a 70% higher odds of having high blood pressure (OR = 1.7, 95% CI 1.0–3.1) than those who had combined concentrations below the 25th percentile after adjustment for age, sex, race, income, cigarette-smoking, serum cotinine, alcohol consumption, and exercise. Those who had high concentrations of the three PCDFs also had a higher prevalence of high blood pressure (OR = 1.9, 95% CI 1.2–3.3), but those who had high concentrations of the four dioxin-like PCBs did not have significantly high blood pressure (OR = 1.4, 95% CI 0.8–2.7). When the individual analytes were examined, only 1,2,3,4,6,7,8-HpCDD and 1,2,3,4,7,8-HxCDF were associated with high blood pressure (OR = 2.6, 95% CI 1.3–5.0 and OR = 2.3, 95% CI 1.3–4.0, respectively); other analytes of these classes with higher dioxin-like toxicity, 1,2,3,6,7,8-HxCDD and 1,2,3,4,7,8-HxCDF, were not so associated. Of the four PCBs with dioxin-like toxicity, high concentrations of only PC-118 and PCB-126 were associated with high blood pressure (OR = 1.8, 95% CI 1.0–3.5; OR = 2.1, 95% CI 1.2–3.7, respectively). There were no associations between any of the five non–dioxin-like PCBs or four other organochlorine pesticides assessed and high blood pressure. The analytic approach makes the data difficult to interpret with respect to the effects of dioxin on blood pressure. The data were analyzed according to their distribution in the sample, not on the basis of measured concentrations. That makes null associations difficult to interpret because, for a given analyte, a reading in a high range of the distribution may still be too low to cause the outcome of interest; this is particularly relevant for assessing dioxin-like activity because the individual chemicals have estimates of dioxin-like activity (toxicity equivalency factors, TEFs) that range over several orders of magnitude.

Everett et al. (2008a) also analyzed the data on people who were at least 20 years old from a one-third stratified subsample of the 1999–2002 NHANES. They focused on 11 PCBs and their relationships with hypertension defined on the basis of a physician diagnosis, the use of antihypertensive medications, or blood pressure above 140/90 mmHg. Of the 11 PCBs, four (PCB-169, PCB-126, PCB-118, and PCB-156) had dioxin-like toxicity. The distribution of serum concentrations of each PCB was partitioned into three ranges, of which the lowest was used as the referent group for those who had intermediate and high readings. The cutpoints for "high" concentrations were defined as concentrations that provided 95% sensitivity for identifying prevalent cases of hypertension. The explanation of how a cutpoint for "low" readings was determined is problematic in that it is said to have minimized *both* false positives and false negatives for hypertension, and this cannot be done simultaneously. In addition, selection of cutpoints that depends on the outcome measure could lead to invalid statistical inference by overstating statistical significance. Estimated ORs were adjusted for age, sex, race and ethnicity, smoking status, BMI, exercise, total cholesterol, and family history of heart attack.

For the 1999–2002 NHANES data analyzed by Everett et al. (2008a), both intermediate and high concentrations of all four dioxin-like PCBs were associated with prevalent hypertension, and the low concentrations were not, but the associations were statistically significant only for the high concentrations of PCB-126 (OR = 2.4, 95% CI 1.5–4.0) and PCB-118 (OR = 2.3; 95% CI 1.3–4.1). It should be noted that high concentrations of five of the seven PCBs that did not have dioxin-like activity were also found to be significantly associated with hypertension. The lack of specificity of the association suggests that there is a nonspecific PCB effect on hypertension rather than one linked specifically to dioxin-like activity. A general PCB effect would not further our understanding of the health effects of Agent Orange because PCBs were not known contaminants of Agent Orange.

Everett et al. (2008b) reported the results obtained when analyses using the methods described earlier (Everett et al., 2008a) were repeated to include an additional 2 years' worth of data. In the committee's evidence database, the more comprehensive results for the 6 years 1999–2004 (presented in Table 9-5) subsume those reported earlier, which are given in the text above for comparison. The new findings did not show any great perturbations from the findings for 1999–2004, but the ORs for the higher concentrations of each congener tended to decrease slightly. The two of the four dioxin-like PCBs that had shown significant associations continued to show them; for five of the seven non–dioxin-like congeners that had been significantly associated for the years 1999–2002, however, only one still was when the additional data were included. That reduces somewhat the concern expressed above regarding the findings for 1999–2002.

Karouna-Renier et al. (2007) gathered health and exposure histories and measured serum concentrations of 17 PCDD and PCDF congeners in 47 people potentially exposed at a Superfund site in Pensacola, Florida, that was contaminated with dioxins and furans. The study sample was selected in a nonsystematic fashion from among former workers, their families, and residents. Dose–response relationships were investigated with logistic analysis of the prevalence of several health problems in terms of TEQs and were adjusted for age, race, sex, BMI, tobacco and alcohol use, and worker status. A significant association was reported between TEQ and hypertension (OR = 1.1, 95% CI 1.1–1.2 [an error is likely inasmuch as the published OR and lower confidence limit were identical to three decimal places]), defined by self-report, use of prescribed medication, or two readings of systolic blood pressure greater than 140 mmHg or diastolic blood pressure greater than 90 mmHg.

Other Reviewed Studies   Wang et al. (2008) reported on the 24-year follow-up of the Yucheng cohort in Taiwan. The cohort was exposed to high concentrations of PCBs and PCDFs (some congeners of both have dioxin-like activity) through contaminated rice oil. A nonexposed referent population was matched on age, sex, and neighborhood. In both men and women, there was no association between being in the Yucheng cohort and having hypertension. The study also contrasted the lifetime prevalence of several medical conditions on the basis of whether the Yucheng cohort member had a history of chloracne. The rate of hypertension was not higher in men (OR = 0.6, 95% CI 0.3–1.1) who had chloracne than in cohort members who did not but it was significantly higher in women who had chloracne than in women who did not (OR = 3.5, 95% CI 1.7–7.2); the rate in those who had chloracne vs the referent population would be more extreme. The results of the study were not reported in terms of dioxin-like activity, so they do not contribute directly to the evidence on Vietnam veterans; however, in light of the well-known association between chloracne and AHR activation and dioxin-like activity, they are consistent with an association between exposure to the chemicals of interest and hypertension in women.

Circulatory Diseases

Vietnam-Veteran Studies Cypel and Kang (2008) analyzed mortality patterns in female Vietnam-era veterans. They linked service files with the master death file from the Social Security Administration and the Department of Veterans Affairs Beneficiary Identification and Records Locator Subsystem to determine vital status as of December 31, 2004. Female veterans who served in Vietnam had lower mortality from circulatory system diseases than female veterans who did not serve in Vietnam after adjustment for duration of military service, age, and race (RR = 0.78, 95% CI 0.6–1.0). The authors considered the subset of veterans who were nurses on the basis of the premise that this group was likely to have been closer to the conflict than women with other job classifications. The results were unchanged when only the mortality experience of nurses was considered. They say little about the potential relationship between dioxin and vascular disease. Circulatory system diseases as an underlying cause of death make up heterogeneous collection of clinical entities with differing constellations of causes and clinical presentations. That heterogeneity may lead to the masking of important health effects if not all the disease entities are related to the exposure of interest. Furthermore, the fact of service in Vietnam says little about exposures to the chemicals of interest. Therefore, the findings cannot be considered to be either contradictory or confirmatory of the hypothesis that Agent Orange exposure increases the occurrence of a specific circulatory disease.

Occupational Studies Peclová and colleagues (2007) assessed vascular function in men who were occupationally exposed to very high concentrations of TCDD while working in the Spolana plant in Noeratovice, Czech Republic, in 1965–1968. In 2004, the authors examined 15 of the exposed workers. Of the 15, nine had hypertension and five had a history of heart attack. The 15 workers were compared with 14 healthy male health-care workers who had no history of occupational exposure to TCDD. Compared with the controls, the exposed workers had lower skin microvascular reactivity in response to a flow-mediated or thermal stimulus. The data are difficult to interpret with respect to the health effects of TCDD. It is unclear how the case series was selected, so the degree to which the participants are representative of all still-living workers, especially with respect to chronic-disease burden, is unclear. Because the exposed group had a large number of metabolic and comorbid conditions of which the control group was largely free, the effects of disease could not be separated from the effects of TCDD. Finally, the relationship between microvascular reactivity and thermal reactivity and clinical cardiovascular events is unclear. Flow-mediated reactivity of brachial arteries can predict clinical disease (Yeboah et al., 2007), but the predictive value of the particular measures used in this study has not been demonstrated.

Environmental Studies   Ha et al. (2007) reported on the cross-sectional association between prevalent CVD and blood concentrations of PCDDs, PCDFs, dioxin-like PCBs, non–dioxin-like PCBs, and organochlorine pesticides in the 1999–2002 NHANES. Within these categories, they presented results on specific chemicals whose concentrations were above the analytic method's lower detection limit in at least 60% of the sample. For each substance, the prevalence of CVD in the lowest quartile was used as the referent for each of the higher quartiles. Participants were classified as having CVD if they reported a physician's diagnosis of coronary heart disease, angina, heart attack, or stroke. Participants who had diabetes were excluded from the analysis. There were 108 cases of CVD in the 899 persons included in the analysis. Results were reported separately for men and women. In men, although the CVD risk for each quartile was elevated compared to the lowest for PCDDs, dioxin-like PCBs, and non-dioxin like PCBs, none of the associations was statistically significant. In women, for dioxin-like PCBs, non–dioxin-like PCBs, and organochlorine pesticides, the adjusted ORs contrasting the prevalence of CVD between those with serum concentrations in the top quartile and those in the lowest quartile were 5.0 (95% CI 1.2–20.4), 3.8 (95% CI 1.1–2.8), and 4.0 (95% CI 1.0–17.1), respectively, and there were significant trends over quartiles ($p < 0.01$, $p = 0.02$, and $p = 0.03$, respectively), but the CVD risk associated with the highest quartile of PCDD concentrations was not significant (OR = 2.0, 95% CI 0.7–6.4) and the PCDFs showed no elevation in risk. The authors also presented data on the three specific TCDDs that were used to form the composite TCDD score (1,2,3,6,7,8-HxCDD, 1,2,3,4,6,7,8-HpCDD, and 1,2,3,4,6,7,8,9-OCDD); in both men and women, there was a dose–response relationship between CVD prevalence and HxCDD ($p = 0.04$ for both sexes), but not HpCDD or OCDD. Individual PCBs were examined only in women; three of five dioxin-like PCBs, three of six non–dioxin-like PCBs, and three of four organochlorine pesticides showed dose–response associations with CVD prevalence. It is intriguing that the PCDD with the strongest dioxin activity was associated with CVD prevalence. However, as discussed above in reference to the articles by Lee DH et al. (2007c) and Everett et al. (2007), the lack of measured concentrations and the lack of specific effects diminish the value of the data in clarifying the role of Agent Orange in CVD risk.

Consonni and colleagues (2008) reported several circulatory-mortality outcomes in their analysis of 25-year mortality in the Seveso cohort. In addition to hypertension deaths, they examined deaths from chronic rheumatic heart disease, ischemic heart disease, and cerebrovascular disease, all of which are in the ICD-9 rubric of circulatory disease. Compared with residents of surrounding localities, residents of the most highly exposed zone (Zone A) had increased mortality from

chronic rheumatic heart disease (RR = 5.7, 95% CI 1.8–18.0) but not from ischemic heart disease (RR = 0.9, 95% CI 0.5–1.4) or cerebrovascular disease (primarily stroke; RR = 0.9, 95% CI 0.5–1.6). Residents of the intermediate-exposure
zone (Zone B) showed only a borderline increase in cerebrovascular disease
(RR = 1.2, 95% CI 1.0–1.5), and residents of the least exposed zone (Zone R)
had an higher rate of cerebrovascular disease (RR = 1.1, 95% CI 1.0–1.2) and
a borderline increase in the rate of ischemic heart disease (RR = 1.06, 95% CI
0.98–1.14). The authors examined mortality patterns by 5-year intervals after
the accidental dioxin release, combining deaths from all circulatory diseases.
The increase in risk in Zone A was restricted to the first 10 years of follow-up.
For residents of Zone B, there was no postaccident interval in which risk was
significantly increased. For residents of Zone R, all intervals showed an increase
in risk except for the period 15–19 years after the incident but the associations
were significant only in the periods 0–4 years and 10–14 years after the incident.
However, the precision of the estimates is such that data are consistent with a
small increase in risk in all study intervals.

Goncharov et al. (2008) investigated associations of PCBs and pesticides
with serum lipids and self-reported cardiovascular disease in 335 adult Akwesasne
Mohawks. The authors used factor analysis to create a latent variable representing PCB concentrations and found that it was related to CVD prevalence but that
the association was confounded by age and either confounded by or mediated by
serum lipid concentrations. The congeners examined included PCBs with and
without dioxin-like activity, and all were associated to a similar extent with the
latent variable. The detailed statistical modeling effort does not have direct utility
in interpreting health risks associated with Agent Orange exposure.

Other Reviewed Studies   Wang et al. (2008) reported on the 24-year follow-up
of the Yucheng cohort in Taiwan. The cohort was exposed to high concentrations
of PCBs and PCDFs (some congeners of both have dioxin-like activity) through
contaminated rice oil. A nonexposed referent population was matched on age,
sex, and neighborhood. In both men and women, there was no association between being in the Yucheng cohort and having CVD. The study also contrasted
the lifetime prevalence of several medical conditions on the basis of whether
the Yucheng cohort members had a history of chloracne. The risk of CVD was
not higher in men (OR = 0.9, 95% CI 0.4–2.2) who had chloracne than in cohort members who did not, but it was significantly higher in women who had
chloracne than in women who did not (OR = 3.0, 95% CI 1.5–8.6); the rate in
women who had chloracne vs the referent population would be more extreme.
The results of the study were not reported in terms of dioxin-like activity, so
they do not contribute directly to the evidence on Vietnam veterans; however, in
light of the well-known association between chloracne and AHR activation and
dioxin-like activity, they are consistent with an association between exposure to
the chemicals of interest and CVD in women.

Biologic Plausibility

It is well established that the vasculature is a target of TCDD toxicity, which leads to significant increases in oxidative stress and induces major changes in expression of genes that regulate numerous signaling pathways (Puga et al., 2004). There is also growing evidence from a variety of experimental models that TCDD induces or promotes CVD in adult animals. For example, chronic exposure of the ApoE knockout mouse to TCDD increased the incidence, severity, and progression of atherosclerotic plaques (Dalton et al., 2001), and rats chronically exposed to TCDD exhibited significant arterial remodeling characterized by endothelial-cell hypertrophy, extensive smooth-muscle cell proliferation, and inflammation (Jokinen et al., 2003). The rats also had dose-related increase in cardiomyopathy. Other studies have shown that TCDD exposure increased myocardial fibrosis (Riecke et al., 2002) and led to cardiac hypertrophy and alteration in control of heart rhythm (Lin et al., 2001; Thackaberry et al., 2005a,b). In one study, acute exposure of mice to a relatively high dose of TCDD significantly increased the release of vasoconstricting eicosanoids and induced hypertension (Dalton et al., 2001). Similarly, constitutive activation of the AHR results in disruption of cardiovascular homeostasis, as shown in expression of a constitutively active AHR in transgenic mice that develop an age-progressive cardiac hypertrophy (Brunnberg et al., 2006). The data show that activation of the AHR, endogenously or by xenobiotics, induces cardiovascular injury and leads to CVD in animal models.

Recently, the role of the AHR in normal cardiovascular function in adult animals has been established with studies of AHR-null mice. The animals develop hypertension, cardiac hypertrophy, and reduction in cardiac function with age; hence, the AHR has a role in cardiovascular function (Lund et al., 2003, 2005, 2006, 2008; Thackaberry et al., 2003; Vasquez et al., 2003). That both the sustained activation of the AHR by TCDD and the genetic deletion of the AHR result in cardiovascular disease suggests that the AHR acts to maintain the physiologic balance of the cardiovascular system and that either its excessive activation or its insufficient activation disrupts this homeostasis.

An additional study in the literature reviewed supports the view that AHR activation may play a role in vascular disease and presumably in ischemic heart disease. The fact that the AHR appears to modulate blood pressure, depending on the partial pressure of oxygen (Lund et al., 2008), is evidence of the relevance of this process to the development of hypertension. Ichihara et al. (2007) found that AHR-null mice had greater vascular endothelial growth factor (VEGF) activity and angiogenesis than wild-type control C57BL/6 mice in a femoral-artery occlusion model. The theory is that the AHR binds to the AHR nuclear translocator (ARNT) protein and this leads to a decrease in the physiologic response to ischemia and hypoxia and then to the induction of hypoxia-inducible factor 1-alpha, binding to ARNT, and activation of VEGF. Thus, there seems to be a consistent effect of AHR and presumably of TCDD on signaling pathways that are known risk factors for ischemic heart disease.

Direct evidence of a vascular effect of TCDD on liver endothelial cells and sinusoids was reported in primates 4 years after subcutaneous injection of TCDD (Korenaga et al., 2007); there was no mention of cardiovascular effects.

The committee believes that the risk factors for ischemic heart disease make it difficult to separate the antiangiogenic effects of TCDD from the glucose and lipid metabolic effects that lead to an increase in atherosclerosis, a known risk factor for ischemic heart disease. TCDD and the related PCB-77 were found to increase adipocyte differentiation and adipokine production in 3T3-L1 adipocytes (Arsenescu et al., 2008); the investigators also found that AHR-null mice and ApoE-null C57/BL/6 mice demonstrated an increase in body weight, serum dyslipidemia, and augmented atherosclerosis. In human vascular endothelial cells, Dabir et al. (2008) found that glucose activates an AHR-associated thrombospondin-1 signaling pathway that is known to have antiangiogenic and proatherosclerotic activities. Finally, AHR-null mice have been shown to have increased angiotensin II production, which leads to hypertension (Lund et al., 2003); the literature reviewed showed that this may be associated with alpha1D-adrenoreceptor expression (Villalobos-Molina et al., 2008). Thus, on the basis of animal models, there appear to be several overlapping and potentially contributing pathways that may interlink AHR activation, TCDD effects, and CVD.

Synthesis

In this section, the committee synthesizes information on circulatory disorders from the new studies described above and reconsiders studies that were reviewed in previous updates. Because circulatory diseases constitute a broad group of diverse conditions, hypertension and ischemic heart disease are discussed separately from other circulatory diseases so that the new studies can be adequately synthesized and integrated with the earlier studies.

Hypertension

Hypertension, typically defined as blood pressure above 140/90 mmHg, affects more than 70 million adult Americans and is a major risk factor for coronary heart disease, myocardial infarction, stroke, and heart and renal failure. The major quantifiable risk factors for hypertension are well established and include age, race, BMI or percentage body fat, and diabetes; the strongest conclusions regarding a potential increase in the incidence of hypertension come from studies that have controlled for these risk factors. The committee responsible for *Update 2006* judged that there was limited or suggestive evidence that Agent Orange exposure is associated with hypertension. The studies published since *Update 2006* are consistent with that conclusion.

The data from the NHANES are broadly consistent with the effect. The NHANES is cross-sectional and so is prone to selection biases that may distort the association between exposure and disease. There is also a concern that reported associations are not limited to compounds that have dioxin-like activity or are not in strict correspondence with TEFs. For example, in the analyses by Everett et al. (2008a,b), the data from 1999–2002 yielded the strongest association for the chemicals with the greatest dioxin-like activity (PCB-126, TEF = 0.1) and showed statistically significant associations with four non–dioxin-like PCBs; when the more extensive data from 1999–2004 were used, however, the increase in risks associated with the four non–dioxin-like PCBs were no longer significant, but the theoretically less potent PCB-118 (TEF = 0.0001) now had the strongest association (although the 95% CIs did remain effectively equivalent). The new data from Karouna-Renier et al. (2007) are from a small survey of a problematic sample, so the association is difficult to interpret. The increased lifetime prevalence of hypertension in women in the Yucheng cohort who had chloracne provides support of the link between doxin-like compounds and hypertension, but the support is diminished by the failure to observe an association in men. There is no clear explanation of the sex difference in the findings, but men may have a lower threshold for the development of hypertension. It is important that those who had chloracne were compared with other (presumably) less exposed persons, not with a nonexposed reference cohort. The cohort experienced a good deal of loss to follow-up, so selection bias cannot be ruled out as a potential explanation of the disparate results. The data from Consonni et al. (2008) also are generally supportive, although there was little ability to control for potentially important confounders. Furthermore, the association was between exposure zone and deaths from hypertension. In the United States, hypertension, although very prevalent, is fairly rarely identified as an underlying cause of death. Most often, deaths associated with hypertension are ascribed to clinical conditions *caused by* hypertension (such as stroke).Thus, the degree of correspondence between death from hypertension and the occurrence of hypertension in the exposed populations is unclear.

Ischemic Heart Disease

Circulatory diseases comprise a group of diverse conditions—of which hypertension, coronary heart disease, and stroke are the most prevalent—that account for 75% of deaths from circulatory diseases in the United States. The major quantifiable risk factors for circulatory diseases are similar to those for hypertension and include age, race, smoking, serum cholesterol, BMI or percentage of body fat, and diabetes.

The committee responsible for *Update 2006* was divided on the weight to be given to the weaknesses of the heart-disease studies and thus remained divided as to whether the evidence related to exposure to the chemicals of interest and ischemic heart disease (ICD-9 410–414) was adequately informative to advance this health outcome from the "inadequate or insufficient" category into the "limited or suggestive" category. The additional data since *Update 2006* are from Ha et al. (2007) on the NHANES data and from Consonni et al. (2008) on the update of the Seveso experience.

The interpretation of the NHANES data is complicated by the same factors that compromise the interpretation of the data with respect to hypertension (for example, the data are from a cross-sectional survey). There seems to be a somewhat more specific effect of dioxin-related compounds and CVD prevalence than the relationships seen for hypertension. Furthermore, the association persisted after statistical adjustment for a large number of potential confounding risk factors for which the information necessary for adjustment is generally not available in other dioxin-exposed populations.

The data on the Seveso incident do not show a dose–response pattern between residence and mortality from ischemic heart disease in that the residential zone with the lowest exposure was the only zone that had a statistically significant increase in mortality. However, the increase was slight (10% excess), and there is a potential for unmeasured confounders to account for it. Consonni et al. (2008) also reported an association with cerebrovascular-disease mortality in the intermediate-exposure and low-exposure zones. The imprecision of the effect estimate for the high-exposure zone was such that the results from that zone do not rule out a small to moderate increase in mortality. Again, the overall mortality increase is small (10–20%) and important confounders were not measured, so the Seveso data do not constitute a firm finding regarding dioxins' role in the risk of stroke.

In light of the inability of the committee responsible for *Update 2006* to reach a consensus, the present committee revisited the entire body of evidence on TCDD exposure and heart disease. More confidence was given to studies that were most rigorously conducted, focused specifically on the chemicals of concern, compared Vietnam veterans with nondeployed era veterans, had individual and reliable measures of exposure that permitted evaluation of dose–response relationships, and so on. Evidence of a dose–response relationship is especially helpful in the interpretation of epidemiologic data. In the context of the TCDD literature, that is reflected in studies in which the disease experience of people whose exposure to TCDD or related compounds (documented in terms of serum concentrations) was compared with that of people whose exposure was similarly documented to have been low. In situations where several alternative analyses were presented, the information from the analyses that had the greatest specificity in the dose–response relationship was given more weight. Nine studies provided such information (AFHS, 2005; Calvert et al., 1998; Consonni et al., 2008; Flesch-Janys, 1995; Ha et al., 2007; Hooiveld et al., 1998; Kang et al., 2006;

Steenland et al., 1999; Vena et al., 1998; these studies are shaded in Table 9-5). The International Agency for Research on Cancer cohort (Vena et al., 1998) is composed of several occupational cohorts that have been studied individually and includes three that are also considered individually here because of their information on serum TCDD: the American NIOSH cohort (Steenland et al., 1999), a German cohort (Flesch-Janys, 1995), and a Dutch cohort (Hooiveld et al., 1998). Six of the reports show strong and statistically significant associations with ischemic heart disease (ORs or RRs ranging from 1.4 to 2.8). The studies include Agent Orange sprayers, occupationally exposed populations, and environmentally exposed populations, and they were either prevalence surveys or mortality follow-up studies. Because of small numbers, the studies that did not report statistically significant associations did not rule out modest increases in ischemic heart disease in those with the strongest evidence of exposure. The committee was impressed by the fact that the studies with the best dose information all showed evidence of risk increases in the highest exposure categories.

Each of the studies has potential limitations. For example, the cross-sectional surveys typically have better measurements of potential confounders, but their design allows for important selection biases. The mortality studies are longitudinal, but fatal cases may not represent all incident cases, so there was a potential for bias in outcome ascertainment. The mortality studies also had little data on potential disease confounders. However, for a potential confounder to explain an observed association completely, the strength of its association with the outcome of interest must be greater than that observed for the exposure under consideration (Rothman and Greenland, 1998). The strongest potential confounder is age, but this was controlled for in most of the mortality studies. BMI is an important potential uncontrolled confounder, but its association with CVD mortality is not strong enough to explain away the high RRs. Although serum dioxin-like chemicals tend to increase with age and BMI in the general population, one would anticipate that half-life decay of the extreme occupational doses would exceed the accumulation attributable to continuing background exposure. Cigarette-smoking is a risk factor for CVD, but for it to be a confounder there would have to be a very strong correlation between smoking and dioxin exposure, which is extremely unlikely to have been the situation in every study. Empirical research also indicates that confounding by smoking could not explain RRs above 1.4 (Siemiatycki et al., 1988).

Previous committees have found that there is limited or suggestive evidence of an association between Agent Orange and both diabetes and hypertension, and the present committee concurs in those conclusions. The present committee considers that both conditions are strong risk factors for ischemic heart disease, and many epidemiologic studies show a dose–response relationship between dioxin and ischemic heart disease.

Finally, toxicologic data support the biologic plausibility of an association between TCDD exposure and vascular disease.

Other Circulatory Disease

Data from Consonni et al. (2008) indicate a relationship between residence in a locality with high dioxin exposure and mortality from chronic rheumatic heart disease. The basis of the association is unclear. Given that this is a single finding from a study of disease mortality rather than incidence and that it lacked control for potentially important confounders, there is little basis for a conclusion regarding an effect of Agent Orange on this outcome.

Conclusion

After extensive deliberation regarding the strengths and weaknesses of the new evidence and evidence from studies reviewed in previous VAO reports, the present committee deemed that the strengths of the evidence related to hypertension outweighed the weaknesses and concluded that there is limited or suggestive evidence of an association between exposure to the chemicals of interest and hypertension (ICD-9 401–405) but that chance, bias, and confounding could not be ruled out. After consideration of the relative strengths and weaknesses of the evidence regarding the chemicals of interest and ischemic heart disease (ICD-9 410–414), which includes a number of studies that showed a strong dose–response relationship and that had good toxicologic data demonstrating biologic plausibility, the committee judged that the evidence was adequately informative to advance this health outcome from the "inadequate or insufficient" category into the "limited or suggestive" category, again acknowledging that bias and confounding could not be ruled out. For all other types of circulatory disease, the committee found that the evidence is inadequate or insufficient to determine whether there is an association with exposure to the chemicals of interest.

THYROID HOMEOSTASIS

Clinical disruptions of thyroid function include various disorders grouped in ICD-9 242.8 and 246.8. The thyroid gland secretes the hormones thyroxine (T4) and triiodothyronine (T3), which stimulate and help to regulate metabolism throughout the body. The thyroid also secretes calcitonin, a hormone that controls calcium concentration in the blood and storage of calcium in bones. Secretion of T4 and T3 is under the control of thyroid-stimulating hormone (TSH), which is secreted by the anterior pituitary gland. Iodine operates in thyroid physiology both as a constituent of thyroid hormones and as a regulator of glandular function. Concentrations of those circulating hormones are regulated primarily by a negative-feedback pathway that involves three organs: the thyroid, the pituitary, and the hypothalamus. In the hypothalamus–pituitary–thyroid feedback scheme, the hypothalamus releases thyrotropin-releasing hormone (TRH), which stimulates the pituitary to produce TSH, which triggers the thyroid to produce T4 and

T3. Cells in the hypothalamus and pituitary respond to concentrations of circulating T4 and T3. When T4 and T3 are low, the pituitary is stimulated to deliver more TSH to the thyroid, which increases T4 and T3 output. When circulating T4 and T3 are high, they signal to reduce the output of TRH and TSH. This negative-feedback loop maintains hormone homeostasis.

Disruption of thyroid homeostasis can be stimulatory (hyperthyroidism) or suppressive (hypothyroidism). Both conditions are diagnosed on the basis of blood concentrations of thyroid hormones, TSH, and other proteins (antithyroid antibodies). The prevalence of thyroid dysfunction in adults in the general population ranges from 1% to 10%, depending on the group, the testing setting, sex, age, method of assessment, and the presence of conditions that affect thyroid function. People with subclinical (biochemical) conditions may or may not show other evidence (signs or symptoms) of thyroid dysfunction.

In *hypothyroidism*, the body lacks sufficient thyroid hormone. Overt hypothyroidism is seen as a high serum concentration of TSH and a low serum concentration of free T4. Subclinical hypothyroidism is defined as a high serum concentration of TSH and a normal serum concentration of free T4. People who have hypothyroidism typically have symptoms of low metabolism. Studies consistently show that subclinical hypothyroidism is common and occurs more frequently in women than in men (Canaris et al., 2000; Hollowell et al., 2002; Sawin et al., 1985). In the Framingham study, for example, among 2,139 people 60 years old or older, 14% of women and 6% of men had subclinical hypothyroidism (Sawin et al., 1985). Subclinical hypothyroidism is a risk factor for overt hypothyroidism. Studies have reported an association of hypothyroidism with a wide variety of other conditions.

The term *hyperthyroidism* may involve any disease that results in overabundance of thyroid hormone. Clinical or overt hyperthyroidism is characterized as a low serum concentration of TSH and high serum concentration of free T4. Subclinical hyperthyroidism is defined as a low serum concentration of TSH and a normal serum concentration of free T4. The prevalence of subclinical hyperthyroidism was estimated at about 1% in men and 1.5% in women over 60 years old (Helfand and Redfern, 1998). Conditions associated with hyperthyroidism include Graves disease and diffuse toxic goiter. Like hypothyroidism, hyperthyroidism is more common in women than in men, and, although it occurs at all ages, it is most likely to occur in people more than 15 years old. A form of hyperthyroidism called neonatal Graves disease occurs in infants born to mothers who have Graves disease. Occult hyperthyroidism may occur in patients more than 65 years old and is characterized by a distinct lack of typical symptoms.

It is important to distinguish between potential effects on adults and effects that may occur during development. In adults, the thyroid is able, within reason, to compensate for mild or moderate disruption (such as that caused by hyperplasia or goiter). In contrast, the fetus is highly sensitive to alterations in thyroid hormones, and alterations in thyroid homeostasis can hamper the development of many organ systems, including the nervous and reproductive systems. Both adult and developmental outcomes are considered here.

Summary of Previous Updates

The thyrotoxic potential of the chemicals of interest was addressed first in *Update 2002* (IOM, 2003). Although several studies have found an association between dioxin-like congeners and markers of thyroid homeostasis, there have been no studies that document an increased risk of thyroid disease in veterans of the Vietnam War. The committee responsible for *Update 2002* concluded that there was inadequate or insufficient information to determine whether there is an association between exposure to the chemicals of interest and adverse effects on thyroid homeostasis in Vietnam veterans. The committee responsible for *Update 2004* concurred.

The committee responsible for *Update 2006* reviewed several environmental studies of the relationship between exposure to dioxin-like compounds and thyroid function. Bloom et al. (2006) found a significant inverse relationship between the sum of dioxin-like compounds and the concentration of free T4 in anglers in New York state, but no association between the sum of dioxin-like compounds and TSH. Significant associations were not found in patients with Yusho disease (Nagayama et al., 2001) or women undergoing amniocentesis (Foster et al., 2005). The committee responsible for *Update 2006* noted that the functional importance of those changes remained unclear because adaptive capacity could be adequate to accommodate them, it retained the previous committees' conclusion that there was inadequate or insufficient evidence of an association.

Update of the Scientific Literature

No Vietnam-veteran or occupational studies concerning the chemicals of interest and thyroid homeostasis have been published since *Update 2006*.

Environmental Studies

Four studies of environmental exposure to PCB congeners and thyroid function in adults have been published since *Update 2006*.

Abdelouahab et al. (2008) reported on a cross-sectional investigation of T3, T4, and TSH in relation to several serum dioxin-like compounds in adult freshwater-fish consumers in two Canadian communities. Fish consumption was measured by self-report. The relationships between fish consumption and serum compound concentrations were adjusted for age, sex, smoking, alcohol consumption, medications, and total lipid concentrations. Analyses were performed with levels of compounds adjusted and unadjusted for lipid concentration to take into account potential TH effects on blood lipid mobilization. Thyroid hormones were within the normal ranges, and biomarkers of exposure were low compared with those in other reports on fish consumers. Non-ortho-substituted (dioxin-like) PCBs (PCB-105, -118, -128, -138, and -170) were among the compounds analyzed. In women, a negative association was found between PCB-138 concentrations and T3, but no association was observed between all dioxin-like congeners combined and T3 or T4. No relationships were observed between any of the chemicals, including the dioxin-like compounds and T4. In men, serum T4 was reported to be inversely related to PCB-138 and dioxin-like congeners (p < 0.05). A positive relationship was found between dioxin-like congeners and TSH (p < 0.001). In men, serum TSH was highest among those in the highest 50th percentile for dioxin-like PCB congeners. No associations with T3 were observed in men. Serum concentration of the dioxin-like congeners ranged from the 25th percentile of lipids at 200 ng/g to a maximum value of 2,810 ng/g. Although those results are based on the sum of dioxin-like compounds, and not TCDD specifically, they augment information that dioxin-like chemicals are associated with changes in some measures of thyroid function, although not to an extent that result in clinically abnormal concentrations of the hormones.

A second study of adults without thyroid disease in the 1999–2002 NHANES examined the association of dioxin-like TEQs with T4 and TSH (Turyk et al., 2007). PCB, PCDD, and PCDF congeners were examined separately in the serum of a nationally representative sample of the US population. TEFs for each PCDD, PCDF, and coplanar PCD and mono-ortho PCB congener were multiplied by the congener's concentration and summed to calculate total TEQs. The total T4 was negatively associated with the serum dioxin-like TEQs in a dose-dependent fashion; associations were stronger in women than in men. In women, mean T4 was 8.2 μg/dL, and T4 concentrations averaged 0.75 μg/dL lower (95% CI 0.04–1.46) in women in the highest quintile of TEQ exposure than in women in the lowest quintiles. Effects were stronger in people over 60 years old.

The committee reviewed two reports concerning thyroid function in adults in the polluted district of Michalovce in East Slovakia compared with neighboring, nonpolluted communities (Langer et al., 2007a,b). Adults were examined for serum TSH, T4, T3, antithyroperoxidase antibodies, and 15 PCBs that included five dioxin-like coplanar congeners. In neither report, however, were the analyses broken out for the dioxin-like congeners alone.

In a study of PCB exposures during pregnancy and thyroid function, Chevrier et al. (2008) measured the dioxin-like congeners PCB-118, -156, -157, -167, -180, and -189 among 34 PCBs measured in samples collected from 334 pregnant women living in Salinas Valley, California. PCB-118 and PCB-156 were among the 19 congeners detected in more than 75% of the study participants. After adjustment for demographic covariates, there was no association between concentrations of those two dioxin-like PCB congeners and free T4, total T4, or TSH concentrations.

Biologic Plausibility

TCDD has been demonstrated to affect concentrations of T4, T3, and TSH in experimental animals, but the effects appear to be species-dependent, and they lack consistency in demonstrating either definite hyperthyroidism or hypothyroidism after exposure to TCDD. Nevertheless, long-term exposure of animals to TCDD usually results in suppressed T4 and T3 and stimulated TSH. The National Toxicology Program reported that female rats exposed chronically to TCDD showed follicular-cell hyperplasia and hypertrophy of thyroid follicles.

TCDD influences the metabolism of thyroid hormones and TSH. Notably, the study by Nishimura et al. (2005) confirmed that induction of the glucuronyl transferase UGT1A6, thought to be involved in the reduction in serum thyroid hormone in mice, depends on the AHR. Thus, some dioxin-like PCB congeners (such as PCB-77) can be metabolized to hydroxy derivatives that more closely resemble the structure of T4 and displace it from thyroid-binding proteins, such as transthyretin—a mechanism not likely with TCDD. Not all mechanisms by which chemicals might affect thyroid homeostasis are understood, and dioxin may act on thyroid function via different mechanisms.

Synthesis

Numerous animal experiments and several epidemiologic studies have shown that TCDD and dioxin-like compounds appear to exert some influence on thyroid homeostasis. An occupational study (Johnson et al., 2001) showed an inverse relationship between TCDD concentrations and T3 and TSH concentrations. The association was strongest when historical, but not current, serum TCDD concentrations were considered. In a paper reviewed in *Update 1998*, Zober et al. (1994) examined workers exposed to TCDD in an industrial incident and reported that thyroid disease was increased ($p < 0.05$) in the exposed population. Other epidemiologic studies have found inverse relationships between dioxin-like compounds and thyroid function after environmental exposures (Bloom et al., 2006). In the AFHS study considered in *Update 2004*, Pavuk et al. (2003) reported a trend toward an increasing concentration of TSH that was not accompanied by changes in circulating T4 or T3 in Vietnam veterans. There was no evidence of changes in clinical thyroid disease. Although the overall assessment of the studies to date suggests some variation in thyroid hormone concentrations in relation to TCDD exposure, the functional importance of those changes remains unclear because adaptive capacity should be adequate to accommodate them.

Conclusions

There is inadequate or insufficient evidence of an association between exposure to the chemicals of interest and clinical or overt adverse effects on thyroid homeostasis. Some effects have been observed in humans, but the functional importance of the changes reported in the studies reviewed remains unclear because adaptive capacity could be adequate to accommodate them.

SUMMARY

On the basis of the occupational, environmental, and veterans studies reviewed and in light of information concerning biologic plausibility, the committee reached one of four conclusions about the strength of the evidence regarding an association between exposure to the chemicals of interest and each of the health outcomes discussed in this chapter. In categorizing diseases according to the strength of the evidence, the committee applied the same criteria (discussed in Chapter 2) that were used in *VAO*, *Update 1996*, *Update 1998*, *Update 2000*, *Update 2002*, *Update 2004*, and *Update 2006*. To be consistent with the charge to the committee by the Secretary of Veterans Affairs in Public Law 102-4 and with accepted standards of scientific reviews, the distinctions between conclusions are based on statistical association.

Health Outcomes with Sufficient Evidence of an Association

For diseases in this category, a positive association between exposure and outcome must be observed in studies in which chance, bias, and confounding can be ruled out with reasonable confidence. The committee regarded evidence from several small studies that were free of bias and confounding and that showed an association that was consistent in magnitude and direction as sufficient to conclude that there is an association.

The committees responsible for *VAO*, *Update 1996*, *Update 1998*, *Update 2000*, *Update 2002*, *Update 2004*, and *Update 2006* concluded that there was sufficient evidence of an association between exposure to at least one chemical of interest and chloracne. The scientific literature continues to support the classification of chloracne in the category of sufficient evidence. On the basis of the literature, no additional health effects discussed in this chapter satisfy the criteria necessary for inclusion in this category.

Health Outcomes with Limited or Suggestive Evidence of an Association

For this category, the evidence must suggest an association between exposure and outcome, although it can be limited because chance, bias, or confounding could not be ruled out with confidence.

The committees responsible for *Update 1996*, *Update 1998*, *Update 2000*, *Update 2002*, *Update 2004*, and *Update 2006* concluded that there was limited or suggestive evidence of an association between exposure to at least one chemical of interest and porphyria cutanea tarda. The scientific literature continues to support the classification of this disorder in the category of limited or suggestive evidence.

On the basis of its evaluation of available scientific evidence, the committee responsible for *Type 2 Diabetes* concluded that there was limited or suggestive evidence of an association between exposure to at least one chemical of interest and type 2 diabetes; the committees responsible for *Update 2000*, *Update 2002*, *Update 2004*, and *Update 2006* reached the same conclusion. New evidence reviewed by the present committee continues to support that conclusion.

The committee for *Update 2006* added the cardiovascular condition hypertension to the list of health outcomes in the category of limited or suggestive evidence. The present committee reached consensus that another cardiovascular outcome, ischemic heart disease, belonged in this category.

Health Outcomes with Inadequate or Insufficient Evidence to Determine Whether There Is an Association

The scientific data on many of the health outcomes reviewed by the present committee were inadequate or insufficient to determine whether there is an association between exposure to the chemicals of interest and the outcomes. For the health outcomes in this category, the available studies are of insufficient quality, consistency, or statistical power to permit a conclusion regarding the presence or absence of an association. Some studies failed to control for confounding or used inadequate exposure assessment. This category includes nonmalignant respiratory disorders, such as asthma in isolation, pleurisy, pneumonia, and tuberculosis; immune-system disorders (immune suppression and autoimmunity); lipid and lipoprotein disorders; gastrointestinal diseases; digestive diseases; liver toxicity; circulatory disorders (except as qualified above); endometriosis; and disorders of thyroid homeostasis.

Health Outcomes with Limited or Suggestive Evidence of *No* Association

To classify outcomes in this category, several adequate studies covering the full range of known human exposure must be consistent in not showing a positive association between exposure and outcome at any magnitude of exposure. The studies also must have relatively narrow confidence intervals. A conclusion of "no association" is inevitably limited to the conditions, magnitudes of exposure, and periods of observation covered by the available studies. The possibility of a very small increase in risk at the exposure studied can never be excluded.

The committees responsible for *VAO*, *Update 1996*, *Update 1998*, *Update 2000*, *Update 2002*, *Update 2004*, and *Update 2006* concluded that none of the health outcomes discussed in this chapter had limited or suggestive evidence of *no* association with exposure to the chemicals of interest. The most recent scientific evidence continues to support that conclusion.

REFERENCES[1]

Abdelouahab N, Mergler D, Takser L, Vanier C, St-Jean M, Baldwin M, Spear PA, Chan HM. 2008. Gender differences in the effects of organochlorines, mercury, and lead on thyroid hormone levels in lakeside communities of Quebec (Canada). *Environmental Research* 107(3):380–392.

ADVA (Australian Department of Veterans Affairs). 2005b. *The Third Australian Vietnam Veterans Mortality Study 2005.* Canberra, Australia: Department of Veterans' Affairs.

ADVA. 2005c. *Australian National Service Vietnam Veterans: Mortality and Cancer Incidence 2005.* Canberra, Australia: Department of Veterans' Affairs.

AFHS (Air Force Health Study). 1984. *An Epidemiologic Investigation of Health Effects in Air Force Personnel Following Exposure to Herbicides. Baseline Morbidity Study Results.* Brooks AFB, TX: USAF School of Aerospace Medicine. NTIS AD-A138 340.

AFHS. 1987. *An Epidemiological Investigation of Health Effects in Air Force Personnel Following Exposure to Herbicides. First Follow-up Examination Results.* Brooks AFB, TX: USAF School of Aerospace Medicine. USAFSAM-TR-87-27.

AFHS. 1990. *An Epidemiologic Investigation of Health Effects in Air Force Personnel Following Exposure to Herbicides.* Brooks AFB, TX: USAF School of Aerospace Medicine. USAFSAM-TR-90-2.

AFHS. 1991b. *An Epidemiologic Investigation of Health Effects in Air Force Personnel Following Exposure to Herbicides. Mortality Update: 1991.* Brooks AFB, TX: Armstrong Laboratory.

AFHS. 1992. *An Epidemiologic Investigation of Health Effects in Air Force Personnel Following Exposure to Herbicides. Reproductive Outcomes.* Brooks AFB, TX: Armstrong Laboratory. AL–TR–1992–0090.

AFHS. 1996. *An Epidemiologic Investigation of Health Effects in Air Force Personnel Following Exposure to Herbicides. Mortality Update 1996.* Brooks AFB, TX: Epidemiologic Research Division, Armstrong Laboratory. AL/AO-TR-1996-0068.

AFHS. 2000. *An Epidemiologic Investigation of Health Effects in Air Force Personnel Following Exposure to Herbicides. 1997 Follow-up Examination and Results.* Reston, VA: Science Application International Corporation. F41624–96–C1012.

AFHS. 2005. *An Epidemiologic Investigation of Health Effects in Air Force Personnel Following Exposure to Herbicides. 1997 Follow-up Examination and Results.* Brooks AFB, TX: Epidemiologic Research Division, Armstrong Laboratory. AFRL-HE-BR-SR-2005-0003.

AHA (American Heart Association). 2009. Heart disease and stroke statistics—2009 update: A report from the American Health Association statistics committee and stroke statistics subcommittee. *Circulation* 119:e21–e181.

Alavanja M, Merkle S, Teske J, Eaton B, Reed B. 1989. Mortality among forest and soil conservationists. *Archives of Environmental Health* 44:94–101.

Anderson H, Hanrahan L, Jensen M, Laurin D, Yick W, Wiegman P. 1986. *Wisconsin Vietnam Veteran Mortality Study: Proportionate Mortality Ratio Study Results.* Madison: Wisconsin Division of Health.

Arsenescu V, Arsenescu RI, King V, Swanson H, Cassis LA. 2008. Polychlorinated biphenyl-77 induces adipocyte differentiation and proinflammatory adipokines and promotes obesity and atherosclerosis. *Environmental Health Perspectives* 116(6):761–768.

Assennato G, Cervino D, Emmett E, Longo G, Merlo F. 1989a. Follow-up of subjects who developed chloracne following TCDD exposure at Seveso. *American Journal of Industrial Medicine* 16:119–125.

---

[1]Throughout the report the same alphabetic indicator following year of publication is used consistently for the same article when there were multiple citations by the same first author in a given year. The convention of assigning the alphabetic indicator in order of citation in a given chapter is not followed.

Assennato G, Cannatelli P, Emmett E, Ghezzi I, Merlo F. 1989b. Medical monitoring of dioxin clean-up workers. *American Industrial Hygiene Association Journal* 50:586–592.

Baccarelli A, Pfeiffer R, Consonni D, Pesatori AC, Bonzini M, Patterson DG Jr, Bertazzi PA. Landi MT. 2005a. Handling of dioxin measurement data in the presence of non-detectable values: Overview of available methods and their application in the Seveso chloracne study. *Chemosphere* 60(7):898–906.

Baccarelli A, Pesatori AC, Consonni D, Mocarelli P, Patterson DG Jr, Caporaso NE, Bertazzi PA, Landi MT. 2005b. Health status and plasma dioxin levels in chloracne cases 20 years after the Seveso, Italy accident. *British Journal of Dermatology* 152(3):459–465.

Becher H, Flesch-Janys D, Kauppinen T, Kogevinas M, Steindorf K, Manz A, Wahrendorf J. 1996. Cancer mortality in German male workers exposed to phenoxy herbicides and dioxins. *Cancer Causes and Control* 7(3):312–321.

Beck H, Eckart K, Mathar W, Wittkowski R. 1989. Levels of PCDDs and PCDFs in adipose tissue of occupationally exposed workers. *Chemosphere* 18:507–516.

Bertazzi P, Zocchetti C, Pesatori A, Guercilena S, Sanarico M, Radice L. 1989a. Mortality in an area contaminated by TCDD following an industrial incident. *Medicina Del Lavoro* 80:316–329.

Bertazzi P, Zocchetti C, Pesatori A, Guercilena S, Sanarico M, Radice L. 1989b. Ten-year mortality study of the population involved in the Seveso incident in 1976. *American Journal of Epidemiology* 129:1187–1200.

Bertazzi PA, Bernucci I, Brambilla G, Consonni D, Pesatori AC. 1998. The Seveso studies on early and long-term effects of dioxin exposure: A review. *Environmental Health Perspectives* 106(Suppl 2):625–633.

Bertazzi PA, Consonni D, Bachetti S, Rubagotti M, Baccarelli A, Zocchetti C, Pesatori AC. 2001. Health effects of dioxin exposure: A 20-year mortality study. *American Journal of Epidemiology* 153(11):1031–1044.

Blair A, Grauman D, Lubin J, Fraumeni JJ. 1983. Lung cancer and other causes of death among licensed pesticide applicators. *Journal of the National Cancer Institute* 71:31–37.

Blair A, Sandler DP, Tarone R, Lubin J, Thomas K, Hoppin JA, Samanic C, Coble J, Kamel F, Knott C, Dosemeci M, Zahm SH, Lynch CF, Rothman N, Alavanja MC. 2005. Mortality among participants in the Agricultural Health Study. *Annals of Epidemiology* 15(4):279–285.

Bleiberg J, Wallen M, Brodkin R, Applebaum IL. 1964. Industrially acquired porphyria. *Archives of Dermatology* 89:793–797.

Bloom M, Vena J, Olson J, Moysich K. 2006. Chronic exposure to dioxin-like compounds and thyroid function among New York anglers. *Environmental Toxicology and Pharmacology* 21(3): 260–267.

Boehmer TK, Flanders WD, McGeehin MA, Boyle C, Barrett DH. 2004. Postservice mortality in Vietnam veterans: 30-year follow-up. *Archives of Internal Medicine* 164(17):1908–1916.

Bohn AA, Harrod KS, Teske S, Lawrence BP. 2005. Increased mortality associated with TCDD exposure in mice infected with influenza A virus is not due to severity of lung injury or alterations in Clara cell protein content. *Chemico-Biological Interactions* 155(3):181–190.

Bond GG, Cook RR, Brenner FE, McLaren EA. 1987. Evaluation of mortality patterns among chemical workers with chloracne. *Chemosphere* 16:2117–2121.

Bond GG, McLaren EA, Brenner FE, Cook RR. 1989a. Incidence of chloracne among chemical workers potentially exposed to chlorinated dioxins. *Journal of Occupational Medicine* 31:771–774.

Bond GG, McLaren EA, Lipps TE, Cook RR. 1989b. Update of mortality among chemical workers with potential exposure to the higher chlorinated dioxins. *Journal of Occupational Medicine* 31:121–123.

Boverhof DR, Burgoon LD, Tashiro C, Chittim B, Harkema JR, Jump DB, Zacharewski TR. 2005. Temporal and dose-dependent hepatic gene expression patterns in mice provide new insights into TCDD-mediated hepatotoxicity. *Toxicological Sciences* 85(2):1048–1063.

Boverhof DR, Burgoon LD, Tashiro C, Sharratt B, Chittim B, Harkema JR, Mendrick DL, Zacharewski TR. 2006. Comparative toxicogenomic analysis of the hepatotoxic effects of TCDD in Sprague Dawley rats and C57BL/6 mice. *Toxicological Sciences* 94(2):398–416.

Brunnnerg S, Andersson P, Lindstam M, Paulson I, Poellinger L, Hanberg A. 2006. The constitutively active Ah receptor (CA-Ahr) mouse as a potential model for dioxin exposure-effects in vital organs. *Toxicology* 224(3):191–201.

Bullman T, Kang H. 1996. The risk of suicide among wounded Vietnam veterans. *American Journal of Public Health* 86(5):662–667.

Burleson GR, Lebrec H, Yang YG, Ibanes JD, Pennington KN, Birnbaum LS. 1996. Effect of 2,3,7,8-tetrachlorodibenzo-*p*-dioxin (TCDD) on influenza virus host resistance in mice. *Fundamental and Applied Toxicology* 29(1):40–47.

Burns C, Beard K, Cartmill J. 2001. Mortality in chemical workers potentially exposed to 2,4-dichlorophenoxyacetic acid (2,4-D) 1945–94: An update. *Occupational and Environmental Medicine* 58:24–30.

Calvert GM, Sweeney MH, Morris JA, Fingerhut MA, Hornung RW, Halperin WE. 1991. Evaluation of chronic bronchitis, chronic obstructive pulmonary disease, and ventilatory function among workers exposed to 2,3,7,8-tetrachlorodibenzo-*p*-dioxin. *The American Review of Respiratory Disease* 144(6):1302–1306.

Calvert GM, Hornung RV, Sweeney MH, Fingerhut MA, Halperin WE. 1992. Hepatic and gastro-intestinal effects in an occupational cohort exposed to 2,3,7,8-tetrachlorodibenzo-*para*-dioxin. *Journal of the American Medical Association* 267:2209–2214.

Calvert GM, Sweeney MH, Fingerhut MA, Hornung RW, Halperin WE. 1994. Evaluation of por-phyria cutanea tarda in US workers exposed to 2,3,7,8-tetrachlorodibenzo-*p*-dioxin. *American Journal of Industrial Medicine* 25(4):559–571.

Calvert GM, Willie KK, Sweeney MH, Fingerhut MA, Halperin WE. 1996. Evaluation of serum lipid concentrations among US workers exposed to 2,3,7,8-tetrachlorodibenzo-*p*-dioxin. *Archives of Environmental Health* 51(2):100–107.

Calvert GM, Wall DK, Sweeney MH, Fingerhut MA. 1998. Evaluation of cardiovascular outcomes among US workers exposed to 2,3,7,8-tetrachlorodibenzo-*p*-dioxin. *Environmental Health Perspectives* 106(Suppl 2):635–643.

Calvert GM, Sweeney MH, Deddens J, Wall DK. 1999. Evaluation of diabetes mellitus, serum glu-cose, and thyroid function among United States workers exposed to 2,3,7,8-tetrachlorodibenzo-*p*-dioxin. *Occupational and Environmental Medicine* 56(4):270–276.

Canaris GJ, Manowitz NR, Mayor G, Ridgway EC. 2000. The Colorado thyroid disease prevalence study. *Archives of Internal Medicine* 160(4):526–534.

Caramaschi F, Del CG, Favaretti C, Giambelluca SE, Montesarchio E, Fara GM. 1981. Chloracne following environmental contamination by TCDD in Seveso, Italy. *International Journal of Epidemiology* 10:135–143.

CDC (Centers for Disease Control and Prevention). 1988. Centers for Disease Control Vietnam Experience Study. Health status of Vietnam veterans. II: Physical health. *Journal of the American Medical Association* 259(18):2708–2714.

CDVA (Commonwealth Department of Veterans' Affairs). 1998a. *Morbidity of Vietnam Veterans: A Study of the Health of Australia's Vietnam Veteran Community. Volume 1: Male Vietnam Veterans Survey and Community Comparison Outcomes.* Canberra, Australia: Department of Veterans' Affairs.

CDVA. 1998b. *Morbidity of Vietnam Veterans: A Study of the Health of Australia's Vietnam Veteran Community. Volume 2: Female Vietnam Veterans Survey and Community Comparison Out-comes.* Canberra, Australia: Department of Veterans' Affairs.

Chen HL, Su HJ, Guo YL, Liao PC, Hung CF, Lee CC. 2006. Biochemistry examinations and health disorder evaluation of Taiwanese living near incinerators and with low serum PCDD/Fs levels. *Science of the Total Environment* 366:538–548.

Chen JW, Wang SL, Liao PC, Chen HY, Ko YC, Lee CC. 2008. Relationship between insulin sensitivity and exposure to dioxin and polychlorinated biphenyls in pregnant women. *Environmental Research* 107:245–253.

Chevrier J, Eskenazi B, Holland N, Bradman A, Barr DB. 2008. Effects of exposure to polychlorinated biphenyls and organochlorine pesticides on thyroid function during pregnancy. *American Journal of Epidemiology* 168(3):298–310.

Codru N, Schymura MJ, Negoita S, Rej R, Carpenter DO. 2007. Diabetes in relation to serum levels of polychlorinated biphenyls and chlorinated pesticides in adult native Americans. *Environmental Health Perspectives* 115(10):1442–1447.

Coggon D, Pannett B, Winter P, Acheson E, Bonsall J. 1986. Mortality of workers exposed to 2-methyl-4-chlorophenoxyacetic acid. *Scandinavian Journal of Work, Environment, and Health* 12:448–454.

Coggon D, Pannett B, Winter P. 1991. Mortality and incidence of cancer at four factories making phenoxy herbicides. *British Journal of Industrial Medicine* 48:173–178.

Consonni D, Pesatori AC, Zocchetti C, Sindaco R, D'Oro LC, Rubagotti M, Bertazzi PA. 2008. Mortality in a population exposed to dioxin after the Seveso, Italy, accident in 1976: 25 years of follow-up. *American Journal of Epidemiology* 167(7):847–858.

Cook RR, Townsend JC, Ott MG, Silverstein LG. 1980. Mortality experience of employees exposed to 2,3,7,8-tetrachlorodibenzo-*p*-dioxin (TCDD). *Journal of Occupational Medicine* 22:530–532.

Cook RR, Bond GG, Olson RA, Ott MG. 1987. Update of the mortality experience of workers exposed to chlorinated dioxins. *Chemosphere* 16:2111–2116.

Cooper GS, Parks CG. 2004. Occupational and environmental exposures as risk factors for systemic lupus erythematosus. *Current Rheumatology Reports* 6(5):367–374.

Crane P, Barnard D, Horsley K, Adena M. 1997a. *Mortality of Vietnam Veterans: The Veteran Cohort Study. A Report of the 1996 Retrospective Cohort Study of Australian Vietnam Veterans.* Canberra, Australia: Department of Veterans' Affairs.

Crane P, Barnard D, Horsley K, Adena M. 1997b. *Mortality of National Service Vietnam Veterans: A Report of the 1996 Retrospective Cohort Study of Australian Vietnam Veterans.* Canberra, Australia: Department of Veterans' Affairs.

Cranmer M, Louie S, Kennedy RH, Kern PA, Fonseca VA. 2000. Exposure to 2,3,7,8-tetrachlorodibenzo-*p*-dioxin (TCDD) is associated with hyperinsulinemia and insulin resistance. *Toxicological Sciences* 56(2):431–436.

Cypel Y, Kang H. 2008. Mortality patterns among women Vietnam-Era veterans: Results of a retrospective cohort Study. *Annals of Epidemiology* 18(3):244–252.

Dabir P, Marinic TE, Krukovets I, Stenina OI. 2008. Aryl hydrocarbon receptor is activated by glucose and regulates the thrombospondin-1 gene promoter in endothelial cells. *Circulation Research* 102(12):1558–1565.

Dahlgren J, Warshaw R, Thornton J, Anderson-Mahoney CP, Takhar H. 2003. Health effects on nearby residents of a wood treatment plant. *Environmental Research* 92(2):92–98.

Dalager MS, Kang HK, Thomas TL. 1995. Cancer mortality patterns among women who served in the military: The Vietnam experience. *Journal of Occupational and Environmental Medicine* 37:298–305.

Dalton TP, Kerzee JK, Wang B, Miller M, Dieter MZ, Lorenz JN, Shertzer HG, Nerbert DW, Puga A. 2001. Dioxin exposure is an environmental risk factor for ischemic heart disease. *Cardiovascular Toxicology* 1(4):285–298.

Doss M, Sauer H, von TR, Colombi AM. 1984. Development of chronic hepatic porphyria (porphyria cutanea tarda) with inherited uroporphyrinogen decarboxylase deficiency under exposure to dioxin. *International Journal of Biochemistry* 16(4):369–373.

Eisen S, Goldberg J, True W, Henderson W. 1991. A co-twin control study of the effects of the Vietnam War on the self-reported physical health of veterans. *American Journal of Epidemiology* 134:49–58.

Everett CJ, Frithsen IL, Diaz VA, Koopman RJ, Simpson WM Jr, Mainous AG 3rd. 2007. Association of a polychlorinated dibenzo-*p*-dioxin, a polychlorinated biphenyl, and DDT with diabetes in the 1999–2002 National Health and Nutrition Examination Survey. *Environmental Research* 103(3):413–418.

Everett CJ, Mainous AG 3rd, Frithsen IL, Player MS, Matheson EM. 2008a. Association of polychlorinated biphenyls with hypertension in the 1999–2002 National Health and Nutrition Examination Survey. *Environmental Research* 108(1):94–97.

Everett CJ, Mainous AG 3rd, Frithsen IL, Player MS, Matheson EM 2008b. Commentary on the associaton of polychlorinated biphenyls with hypertension. *Environmental Research* 108(3): 428–429.

Fierens S, Mairesse H, Heilier JF, De Burbure C, Focant JF, Eppe G, De Pauw E, Bernard A. 2003. Dioxin/polychlorinated biphenyl body burden, diabetes and endometriosis: Findings in a population-based study in Belgium. *Biomarkers* 8(6):529–534.

Flesch-Janys D. 1997/1998. Analyses of exposure to polychlorinated dibenzo-*p*-dioxins, furans, and hexachlorocyclohexane and different health outcomes in a cohort of former herbicide-producing workers in Hamburg, Germany. *Teratogenesis Carcinogenesis and Mutagenesis* 17(4-5): 257–264.

Flesch-Janys D, Berger J, Gurn P, Manz A, Nagel S, Waltsgott H, Dwyer. 1995. Exposure to polychlorinated dioxins and furans (PCDD/F) and mortality in a cohort of workers from a herbicide-producing plant in Hamburg, Federal Republic of Germany. *American Journal of Epidemiology* 142:1165–1175.

Flesch-Janys D, Becher H, Berger J, Dwyer JH, Gurn P, Manz A, Nagel S, Steindorf K, Waltsgott H. 1998. [Aspects of dose–response relationship of mortality due to malignant regeneration and cardiovascular diseases and exposure to polychlorinated dibenzodioxins and furans (PCDD/F) in an occupational cohort study—German]. *Arbeitsmedizin Sozialmedizin Umweltmedizin* 24:54–59.

Foster WG, Holloway AC, Hughes CL Jr. 2005. Dioxin-like activity and maternal thyroid hormone levels in second trimester maternal serum. *American Journal of Obstetrics and Gynecology* 193(6):1900–1907.

Fujiyoshi PT, Michalek JE, Matsumura F. 2006. Molecular epidemiologic evidence for diabetogenic effects of dioxin exposure in US Air Force veterans of the Vietnam war. *Environmental Health Perspectives* 114(11):1677–1683.

Funatake CJ, Marshall NB, Kerkvliet NI. 2008. 2,3,7,8-Tetrachlorodibenzo-*p*-dioxin alters the differentiation of alloreactive CD8+ T cells toward a regulatory T cell phenotype by a mechanism that is dependent on aryl hydrocarbon receptor in CD4+ T cells. *Journal of Immunotoxicology* 5(1):81–91.

Gambini G, Mantovani C, Pira E, Piolatto P, Negri E. 1997. Cancer mortality among rice growers in Novara Province, Northern Italy. *American Journal of Industrial Medicine* 31:435–441.

Geusau A, Khorchide M, Mildner M, Pammer J, Eckhart L, Tschachler E. 2005. 2,3,7,8-tetrachlorodibenzo-*p*-dioxin impairs differentiation of normal human epidermal keratinocytes in a skin equivalent model. *Journal of Investigative Dermatology* 124(1):275–277.

Goldman P. 1972. Critically acute chloracne caused by trichlorophenol decomposition products. *Arbeitsmedizen Sozialmedizen Arbeitshygiene* 7:12–18.

Goncharov A, Haase RF, Santiago-Rivera A, Morse G, Akwesasne Task Force on the E, McCaffrey RJ, Rej R, Carpenter DO. 2008. High serum PCBs are associated with elevation of serum lipids and cardiovascular disease in a Native American population. *Environmental Research* 106(2):226–239.

Ha MH, Lee DH, Jacobs DR Jr. 2007. Association between serum concentrations of persistent organic pollutants and self-reported cardiovascular disease prevalence: Results from the National Health and Nutrition Examination Survey, 1999–2002. *Environmental Health Perspectives* 115(8):1204–1209.

Harrigan JA, McGarrigle BP, Sutter TR, Olson JR. 2006. Tissue specific induction of cytochrome P450 (CYP) 1A1 and 1B1 in rat liver and lung following in vitro (tissue slice) and in vivo exposure to benzo(a)pyrene. *Toxicology in Vitro* 20(4):426–438.

Helfand M, Redfern CC. 1998. Clinical guidelines part 2. Screening for thyroid disease. *Annals of Internal Medicine* 129:144–158.

Henneberger PK, Ferris BG Jr, Monson RR. 1989. Mortality among pulp and paper workers in Berlin, New Hampshire. *British Journal of Industrial Medicine* 46:658–664.

Henriksen GL, Ketchum NS, Michalek JE, Swaby JA. 1997. Serum dioxin and diabetes mellitus in veterans of Operation Ranch Hand. *Epidemiology* 8(3):252–258.

Hoffman RE, Stehr-Green PA, Webb KB, Evans RG, Knutsen AP, Schramm WF, Staake JL, Gibson BB, Steinberg KK. 1986. Health effects of long-term exposure to 2,3,7,8-tetrachlorodibenzo-*p*-dioxin. *Journal of the American Medical Association* 255:2031–2038.

Hollowell JG, Staehling NW, Flanders WD, Hannon WH, Gunter EW, Spencer CA, Braverman LE. 2002. Serum TSH, T(4), and thyroid antibodies in the United States population (1988 to 1994): National Health and Nutrition Examination Survey (NHANES III). *The Journal of Clinical Endocrinology and Metabolism* 87(2):489–499.

Hooiveld M, Heederik DJ, Kogevinas M, Boffetta P, Needham LL, Patterson DG Jr, Bueno de Mesquita HB. 1998. Second follow-up of a Dutch cohort occupationally exposed to phenoxy herbicides, chlorophenols, and contaminants. *American Journal of Epidemiology* 147(9):891–901.

Hoppin JA, Umbach DM, London SJ, Lynch CF, Alavanja MC, Sandler DP. 2006a. Pesticides associated with wheeze among commercial pesticide applicators in the Agricultural Health Study. *American Journal of Epidemiology* 163(12):1129–1137.

Hoppin JA, Umbach DM, London SJ, Lynch CF, Alavanja MC, Sandler DP. 2006b. Pesticides and adult respiratory outcomes in the Agricultural Health Study. *Annals of the New York Academy of Sciences* 1076:343–354.

Hoppin JA, Umbach DM, Kullman GJ, Henneberger PK, London SJ, Alavanja MC, Sandler DP. 2007a. Pesticides and other agricultural factors associated with self-reported farmer's lung among farm residents in the Agricultural Health Study. *Occupational and Environmental Medicine* 64(5):334–341.

Hoppin JA, Valcin M, Henneberger PK, Kullman GJ, Limbach DM, London SJ, Alavanja MCR, Sandler DP. 2007b. Pesticide use and chronic bronchitis among farmers in the Agricultural Health Study. *American Journal of Industrial Medicine* 50(12):969–979.

Hoppin JA, Umbach DM, London SJ, Henneberger PK, Kullman GJ, Alavanja MC, Sandler DP. 2008. Pesticides and atopic and nonatopic asthma among farm women in the Agricultural Health Study. *American Journal of Respiratory and Critical Care Medicine* 177(1):11–18.

Hu SW, Cheng TJ, ChangChien GP, Chan CC. 2003. Association between dioxins/furans exposures and incinerator workers' hepatic function and blood lipids. *Journal of Occupational and Environmental Medicine* 45(6):601–608.

Ichihara S, Yamada Y, Ichihara G, Nakajima T, Li P, Kondo T, Gonzalez FJ, Murohara T. 2007. A role for the aryl hydrocarbon receptor in regulation of ischemia-induced angiogenesis. *Arteriosclerosis, Thrombosis and Vascular Biology* 27(6):1297–1304.

IOM (Institute of Medicine). 1994. *Veterans and Agent Orange: Health Effects of Herbicides Used in Vietnam.* Washington, DC: National Academy Press.

IOM. 1996. *Veterans and Agent Orange: Update 1996.* Washington, DC: National Academy Press.

IOM. 1999. *Veterans and Agent Orange: Update 1998.* Washington, DC: National Academy Press.

IOM. 2000. *Veterans and Agent Orange: Herbicide/Dioxin Exposure and Type 2 Diabetes.* Washington, DC: National Academy Press.

IOM. 2001. *Veterans and Agent Orange: Update 2000.* Washington, DC: National Academy Press.

IOM. 2003. *Veterans and Agent Orange: Update 2002.* Washington, DC: The National Academies Press.

IOM. 2005. *Veterans and Agent Orange: Update 2004.* Washington, DC: The National Academies Press.

IOM. 2007. *Veterans and Agent Orange: Update 2006.* Washington, DC: The National Academies Press.

Johnson ES, Shorter C, Bestervelt LL, Patterson DG, Needham LL, Piper WN, Lucier G, Nolan CJ. 2001. Serum hormone levels in humans with low serum concentrations of 2,3,7,8-TCDD. *Toxicology and Industrial Health* 17(4):105–112.

Jokinen MP, Walker NJ, Brix AE, Sells DM, Haseman JK, Nyska A. 2003. Increase in cardiovascular pathology in female Sprague-Dawley rats following chronic treatment with 2,3,7,8-tetrachlorodibenzo-*p*-dioxin and 3,3',4,4',5-pentachlorobiphenyl. *Cardiovascular Toxicology* 3(4):299–310.

Jung D, Konietzko J, Reill-Konietzko G, Muttray A, Zimmermann-Holz HJ, Doss M, Beck H, Edler L, Kopp-Schneider A. 1994. Porphyrin studies in TCDD-exposed workers. *Archives of Toxicology* 68:595–598.

Kang HK, Dalager NA, Needham LL, Patterson DG, Lees PSJ, Yates K, Matanoski G.M. 2006. Health status of Army Chemical Corps Vietnam veterans who sprayed defoliant in Vietnam. *American Journal of Industrial Medicine* 49(11):875–884.

Karouna-Renier NK, Rao KR, Lanza JJ, Davis DA, Wilson PA. 2007. Serum profiles of PCDDs and PCDFs in individuals near the Escambia Wood Treating Company Superfund site in Pensacola, FL. *Chemosphere* 69:1312–1319.

Kern PA, Dicker-Brown A, Said ST, Kennedy R, Fonseca VA. 2002. The stimulation of tumor necrosis factor and inhibition of glucose transport and lipoprotein lipase in adipose cells by 2,3,7,8-tetrachlorodibenzo-*p*-dioxin. *Metabolism: Clinical and Experimental* 51(1):65–68.

Kern PA, Said S, Jackson WG Jr, Michalek JE. 2004. Insulin sensitivity following Agent Orange exposure in Vietnam veterans with high blood levels of 2,3,7,8-tetrachlorodibenzo-*p*-dioxin. *Journal of Clinical Endocrinology and Metabolism* 89(9):4665–4672.

Ketchum NS, Michalek JE. 2005. Postservice mortality of Air Force veterans occupationally exposed to herbicides during the Vietnam War: 20-year follow-up results. *Military Medicine* 170(5):406–413.

Kim J-S, Lim HS, Cho SI, Cheong HK, Lim MK. 2003. Impact of Agent Orange exposure among Korean Vietnam veterans. *Industrial Health* 41(3):149–157.

Kitamura K, Kikuchi Y, Watanabe S, Waechter G, Sakurai H, Takada T. 2000. Health effects of chronic exposure to polychlorinated dibenzo-*p*-dioxins (PCDD), dibenzofurans (PCDF) and coplanar PCB (Co-PCB) of municipal waste incinerator workers. *Journal of Epidemiology* 10(4):262–270.

Kogan M, Clapp R. 1985. Mortality Among Vietnam Veterans in Massachusetts, 1972–1983. *Massachusetts Office of the Commissioner of Veterans Services, Agent Orange Program.*

Kogevinas M, Becher H, Benn T, Bertazzi P, Boffetta P, Bueno de Mesquita H, Coggon D, Colin D, Flesch-Janys D, Fingerhut M, Green L, Kauppinen T, Littorin M, Lynge E, Mathews J, Neuberger M, Pearce N, Saracci R. 1997. Cancer mortality in workers exposed to phenoxy herbicides, chlorophenols, and dioxins. An expanded and updated international cohort study. *American Journal of Epidemiology* 145(12):1061–1075.

Korenaga T, Fukusato T, Ohta M, Asaoka K, Murata N, Arima A, Kubota S. 2007. Long-term effects of subcutaneously injected 2,3,7,8-tetrachlorodibenzo-*p*-dioxin on the liver of rhesus monkeys. *Chemosphere* 67(9):S399–S404.

Langer P, Kocan A, Tajtakova M, Radikova Z, Petrik J, Koska J, Ksinantova L, Imrich R, Huckova M, Chovancova J, Drobna B, Jursa S, Bergman A, Athanasiadou M, Hovander L, Gasperikova D, Trnovec T, Sebokova E, Klimes I. 2007a. Possible effects of persistent organochlorinated pollutants cocktail on thyroid hormone levels and pituitary-thyroid interrelations. *Chemosphere* 70(1):110–118.

Langer P, Tajtakova M, Kocan A, Petrik J, Koska J, Ksinantova L, Radikova Z, Ukropec J, Imrich R, Huckova M, Chovancova J, Drobna B, Jursa S, Vlcek M, Bergman A, Athanasiadou M, Hovander L, Shishiba Y, Trnovec T, Sebokova E, Klimes I. 2007b. Thyroid ultrasound volume, structure and function after long-term high exposure of large population to polychlorinated biphenyls, pesticides and dioxin. *Chemosphere* 69(1):118–127.

Lee DH, Lee IK, Song K, Steffes M, Toscano W, Baker BA, Jacobs DR, Jr. 2006. A strong dose–response relation between serum concentrations of persistent organic pollutants and diabetes: Results from the National Health and Examination Survey 1999–2002. *Diabetes Care* 29(7):1638–1644.

Lee DH, Steffes M, Jacobs DR Jr. 2007a. Positive associations of serum concentration of polychlorinated biphenyls or organochlorine pesticides with self-reported arthritis, especially rheumatoid type, in women. *Environmental Health Perspectives* 115(6):883–888.

Lee DH, Lee IK, Jin SH, Steffes M, Jacobs DR Jr. 2007b. Association between serum concentrations of persistent organic pollutants and insulin resistance among nondiabetic adults: Results from the National Health and Nutrition Examination Survey 1999–2002. *Diabetes Care* 30(3):622–628.

Lee DH, Lee IK, Porta M, Steffes M, Jacobs DR Jr. 2007c. Relationship between serum concentrations of persistent organic pollutants and the prevalence of metabolic syndrome among nondiabetic adults: Results from the National Health and Nutrition Examination Survey 1999–2002. *Diabetologia* 50(9):1841–1851.

Lin TM, Ko K, Moore RW, Buchanan DL, Cooke PS, Peterson RE. 2001. Role of the aryl hydrocarbon receptor in the development of control and 2,3,7,8-tetrachlorodibenzo-*p*-dioxin-exposed male mice. *Journal of Toxicology and Environmental Health, Part A* 64(4):327–342.

Longnecker MP, Michalek JE. 2000. Serum dioxin level in relation to diabetes mellitus among Air Force veterans with background levels of exposure. *Epidemiology* 11(1):44–48.

Lund AK, Goens MB, Kanagy NL, Walker MK. 2003. Cardiac hypertrophy in aryl hydrocarbon receptor null mice is correlated with elevated angiotensin II, endothelin-1, and mean arterial blood pressure. *Toxicology and Applied Pharmacology* 193(2):177–187.

Lund AK, Peterson SL, Timmins GS, Walker MK. 2005. Endothelin-1-mediated increase in reactive oxygen species and NADPH oxidase activity in hearts of aryl hydrocarbon receptor (AhR) null mice. *Toxicological Sciences* 88(1):265–273.

Lund AK, Goens MB, Nunez BA, Walker MK. 2006. Characterizing the role of endothelin-1 in the progression of cardiac hypertrophy in aryl hydrocarbon receptor (AhR) null mice. *Toxicology and Applied Pharmacology* 212(2):127–135.

Lund AK, Agbor LN, Zhang N, Baker A, Zhao H, Fink GD, Kanagy NL, Walker MK. 2008. Loss of the aryl hydrocarbon receptor induces hypoxemia, endothelin-1, and systemic hypertension at modest altitude. *Hypertension* 51(3):803–809.

Marshall N, Vorachek W, Steppan L, Mourich D, Kerkvliet N. 2008. Functional characterization and gene expression analysis of CD4+ CD25+ regulatory T cells generated in mice treated with 2,3,7,8-tetrachlorodibenzo-*p*-dioxin. *Journal of Immunology* 181(4):2382–2391.

Martin JV. 1984. Lipid abnormalities in workers exposed to dioxin. *British Journal of Industrial Medicine* 41:254–256.

Masley ML, Semchuk KM, Senthilselvan A, McDuffie HH, Hanke P, Dosman JA, Cessna AJ, Crossley MFO, Irvine DG, Rosenberg AM, Hagel LM. 2000. Health and environment of rural families: Results of a community canvass survey in the Prairie Ecosystem Study (PECOS). *Journal of Agricultural Safety and Health* 6(2):103–115.

Matsumura F. 2003. On the significance of the role of cellular stress response reactions in the toxic actions of dioxin. *Biochemical and Pharmacology* 66:527–540.

May G. 1973. Chloracne from the accidental production of tetrachlorodibenzodioxin. *British Journal of Industrial Medicine* 30:276–283.

May G. 1982. Tetrachlorodibenzodioxin: A survey of subjects ten years after exposure. *British Journal of Industrial Medicine* 39(2):128–135.

McKinney WP, McIntire DD, Carmody TJ, Joseph A. 1997. Comparing the smoking behavior of veterans and nonveterans. *Public Health Reports* 112(3):212–217.

McLean D, Pearce N, Langseth H, Jappinen P, Szadkowska-Stanczyk I, Persson B, Wild P, Kishi R, Lynge E, Henneberger P, Sala M, Teschke K, Kauppinen T, Colin D, Kogevinas M, Boffetta P. 2006. Cancer mortality in workers exposed to organochlorine compounds in the pulp and paper industry: An international collaborative study. *Environmental Health Perspectives* 114(7):1007–1012.

Michalek JE, Pavuk M. 2008. Diabetes and cancer in veterans of operation Ranch Hand after adjustment for calendar period, days of spraying, and time spent in Southeast Asia. *Journal of Occupational and Environmental Medicine* 50(3):330–340.

Michalek J, Wolfe W, Miner J. 1990. Health status of Air Force veterans occupationally exposed to herbicides in Vietnam. II. Mortality. *Journal of the American Medical Association* 264:1832–1836.

Michalek J, Ketchum N, Tripathi RC. 2003. Diabetes mellitus and 2,3,7,8-tetrachlorodibenzo-*p*-dioxin elimination in veterans of Operation Ranch Hand. *Journal of Toxicology and Environmental Health. Part A* 66(3):211–221.

Mitchell KA, Lawrence BP. 2003. Exposure to 2,3,7,8–tetrachlorodibenzo-*p*-dioxin (TCDD) renders influenza virus-specific CD8$^+$ T cells hyporesponsive to antigen. *Toxicological Sciences* 74:74–84.

Mocarelli P, Marocchi A, Brambilla P, Gerthoux P, Young DS, Mantel N. 1986. Clinical laboratory manifestations of exposure to dioxin in children. A six-year study of the effects of an environmental disaster near Seveso, Italy. *Journal of the American Medical Association* 256:2687–2695.

Mocarelli P, Needham LL, Marocchi A, Patterson DG Jr, Brambilla P, Gerthoux PM, Meazza L, Carreri V. 1991. Serum concentrations of 2,3,7,8-tetrachlorodibenzo-*p*-dioxin and test results from selected residents of Seveso, Italy. *Journal of Toxicology and Environmental Health* 32:357–366.

Montgomery MP, Kamel F, Saldana TM, Alavanja MC, Sandler DP. 2008. Incident diabetes and pesticide exposure among licensed pesticide applicators: Agricultural Health Study, 1993–2003. *American Journal of Epidemiology* 167(10):1235–1246.

Moses M, Lilis R, Crow KD, Thornton J, Fischbein A, Anderson HA, Selikoff IJ. 1984. Health status of workers with past exposure to 2,3,7,8-tetrachlorodibenzo-*p*-dioxin in the manufacture of 2,4,5-trichlorophenoxyacetic acid: Comparison of findings with and without chloracne. *American Journal of Industrial Medicine* 5:161–182.

Nagayama J, Tsuji H, Iida T, Hirakawa H, Matsueda T, Ohki M. 2001. Effects of contamination level of dioxins and related chemicals on thyroid hormone and immune response systems in patients with "Yusho." *Chemosphere* 43(4-7):1005–1010.

Neuberger M, Kundi M, Jäger R. 1998. Chloracne and morbidity after dioxin exposure (preliminary results). *Toxicology Letters* 96, 97:347–350.

Nishimura N, Yonemoto J, Miyabara Y, Fujii-Kuriyama Y, Tohyama C. 2005. Altered thyroxin and retinoid metabolic response to 2,3,7,8-tetrachlorodibenzo-*p*-dioxin in aryl hydrocarbon receptor-null mice. *Archives of Toxicology* 79(5):260–267.

NTP (National Toxicology Program). 2004. *NTP Technical Report on the Toxicology and Carcinogenesis Studies of 2,3,7,8-Tetrachlorodibenzo-[rho]-dioxin (TCDD) (CAS no. 1746-01-6) in Female Harlan Sprague-Dawley Rats (Gavage Studies).* National Toxicology Program, Research Triangle Park, NC, and US Department of Health and Human Services, Public Health Service, National Institutes of Health.

Oliver RM. 1975. Toxic effects of 2,3,7,8 tetrachlorodibenzo 1,4-dioxin in laboratory workers. *British Journal of Industrial Medicine* 32:49–53.

Orchard TJ, LaPorte RE, Dorman JS. 1992. Diabetes. In: Last JM, Wallace RB, eds, *Public Health and Preventive Medicine*, 13th ed., Norwalk, CT: Appleton and Lange. Chapter 51:873–883.

O'Toole BI, Marshall RP, Grayson DA, Schureck RJ, Dobson M, Ffrench M, Pulvertaft B, Meldrum L, Bolton J, Vennard J. 1996. The Australian Vietnam Veterans Health Study: II. Self-reported health of veterans compared with the Australian population. *International Journal of Epidemiology* 25(2):319–330.

Ott MG, Zober A. 1996. Morbidity study of extruder personnel with potential exposure to brominated dioxins and furans. II. Results of clinical laboratory studies. *Occupational and Environmental Medicine* 53(12):844–846.

Ott MG, Zober A, Germann C. 1994. Laboratory results for selected target organs in 138 individuals occupationally exposed to TCDD. *Chemosphere* 29:2423–2437.

Panteleyev AA, Bickers DR. 2006. Dioxin-induced chloracne—reconstructing the cellular and molecular mechanisms of a classic environmental disease. *Experimental Dermatology* 15(9): 705–730.

Parks CG, Cooper GS. 2005. Occupational exposures and risk of systemic lupus erythematosus. *Autoimmunity* 38(7):497–506.

Pavuk M, Schecter AJ, Akhtar FZ, Michalek JE. 2003. Serum 2,3,7,8-tetrachlorodibenzo-*p*-dioxin (TCDD) levels and thyroid function in Air Force veterans of the Vietnam War. *Annals of Epidemiology* 13(5):335–343.

Pazderova-Vejlupkova J, Lukáš E, Nemcova M, Pickova J, Jirasek L. 1981. The development and prognosis of chronic intoxication by tetrachlorodibenzo-*p*-dioxin in men. *Archives of Environmental Health* 36:5–11.

Pelclová D, Fenclová Z, Preiss J, Procházka B, Spácil J, Dubská Z, Okrouhlík B, Lukáš E, Urban P. 2002. Lipid metabolism and neuropsychological follow-up study of workers exposed to 2,3,7,8-tetrachlordibenzo-*p*-dioxin. *International Archives of Occupational and Environmental Health* 75(Supplement l):S60–S66.

Pelclová D, Prazny M, Skrha J, Fenclová Z, Kalousova M, Urban P, Navratil T, Senholdova Z, Smerhovsky Z. 2007. 2,3,7,8-TCDD exposure, endothelial dysfunction and impaired microvascular reactivity. *Human and Experimental Toxicology* 26(9):705–713.

Pesatori AC, Zocchetti C, Guercilena S, Consonni D, Turrini D, Bertazzi PA. 1998. Dioxin exposure and non-malignant health effects: A mortality study. *Occupational and Environmental Medicine* 55:126–131.

Poland AP, Smith D, Metter G, Possick P. 1971. A health survey of workers in a 2,4-D and 2,4,5-T plant with special attention to chloracne, porphyria cutanea tarda, and psychologic parameters. *Archives of Environmental Health* 22:316–327.

Puga A, Sartor MA, Huang MY, Kerzee JK, Wei YD, Tomlinson CR, Baxter CS, Medvedovic M. 2004. Gene expression profiles of mouse aorta and cultured vascular smooth muscle cells differ widely, yet show common responses to dioxin exposure. *Cardiovascular Toxicology* 4(4):385–404.

Quintana FJ, Basso AS, Iglesias AH, Korn T, Farez MF, Bettelli E, Caccamo M, Oukka M, Weiner HL. 2008. Control of T(reg) and T(H)17 cell differentiation by the aryl hydrocarbon receptor. *Nature* 453(7191):65–71.

Ramlow JM, Spadacene NW, Hoag SR, Stafford BA, Cartmill JB, Lerner PJ. 1996. Mortality in a cohort of pentachlorophenol manufacturing workers, 1940–1989. *American Journal of Industrial Medicine* 30(2):180–194.

Riecke K, Grimm D, Shakibaei M, Kossmehl P, Schulze-Tanzil G, Paul M, Stahlmann R. 2002. Low doses of 2,3,7,8-tetrachlorodibenzo-*p*-dioxin increase transforming growth factor beta and cause myocardial fibrosis in marmosets (*Callithrix jacchus*). *Archives of Toxicology* 76(5-6): 360–366.

Rier SE, Martin DC, Bowman RE, Dmowski WP, Becker JL. 1993. Endometriosis in rhesus monkeys (*Macaca mulatta*) following chronic exposure to 2,3,7,8-tetrachlorodibenzo-*p*-dioxin. *Fundamental and Applied Toxicology* 21:433–441.

Roberts W. 2000. Twenty questions on atherosclerosis. *Baylor University Medical Center Proceedings* 13(2):139–143.

Robinson SW, Clothier B, Akhtar RA, Yang AL, Latour I, Van Ijperen C, Festing MF, Smith AG. 2002. Non-ahr gene susceptibility Loci for porphyria and liver injury induced by the interaction of 'dioxin' with iron overload in mice. *Molecular Pharmacology* 61(3):674–681.

Rothman K, Greenland S. 1998. *Modern Epidemiology 2nd ed.* Philadelphia Pa: Lippincott-Raven.

Saldana TM, Basso O, Hoppin JA, Baird DD, Knott C, Blair A, Alavanja MC, Sandler DP. 2007. Pesticide exposure and self-reported gestational diabetes mellitus in the Agricultural Health Study. *Diabetes Care* 30(3):529–534.

Sato S, Shirakawa H, Tomita S, Ohsaki Y, Haketa K, Tooi O, Santo N, Tohkin M, Furukawa Y, Gonzalez FJ, Komai M. 2008. Low-dose dioxins alter gene expression related to cholesterol biosynthesis, lipogenesis, and glucose metabolism through the aryl hydrocarbon receptor-mediated pathway in mouse liver. *Toxicology and Applied Pharmacology* 229(1):10–19.

Sawin CT, Castelli WP, Hershman JM, McNamara P, Bacharach P. 1985. The aging thyroid. Thyroid deficiency in the Framingham Study. *Archives of Internal Medicine* 145(8):1386–1388.

Senthilselvan A, McDuffie HH, Dosman JA. 1992. Association of asthma with use of pesticides. Results of a cross-sectional survey of farmers. *The American Review of Respiratory Disease* 146(4):884–887.

Siemiatycki J, Wacholder S, Dewar R, Wald L, Bégin D, Richardson L, Rosenman K, Gérin M. 1988. Smoking and degree of occupational exposure: Are internal analyses in cohort studies likely to be confounded by smoking status? *American Journal of Industrial Medicine* 13(1):59–69.

Smith AG, Clothier B, Carthew P, Childs NL, Sinclair PR, Nebert DW, Dalton TP. 2001. Protection of the Cyp1a2 (−/−) null mouse against uroporphyria and hepatic injury following exposure to 2,3,7,8-tetrachlorodibenzo-*p*-dioxin. *Toxicology and Applied Pharmacology* 173(2):89–98.

Smith AG, Hansson M, Rodriguez-Pichardo A, Ferrer-Dufol A, Neubert RT, Webb JR, Rappe C, Neubert D. 2008. Polychlorinated dibenzo-*p*-dioxins and the human immune system: 4 studies on two Spanish families with increased body burdens of highly chlorinated PCDDs. *Environment International* 34(3):330–344.

Steenland K, Nowlin S, Ryan B, Adams S. 1992. Use of multiple-cause mortality data in epidemiologic analyses: US rate and proportion files developed by the National Institute for Occupational Safety and Health and the National Cancer Institute. *American Journal of Epidemiology* 136(7):855–862.

Steenland K, Piacitelli L, Deddens J, Fingerhut M, Chang LI. 1999. Cancer, heart disease, and diabetes in workers exposed to 2,3,7,8-tetrachlorodibenzo-*p*-dioxin. *Journal of the National Cancer Institute* 91(9):779–786.

Steenland K, Calvert G, Ketchum N, Michalek J. 2001. Dioxin and diabetes mellitus: An analysis of combined NIOSH and Ranch Hand data. *Occupational and Environmental Medicine* 58(10):641–648.

Stehr-Green P, Hoffman R, Webb K, Evans RG, Knutsen A, Schramm W, Staake J, Gibson B, Steinberg K. 1987. Health effects of long-term exposure to 2,3,7,8-tetrachlorodibenzo-*p*-dioxin. *Chemosphere* 16:2089–2094.

Stellman S, Stellman J, Sommer JJ. 1988. Health and reproductive outcomes among American Legionnaires in relation to combat and herbicide exposure in Vietnam. *Environmental Research* 47:150–174.

Suskind RR, Hertzberg VS. 1984. Human health effects of 2,4,5-T and its toxic contaminants. *Journal of the American Medical Association* 251(18):2372–2380.

Suskind R, Cholak J, Schater LJ, Yeager D. 1953. *Reports on Clinical and Environmental Surveys at Monsanto Chemical Co., Nitro, West Virginia, 1953.* Cincinnati, OH: Department of Environmental Health, University of Cincinnati (unpublished).

Svensson BG, Nilsson A, Jonsson E, Schutz A, Akesson B, Hagmar L. 1995. Fish consumption and exposure to persistent organochlorine compounds, mercury, selenium and methylamines among Swedish fishermen. *Scandinavian Journal of Work, Environment, and Health* 21(2):96–105.

Swaen GM, van VC, Slangen J, Sturmans F. 1992. Cancer mortality among licensed herbicide applicators. *Scandinavian Journal of Work, Environment, and Health* 18:201–204.

Swaen GM, van Amelsvoort LG, Slangen JJ, Mohren DC. 2004. Cancer mortality in a cohort of licensed herbicide applicators. *International Archives of Occupational and Environmental Health* 77(4):293–295.

Sweeney MH, Mocarelli P. 2000. Human health effects after exposure to 2,3,7,8-TCDD. *Food Additives and Contaminants* 17(4):303–316.

Sweeney MH, Hornung RW, Wall DK, Fingerhut MA, Halperin WE. 1992. *Diabetes and serum glucose levels in TCDD-exposed workers.* Abstract of a paper presented at the 12th International Symposium on Chlorinated Dioxins (Dioxin '92), Tampere, Finland, August 24–28.

Sweeney MH, Calvert GM, Egeland GA, Fingerhut MA, Halperin WE, Piacitelli LA. 1997/98. Review and update of the results of the NIOSH medical study of workers exposed to chemicals contaminated with 2,3,7,8-tetrachlorodibenzodioxin. *Teratogenesis, Carcinogenesis, and Mutagenesis* 17(4–5):241–247.

't Mannetje A, McLean D, Cheng S, Boffetta P, Colin D, Pearce N. 2005. Mortality in New Zealand workers exposed to phenoxy herbicides and dioxins. *Occupational and Environmental Medicine* 62(1):34–40.

Tauchi M, Hida A, Negishi T, Katsuoka F, Noda S, Mimura J, Hosoya T, Yanaka A, Aburatani H, Fujii-Kuriyama Y, Motohashi H, Yamamoto M. 2005. Constitutive expression of aryl hydrocarbon receptor in keratinocytes causes inflammatory skin lesions. *Molecular and Cellular Biology* 25(21):9360–9368.

Teske S, Bohn AA, Regal JF, Neumiller JJ, Lawrence BP. 2005. Activation of the aryl hydrocarbon receptor increases pulmonary neutrophilia and diminishes host resistance to influenza A virus. *American Journal of Physiology—Lung Cellular and Molecular Physiology* 289(1): L111–L124.

Teske S, Bohn AA, Hogaboam JP, Lawrence BP. 2008. Aryl hydrocarbon receptor targets pathways extrinsic to bone marrow cells to enhance neutrophil recruitment during influenza virus infection. *Toxicological Sciences* 102(1):89–99.

Thackaberry EA, Bedrick EJ, Goens MB, Danielson L, Lund AK, Gabaldon D, Smith SM, Walker MK. 2003. Insulin regulation in AhR-null mice: Embryonic cardiac enlargement, neonatal macrosomia, and altered insulin regulation and response in pregnant and aging AhR-null females. *Toxicological Sciences* 76(2):407–417.

Thackaberry EA, Jiang Z, Johnson CD, Ramos KS, Walker MK. 2005a. Toxicogenomic profile of 2,3,7,8-tetrachlorodibenzo-*p*-dioxin in the murine fetal heart: Modulation of cell cycle and extracellular matrix genes. *Toxicological Sciences* 88(1):231–241.

Thackaberry EA, Nunez BA, Ivnitski-Steele ID, Friggins M, Walker MK. 2005b. Effect of 2,3,7,8-tetrachlorodibenzo-*p*-dioxin on murine heart development: Alteration in fetal and postnatal cardiac growth, and postnatal cardiac chronotropy. *Toxicological Sciences* 88(1):242–249.

Thomas TL, Kang H. 1990. Mortality and morbidity among Army Chemical Corps Vietnam veterans: A preliminary report. *American Journal of Industrial Medicine* 18:665–673.

Thomas TL, Kang H, Dalager N. 1991. Mortality among women Vietnam veterans, 1973–1987. *American Journal of Epidemiology* 134:973–980.

Turyk ME, Anderson HA, Persky VW. 2007. Relationships of thyroid hormones with polychlorinated biphenyls, dioxins, furans, and DDE in adults. *Environmental Health Perspectives* 115(8):1197–1203.

Uemura H, Arisawa K, Hiyoshi M, Satoh H, Sumiyoshi Y, Morinaga K, Kodama K, Suzuki TI, Nagai M, Suzuki T. 2008a. Associations of environmental exposure to dioxins with prevalent diabetes among general inhabitants in Japan. *Environmental Research* 108(1):63–68.

Uemura H, Arisawa K, Hiyoshi M, Satoh H, Sumiyoshi Y, Morinaga K, Kodama K, Suzuki TI, Nagai M, Suzuki T. 2008b. PCDDs/PCDFs and dioxin-like PCBs: Recent body burden levels and their determinants among general inhabitants in Japan. *Chemosphere* 73(1):30–37.

Uno S, Dalton TP, Sinclair PR, Gorman N, Wang B, Smith AG, Miller ML, Shertzer HG, Nebert DW. 2004. Cyp1a1(−/−) male mice: Protection against high-dose TCDD-induced lethality and wasting syndrome, and resistance to intrahepatocyte lipid accumulation and uroporphyria. *Toxicology and Applied Pharmacology* 196(3):410–421.

Valcin M, Henneberger PK, Kullman GJ, Umbach DM, London SJ, Alavanja MC, Sandler DP, Hoppin JA. 2007. Chronic bronchitis among nonsmoking farm women in the Agricultural Health Study. *Journal of Occupational and Environmental Medicine* 49(5):574–583.

Vasquez A, Atallah-Yunes N, Smith FC, You X, Chase SE, Silverstone AE, Vikstrom KL. 2003. A role for the aryl hydrocarbon receptor in cardiac physiology and function as demonstrated by AhR knockout mice. *Cardiovascular Toxicology* 3(2):153–163.

Vena J, Boffeta P, Becher H, Benn T, Bueno de Mesquita HB, Coggon D, Colin D, Flesch-Janys D, Green L, Kauppinen T, Littorin M, Lynge E, Mathews JD, Neuberger M, Pearce N, Pesatori AC, Saracci R, Steenland K, Kogevinas M. 1998. Exposure to dioxin and nonneoplastic mortality in the expanded IARC international cohort study of phenoxy herbicide and chlorophenol production workers and sprayers. *Environmental Health Perspectives* 106(Supplement 2):645–653.

Vergés B. 2005. New insight into the pathophysiology of lipid abnormalities in type 2 diabetes. *Diabetes and Metabolism* 31(5):429–439.

Villalobos-Molina R, Vazquez-Cuevas FG, Lopez-Guerrero JJ, Figueroa-Garcia MC, Gallardo-Ortiz IA, Ibarra M, Rodriguez-Sosa M, Gonzalez FJ, Elizondo G. 2008. Vascular alpha-1D-adrenoceptors are overexpressed in aorta of the aryl hydrocarbon receptor null mouse: Role of increased angiotensin II. *Autonomic and Autacoid Pharmacology* 28(2-3):61–67.

Von Benner A, Edler L, Mayer K, Zober A. 1994. "Dioxin" investigation program of the chemical industry professional association. *Arbeitsmedizin Sozialmedizin Praventivmedizin* 29:11–16.

Wang SL, Tsai PC, Yang CY, Guo YL. 2008. Increased risk of diabetes and polychlorinated biphenyls and dioxins: A 24-year follow-up study of the Yucheng cohort. *Diabetes Care* 31(8):1574–1579.

Watanabe K, Kang H. 1996. Mortality patterns among Vietnam veterans: A 24-year retrospective analysis. *Journal of Occupational and Environmental Medicine* 38(3):272–278.

Webb K, Evans RG, Stehr P, Ayres SM. 1987. Pilot study on health effects of environmental 2,3,7,8-TCDD in Missouri. *American Journal of Industrial Medicine* 11:685–691.

Wolfe WH, Michalek JE, Miner JC, Rahe A, Silva J, Thomas WF, Grubbs WD, Lustik MB, Karrison TG, Roegner RH, Williams DE. 1990. Health status of Air Force veterans occupationally exposed to herbicides in Vietnam. I. Physical health. *Journal of the American Medical Association* 264:1824–1831.

Wolfe W, Michalek J, Miner J, Roegner R, Grubbs W, Lustik M, Brockman A, Henderson S, Williams D. 1992. The Air Force Health Study: An epidemiologic investigation of health effects in Air Force personnel following exposure to herbicides, serum dioxin analysis of 1987 examination results. *Chemosphere* 25: 213–216.

Yeboah J, Crouse J, Hsu F, Burke G, Herrington D. 2007. Brachial flow-mediated dilation predicts incident cardiovascular events in older adults: The Cardiovascular Health Study. *Circulation* 115(18):2390–2397.

Zack J, Gaffey W. 1983. A mortality study of workers employed at the Monsanto company plant in Nitro, West Virginia. *Environmental Science Research* 26:575–591.

Zack J, Suskind R. 1980. The mortality experience of workers exposed to tetrachlorodibenzodioxin in a trichlorophenol process accident. *Journal of Occupational Medicine* 22:11–14.

Zober A, Messerer P, Huber P. 1990. Thirty-four-year mortality follow-up of BASF employees exposed to 2,3,7,8-TCDD after the 1953 accident. *International Archives of Occupational and Environmental Health* 62:139–157.

Zober A, Ott MG, Messerer P. 1994. Morbidity follow up study of BASF employees exposed to 2,3,7,8-tetrachlorodibenzo-*p*-dioxin (TCDD) after a 1953 chemical reactor incident. *Occupational and Environmental Medicine* 51:479–486.

10

Conclusions and Recommendations

SYNOPSIS OF COMMITTEE CONCLUSIONS

The committee weighed the strengths and limitations of the epidemiologic evidence reviewed in this report and in previous *Veterans and Agent Orange* (VAO) reports. Although the studies published since *Update 2006* are the subject of detailed evaluation here, the committee drew its conclusions in the context of the entire body of literature. The contribution of recent publications to the evidence database was substantial, but the committee did not weigh them more heavily merely because they were new. Epidemiologic methods and analytic capabilities have improved, but many of the recent studies were also particularly useful for the committee's purpose because they produced results in terms of serum TCDD concentrations or because their findings consisted of observations on the aging population of primary concern, Vietnam veterans. The committee also notes that experimental data related to biologic plausibility of health conditions statistically associated with exposure to the components of Agent Orange has gradually emerged since the beginning of this series of VAO reports. These findings now better inform decisions about how to categorize the degree of association for individual conditions; a footnote to this effect has been added to Table 10-1.

On the basis of its evaluation of veterans, occupational, and environmental studies, the committee assigned each health outcome to one of four categories of relative certainty of association with exposure to the herbicides that were used in Vietnam or to any of their components or contaminants (with no intention of specifying particular chemicals). Changes made by the current committee to the

TABLE 10-1 Summary from *Seventh Biennial Update* of Findings in Occupational, Environmental, and Veterans Studies Regarding the Association Between Specific Health Outcomes and Exposure to Herbicides[a]

Sufficient Evidence of an Association
Epidemiologic evidence is sufficient to conclude that there is a positive association. That is, a positive association has been observed between exposure to herbicides and the outcome in studies in which chance, bias, and confounding could be ruled out with reasonable confidence.[b] For example, if several small studies that are free of bias and confounding show an association that is consistent in magnitude and direction, there could be sufficient evidence of an association. There is sufficient evidence of an association between exposure to the chemicals of interest and the following health outcomes:

> Soft-tissue sarcoma (including heart)
> Non-Hodgkin's lymphoma
> Chronic lymphocytic leukemia (including **hairy cell leukemia and other chronic
>   B-cell leukemias**) (**category clarification since** *Update 2006*)
> Hodgkin's disease
> Chloracne

Limited or Suggestive Evidence of an Association
Epidemiologic evidence suggests an association between exposure to herbicides and the outcome, but a firm conclusion is limited because chance, bias, and confounding could not be ruled out with confidence.[b] For example, a well-conducted study with strong findings in accord with less compelling results from studies of populations with similar exposures could constitute such evidence. There is limited or suggestive evidence of an association between exposure to the chemicals of interest and the following health outcomes:

> Laryngeal cancer
> Cancer of the lung, bronchus, or trachea
> Prostate cancer
> Multiple myeloma
> AL amyloidosis
> Early-onset transient peripheral neuropathy
> **Parkinson's disease (category change from** *Update 2006*)
> Porphyria cutanea tarda
> Hypertension
> **Ischemic heart disease (category change from** *Update 2006*)
> Type 2 diabetes (mellitus)
> Spina bifida in offspring of exposed people

Inadequate or Insufficient Evidence to Determine an Association
The available epidemiologic studies are of insufficient quality, consistency, or statistical power to permit a conclusion regarding the presence or absence of an association. For example, studies fail to control for confounding, have inadequate exposure assessment, or fail to address latency. There is inadequate or insufficient evidence to determine association between exposure to the chemicals of interest and the following health outcomes that were explicitly reviewed:

> Cancers of the oral cavity (including lips and tongue), pharynx (including tonsils), or
>   nasal cavity (including ears and sinuses)
> Cancers of the pleura, mediastinum, and other unspecified sites in the respiratory system
>   and intrathoracic organs

continued

TABLE 10-1 Continued

Esophageal cancer

Stomach cancer

Colorectal cancer (including small intestine and anus)

Hepatobiliary cancers (liver, gallbladder, and bile ducts)

Pancreatic cancer

Bone and joint cancer

Melanoma

Nonmelanoma skin cancer (basal cell and squamous cell)

Breast cancer

Cancers of reproductive organs (cervix, uterus, ovary, testes, and penis; excluding prostate)

Urinary bladder cancer

Renal cancer (kidney and renal pelvis)

Cancers of brain and nervous system (including eye)

Endocrine cancers (thyroid, thymus, and other endocrine organs)

Leukemia (**other than all chronic B-cell leukemias**, including chronic lymphocytic leukemia and hairy cell leukemia)

Cancers at other and unspecified sites

Infertility

Spontaneous abortion (other than after paternal exposure to TCDD, which appears *not* to be associated)[b]

Neonatal or infant death and stillbirth in offspring of exposed people

Low birth weight in offspring of exposed people

Birth defects (other than spina bifida) in offspring of exposed people

Childhood cancer (including acute myelogenous leukemia) in offspring of exposed people

Neurobehavioral disorders (cognitive and neuropsychiatric)

Neurodegenerative diseases, excluding Parkinson's disease

Chronic peripheral nervous system disorders

Respiratory disorders (wheeze or asthma, chronic obstructive pulmonary disease, and farmer's lung)

Gastrointestinal, metabolic, and digestive disorders (changes in hepatic enzymes, lipid abnormalities, and ulcers)

Immune system disorders (immune suppression, allergy, and autoimmunity)

Circulatory disorders (other than hypertension and ischemic heart disease)

Endometriosis

Effects on thyroid homeostasis

This committee used a classification that spans the full array of cancers. However, reviews for nonmalignant conditions were conducted only if they were found to have been the subjects of epidemiologic investigation or at the request of the Department of Veterans Affairs. *By default, any health outcome on which no epidemiologic information has been found falls into this category.*

Limited or Suggestive Evidence of *No* Association
Several adequate studies, which cover the full range of human exposure, are consistent in not showing a positive association between any magnitude of exposure to the herbicides of interest and the outcome. A conclusion of "no association" is inevitably limited to the conditions, exposures, and length of observation covered by the available studies. *In addition, the possibility of a very small increase in risk at the exposure studied can never be excluded.* There is limited or suggestive

TABLE 10-1 Continued

evidence of *no* association between exposure to the herbicides of interest and the following health outcomes:

        Spontaneous abortion after paternal exposure to TCDD

---

[a] *Herbicides* indicates the following chemicals of interest: 2,4-dichlorophenoxyacetic acid (2,4-D), 2,4,5-trichlorophenoxyacetic acid (2,4,5-T) and its contaminant 2,3,7,8-tetrachlorodibenzo-*p*-dioxin (TCDD, or dioxin), cacodylic acid, and picloram. The evidence regarding association was drawn from occupational, environmental, and veteran studies in which people were exposed to the herbicides used in Vietnam, to their components, or to their contaminants.

[b] Evidence for an association is strengthened by experimental data supporting biologic plausibility, but its absence would not detract from the epidemiologic evidence.

categorizations determined by the committee for *Update 2006* (as presented in Table 1-1) are noted in boldface in Table 10-1.

    After considering information related to the Department of Veterans Affairs (VA) question about hairy cell leukemia, the committee concluded that not just hairy cell leukemia—like chronic lymphoid leukemia (CLL)—but all chronic B-cell leukemias belong in the category of "sufficient evidence of an association" with Hodgkin's disease and non-Hodgkin's lymphoma (NHL). Because the committee for *Update 2006* could not reach consensus, ischemic heart disease had remained in the category of "inadequate or insufficient evidence to determine an association," but accruing evidence convinced the present committee to move ischemic heart disease from the category of "inadequate or insufficient evidence to determine an association" to the category of "limited or suggestive evidence of an association" with hypertension. The committee for *Update 2006* had also been unable to reach consensus about whether the evidence of an association with herbicide exposure reached the level of "limited or suggestive," but the present committee did not find new evidence to justify moving either melanoma or breast cancer out of the category of "inadequate or insufficient evidence." Several pieces of new information specifically about the chemicals of interest led the committee to decide that there is now "limited or suggestive" evidence of association for Parkinson's disease (PD).

    As mandated by Public Law (PL) 102-4, the distinctions among categories are based on statistical association, not on strict causality. The committee was directed to review the scientific data, not to recommend VA policy; therefore, conclusions reported in Table 10-1 are not intended to imply or suggest policy decisions. The conclusions are related to associations between exposure and outcomes in human populations, not to the likelihood that any individual's health problem is associated with or caused by the chemicals in question.

COMMITTEE RECOMMENDATIONS

As part of its charge, the committee was asked to make recommendations concerning the need, if any, for additional scientific studies to resolve uncertainties concerning the health effects of the chemicals of interest sprayed in Vietnam: 2,4-dichlorophenoxyacetic acid (2,4-D), 2,4,5-trichlorophenoxyacetic acid (2,4,5-T) and its contaminant 2,3,7,8-tetrachlorodibenzo-p-dioxin (TCDD), picloram, and cacodylic acid. This chapter summarizes the committee's recommendations.

Although great strides have been made over the last several years in understanding the health effects of exposure to the chemicals of interest and in elucidating the mechanisms underlying them, gaps in our knowledge remain. The scope of potential research on the chemicals is wide, and what follows here is not an exhaustive list of future research that might have value. There are many additional opportunities for progress in such subjects as toxicology, exposure assessment, the conduct of continuing or additional epidemiologic studies, and systematic and comprehensive integration of existing data that have not been explicitly noted here. It is the committee's conviction, however, that work needs to be undertaken promptly, particularly to address questions regarding several health outcomes, most urgently tonsil cancer, melanoma, paternally mediated transgenerational effects, and PD.

- **The current definition of *Vietnam service* is not supported by existing data.**

The evidence that this committee has reviewed makes limiting *Vietnam service* to those who set foot on Vietnamese soil seem inappropriate. The ongoing series of hearings and appeals in the US Court of Appeals for Veterans Claims (*Haas v. Nicholson*) reflect the controversy. As discussed in Chapter 3, there is little reason to believe that exposure of US military personnel to the herbicides sprayed in Vietnam was limited to those who actually set foot in the Republic of Vietnam. Having reviewed the Australian report (NRCET, 2002) on the fate of TCDD when seawater is distilled to produce drinking water, the committee is convinced that this use of seawater would provide a feasible route of exposure of personnel in the Blue Water Navy, which might have been supplemented by drift from herbicide spraying.

The epidemiologic evidence itself supports a broader definition of *Vietnam service* to serve as a surrogate for presumed exposure to Agent Orange or other herbicides sprayed in Vietnam. For instance, the Centers for Disease Control and Prevention (CDC, 1990) study of selected cancers in Vietnam veterans found that the risk of the "classic AO cancer" NHL was highest and most significant in Blue Water Navy veterans. More recently, the Air Force Health Study (AFHS) has demonstrated that TCDD concentrations in Vietnam-era veterans deployed to Southeast Asia, not just the "Vietnam veteran" Ranch Hand subjects, are generally higher than US background concentrations (although notably lower than in Ranch Hand sprayers themselves).

The present committee notes that all previous VAO committees have considered information on naval Vietnam veterans to pertain to possible Agent Orange exposure when evaluating the full spectrum of health outcomes. The present committee finds that exposure assignment to be appropriate. No new studies considered in this update contained Navy-specific information, but such information has been factored into the evolving conclusions of VAO committees.

Given the available evidence, the committee recommends that members of the Blue Water Navy should not be excluded from the set of Vietnam-era veterans with presumed herbicide exposure.

- **VA should evaluate possibilities for studying health outcomes in Vietnam-era veterans by using the existing administrative and health-services databases.**

The original *VAO* committee recommended that the Department of Defense (DOD) and VA identify Vietnam service in the computerized index of records. Linking that information with the VA electronic medical-record and associated administrative databases, such as discharge-diagnosis and pharmacy-use records, should make it possible to assemble epidemiologic information on common health conditions for evaluation of possible associations with military service in Vietnam.

Particular attention should be paid to the feasibility of conducting epidemiologic studies of conditions that have been noted to be of special interest but on which the current evidence is inadequate or insufficient to determine whether there is an association with herbicide exposure (such as tonsil and breast cancers, melanoma, amyotrophic lateral sclerosis, lupus, ischemic heart disease, and stroke). For very uncommon health outcomes, a case–control design would probably be most appropriate.

Although applications for compensation and appeals constitute a nonrepresentative, self-selected sample that is influenced by which conditions are already judged to be service-related, an effort to use existing VA information should include a more systematic review of the distribution of health outcomes in the database.

To evaluate whether Vietnam veterans actually have experienced an increase in tonsil cancer, the next logical step would be for VA to identify the veterans with tonsil cancer that are already in the system and examine the biopsy results to classify the form (origin) of tonsil cancer better. Given the low incidence of this rare condition, a typical epidemiologic study in the general population would not be useful. Determining whether the lymphatic nature of the tonsil plays a role in a substantial proportion of tonsil cancers would guide planning of the next steps for research.

A portion of the Neurotoxin Exposure Treatment Research Program (NETRP) is related to the pathogenesis and etiology of several conditions, including PD, and has been funded since 1997. Originally housed in the US Army Military

Operational Medicine Research Program, the NETRP has recently moved to the Telemedicine and Advanced Technology Research Center under the US Army Medical Research and Materiel Command. Perhaps coordination with that effort and with the resources of VA's appeals and medical records would be a productive means of addressing whether an increased risk of PD is being manifested in Vietnam veterans.

- **Available information should be gleaned from existing cohort studies.**

The present committee joins the committee for *Update 2006* in concurring with the recommendations of the Committee on the Disposition of the Air Force Health Study (IOM, 2006). The latter committee made strong recommendations regarding the retention of all data from the AFHS and suggested mechanisms by which the data could be made available to researchers. We reiterate that committee's statement that "no other epidemiologic dataset on Vietnam veterans contains as detailed information over as long a time period, the data appear to be of high quality and the specimens well preserved, and analysis of the assets has contributed to the literature addressing the health of Vietnam veterans." Congress directed the Institute of Medicine (IOM) Medical Follow-up Agency (MFUA) to become custodian of the data and biologic specimens in 2006 (PL 109-364; 120 Stat. 2290); the specimens are now in storage at the Wright-Patterson Air Force Base under the MFUA's aegis. The MFUA is pursuing the funding that PL 110-389, §803 directed VA to provide to IOM to maintain and manage the materials and make them available as a resource for research. What is required is a strong commitment by the federal government to provide sufficient funds to develop the infrastructure necessary to meet the goals of further research using this invaluable database. Moreover, dedicated funding is required so that focused analyses can be carried out by independent investigators, especially as related to the research questions that concerns the present committee. The investment would be a small fraction of the $143 million invested to date in the AFHS. Such research could clarify the various issues and would reap substantial benefits in the understanding of health issues of Vietnam veterans exposed to herbicides. Comprehensive longitudinal analysis of the data collected in the various medical-cycle examinations, data on medical interventions (such as hospitalizations and emergency-department visits), data on cancer incidence, data on mortality, and other data on exposure could be used profitably to investigate further some of or all of the health outcomes that may be associated with the exposures under consideration in this report. The present committee believes strongly that a complete analysis of the melanoma findings should be performed because an unambiguous interpretation is not possible on the basis of the papers published to date (Akhtar et al., 2004; Pavuk et al., 2005).

Members of the Army Chemical Corps (ACC) constitute the largest cohort of Vietnam veterans exposed directly to herbicides and TCDD. They were involved in the handling and distribution of the chemicals in Vietnam. ACC veterans who reported spraying herbicides as part of their duties have been shown to have increased serum TCDD concentrations; this highly exposed population has also been shown to be at increased risk for several diseases. The population should be the focus of additional study, with new resources devoted to it, because it represents our best opportunity to understand the health effects of exposure to TCDD and the herbicides used in Vietnam.

Few data on the women who served in Vietnam are available. The cohort of nurses studied by Kang et al. (2000) largely exhausted the source population. The mortality study of the population (Cypel and Kang, 2008) reviewed in the present update was helpful, but additional follow-up of the health status of the group and determination of their TCDD concentrations would be worthwhile.

At the direction of Congress, the National Vietnam Veterans Readjustment Study (1986–1988) investigated primarily psychiatric sequelae in a representative cohort of about 1,600 men and women. In 2000, Congress mandated (PL 106-419) that VA assess the current physical and mental well-being of the members of that cohort. In 2001, VA contracted for the work, named the National Vietnam Veterans Longitudinal Study (NVVLS), but progress ceased within 2 years. VA's Inspector General (VAOIG, 2005) ruled that "the Study was not properly, planned, procured, or managed," but directed that it be completed and that provisions be made to avoid the previous problems. Because baseline information is available on symptoms and chronic health problems in the original cohort, the committee thinks that completion of the NVVLS could generate useful information for future updates and concurs that serious consideration should be given to restarting the study.

Starting in 1978, the National Institute for Occupational Safety and Health (NIOSH) began to study US workers potentially exposed to TCDD. A total of 5,132 workers in 12 large manufacturing companies were included in the NIOSH cohort. The cohort has been a source of data extremely valuable in assessing the health effects associated with TCDD exposure. The studies have included high-quality exposure assessment, and evaluations of a wide array of health outcomes have been published. Given its value as an important source of epidemiologic data, the committee recommends that studies of the NIOSH cohort be extended.

Although the committee concluded that there is limited or suggestive evidence that the occurrence of Parkinson's disease is associated with the chemicals of interest, it would still be desirable to investigate whether the apparent inconsistencies in the results for incident and prevalent cases in the Agricultural Health Study (Kamel et al., 2007b) could be resolved. The committee recommends that the researchers conducting that ongoing study apply the analytic method described in Copas and Farewell (2008) to this dataset.

The committee also notes that future analyses of health outcomes in those and other important study populations should be as specific as possible because generic findings, such as those for "all respiratory outcomes," are not useful in addressing the committee's charge of determining associations of herbicide exposures with specific health conditions.

- **The exposure-reconstruction study should be put to use.**

IOM's Committee on the Assessment of Wartime Exposure to Herbicides in Vietnam oversaw the development of a model of herbicide exposure of Vietnam veterans (the "Stellman model"), which has been described in detail (IOM, 2003a,b). The present committee endorses the finding in the recent report (IOM, 2008) of the Committee on Making Best Use of the Agent Orange Reconstruction Model that the model should be incorporated into new epidemiologic studies where feasible.

- **Studies of the Vietnamese population would be worthwhile.**

As discussed in earlier updates, the Vietnamese are an under studied population. Although there are likely to be serious logistical challenges, the many Vietnamese people who had substantial exposure constitute a potentially informative study sample. It will be important to include appropriate exposure measures, such as tissue TCDD concentrations, in studying Vietnamese residents. Because such research has the potential to close a number of gaps in the understanding of the long-term health consequences of exposure to TCDD and the herbicides used in Vietnam, the committee endorses action toward developing collaborative programs of research.

- **Possible effects in offspring of exposed people merit further investigation.**

The assessment of any link between exposure of Vietnam veterans to the chemicals of interest and birth defects or developmental disease in their offspring presents distinct challenges. VA should review all the possible cognitive and developmental effects in offspring of veterans. Such a review should include the possibility of effects in grandchildren, which are of growing concern to veterans and their families. A recent meta-analysis of Agent Orange exposure and birth defects in both Vietnamese and non-Vietnamese populations (Ngo et al., 2006) found the studies of non-Vietnamese subjects (that is, Vietnam veterans) overall showed significant association, pointing to the need to examine closely both the biologic plausibility of paternally mediated birth defects and the existing epidemiologic evidence. Reviews have also focused on epidemiologic studies of data from birth-defects registries and from parental reports of birth defects. Those studies often exclude alterations in function that could appear later in a child's life, such as alterations in neurologic function, endocrine function, or reproductive capacity. The findings of the AFHS on birth defects in veterans' offspring have not yet been (and, if funding is not provided, may never be) formally and systematically integrated and analyzed in a longitudinal fashion.

Most etiologic research has focused on the effects of maternal and fetal exposures, but some work addressing paternal exposures has been discussed in previous reviews. With increasing concern about male reproductive function, increasing numbers of epidemiologic studies of the role of paternal exposures in the risk of birth defects are being published. This work is particularly relevant in assessing health outcomes in offspring of a largely male service population. The plausibility of birth defects arising from parental exposure, especially from paternal exposure, merits careful review in light of newly hypothesized epigenetic mechanisms (such as heritable forms of gamete imprinting) that might make paternal transmission of a TCDD effect more plausible. The committee recommends that an ad hoc group be established to review current mechanistic studies that could further knowledge of a possible paternally mediated link between exposure to the chemicals of interest and health conditions (including birth defects) in offspring. Given the sparseness of the data on birth defects in the children of Vietnam veterans, the committee also recommends that the ad hoc group conduct meta-analyses of existing epidemiologic studies of male populations exposed to TCDD, 2,4-D, or 2,4,5-T and the risk of birth defects in their offspring.

- **Potential emergence of metabolic syndrome should be analyzed.**

Within the study populations reviewed, the committee recognized a possible interrelationship among the reported associations of serum concentrations of dioxin-like compounds with certain health outcomes, including hypertriglyceridemia, type 2 diabetes, hypertension, and ischemic heart disease. The first three of those outcomes are key criteria for the diagnosis of metabolic syndrome, and the fourth is a major consequence of it. Thus, the committee recommends that—in addition to analysis of the association of exposure to the chemicals of interest with individual health outcomes—the incidence of multiple health outcomes that define metabolic syndrome should be analyzed as a group.

- **There is a need for new animal models to elucidate mechanisms of diseases and disease progression.**

The committee believes that experimental research in the mechanisms that underlie human health outcomes (particularly cardiovascular disease and transgenerational effects) could provide valuable information related to the risk of disease in Vietnam veterans. The central role of the aryl hydrocarbon receptor (AHR) in animal models is clear, and AHR gene differences in animals clearly affect susceptibility to the effects of TCDD. Although work on the AHR in humans has been sparse, variations in this specific genetic factor alone are likely to affect human susceptibility to the toxic effects of TCDD, dioxin-like chemicals, and herbicide formulations that contain these chemicals. In addition, recent research makes it clear that variations in the genetic regulation of the expression or activity of other factors, including proteins that interact with the AHR and the gene products that are regulated by the AHR, are critical in determining susceptibility to the effects of TCDD and the types of toxic effects observed. Studies addressing the identification, distribution, and functional consequences of polymorphisms of the AHR and the other cofactors in human populations should be pursued. The committee expects that investigations of mitochondrial disease and epigenetic mechanisms will have important implications for health effects of concern in Vietnam veterans.

The committee notes that although its predecessors have made similar recommendations, there has been little or no action toward implementing several investigations that the committee regards as imperative. Those projects need to be undertaken to address veterans concerns and to meet the scientific needs of future VAO committees to resolve outstanding questions, particularly with regard to PD, tonsil cancer, and melanoma. VA and DOD are in the unique position of being able to study the very population that is of concern. Focused study of Vietnam veterans themselves would be especially appropriate for extremely rare conditions, such as tonsil cancer, which appears anecdotally to be occurring at an unusual rate in Vietnam veterans and in connection with which the study of surrogate populations (even with a case–control design) might exclude factors that are important for the military situation.

REFERENCES[1]

Akhtar FZ, Garabrant DH, Ketchum NS, Michalek JE. 2004. Cancer in US Air Force veterans of the Vietnam war. *Journal of Occupational and Environmental Medicine* 46(2):123–136.

CDC (Centers for Disease Control and Prevention). 1990. The association of selected cancers with service in the US military in Vietnam. I. Non-Hodgkin's lymphoma. *Archives of Internal Medicine* 150:2473–2483.

Copas AJ, Farewell VT. 2008. Incorporating retrospective data into an analysis of time to illness. *Biostatistics* 2(1):1–12.

Cypel Y, Kang H. 2008. Mortality patterns among women Vietnam-era veterans: Results of a retrospective cohort study. *Annals of Epidemiology* 18(3):244–252.

IOM (Institute of Medicine). 2003a. *Characterizing Exposure of Veterans to Agent Orange and Other Herbicides Used in Vietnam: Interim Findings and Recommendations.* Washington, DC: The National Academies Press.

IOM. 2003b. *Characterizing Exposure of Veterans to Agent Orange and Other Herbicides Used in Vietnam: Final Report.* Washington, DC: The National Academies Press.

IOM. 2006. *Disposition of the Air Force Health Study.* Washington, DC: The National Academies Press.

IOM. 2008. *The Utility of Proximity-Based Herbicide Exposure Assessment in Epidemiologic Studies of Vietnam Veterans.* Washington, DC: The National Academies Press.

Kamel F, Tanner C, Umbach D, Hoppin J, Alavanja M, Blair A, Comyns K, Goldman S, Korell M, Langston J, Ross G, Sandler D. 2007b. Pesticide exposure and self-reported Parkinson's disease in the Agricultural Health Study. *American Journal of Epidemiology* 165(4):364–374.

Kang HK, Mahan CM, Lee KY, Magee CA, Mather SH, Matanoski G. 2000. Pregnancy outcomes among US women Vietnam veterans. *American Journal of Industrial Medicine* 38(4): 447–454.

---

[1]Throughout the report the same alphabetic indicator following year of publication is used consistently for the same article when there were multiple citations by the same first author in a given year. The convention of assigning the alphabetic indicator in order of citation in a given chapter is not followed.

Ngo AD, Taylor R, Roberts CL, Nguyen TV. 2006. Association between Agent Orange and birth defects: Systematic review and meta-analysis. *International Journal of Epidemiology* 35(5): 1220–1230.

NRCET (National Research Centre for Environmental Toxicology). 2002. *Examination of the Potential Exposure of Royal Australian Navy (RAN) Personnel to Polychlorinated Dibenzodioxins and Polychlorinated Dibenzofurans Via Drinking Water*. Brisbane, Australia.

Pavuk M, Michalek JE, Schecter A, Ketchum NS, Akhtar FZ, Fox KA. 2005. Did TCDD exposure or service in Southeast Asia increase the risk of cancer in Air Force Vietnam veterans who did not spray Agent Orange? *Journal of Occupational and Environmental Medicine* 47(4):335–342.

VAOIG (Department of Veterans' Affairs Office of Inspector General). 2005. *Audit of VA Acquisition Practices for the National Vietnam Veterans Longitudinal Study* (Report No. 04-02330-212). Washington, DC.

APPENDIX
A

Agendas of Public Meetings Held by the Committee to Review the Health Effects in Vietnam Veterans of Exposure to Herbicides (Seventh Biennial Update)

FIRST PUBLIC MEETING

Thursday, March 27, 2008
National Academies of Science, Room 150
2101 Constitution Avenue, NW
Washington, DC 20418

Presentations

- **Welcome; Goals and Conduct of the Public Meeting; Introduction**
  Richard Fenske, PhD, Committee Chair

- **Charge to the Committee**
  Mark Brown, PhD, US Department of Veterans Affairs

- **IOM Veterans and Agent Orange Reports: A Brief History**
  David Butler, PhD, Institute of Medicine

- **Report of the Committee on Making Best Use of the Agent Orange Reconstruction Model**
  Lois Joellenbeck, PhD, Institute of Medicine

- **Possibility of Epigenetic Mechanisms for Dioxin, Particularly for Transgenerational Effects**
  Barbara R. Migeon, MD, Institute of Genetic Medicine, Johns Hopkins Hospital
  Michael K. Skinner, PhD, Washington State University (by phone)

- **Activities Involving the Vietnamese Population**
  Vaughan C. Turekian, PhD, Chief International Officer, AAAS and
  representative to US-Vietnam Dialogue Group on Agent Orange/Dioxin

SECOND PUBLIC MEETING

Thursday, June 19, 2008
Hyatt Regency San Antonio
123 Losoya Street
San Antonio, TX 78205

Presentations

- **Welcome; Goals and Conduct of the Public Meeting; Introduction**
  Richard Fenske, PhD, Committee Chair

- **Toxicity of Organic Arsenic**
  Samuel Cohen, MD, PhD, University of Nebraska Medical Center
  Placido Salazar, State Veterans' Affairs Officer, American GI Forum
  Alberto Zambrano, Colonel USAF (retired)

- **Possible Association Between Parkinson's Disease and the Herbicides
  Sprayed in Vietnam**
  Steve Fiscus, President, US Military Veterans with Parkinson's (USMVP)
  Alan Oates, Director Special Projects, USMVP
  Lorenzo Gonzalez, VP, USMVP
  Christopher Reid, MD, PhD, Charles Drew University of Medicine and
  Science

- **Genetic Implications**
  Isaac D. Brown, III, PhD, AMVETS & DAV

- **Delayed Onset of Symptoms**
  Don Wilson, Military Order of the Purple Heart

- **Conditions Not Covered**
  Alexander Hill, Vietnam Veterans of America

- **Blue Water Navy Issue**
  John Wells, Esq., Commander USN (retired)

- **Air Force Health Study**
  Joel E. Michalek, PhD, University of Texas Health Center at San Antonio

- **Written Statements Received**
  Jon Anderson, Concerning PD and use of dieldrin in Vietnam

Ronald Denbow, Concerning possible role of compromised immune system increasing sensitivity to dioxin toxicity
Jerry Dittmer, Concerning renal cell carcinoma
Michael Eckstein, Concerning nerve disorders and birth defects
Michael J. Harris, Concerning child with fascioscapular humeral dystrophy

THIRD PUBLIC MEETING

December 8, 2008
Beckman Center
100 Academy Rd.
Irvine, CA

Presentations

- **Welcome; Goals and Conduct of the Public Meeting; Introduction**
  Richard Fenske, Committee Chair

- **Effects of Dioxin on Mitochondria and What the Implications Might Be for Dioxin's Carcinogenic Potential and for Inducing Other Chronic or Transgenerational Adverse Health Outcomes**
  Doug Wallace, University of California, Irvine

APPENDIX

B

Clarification of Cancer Groupings
Used in Reporting Results, with
Correspondence to NIOSH Cause-of-
Death Codes and ICD Codes for Cancers

In response to a request from the Department of Veterans Affairs (VA), the
committee responsible for the last report in this series (*Update 2006*) prepared
Table B-1 to demonstrate how conclusions provided for the full range of cancer
types and to clarify into which groupings any specific cancer diagnosis falls.

The major portion of evidence compiled for review in the *Veterans and Agent
Orange* (*VAO*) series comes from cohort studies, primarily of mortality but some
of incidence. Other data have been generated by case–control studies, which follow the only design amenable to studying very infrequent or very specific health
outcomes. How researchers are able to group, analyze, and report their findings
is influenced by the distribution of cases that they observe, so the data that *VAO*
committees have had available for review reflect mortality experience at a level
of specificity concordant with statistical analysis.

The International Classification of Diseases (ICD) system is used by physicians and researchers around the world to group related diseases and procedures
so that morbidity and mortality information can be classified for statistical purposes in a standard form amenable to data storage and retrieval. It is a comprehensive hierarchic system that permits great detail, but that can be collapsed into
broad categories. Codes mentioned in *VAO* reports are stated in terms of ICD,
Version 9 (ICD-9). ICD-7, ICD-8, and ICD-9 were in effect for deaths that occurred in 1960–1967, 1968–1978, and 1979–1998, respectively; the differences
among them are fairly subtle. Although ICD-10, which went into effect for coding
causes of deaths that occurred from 1999 on, appears radically different from the
earlier versions, it corresponds in large part to basically the same disease entities
(see Table B-2). To date, most published epidemiologic studies considered in the

TABLE B-1 Mapping of Groupings of Malignant Neoplasms That Are the Subjects of Conclusions in Veterans and Agent Orange Series with ICD-9 Codes

NIOSH Category for Cause of Death			"VAO Characterization of Grouping"[a]	
Major	Minor	NIOSH Groupings of Cancer Sites	Subsites	ICD-9 codes
02		Buccal cavity and pharynx	**"Oral, nasal, and pharyngeal"**	
	004	Lip		140
	005	Tongue		141
	006	Other parts of buccal cavity		
			Salivary glands	142
			Floor of mouth	144
			Gum and other mouth	143, 145
	007	Pharynx		
			Oropharynx	146
			Tonsil	146.0–146.2
			Nasopharynx	147
			Hypopharynx	148
			Other buccal cavity and pharynx	149
				(160 = nasal below)
03		Digestive organs and peritoneum		
	008	Esophagus	**"Esophagus"**	150
	009	Stomach	**"Stomach"**	151
	010	Intestine except rectum	**"Colorectal"**	
			Small intestine	152
			Colon (large intestine)	153
	011	Rectum		154

continued

TABLE B-1 Continued

NIOSH Category for Cause of Death		NIOSH Groupings of Cancer Sites	"VAO Characterization of Grouping"ᵃ Subsites	ICD-9 codes
Major	Minor			
	012	Biliary passages, liver, and gall bladder	**"Hepatobiliary"**	
			Liver and intrahepatic bile ducts	155
			Gallbladder and extrahepatic bile ducts	156
	013	Pancreas		157
	014	Retroperitoneum and other and unspecified digestive organs		158–159
04		Respiratory system	**"Respiratory"**	
	015	Larynx	**"Larynx"**	161
	016	Trachea, bronchus, and lung	**"Lung"**	162
			Trachea	162.0 (there is no ICD 162.1)
			Lung and bronchus	162.2–162.9
	017	Pleura		163
	018	Other respiratory	Nasal cavity, middle ear, and accessory sinuses	(160, above with oral and pharyngeal)
			Thymus, heart, and mediastinum	164 (164.0, below with endocrine; 164.1, below with soft tissue sarcoma)
			Other respiratory, unspecified	165
				(discontinuity with ICD codes)
05	019	Breast (male and female)	**"Breast"**	174, 175
06	020	Female genital organs	**"Female reproductive"**	
		Cervix uteri		180

			ICD codes
021	Other unspecified parts of uterus	Uterus, parts unspecified	179, 181, 182
		Placenta	179
		Body of uterus	181
			182
022	Ovary, fallopian tube, and broad ligament		183
			183.0 (there is no ICD 183.1)
		Ovary	183.2–183.9
		Fallopian tube and other uterine adnexa	184
023	Other female genital organs		
07	Male genital system	**"Prostate"**	185, 186
024	Prostate	**"Testicular"**	185
025	Testis		186
	Penis and other male genital organs	[for NIOSH in minor group 036]	187
08	Urinary system	**"Renal"**	
026	Kidney (including renal pelvis and ureter)	**"Urinary bladder"**	189.0–189.2
027	Bladder and other urinary organs	Bladder	188, 189.3–189.9
		Urethra, paraurethral glands, other and unspecified urinary	188
			189.3–189.9
			(discontinuity with ICD codes)
09	Other and unspecified sites	**"Bone and joint"**	170
028	Bone ("and articular cartilage" in ICD nomenclature)	**"Melanoma"**	172
029	Melanoma	**"Non-melanoma skin"**	173
030	Other malignant skin neoplasm		No codes (new minor code, above with lung)
031	Mesothelioma	**"Soft-tissue sarcoma"**	171
032	Connective ("and other soft" in ICD nomenclature) tissue		
		(heart)	(164.1)

continued

TABLE B-1 Continued

NIOSH Category for Cause of Death			"VAO Characterization of Grouping"[a]	
Major	Minor	NIOSH Groupings of Cancer Sites	Subsites	ICD-9 codes
	033	Brain and other parts of nervous system (ICD "soft tissue" includes peripheral nerves and autonomic nervous system)	**"Brain"**	191–192
	034	Eye		190
	035	Thyroid		193
			(thymus)	164.0
	036	Other and unspecified sites	Other endocrine cancers	194
			Other and ill-defined sites	195
			Stated or assumed to be secondary of specified sites	196–198
			Site unspecified	199
10		Lymphatic and hematopoietic tissue		
		Lymphoma		
	037	**Hodgkin's disease**		201
	038	**Non-Hodgkin's lymphoma**		200, 202 (excluding 202.4), 273.3
	039	**Multiple myeloma**		203 (excluding 203.1)
	040	Leukemia and aleukemia	**"Leukemia (other than chronic B-cell leukemias)"**	204–208
		Lymphocytic	Acute lymphocytic	204.0
			"Chronic lymphocytic (including hairy cell leukemia)"	204.1
			Other lymphocytic	202.4; 204.2–204.9

Myeloid (granulocytic)		
	Acute myeloid	
	Acute	205.0
	Acute erythremia and erythroleukemia	207.0
	Megakaryocytic leukemia	207.2
	Chronic myeloid	205.1
	Other myeloid	205.2–205.3, 205.8–205.9
Monocytic		
	Acute monocytic	206.0
	Chronic monocytic	206.1
	Other monocytic	206.2–206.9
Other leukemia		
	Other acute	208.0
	Other chronic	207.1, 208.1
	Aleukemic, subleukemia and "not otherwise specified"	203.1, 207.2, 207.8, 208.2–208.9

[a]**Boldface cancer (sub)site:** most comprehensive grouping for which a conclusion has been drawn.

VAO series have been related to health outcomes that occurred and were encoded before ICD-10 went into effect.

Since 1983, the National Institute for Occupational Safety and Health (NIOSH) has maintained software for generating standardized expectations, as derived from US mortality data assembled by the National Center for Health Statistics, for ICD-encoded mortality datasets. An article by Robinson et al. (2006) discusses revisions to that standard software to incorporate deaths coded according to ICD-10 and includes conversions and equivalencies between ICD-7, -8, -9, and -10 for 119 exhaustive categories for cause of death. Codes for malignant neoplasms span the ICD-9 range 140.0–208.9, NIOSH's major categories 02–10, or NIOSH's more specific minor categories 004–040.

The NIOSH death codes for neoplasms provide comprehensive scaffolding for organizing the committee's reviews and conclusions by cancer type that is somewhat simpler than ICD classifications, but maps completely to the ICD system as it has evolved. Because the NIOSH system has been used to mediate analysis of many sets of cohort data, its groupings correspond quite closely with the published research findings available for *VAO* review. In general cohort studies, one is unlikely to encounter results on more specific groupings than NIOSH's minor categories.

As discussed in Chapter 2, this committee has not framed its conclusions strictly in terms of ICD codes, but the ICD system has been a valuable tool for the work of *VAO* committees. There can be coding errors on hospital records or death certificates, but when researchers present their results labeled with ICD codes, there can be little ambiguity about what they intended. When their most definitive indication is something like "respiratory cancers," however, there can be uncertainty about where the evidence should be considered. In such cases, the committee has done its best to follow the hierarchy laid out in Table B-1.

As indicated above, many of the studies reviewed by the committee use or were written at a time when ICD-9 was in place. Accordingly, ICD references in this report use that scheme. ICD-10 began to be implemented in the United States in 1999. It differs from ICD-9 in level of detail (about 8,000 categories versus about 5,000 in ICD-9) and nomenclature (alphanumeric versus the numeric codes of ICD-9); additions and modifications were also made with regard to some coding rules and the rules for selecting an underlying cause of death (Anderson et al., 2001). Table B-2 lists the ICD-9 and ICD-10 codes for the various forms of malignant neoplasm addressed in this report. In situ neoplasms, benign neoplasms, neoplasms of uncertain behavior, and neoplasms of unspecified behavior have separate codes in both schemes.

TABLE B-2 Surveillance, Epidemiology, and End Results (SEER) Program Malignant Neoplasm Site Groupings for ICD-9 and ICD-10

Cancer Site	ICD-9 codes	ICD-10 codes
Buccal cavity and pharynx		
Lip	140.0–140.9	C00.0–C00.9
Tongue	141.0–141.9	C01, C02.1–C02.9
Salivary glands	142.0–142.9	C07, C08.0–C08.9
Floor of mouth	144.0–144.9	C04.0–C04.9
Gum and other mouth	143.0–143.9, 145.0–145.6, 145.8–145.9	C03.0–C03.9, C05.0–C05.9, C06.0–C06.9
Nasopharynx	147.0–147.9	C11.1–C11.9
Tonsil	146.0–146.2	C09.0–C09.9
Oropharynx	146.3–146.9	C10.1–C10.9
Hypopharynx	148.0–148.9	C12, C13.0–C13.9
Other buccal cavity and pharynx	149.0–149.9	C14.0–C14.9
Digestive system		
Esophagus	150.0–150.9	C15.0–C15.9
Stomach	151.0–151.9	C16.0–C16.9
Small intestine	152.0–152.9	C17.0–C17.9
Colon excluding rectum	153.0–153.9, 159.0	C18.0–C18.9, C26.0
Rectum and rectosigmoid junction	154.0–154.1	C19, C20
Anus, anal canal, and anorectum	154.2–154.3, 154.8	C21.0–C21.9
Liver and intrahepatic bile duct		
Liver	155.0,155.2	C22.0, C22.2–C22.4, C22.7–C22.9
Intrahepatic bile duct	155.1	C22.1
Gallbladder	156.0	C23
Other biliary	156.1–156.9	C24.0–C24.9
Pancreas	157.0–157.9	C25.0–C25.9
Retroperitoneum	158.0	C48.0
Peritoneum, omentum, and mesentery	158.8–158.9	C48.1–C48.2
Other digestive organs	159.8–159.9	C26.8–26.9, C48.8
Respiratory system		
Nasal cavity, middle ear, and accessory sinuses	160.0–160.9	C30.0, C30.1, C31.0–C31.9
Larynx	161.0–161.9	C32.0–C32.9
Lung and bronchus	162.2–162.9	C34.0–C34.9
Pleura	163.0–163.9	C38.4
Trachea, mediastinum, and other respiratory organs	162.0, 164.2–165.9	C33, C38.1–C38.3, C38.8, C39
Bones and joints	170.0–170.9	C40.0–C40.9, C41.0–C41.9
Soft tissue (including heart)	171.0–171.9, 164.1	C38.0, C47.0–C47.9, C49.0–C49.9

continued

TABLE B-2 Continued

Cancer Site	ICD-9 codes	ICD-10 codes
Skin		
Malignant melanomas	172.0–172.9	C43.0–C43.9
Other malignant skin neoplasms	173.0–173.9	C44.0–C44.9
Breast (male and female)	174.0–174.9, 175	C50.0–C50.9
Female genital system		
Cervix	180.0–180.9	C53.0–C53.9
Corpus	182.0–182.1, 182.8	C54.0–C54.9
Uterus, not otherwise specified	179	C55
Ovary	183.0	C56.0–C56.9
Vagina	184.0	C52
Vulva	184.1–184.4	C51.0–C51.9
Other female genital organs	181, 183.2–183.9, 184.8, 184.9	C57.0–C57.9, C58
Male genital system		
Prostate	185	C61
Testis	186.0–186.9	C62.0–C62.9
Penis	187.1–187.4	C60.0–C60.9
Other male genital organs	187.5–187.9	C63.0–C63.9
Urinary system		
Urinary bladder	188.0–188.9	C67.0–C67.9
Kidney and renal pelvis	189.0, 189.1	C64.0–C64.9, C65.0–C65.9
Ureter	189.2	C66.0–C66.9
Other urinary organs	189.3–189.4, 189.8–189.9	C68.0–C68.9
Eye and orbit	190.0–190.9	C69.0–C69.9
Brain and other nervous system		
Brain	191.0–191.9	C71.0–C71.9
Meninges	192.1	C70.0–C70.9
Other nervous system[a]	192.0, 192.2–192.9	C72.0–C72.9
Endocrine system		
Thyroid	193	C73
Other endocrine (including thymus)	164.0, 194.0–194.9	C37, C74.00–C74.92, C75.0–C75.9
Lymphomas		
Hodgkin's disease	201.0–201.9	C81.0–81.9
Non-Hodgkin's lymphomas	200.0–200.8, 202.0–202.2, 202.8–202.9	C82.0–C82.9, C83.0–C83.9, C84.0–C84.5, C85.0–C85.9, C96.3
Multiple myeloma	203.0, 238.6	C90.0, C90.2
Leukemias		
Lymphocytic		
Acute lymphocytic	204.0	C91.0
Chronic lymphocytic	204.1	C91.1
Other lymphocytic	202.4, 204.2–204.9	C91.2–C91.4, C91.7, C91.9

TABLE B-2 Continued

Cancer Site	ICD-9 codes	ICD-10 codes
Myeloid (granulocytic)		
Acute myeloid	205.0, 207.0, 207.2	C92.0, C92.4–C92.5, C94.0, C94.2
Chronic myeloid	205.1	C92.1
Other myeloid	205.2–205.3, 205.8–205.9	C92.2–C92.3, C92.7, C92.9
Monocytic		
Acute monocytic	206.0	C93.0
Chronic monocytic	206.1	C93.1
Other monocytic	206.2–206.9	C93.2, C93.7, C93.9
Other leukemia		
Other acute	208.0	C94.4, C94.5, C95.0
Other chronic	207.1, 208.1	C94.1, C95.1
Aleukemic, subleukemic and "not otherwise specified"	203.1, 207.2, 207.8, 208.2–208.9	C90.1, C91.5, C94.3, C94.7, C95.2, C95.7, C95.9
Miscellaneous malignant neoplasms	159.1, 195.0–195.8, 196.0–196.9, 199.0–199.1, 202.3, 202.5–202.6, 203.8	C26.1, C76.0–C76.8, C77.0–C77.9, C78.0–C78.8, C79.0–C79.8, C80, C88.0–C88.9, C96.0–C96.2, C96.7, C96.9, C97

[a]Cancers of the peripheral nerves and the autonomic nervous system are classified as "soft tissue" in ICD.
Adapted from Ries et al. (2003), Table A-4.

REFERENCES

Anderson RN, Minino AM, Hoyert DL, Rosenberg HM. 2001. Comparability of cause of death between ICD-9 and ICD-10: Preliminary estimates. *National Vital Statistics Reports* 49(2):1–32.

Ries LAG, Eisner MP, Kosary CL, Hankey BF, Miller BA, Clegg L, Mariotto A, Fay MP, Feuer EJ, Edwards BK (eds). 2003. *SEER Cancer Statistics Review, 1975–2000*. Bethesda, MD: National Cancer Institute.

Robinson CF, Schnorr TM, Cassinelli RT, Calvert GM, Steenland K, Gersic CM, Schubauer-Berigan MK. 2006. Tenth revision US mortality rates for use with the NIOSH Life Table Analysis System. *Journal of Occupational and Environmental Medicine* 48(7):662–667.

APPENDIX
C

Committee to Review the Health Effects in Vietnam Veterans of Exposure to Herbicides (Seventh Biennial Update) and Staff Biographies

Richard A. Fenske, Ph.D., M.P.H. (*Chair*), is a Professor and Associate Chair of Environmental and Occupational Health Sciences at the University of Washington School of Public Health and Community Medicine, and is the Director of the Pacific Northwest Agricultural Safety and Health Center at the University of Washington in Seattle. Dr. Fenske's work has focused on the evaluation of environmental health risks in special populations. Specialty areas include health risks of pesticide exposures, development of new exposure assessment methods, children's exposure to hazardous chemicals, and investigation of the role of dermal exposure for workers. Dr. Fenske serves on the Science Advisory Board of the US Environmental Protection Agency, and also serves as a member of EPA's Human Studies Review Board. He had previously served on the committees for *Veterans and Agent Orange: Update 2002, Update 2004*, and *Update 2006*.

Erin M. Bell, Ph.D., is Assistant Professor in the Departments of Epidemiology and Biostatistics and of Environmental Health Sciences at the State University of New York's School of Public Health in Albany. She received her undergraduate degree in biology with honors from Hartwick College and her M.S. and Ph.D. degrees in epidemiology from the University of Massachusetts, Amherst, and the University of North Carolina, Chapel Hill, respectively. Between her master's and doctoral studies, she was a Research Associate at IOM's Medical Follow-up Agency. Her epidemiology research focuses on environmental exposures, particularly to pesticides, especially as they are related to reproductive, immune, and cancer outcomes.

Scott W. Burchiel, Ph.D., holds the Nunzio and Sherolyn DeSantis Endowed Chair in Pharmaco-genomics and is Associate Dean for Research at the University of New Mexico (UNM) College of Pharmacy in Albuquerque. He has served at UNM in numerous capacities since receiving his Ph.D. in pharmacology in 1977 from the University of California at San Francisco School of Medicine. His continuing research interests include monoclonal antibody production and radiolabeled imaging, lymphocyte activation and signal transduction mechanisms, and development of biomarkers for immunotoxicity. He has previously served on NAS committees addressing Beryllium Alloy Exposures and Human Health Risks of Trichloroethylene and the subcommittee on jet propulsion fuel 8.

Janice Chambers, Ph.D., is a William L. Giles Distinguished Professor and Director at the Center for Environmental Health Sciences, and Professor at the Department of Basic Sciences at Mississippi State University. Dr. Chambers directs several research projects that deal with the effects of pesticides in mammalian systems to determine the potential human health effects of pesticide exposures. Specifically, she leads projects related to the metabolism of pesticides and their neurochemical and behavioral effects in developing organisms to yield predictions about potential effects of pesticides in infants and children. Her other projects are involved in developing mathematical predictions of the effects of mixtures of pesticides on the nervous system so that predictive models can be generated to potentially describe the effects of future uncharacterized mixtures, and the development of more effective antidotes to nerve agent poisoning. Dr. Chambers has been the principal investigator for numerous federally funded competitive grants in the field of toxicology. Because of her expertise, she has been asked to serve on a number of advisory boards and prestigious committees. Dr. Chambers is board certified as a toxicologist by the American Board of Toxicology and the Academy of Toxicological Sciences. As Director of the Center for Environmental Health Sciences, she has developed an interdisciplinary research center specializing in pesticide toxicology and funded primarily by NIH. The center comprises the areas of neurotoxicology, biochemical toxicology, analytical chemistry, biostatistics, epidemiology, computational chemistry, computational simulation, biochemistry, and endocrinology. Dr. Chambers is a member of the EPA FIFRA Scientific Advisory Panel, the EPA Human Studies Review Board, and the NCEH/ATSDR Board of Scientific Counselors.

Naihua Duan, Ph.D., M.A., is a Professor of Biostatistics at Columbia University and Director of the Division of Biostatistics at the New York State Psychiatric Institute in New York City. He received a B.S. in mathematics from National Taiwan University, an M.A. in mathematical statistics from Columbia University, and a Ph.D. in statistics from Stanford University. His primary research interest is study design, particularly for investigations with multilevel data structures. He previously served on the NAS committees on Advances in Assessing Human Exposure to Airborne Pollutants, Organ Procurement and Transplantation Policy, Carbon Monoxide Episodes in Meteorological and Topographical Problem Areas, and Assessing the Medical Risks of Human Oocyte Donation for Stem Cell Research.

Peter H. Gann, M.D., Sc.D., is a Professor and Director of Pathology Research at the University of Illinois at Chicago. A physician-epidemiologist by training, his research work focuses on the causes of breast and prostate cancer, with particular emphasis on the development and application of novel biological markers. His interest in biological markers actually originates with his service as a Project Director at the National Academy of Sciences in the 1980s. Prior to his current position, Dr. Gann spent 13 years in the Department of Preventive Medicine at Northwestern University Medical School. He received a B.A. degree from Swarthmore College, M.D. and M.S. (epidemiology/biostatistics) degrees from the University of Pennsylvania, and his doctorate in epidemiology from Harvard University. Dr. Gann serves on a number of national and international advisory and peer review panels in the field of cancer prevention. He previously served on the committee for *Veterans and Agent Orange: Update 2006.*

Mark S. Goldberg, Ph.D., is a Professor in the Department of Medicine, McGill University, Montreal, associate member in the Joint Departments of Epidemiology and Biostatistics and Occupational Health, the Department of Oncology, and Medical Scientist, Royal Victoria Hospital, McGill University Health Centre. Dr. Goldberg is an occupational and environmental epidemiologist and holds an Investigator Award from the Canadian Institute for Health Research. His current research interests include the investigation of occupational and environmental risk factors for breast cancer and the health effects associated with exposures to ambient air pollution. In addition to being a member of grant review panels, Dr. Goldberg is also a member of Health Canada's Science Advisory Board. He has served on the committee for *Disposition of the Air Force Health Study*; the Division of Earth and Life Sciences (DELS) committee for *Assessing the Human Health Risks of Trichloroethylene: Key Scientific Issues;* and *Veterans and Agent Orange: Update 2006.*

Nancy I. Kerkvliet, Ph.D., is a Professor in the Department of Environmental and Molecular Toxicology at Oregon State University, Corvallis, Oregon. Dr. Kerkvliet's research is focused on using animal models to understand how chemicals of environmental concern alter immune function. Her primary interest is focused on understanding how activation of the Ah receptor by TCDD and other ligands suppresses immune responses. She previously served on the Committee on Toxicology, the Subcommittee of Jet Propulsion Fuel 8, and the committee for *Veterans and Agent Orange: Update 2004* and *Update 2006.*

Stephen B. Kritchevsky, Ph.D., M.S.P.H., is Professor of Internal Medicine in the Section on Gerontology and Geriatric Medicine and Director of the J. Paul

Sticht Center on Aging and Rehabilitation at Wake Forest University School of Medicine in Winston-Salem, NC. After receiving both his M.S.P.H. and Ph.D. degrees in epidemiology from the University of North Carolina, Chapel Hill, he joined the Departments of Biostatistics and of Epidemiology at the University of Tennessee Health Science Center. Dr. Kritchevsky's research interests are related to conditions compromising the health of aging populations, particularly inflammation, obesity, metabolic syndrome, and cardiovascular disease.

Michele Marcus, Ph.D., is a Professor in the Departments of Epidemiology and Environmental and Occupational Health of Emory University in Atlanta. She is also Director of Graduate studies for the Department of Epidemiology and a Fellow with the Centers for Disease Control and Prevention. Previously, she was a faculty member in the Department of Environmental and Occupational Medicine at the Mount Sinai School of Medicine in New York City. She received her M.P.H., M.Phil., and Ph.D. degrees from Columbia University and her research interests include environmental and genetic contributions to reproduction and investigation of the human health effects of endocrine disruptors. She is also a member of the Southeast Pediatric Environmental Health Specialty Unit.

Linda A. McCauley, Ph.D., FAAN, R.N., is Dean of Emory University's Nell Hodgson Woodruff School of Nursing in Atlanta. She was previously the Associate Dean for Research and the Nightingale Professor in Nursing at the University of Pennsylvania School of Nursing. Dr. McCauley received her doctoral degree in environmental health/epidemiology from the University of Cincinnati. Dr. McCauley has special expertise in the design of epidemiological investigations of occupational and environmental hazards and is nationally recognized for her expertise in occupational and environmental health nursing. Dr. McCauley's research interests are in the areas of chemical exposure among working populations and young children. Dr. McCauley is a member of the Institute of Medicine. She previously served on the committees for *Veterans and Agent Orange: Update 2006.*

Alvaro Puga, Ph.D., is a Professor of Molecular Biology and Environmental Health, Deputy Director of the NIEHS Center for Environmental Genetics, and Associate Director of the Superfund Basic Research Program at the University of Cincinnati Medical Center. Following studies of biology at Universidad de Madrid, Spain, and of molecular cytogenetics at the University of Lund, Sweden, he received a Ph.D. in molecular biology and biophysics from Purdue University. Before going to the University of Cincinnati, Dr. Puga served for 15 years in several capacities at NIH in the Institute of Dental Research and the Institute of Child Health and Human Development. Study of the AH receptor has been a major theme of his research. He recently served on the NRC committee that reviewed EPA's exposure and human health assessment of dioxin.

Jeremy Shefner, M.D., Ph.D., is a Professor and Chair of Neurology at Upstate Medical University, and Director of the Clinical Neurophysiology Laboratory and the MDA/ALS Research and Treatment Center at University Hospital, in Syracuse, New York. He is trained in neurology and clinical neurophysiology, and has devoted his clinical and research efforts to ALS. After receiving an M.D. with distinction from Northwestern University, he completed residency and fellowship training in neurology and clinical neurophysiology at the Harvard-Longwood Neurological training program. After fellowship, he joined the faculty at Brigham and Women's Hospital and Harvard Medical School. While at the Brigham and Women's Hospital, Dr. Shefner directed the ALS Clinic and participated in multiple industry-sponsored ALS clinical trials. He founded the Northeast ALS Clinical Trials Consortium in 1995, which has grown to become the largest ALS clinical trials group in North America. Since moving to Syracuse, he established the multidisciplinary ALS clinic there, and continues to hold leadership positions in both industry- and investigator-initiated clinical trials. Dr. Shefner is the recipient of numerous research grants from NIH and industry sponsors, as well as the author of more than 100 original research articles and book chapters on neurophysiology. Dr. Shefner previously served the IOM Committee on the Review of Scientific Literature on Amyotrophic Lateral Sclerosis in Veterans.

Hollie I. Swanson, Ph.D., is an Associate Professor in the Department of Molecular and Biomedical Pharmacology with a joint position with the Toxicology Department at the University of Kentucky College of Medicine. She received her M.S. from Oregon State University, Ph.D. from Purdue University, and post-doctoral training from Michigan State University and Northwestern University. Her research focuses on the study of the aryl hydrocarbon pathway and its role in altering cell fate. She currently serves as Councilor of the Drug Metabolism Specialty Section of the National Chapter of the American Society for Pharmacology and Experimental Therapeutics, and she is a member of the National and Ohio Valley Chapters of the Society of Toxicology. She is an editorial board member of *Toxicology and Applied Pharmacology*. Dr. Swanson has published numerous articles pertaining to the molecular and cellular aspects of the AH receptor and dioxin. She previously served on the committee for *Veterans and Agent Orange: Update 2006*.

Staff

Mary Burr Paxton, Ph.D., is a Senior Program Officer in the Institute of Medicine Board on Population Health and Public Health Practice. Before joining IOM, she worked as a consultant on the regulation of toxic substances and managed the conduct and analysis of several epidemiology studies on veterans' health. She received a master's of science in biostatistics from the Johns Hopkins School of Hygiene and Public Health and a doctorate in genetics from the George Washington University. She is a diplomate of the American Board of Toxicology. Dr. Paxton has worked on several National Academies reports, including *Issues in Risk Assessment*; *Environmental Neurotoxicology*; *Gulf War and Health: Insecticides and Solvents*; *Gulf War and Health: Fuels, Combustion Products, and Propellants*; *Asbestos: Selected Cancers*; *Veterans and Agent Orange: Update 2004*, and *Veterans and Agent Orange: Update 2006*.

Jennifer A. Cohen, M.P.H., is a Program Officer in the Institute of Medicine Board on Population Health and Public Health Practice. She has been involved with the IOM committees that produced *Organ Procurement and Transplantation*; *Clearing the Air: Asthma and Indoor Air Exposures*; *Veterans and Agent Orange: Herbicide/Dioxin Exposure and Type 2 Diabetes*; *Veterans and Agent Orange: Update 2000*; *Veterans and Agent Orange: Herbicide/Dioxin Exposure and Acute Myelogenous Leukemia in the Children of Vietnam Veterans*; *Veterans and Agent Orange: Update 2004*; and *Veterans and Agent Orange: Update 2006*.

Rose Marie Martinez, Sc.D., is Director of the Institute of Medicine Board on Population Health and Public Health Practice. Before joining the IOM, she was Senior Health Researcher at Mathematica Policy Research, where she studied the effects of health-system change on the public-health infrastructure, access to care for vulnerable populations, managed care, and the health-care workforce. Dr. Martinez is former Assistant Director for Health Financing and Policy with the US General Accounting Office, for which she directed evaluations and policy analysis on national and public-health issues. Dr. Martinez received her doctorate from the Johns Hopkins School of Hygiene and Public Health.

Tia S. Carter is a Senior Program Assistant in the IOM Board on Population Health and Public Health Practice. In December 2008, she graduated with her masters in health-care administration from the University of Maryland University College. She received her undergraduate degree in community health from the University of Maryland, College Park. Before coming to the IOM, she worked at the Greater Washington Urban League in the Division of Aging and Health Services as the Health Promotions Coordinator, where she was responsible for health-promotion and disease-prevention education services and activities among the elderly. She has been involved with the IOM committees on *Asbestos: Selected Cancers*, *Veterans and Agent Orange: Updates 2004*, and *Veterans and Agent Orange: Update 2006*.

Norman Grossblatt, ELS(D), is a Senior Editor at the National Academies. Before joining the National Research Council Division of Medical Sciences in 1963, he worked as an analyst in information storage and retrieval at Documentation Incorporated and as a technical editor at the Allis-Chalmers Manufacturing Co., Nuclear Power Department, in Washington, DC. He received a B.A. in English from Haverford College. Mr. Grossblatt is a diplomate editor in the life sciences and was the founding president of the Board of Editors in the Life Sciences. He is a fellow of the American Medical Writers Association and a recipient of its President's Award; a member of the Council of Science Editors and since 1997 the manuscript editor of its journal, *Science Editor*; and a member of the European Association of Science Editors. At the National Academies, he has edited over 300 reports.